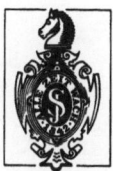

S. Matsumoto · N. Tamaki (Eds.)

Hydrocephalus

Pathogenesis and Treatment

With 341 Illustrations and 14 in Color

Springer-Verlag
Tokyo Berlin Heidelberg
New York London Paris
Hong Kong Barcelona

Satoshi Matsumoto, M.D.
Professor Emeritus

Norihiko Tamaki, M.D.
Professor and Chairman
Department of Neurosurgery
Kobe University
Kobe, 650 Japan

ISBN-13: 978-4-431-68158-8   e-ISBN-13: 978-4-431-68156-4
DOI: 10.1007/ 978-4-431-68156-4

Library of Congress Cataloging-in-Publication Data
Hydrocephalus: pathogenesis and treatment / S. Matsumoto, N. Tamaki (eds.). p.   cm.
Includes bibliographical references and index. ISBN-13: 978-4-431-68158-8 ISBN-13: 978-4-431-70080-7
                1. Hydrocephalus. I. Matsumoto, Satoshi, 1927– . II. Tamaki, Norihiko.
[DNLM: 1. Hydrocephalus—pathology. 2. Hydrocephalus-physiopathology. 3. Hydrocephalus—
therapy.] RC391.H96   1991. 616.85′8843—dc20. DNLM/DLC. for Library of Congress.
                                                                                    91–5009

© Springer-Verlag Tokyo 1991
Softcover reprint of the hardcover 1st edition 1991

Preface

During the past ten years, technology has been progressing at a rapid pace in the field of medical science, and there have been great improvements in the basic understanding, diagnosis, and treatment of hydrocephalus.

The present volume contains the proceedings of the International Symposium on "Hydrocephalus" that was held in Kobe, Japan, from November 12–14, 1990. The purpose of the symposium was to highlight the recent advances in this field and to provide a unique opportunity for exchange of basic and clinical knowledge among experts in this field. During the symposium, 84 papers were presented by 240 contributors from 14 countries. This volume is a comprehensive description of the current knowledge in this area, and it may help to define what is known and to find new strategies to understand the pathogenesis, pathophysiology, diagnosis, and treatment of the hydrocephalic process.

The editors take great pleasure in expressing their thanks to the contributors for their participation and cooperation, and to Springer Verlag for personal and technical assistance in publishing the proceedings.

We sincerely hope that this volume will contribute to improving the treatment for hydrocephalus.

August 1991   The Editors

Contents

III. CSF Hydrodynamics

Treatment of Hydrocephalus

I. *Hydrocephalus of Various Etiologies*

II. *Shunt Systems*

III. Shunt Complications

VI. New Concepts and Future Aspects

List of Contributors

Special Exhibition

1 — Hydrocephalus: Historical Review

Hiromi Sato[1] and Satoshi Matsumoto[2]

Historical Summary and Future Perspectives

Although the history of hydrocephalus can be traced back to Hippocrates' description of external hydrocephalus, the prevailing humoral theory, later institutionalized as Galenism, hindered the recognition of internal hydrocephalus for nearly 2000 years.

Internal hydrocephalus was first recognized by Vesalius in 1543, after which a great deal of interest was focused on the anatomy of the cerebrospinal fluid (CSF) pathway. In the 18th century, Contugno (1764) and Haller (1768) gave fairly accurate accounts of the cerebrospinal fluid and Monro formulated a revolutionary theory on the nature of the intracranial volume (1783). In the 19th century, Magendie constructed a comprehensive picture of CSF circulation (1842) and in 1875, Key and Retzius compiled a superb atlas of the CSF system. This, then, was "the third circulation" to be described, more than a century after the blood and lymphatic circulation systems had been established by Willis and Bartholin, respectively. The basis of modern research, therefore, was established in the fields of the physiology of CSF and the anatomy of its pathway.

With respect to pathology, with the exception of Morgagni's description (1761) of the organ pathology of hydrocephalus related to myelomeningocele, only a little knowledge was gained until the mid-1900s, when tissue pathology was established. Until the 19th century, such congenital malformations were regarded as untreatable and high infant mortality was accepted as inevitable. The surgical implications of congenital malformations were first recognized in the late 19th century. The clinical entity of the Chiari malformation was established and arachnoid cysts and dysgenetic hydrocephalus, including the Dandy-Walker syndrome, holoprosencephaly, and hydroanencephaly were recognized.

[1] Department of Neurosurgery, Shizuoka Children's Hospital, Shizuoka, 420 Japan
[2] Department of Neurosurgery, Kobe University School of Medicine, 650 Japan

Traditional medical treatment for hydrocephalus, which was essentially the same as that of the Hippocratic era, prevailed until the 18th century. In the early 1900s, the first new treatment, ventricular puncture, was attempted. This operation, based on the obstructive hypothesis, attempted a modification of the flow of the CSF. However, it was almost always fatal, despite the aid of newly invented listerism and ether anesthesia.

From the beginning of the 20th century until the 1950s, the aim of the many clinical and pathological studies was to demonstrate an anatomical obstruction to the major pathway of CSF. *The concept of obstruction* was formulated and published by Penfield and Elvidge (1932) and Russell (1942). Dandy and Blackfan's conclusion (1918) that CSF was derived mainly from the choroid plexus strongly influenced future surgical treatment. They developed and performed choroid plexectomy, third ventriculostomy and aqueductal canalization. Their classification of hydrocephalus into communicating and non-communicating types has since been used clinically without major modifications. Dandy developed the phenol-sulfonphthalein test, airencephalography, and airventriculography to diagnose communicating hydrocephalus. In the same era, Cushing proposed a distinguished theory on the biological role of CSF (1925), although until recently this theory could not be tested.

Although internal shunting had been attempted in the early 1900s, it was Nulsen and Spitz' work, in 1949, on the introduction of a one-way valve, which opened the modern era of treatment. Shunt procedures soon became widely accepted as an effective diversion method, which was regarded as bringing hydrocephalus to a surgically arrested state. At the same time, it was the beginning of an era of painful battles against shunt complications. Much effort was devoted to revising and upgrading the shunt system to a more physiological one with less risk of complications.

The introduction of radioactive tracers in the 1950s enabled the dynamics of the circulatory pattern of the CSF to be evaluated in detail. Since the 1960s, new research methods have updated earlier work. Papenheimer's perfusion method (1962), using various tracers, enabled not only the rate of formation and absorption at various pressure levels to be measured, but also contributed to the entire field of CSF physiology and pharmacology. With this method, the extrachoroidal formation of CSF was established. However, Katzman's infusion manometric test, developed in 1970, demonstrated various patterns of reduced absorption capacity or increased outflow resistance in hydrocephalus, which led to *the concept of defective absorption.*

Although useful data have been collected on the interaction of pharmacological agents on the formation of CSF, and on the pressure factors involved in its absorption, we have, as yet, no drugs available and no other more effective method than shunting.

The development of teratological induction methods and the introduction of hereditary models, established in the 1960s, enabled the pathology of congenital hydrocephalus to be studied. These experimental studies were predicted to, and in fact did, provide data on the pathological cerebral changes which occur in hydrocephalus. Many experimental studies demonstrated secondary aqueductal stenosis; these findings were also supported clinically by Folz' reports of functional aqueductal stenosis which occurred after shunting, and by Raimondi's studies on Dandy-Walker cysts. Then Epstein proposed the existence of slit ventricle syndrome and the isolated fourth ventricle, which later led to *the concept of isolation*, or compartmentalization of the CSF space, which encompassed unilateral hydrocephalus and the isolated temporal horn. This concept emphasized the significance of the pressure differences between each isolated compartment in the pathogenesis of functional stenosis of the CSF pathway.

The description of normal pressure hydrocephalus by Adams and his colleagues, in 1965, prompted and then advanced further research, especially on analysis of the correlation of intracranial pressure and pulse pressure with related physiological parameters and studies on biomechanics and their role in hydrocephalus.

Thereafter, as clinical experience with normal pressure, slowly progressive, and arrested hydrocephalus accumulated, insight was gained into these conditions. This led to *the concept of chronological change* in hydrocephalus, proposed by Matsumoto in 1976. This concept proposes that hydrocephalus should be regarded as a dynamic process with a chronological sequence of events, which may be comparable to the life-cycle. Experimental studies with hereditary and teratologically induced models support the concept.

The interaction between CSF and cerebral extracellular fluid, originally suggested in the early 1900s, was further clarified. Ultrastructural studies defined the brain barrier systems, that is, the blood-brain, blood-CSF, and brain-CSF barriers. In 1965, Brightman and Reese demonstrated that the communication between cerebral extracellular fluid and CSF was relatively free. Milhorat (1970) showed that periventricular permeability was increased in experimental hydrocephalus. Later this was found to correlate with periventricular low density in X-ray CT and periventricular hyperintensity on MR-CT. Cserr (1974) demonstrated the bulk flow of cerebral interstitial fluid, and Reulen (1977) demonstrated the bulk flow of edema fluid through the cerebral extracellular space. Thus, the accumulated data led to *the concept of compensation* via transependymal and intraparenchymal absorption of CSF. If compensation is insufficient then the result is parenchymal damage. Thus, our attention was refocused on changes occurring in the brain in hydrocephalus.

In any era, the definition of hydrocephalus is a summary of the leading concepts of that era, based on each author's insights. Several definitions have been proposed in our era. In 1977, Raimondi classified intraparenchymal, extraparenchymal, and combined hydrocephalus according to their pathophysiologies. In 1976, Matsumoto classified hydrocephalus based on changes in the flow dynamics of CSF, the degree of cerebral damage, and chronological change; he emphasized the necessity of considering changes in the cerebral parenchyma. At this stage, his new concept of dynamic changes and their chronological sequence in hydrocephalus was introduced. From its onset, hydrocephalus progresses, first, to the stage of pressure hydrocephalus, then through a normal pressure stage or, in some patients, slowly progressive hydrocephalus, and finally to the stage of arrested or compensated hydrocephalus with varying degrees of cerebral damage. This concept led to the definition of intractable hydrocephalus used by the Research Group of the Japanese Ministry of Health and Welfare.

Now, we are at a turning point in the history of hydrocephalus. Most of the 20th century was devoted to studying the altered physiology of CSF. As the 21st century approaches, the recognition of hydrocephalus as a brain disease should be reemphasized, which should lead to new treatment methods. Updating of early work should be done with this in mind. Rapidly advancing technology, including positron emission CT, Magnetic Resonance Imaging, spectroscopy, and other sophisticated methods, should provide more advanced knowledge of the pathophysiology of the brain and should open a new era in the management of hydrocephalus. There is much promising data already. For instance, increased knowledge of nerve regeneration and remyelination may lead to drug therapy aimed at regrowth with functional recovery. The extravillous drainage mechanism, as represented by the supposed lymphatic route, and further clarification of the intraparenchymal absorption mechanism may lead to new methods which will reduce outflow resistance. Moreover, advanced research into the interaction of the brain-CSF interface should demand revision of diversion surgery to more physiological procedures which will allow the CSF to maintain its role as a biological fluid. Furthermore, in the near future, the concept of the isolated cerebrospinal fluid space, based on a pressure-difference mechanism, may prompt the invention of new treatments. We have already waited too long for the advent of more appropriate treatments to replace shunting. Future treatment of hydrocephalus should be aimed at including effective functional recovery, and not simply at producing a surgically arrested state with brain damage.

Pathogenesis of Hydrocephalus

I. Morphological and Biochemical Aspects

2 — Early Vs Delayed Ventriculoperitoneal Shunt-Effects on the Impairment of the Developing Brain in Congenitally Hydrocephalic HTX-Rats

Kikuo Suda, Kiyoshi Sato, Nobuaki Takeda, Mitsuru Wada, Takahito Miyazawa, Hajime Arai, Masanori Ito, and Makoto Miyaoka

Summary. In the present investigation, we report on the effects of the early placement of a ventriculoperitoneal shunt (V-P shunt) on the development of cerebral synapses by counting spine density of the cortical pyramidal neurons (stained by rapid Golgi method) and measuring one of the synaptic vesicle proteins, SVP-38. The techniques used were quantitative histochemical and immunoblot analysis. The learning ability of congenitally hydrocephalic HTX-rats whose hydrocephalus had been arrested by insertion of a V-P shunt 7–9 days after birth (Early Shunt) was assessed by the light-darkness discrimination test. When a V-P shunt was inserted into the hydrocephalic animals approximately 4 weeks after birth (Delayed Shunt), not only was there no reduction in the size of the abnormally enlarged ventricles, but also there was no increase in cortical mantle thickness. Furthermore, spine density in the cerebral cortex in such animals was found to be decreased. Learning disability could not be corrected by the delayed shunt procedure. Contrary to these observations, early shunt placement was found to result in normalization of the abnormally enlarged ventricles, concomitant with simultaneous cortical mantle thickening and prevention of both decreased spine density and decay of SVP-38 in the affected cerebral cortex. The learning disability of such animals was not found to be disturbed, compared with that of the sham-operation group. From these observations, it is concluded that early shunt placement may have a beneficial role not only in repairing, but also in preventing the impairment of synaptogenesis caused by the progression of congenital hydrocephalus.

Keywords. Congenital hydrocephalus — Rat — Ventriculoperitoneal shunt synaptogenesis — Learning ability

[1] Department of Neurosurgery, The Juntendo University School of Medicine, Bunkyo-ku, Tokyo, 113 Japan

Introduction

In previous experiments using congenitally hydrocephalic HTX-rats (Kohn et al. 1981, 1984), we reported that congenital hydrocephalus impaired the development of dendrites and spines of neurons in the affected cerebral cortex (Miyazawa et al. 1988). Such impairment of neuronal development in the hydrocephalic brain of HTX-rats may not be completely corrected by insertion of a ventriculoperitoneal shunt approximately 4 weeks after birth (Delayed Shunt). We also suggested that the learning disability found in mature HTX-rats whose hydrocephalus had been arrested by delayed shunt insertion could be related to the aforementioned disturbance of neuronal development, especially synaptogenesis of the brain (Miyazawa and Sato 1991).

In the present study, we report on the beneficial effects of early placement of a ventriculoperitoneal shunt (Early Shunt) in HTX-rats whose hydrocephalus was arrested by insertion of a ventriculoperitoneal shunt 7–9 days after birth. The beneficial effects on the development of cerebral synapses, and also on the learning ability of these animals, were examined.

Materials and Methods

Congenitally hydrocephalic male HTX-rats (HTX) were used, and non-hydrocephalic male HTX-rats served as controls with and without sham operations.

Preparation of HTX with Early and Delayed Shunts

HTX manifesting hydrocephalus were divided into two groups in accordance with the time of ventriculoperitoneal (V-P) shunt insertion, that is, the Early Shunt Group in which a V-P shunt was intially inserted 7–9 days after birth, and the Delayed Shunt Group in which the V-P shunt was inserted approximately 4 weeks after birth. Non-hydrocephalic HTX were also divided into two groups, in one of which sham operations were carried out at the same times as the shunt operations in the experimental groups.

The HTX were anesthetized in the prone position by inhalation of 1.0% halothane. The scalp was incised to expose the parietal bone on the left side, and a hole approximately 2 mm in diameter was bored in the skull in an area 2 mm anterior to the left lambdoid suture and 4–5 mm to the left of the sagittal suture. After the dura matter was exposed and coagulated, a laparatomy was performed at the right dorsal flank to expose the peritoneal space. A shunt passer was inserted into the subcutaneous tissue, and then a V-P shunt tube without pressure regulation valve (Dow Corning Co., silastic catheter, inside diameter 0.025 in, length 12 cm) was passed from the left parietal area to the right flank. The tip of the ventricular catheter was inserted into the left lateral ventricle 4–5 mm from the inner table of the calvaria. After the flow of the cerebrospinal fluid (CSF) from the abdominal catheter was confirmed, the ventricular catheter was fixed to the skull using Aron Alpha. The abdominal catheter was then inserted into the peritoneal space, and the skin incision was closed.

Ventriculography and Magnetic Resonance Imaging (MRI)

The chronological change in ventricular size and thickness of the cortical mantle of the brains of animals subjected to a V-P shunt was assessed at random times after the surgery by ventriculography and by MRI (installed at the National Institute for Physiological Science in Okazaki). During ventriculography under Halothane general anesthesia, 0.2–0.3 ml of Iotroran was slowly injected into the lateral ventricle via V-P shunt abdominal catheter or via 27 G scalp needle inserted directly into the lateral ventricle. Softex X-ray films (Softex Corp., Tokyo) were used to obtain ventriculograms, and the lateral ventricular size visualized on the Softex film was measured by planimetry using a computer-assisted image analyzer (IBASS 2000, Zeiss). The MRI used in this study was Hitachi 2.114 T, and T1 weighted images were obtained.

Light-Darkness Discrimination using Y-Maze Test (Takiguchi et al. 1988)

When the experimental and sham-operated animals subjected either to an early or a delayed V-P shunt became sexually mature, their learning ability was assessed by the Y-maze test, as described elsewhere (Miyazawa and Sato 1991). A mean correct response rate and a mean response latency time were calculated for each set of 10 trials for each respective animal. Different conditions in the animals were compared statistically, using three-way analysis of variance (ANOVA) and the Wilcoxon *t*-test.

Measurement of Locomotor Activity

All animals subjected to the Y-maze test were individually placed on an Automex-II in order to count their motions in a 12-hour period from 19:00 to 07:00. The statistical differences in motion counts among the different experimental animal groups were evaluated using the Wilcoxon *t*-test.

Neuropathological Study

Animals which had completed the Y-maze test and assessment of locomotor activity were anesthetized by ethyl inhalation. They were sacrificed by transcardial perfusion with a 4% paraformaldehyde solution for conventional light microscope and histochemical examinations, and with a perfusate containing 3% potassium dichromate and 0.2% osmium tetroxide for quantitative Golgi study (Millhouse 1981). In the latter study, the spines of the apical and basal dendrites of the pyramidal neurons in layers II and III of the fronto-parietal cortex (Zilles and Wree 1985) were quantitatively measured, as described elsewhere (Sholl 1953; Miyazawa et al. 1988). In brief, the number of spines on 20 µm segments of, apical and basal dendrites respectively, at a distance of 100 µm from the cell body of a neuron were counted. The number of dendritic spines obtained from 30 pyramidal neurons of one aminal was considered to represent spine density. Student's *t*-test was used for the statistical comparison of spine densities among different experimental groups (Miyazawa and Sato 1991).

Histochemical Quantification of Synaptic Vesicle Protein (SVP-38)

Paraffin-embedded sections of the brain were stained by an indirect immuno-histochemical technique, with mouse monoclonal antibody (MAb) against synaptic vesicle protein (SVP-38) purified from guinea-pig cerebrum (Obata et al. 1986, 1987); histochemical quantification of SVP-38 was then carried out. In brief, the sections were incubated with MAb and FITC-conjugated sheep anti-mouse IgG, after which the fluorescence intensity of the immunoreactive products in a 5-µm spot in the molecular layer of the parieto-occipital cortex was measured with a microphotometer. The fluorescence intensity values were expressed as the mean standard error of the 60 measurements of four rats in each experimental group, and the results were statistically compared by Student's *t*-test (T. Miyazawa et al., unpublished data).

Immunoblot Analysis of Synaptic Vesicle Protein (SVP-38)

For electrophoresis, animals in each experimental group were sacrificed by decapitation at 4 weeks of age. The isolated brain tissues were homogenized in 10 volumes of electrophoresis-sample buffer and subjected to immunoblot analysis. Sodium dodecyl sulfate polyacrylamide gel electrophoresis (SDS-PAGE) was performed by Laemmli's method (1970). The gels were then electroblotted onto nitrocellulose sheets and the blots were reacted successively with MAb, HRP-conjugated goat anti-mouse IgG, and 3,3'-diaminobenzidine (DAB).

Results

Sequelae of Early Ventriculoperitoneal Shunt

The survival rates of 4-week and 8-week-old hydrocephalic HTX treated with early shunts were approximately 80% and 40%, respectively. Because of animal death due to shunt malfunction, shunt infection, and subdural hematoma, only 32% of the animals thus treated grew to a sexually mature age and could be subjected to the Y-maze test. The survival rate of 8-week-olds in the delayed shunt group was approximately 20%.

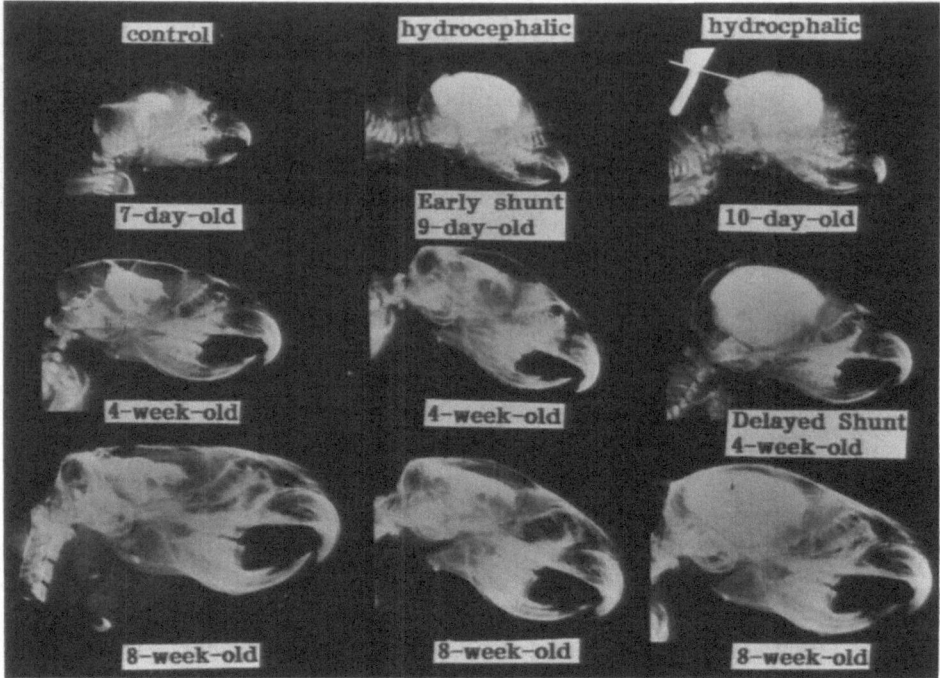

Fig. 1. Ventriculographic follow-up of HTX-rat. *Left*, non-hydrocephalic HTX-rat with sham-operation (control); *Center*, hydrocephalic HTX-rat with early shunt insertion at 9 days after birth; *Right*, hydrocephalic HTX-rat with delayed shunt insertion at 4 weeks after birth

Ventriculography and MRI

The early shunt and delayed shunt groups of hydrocephalic animals displayed distinct differences in the chronological changes in size of their lateral ventricles. In the former group, the size of the lateral ventricle, as assessed by venticulography early during shunt procedure, was abnormally enlarged. However, follow-up ventriculography approximately 4 and 8 weeks after birth revealed that early shunt resulted in normalization not only of enlarged ventricles, but also of cranial vault bulging (Figs. 1 and 2). Normalization of abnormally enlarged ventricles concomitant with increase in cortical mantle thickness following early shunt placement was clearly demonstrated by MRI (Fig. 3). Contrary to these findings, little reduction in the size of abnormally enlarged ventricles was observed in the delayed shunt group (Figs. 1 and 2).

Y-Maze Test: Early Shunt Group

The learning ability of sexually mature HTX whose congenital hydrocephalus had been arrested by an early shunt was assessed by the Y-Maze test and compared with that of sham-operated animals. In both groups, the correct

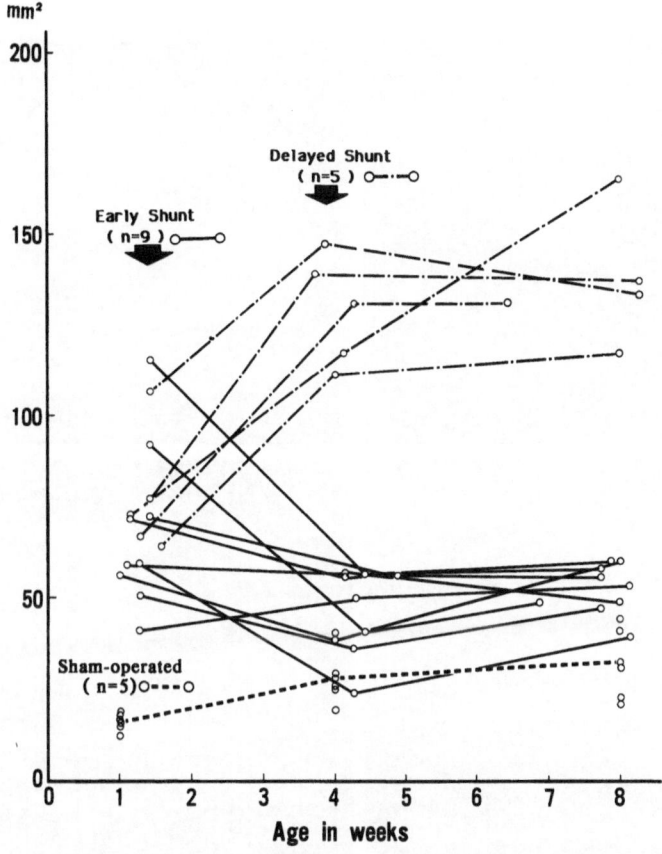

Fig. 2. Comparison of chronological changes in ventricular size of hydrocephalic rats after early and delayed ventriculoperitoneal shunt insertions

response rate increased progressively with advancing sessions, as demonstrated by the significant session effect of analysis of variance [$F(23,552) = 23.38$, $P < 0.01$ ANOVA]. Although a statistically significant difference of mean correct response could be found in 2 out of 24 sessions, the group effect of analysis of variance [$F(1,23) = 1.43$ N.S. ANOVA] did not show any statistically significant difference between the two groups. In addition, there was interaction between the two factors of group and session [$F(23,552) = 1.77$, $P < 0.05$ ANOVA] (Fig. 4a). The response latency time of both groups was progressively shortened with advancing sessions, as demonstrated by the significant session effect of analysis of variance [$F(23,552) = 6.75$, $P < 0.01$ ANOVA]. Comparisons of mean response latency time in each session with Wilcoxon t-test did not demonstrate significant differences between the two groups in all sessions. And then, there was no significant difference between the two groups as demonstrated by group effect of analysis of variance [$F(1,23) = 0.06$ N.S. ANOVA]. In addition, no interaction between the two factors of group and session was found [$F(1,23) = 0.55$, N.S. ANOVA] (Fig. 4b).

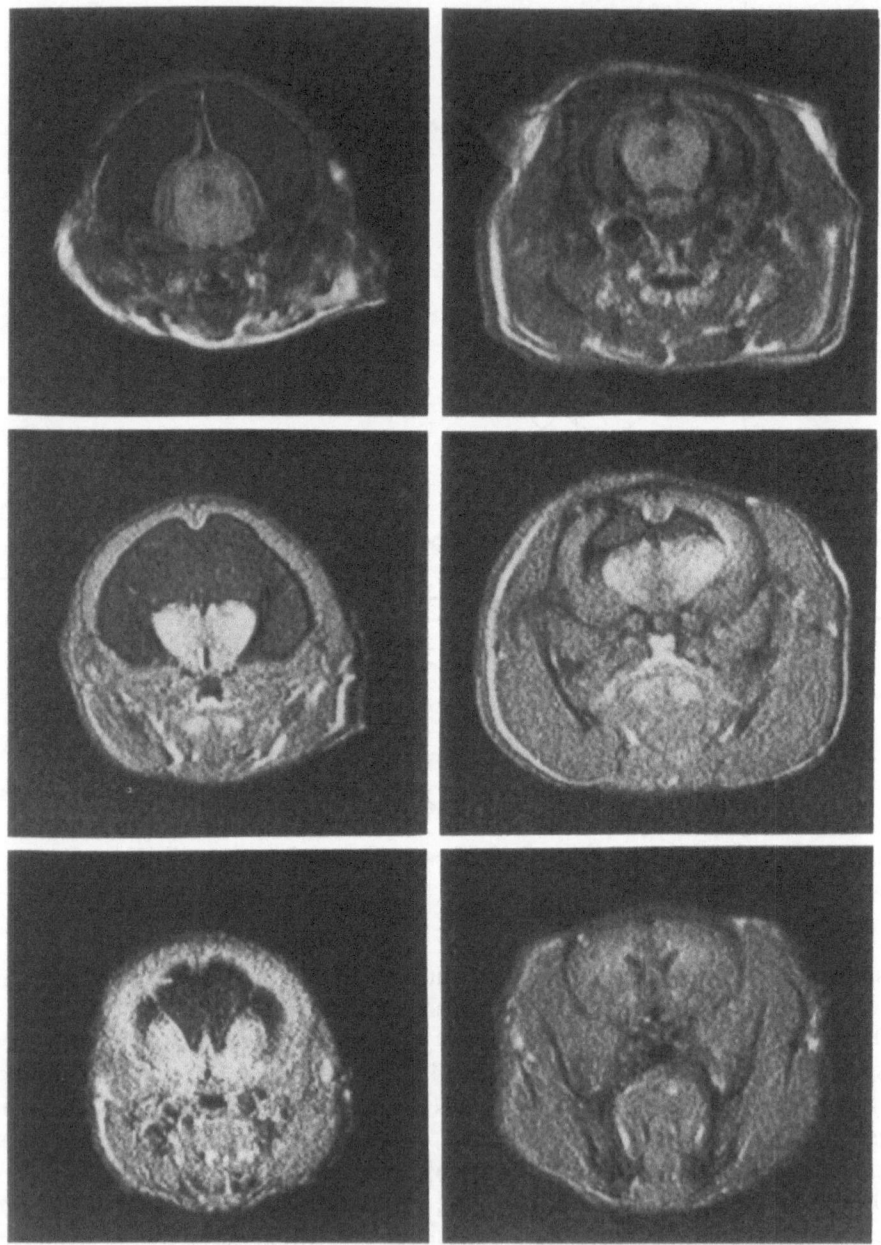

Fig. 3. *Left*, MRI findings of 4-week-old hydrocephalic HTX-rat without ventriculoperitoneal shunt; *Right*, 12-week-old hydrocephalic HTX-rat with early shunt insertion

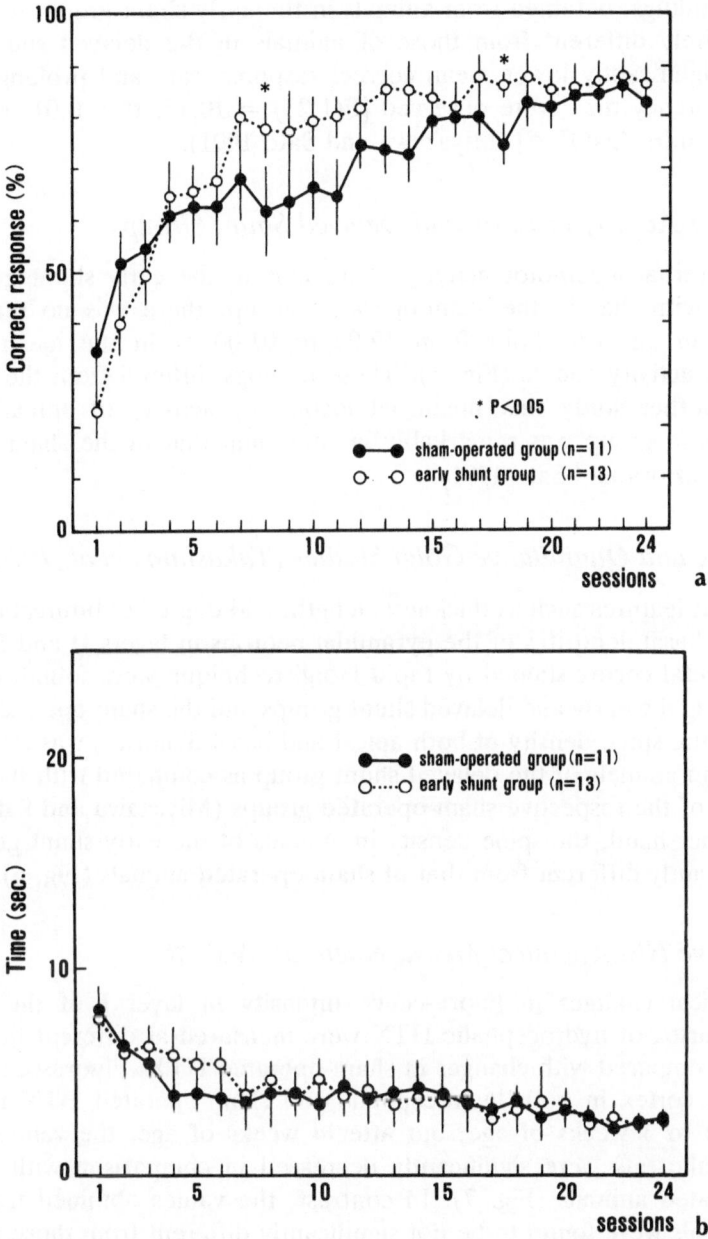

Fig. 4. Light-darkness discrimination test (Y-maze test): **a** Comparison of correct response rate between early shunt and sham-operated groups, and **b** comparison of response latency time between early shunt and sham-operated groups. *Vertical bars* indicate standard errors of the mean

These findings, obtained from animals in the early shunt group, were found to be entirely different from those of animals in the delayed shunt group, where a significantly lower mean correct response rate and prolonged mean response latency time were observed [$F(1,23) = 10.16$, $P < 0.01$, $F(1,23) = 10.35$, $P < 0.01$ ANOVA] (Miyazawa and Sato 1991).

Locomotor Activity in Early and Delayed Shunt Groups

When nocturnal locomotor activity of animals in the early shunt group was compared with that in the sham-operated group, there was no remarkable difference in any one hour from 19:00 to 07:00 or in the mean 12-hour cumulative activity counts (Fig. 5). These findings differed from the observation of another study that nocturnal locomotor activity of animals in the delayed shunt group was remarkably greater than that in the sham-operated group (Miyazawa and Sato 1991).

Qualitative and Quantitative Golgi Studies (Takashima et al. 1978)

Histological features such as thickness, length, and degree of bifurcation of the apical and basal dendrites of the pyramidal neurons in layers II and III of the fronto-parietal cortex stained by rapid Golgi technique were found not to be differ among the early and delayed shunt groups and the sham-operated group. However, the spine density of both apical and basal dendrites was remarkably decreased in animals of the delayed shunt group as compared with the density in animals of the respective sham-operated groups (Miyazawa and Sato 1991). On the other hand, the spine density in animals of the early shunt group was not significantly different from that of sham-operated animals (Fig. 6).

Quantitative Histochemical Measurement of SVP-38

Chronological changes in fluorescence intensity in layer I of the parieto-occipital cortex of hydrocephalic HTX were measured at different times after birth and compared with changes in sham-operated HTX. Fluorescence intensity of the cortex in both hydrocephalic and sham-operated HTX increased linearly up to 3 weeks of age, but after 4 weeks of age, the values for the hydrocephalic rats were significantly decreased in comparison with those of sham-operated animals (Fig. 7). In contrast, the values obtained from early shunt animals were found to be not significantly different from those of sham-operated animals (Fig. 8).

Immunoblot Analysis of SVP-38

In the cerebrum of 4-week-old non-hydrocephalic HTX, SVP-38 was detected by immunoblot analysis as an intense band with a molecular weight of 38 kilodalton. In contrast, in the cerebrum of 4-week-old hydrocephalic HTX, SVP-38 decayed in parallel with the progression of hydrocephalus. Such decay

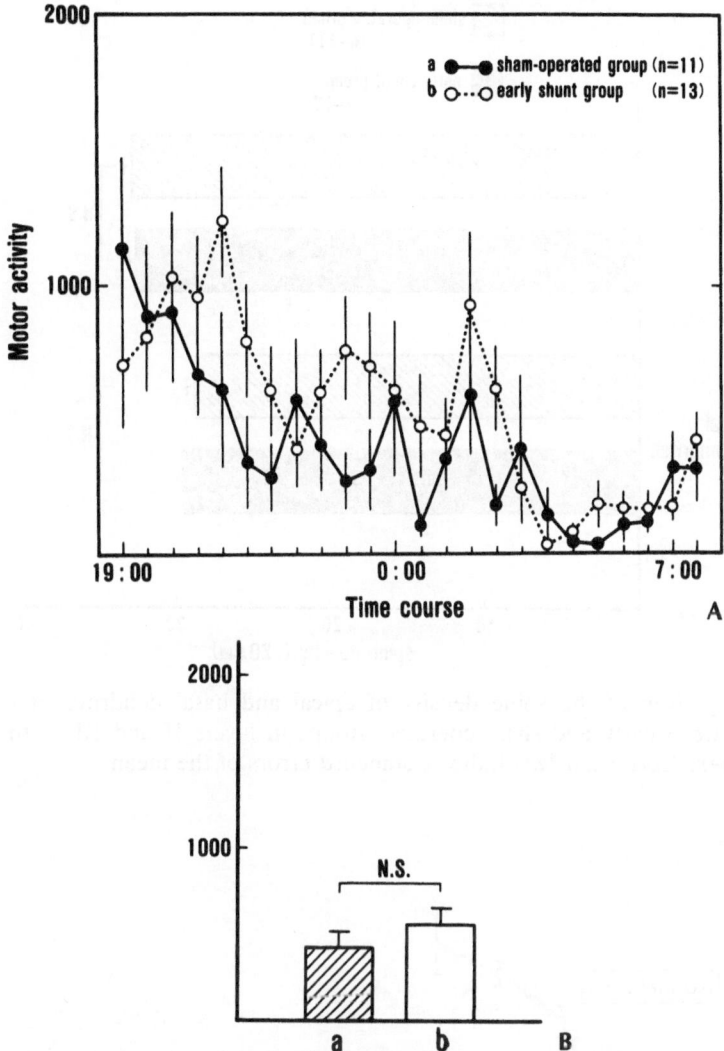

Fig. 5. Locomotor activity assessed with Automex II: **A** Comparison of nocturnal activity between early shunt and sham-operated groups, and **B** comparison of mean 12-hour cumulative activity between early shunt and sham-operated groups

of SVP-38 was not observed when progression of hydrocephalus had been arrested by early shunt insertion (Fig. 9)

Discussion

In earlier studies, large animals such as cats and rabbits, in which aquired hydrocephalus was induced by such techniques as intracisternal injection of kaolin, were used as hydrocephalic animal models for experimental shunt oper-

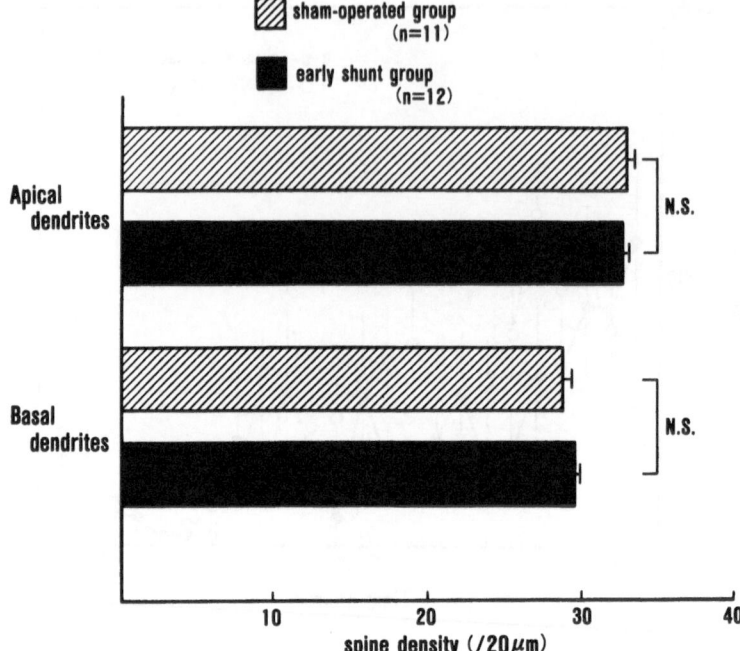

Fig. 6. Comparison of the spine density of apical and basal dendrites of pyramidal neurons between early and sham-operated groups in layers II and III of the fronto-parietal cortex. *Horizontal bars* indicate standard errors of the mean

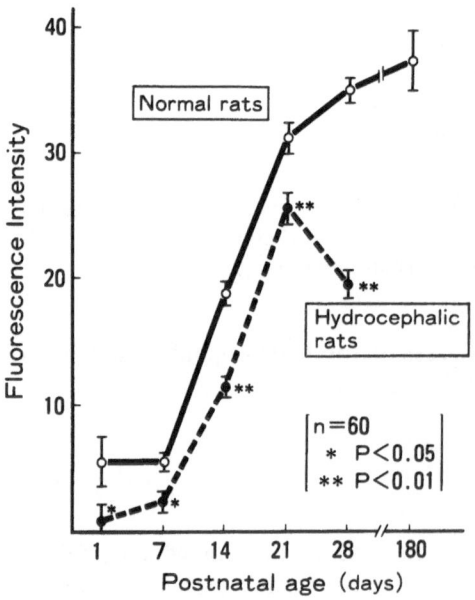

Fig. 7. Fluorescence intensity of SVP-38 throughout postnatal development of non-hydrocephalic and hydrocephalic HTX-rats in layer I of the cerebral cortex. Values are expressed as mean standard error of the 60 measurements of 4 rats in each group. *Vertical bars* indicate standard errors of the mean

Fig. 8. Fluorescence intensity of SVP-38 in layers I and II of the parieto-occipital cortex of 4-week-old HTX-rats. **A**, non-hydrocephalic HTX-rats with sham-operation (n = 4); **B**, hydrocephalic HTX-rats with early shunt insertion (n = 4); **C**, hydrocephalic HTX-rats without ventriculoperitoneal shunt (n = 4). *Vertical bars* indicate standard errors of the mean

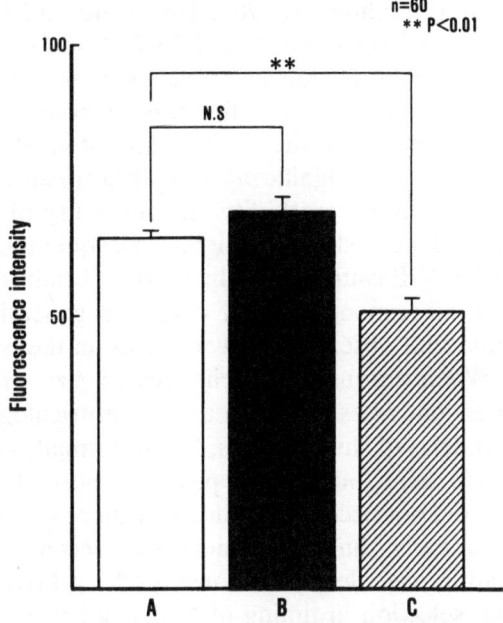

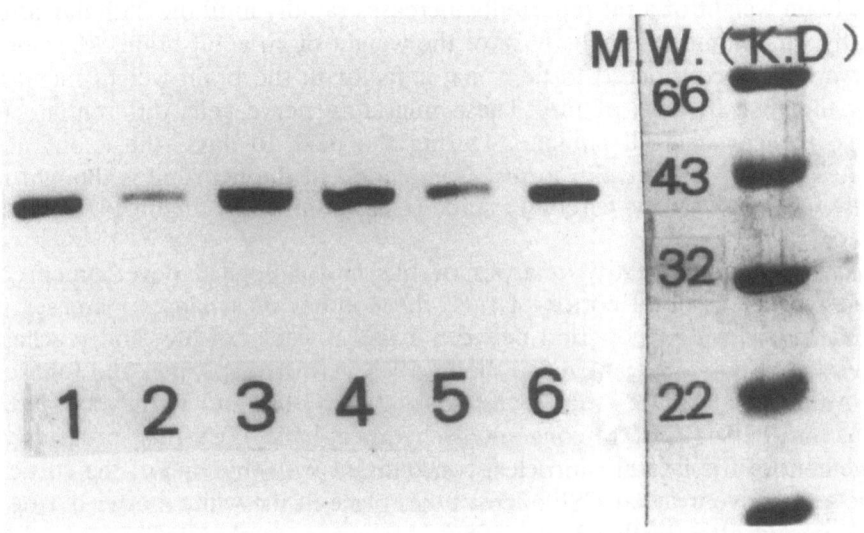

Fig. 9. Immunoblot analysis of SVP-38 in the cerebral cortex of 4-week-old HTX-rats. *Lanes 1 and 4*, non-hydrocephalic HTX-rats with sham-operation; *Lanes 2 and 5*, hydrocephalic HTX-rats without ventriculoperitoneal shunt; *Lanes 3 and 6*, hydrocephalic HTX-rats with early shunt insertion

ation (Granholm L 1966; Hochwald and Epstain 1973; Rubin and Hochwald 1976; Del Bigio and Bruni 1980; Fried et al. 1987). It has, however, become increasingly difficult in recent years to use such large animals in experiments. Such being the case, the use of congenitally hydrocephalic HTX-rats and development of the ventriculoperitoneal shunt technique in small animals appear to be significant in hydrocephalus research. As was reported in the present study, morbidity and mortality of HTX to which the V-P shunt was applied were still very high. Consequently, we felt that techical improvement of the V-P shunt would have to be established before the universal validity of this experimental model could be generally accepted. Nevertheless, various important observations were made in the present investigation.

When chronological changes in size of the lateral ventricles after shunt insertion, assessed by means of ventriculography, were compared in the early and delayed shunt groups, the abnormally enlarged ventricles in the early shunt group were found to be promptly normalized after V-P shunt placement, but this did not occur in the delayed shunt group. That reduction in ventricular size after early shunt placement was accompanied by thickening of the cortical mantle was clearly demonstrated by MRI. These observations may indicate that selection in timing of V-P shunt placement is one crucial factor in regard to prevention of functional and morphological disturbances of the developing brain caused by congenital hydrocephalus in HTX-rats.

The brain weight of a rat reportedly increases rapidly until the 25th day after birth, by which time it may be 85% of the weight of an adult brain. Migration of nerve cells is considered to be a major factor in the brain weight increase during the first 10 days of life. These migrating nerve cells differentiate to produce the cortical cell laminae. During the next 10 days, the axons and dendrites develop and myelin forms. Completion of the neuropil is thought to increase the weight of the cerebral mantle (Haas et al. 1970; Sugita 1971; Wada 1988).

According to quantitative analysis of the morphological development of synapses in the cerebral cortex of rats, the number of synapses increases in linear fashion during the period between 1 and 3 weeks of life, and reachesa plateau thereafter (Aghajanian and Bloom 1967; Armstrong-James and Johnson 1970; Miller et al. 1988; Adams and Jones 1982; Blue and Parnavelas 1983; Markus and Petit 1987). In congenitally hydrocephalic HTX-rats, progressive enlargement of the lateral ventricles, concomitant with thinning of the cortical mantle and periventricular CSF edema takes place in the white matter during a 3-week period after birth (Wada: 1988). Miyazawa et al. (1988), when they investigated cortical pyramidal neurons of such hydrocephalic brains by qualitative and quantitative Golgi technique at 2 weeks after birth, found that the neuronal soma remained morphologically intact, although such drastic changes as winding, tortuosity, and varicosity were noted in the apical and basal dendrites, in association with marked reduction in the spine density (Borit and Sidmann 1972; Marin-Padilla 1972; Purpura et al. 1982; McAllister et al. 1985). Since dendritic spines are now recognized as representing "specific postsynaptic receptive structures" on the dendrites, it was assumed by us that presynaptic structures also may be affected by hydrocephalic pathology. Consequently Miyazawa et al. (unpublished data) demonstrated, by using quantitative histochemical measurement of the synaptic vesicle protein, SVP-38, that in the cerebral cortex of hydrocephalic HTX-rats, a progressive increase in the amount of SVP-38 occurs during a 3-week period after birth, followed by a marked drop in its amount at 4 weeks after birth. The age-related increase of SVP-38 observed in both hydrocephalic and control HTX-rats up to 3 weeks after birth seemed to be reflected by a progressive increase of the synaptic vesicle protein occurring in association with synaptogenesis. In this regard, we felt that the age-related changes of synaptic density, assessed by quantitative electronmicroscopic analysis of synaptogenesis of the rat cerebral cortex, and reported by several investigators such as Aghajanian et al. (1967), Blue and Parnavelas (1983), and Markus and Petit (1987), lent support to our observation. The sudden decay of SVP-38 4 weeks after birth is considered to be one of the direct effects of the progression of hydrocephalus. This observation, obtained by quantitative histochemical methods, was also confirmed by immunoblot analysis in the present investigation. Since reduced spine density was noted in the hydrocephalic animals as early as 2 weeks after birth, we speculated that a dissociation of pre- and post-synaptic structures may be present in the disturbance of synaptogenesis.

According to the observations of Jones and Bucknall (1987, 1988), the resting pressure of cerebrospinal fluid in the lateral ventricles of hydrocephalic HTX-rats was not elevated above normal for up to 10 days after birth, but by 21 days the pressure was nearly twice that of normal rats. Miyaoka et al. (1988) reported that local cerebral glucose utilization (LCGU) of severely affected hydrocephalic HTX-rats was decreased throughout the brain and that application of a delayed shunt to such animals at 4 weeks of age could not completely correct the impairment of LCGU. Therefore, the significance of early shunt insertion in these HTX is believed to lie in eradicating the pathological processes, which occur secondary to increased intracranial pressure, that affect cerebral blood flow and metabolism in the developing brain. As was demonstrated in the present investigation, when a ventriculoperitoneal shunt was inserted into animals with progressive hydrocephalus at approximately 4 weeks after birth, not only was there no reduction in size of the abnormally enlarged ventricles, but there was also no increase in cortical mantle thickness. Furthermore, spine density in the cerebral cortex in such animals also was found to be decreased when compared with that in sham-operated animals, and learning disability could not be corrected which differed from results in with sham operated animals. Contrary to these observations, in the present investigation in HTX-rats we found that insertion of a V-P shunt as early as 7−9 days after birth prevented most of the unfavorable effects inflicted by hydrocephalus upon the morphological and biochemical development of the brain. In fact, early shunt placement was found to result in normalization of the abnormally enlarged ventricles, in association with simultaneous thickening of the cerebral cortical mantle and preservation of normal spine density in the dendrites of cortical pyramidal neurons. The learning ability of such animals was not found to be disturbed compared with that of the sham-operated group.

We assume, based on these observations, that early shunt placement may have a beneficial role both in repairing and in preventing the impairment of synaptogenesis which occurs in association with the progression of congenital hydrocephalus. Whether or not there is a close correlation between learning disability and impairment of synaptogenesis, as observed in the experiment with the delayed shunt, is still not clear. However, such a correlation seems to plausible, since the prevention of disturbance of synaptogenesis and lack of learning disability in the early shunt experiment were confirmed in the present investigation.

During human fetal brain development, differentiation of the neocortex extends from the beginning of the 3rd month to the end of the 6th month at gestational age (Tuchmann-Duplessis et al., 1980). Synaptogenesis of the cerebral cortex begins from the 7th month of gestation and reaches a maximum at the age of one year (Huttenlocher 1979). Although direct correlation in cerebral development between human and rat is difficult to define, the early and delayed shunts applied to HTX-rats by ourselves may be regarded as a model for treatment of human congenital hydrocephalus in utero and in late infancy. Many investigators have reported that learning disability was found in children whose congenital hydrocephalus was treated during the postnatal period (Milhorat 1972; Dennis et al. 1981; Pretorius et al. 1985). In regard to this, treatment of congenital hydrocephalus in utero, namely, a ventriculoamniotic shunt, was thought to be most promising (Clewell et al. 1982); however the evolution of this new method has been became slowed by the high morbidity and mortality of the fetuses and/or children thus treated (Michejda et al. 1986).

At present, pediatric neurosurgeons generally consider that when congenital hydrocephalus is diagnosed in utero by ultrasound, the affected fetus should be delivered after 33 weeks of gestation and treated by prompt cerebrospinal fluid diversion, when the respiratory distress syndrome can be overcome by medical treatment (Edwards et al. 1986). However, the sequelae of prompt cerebrospinal fluid diversion in premature infants cannot be ignored. Considering our experimental observations presented here, the development of new treatments for congenital hydrocephalus in utero seems to be one of the tasks required of pediatric neurosurgeons.

References

Adams I, Jones DG (1982) Quantitative ultrastructual changes in rat cortical synapses during early-, mid- and late-adulthood. Brain Res 239: 349–363

Aghajanian GK, Bloom FE (1967) The formation of synaptic junctions in developing rat brain: A quantitative electron microscopic study. Brain Res 6: 716–727

Armstrong-James M, Johnson R (1970) Quantitative studies of postnatal changes in synapses in rat superficial motor cerebral cortex: An electron microscopical study Z Zellforsch 110: 559–568

Blue ME, Parnavelas JG (1983) The formation and maturation of synapses in the visual cortex of the rat. II. Quantitative analysis. J Neurocytol 12: 697–712

Borit A, Sidman RL (1972) New mutant mouse with communicating hydrocephalus and secondary aqueductal stenosis. Acta Neuropathol (Berl) 21: 316–331

Clewell WH, Johnson ML, Meier PR, et al. (1982) A surgical approach to the treatment of fetal hydrocephalus. N Engl J Med 306: 1320–1325

Del Bigio MR, Bruni JE (1980) Changes in periventricular vasculature of rabbit brain following induction of hydrocephalus and after shunting. J Neurosurg 69: 115–120

Dennis M, Fitz CR, Netley CT, Sugar J , Hoffman HJ (1981) The intelligence of hydrocephalic children. Arch Neurol 38: 607–615

Edwards MS (1986) An evaluation of the in utero neurosurgical treatment of ventriculomegaly. Clin Neurosurg 33: 341–357

Freid A, Schapiro K, Takei F (1987) A laboratory model of shunt-dependent hydrocephalus. Development and biochemical characterization. J Neurosurg 66: 734–740

Granholm L (1966) Induced reversibility of ventricular dilatation on experimental hydrocephalus. Acta Neurol Scand 42: 581–588

Haas RJ, Werner J, Fliedner TM (1970) The cytokinetics of neonatal brain cell development in rats as studied by the complete labeling tritiated thymidine method. J Anat 107: 421–437

Hochwald GM, Epstain F (1973) The relationship of compensated to decompensated hydrocephalus in the cat. J Neurosurg 39: 694–697

Huttenlocher PR (1979) Synaptic density in human frontal cortex. Developmental changes and effects of aging. Brain Res 163: 195–205

Jones HC, Bucknall RM (1987) Changes in cerebrospinal fluid pressure and outflow from the lateral ventricles during development of congenital hydrocephalus in the HTX Rat. Exp Neurol 98: 573–583

Jones HC, Bucknall RM (1988) Inherited prenatal hydrocephalus in the HTX rat: a morphological study. Neuropathol Appl Neurobiol 14: 263–274

Kohn DF, Chinookoswong N, Chou SM (1981) A new model of congenital hydrocephalus in the rat. Acta Neuropathol (Berl) 54: 211–218

Kohn DF, Chinookoswong N, Chou SM (1984) Animal models of human disease. Congenital hydrocephalus. Am J Pathol 114: 184–185

Laemmli UK (1970) Cleavage of structual proteins during the assembly of the head of bacteriophage T4. Nature 227: 680–685

Marin-Padilla M (1972) Structual abnormalities of the cerebral cortex in human chromosomal abserrations: a Golgi study. Brain Res 44: 625–629

Markus EJ, Petit TL (1987) Neocortical synaptogenesis, aging, and behavior: lifespan development in the motor-sensory system of the rat. Exp Neurol 96: 262–278

McAllister JP, Maugans TA, Shah MV, et al. (1985) Neuronal effects of experimentally induced hydrocephalus in newborn rats. J Neurosurg 63: 776–783

Michejda M, Queenan JT, McCullough D (1986) Present status of intrauterine treatment of hydrocephalus and its future. Am J Obstet Gynecol 155: 873–882

Milhorat TH (1972) Hydrocephalus and the cerebrospinal fluid. Williams and Wilkins, Baltimore, pp 177–199

Miller M (1981) Maturation of rat visual cortex. I. A quantitative study of Golgi-impregnated pyramidal neurons. J Neurocytol 10: 859–878

Millhouse OE (1981) The Golgi methods. In: Heimer L, Robards MJ (eds) Neuroanatomical tract-tracing methods. Plenum, New York, pp 311–344

Miyaok M, Ito M, Sato K, Ishii S (1988) Measurement of local cerebral glucose utilization before and after V-P shunt in congenital hydrocephalus in rats. Metab Brain Dis 3: 125–132

Miyazawa T, Sato K (to be published) Learning disability and impairment of synaptogene in the HTX-rats with arrested shunt-dependent hydrocephalus. Nerv Syst Child

Miyazawa T, Wada M, Sato K (1988) A quantitative Golgi study of cortical pyramidal neurons in congenitally hydrocephalic HTX-rats — Golgi study. Nerv Syst Child 13(4): 263–270

Obata K, Nishiye H, Fujita SC, Shirao T, Uchizono K (1986) Identification of a synaptic vesicle-specific 38000-dalton protein by monoclonal antibodies. Brain Res 375: 37–48

Obata K, Kojima N, Nishiye H, Inoue H, Shirao T, Uchizono K (1987) Four synaptic vesicle-specific proteins: identification by monoclonal antibodies and distribution in the nervous tissue and the adrenal medulla. Brain Res 404: 167–179

Pretorius DH, Davis K, Manco-Johnson ML (1985) Cinical course of fetal hydrocephalus: 40 cases. AJNR 144: 827–831

Purpura RC, Bodick N, Suzuki K, Rapin I, Wurzelmann S (1982) Microtubule disarray in cortical dendrites and neurobehavioral failure. I. Golgi and electron microscopic study. Dev Brain Res 5: 287–297

Rubin RC, Hochwald GM (1976) Hydrocephalus III. Reconstitution of the cerebral cortical mantle following ventricular shunting. Surg Neurol 5: 179–183

Sholl DA (1953) Dendritic organization in the neurons of the visual and motor cortices of the cat. J Anat 87: 387–406

Sugita N (1972) Comparative studies on the growth of the cerebral cortex. II On the increase in the thickness of the cerebral cortex during the postnatal growth of the brain in the albino rat. J Comp Neurol 28: 511–591

Takashima S, Chan F, Becker LE, Armstrong DL (1978) Morphology of the developing visual cortex of the human infant: A quantitative and qualitative Golgi study J Neuropathol Exp Neurol 39: 487–501

Takiguchi H, Ishizuka A, Ikeda Y (1988) The effects of a dibenzoxazepine derivative on learning ability and local cerebral glucose utilization in aged rats. Jpn J Neuropsychopharmacol 10: 459–469

Tuchmann-Duplessis H, Auroux M, Haegel P (1980) Illustrated human embryology. pp 72–74

Wada M (1988) Congenital hydrocephalus in HTX rats: Incidence, pathophysiology and developmental impairment. Neurol Med Chir (Tokyo) 28: 955–964

Zilles K, Wree A (1985) Cortex: A real and laminar structure. In: George P (ed) The rat nervous system, Vol. 1. Academic, pp 375–415

3 — Embryopathoetiology of Congenital Hydrocephalus in Experimental Models: A Comparative Morphological Study in Two Different Models

Hiroshi Yamada, Shizuo Oi, Norihiko Tamaki, Satoshi Matsumoto[1], and Katsushi Taomoto[2]

Summary. We studied the morphological aspects of two different kinds of exerimental hydrocephalic model in rats. LEW/Jms rats were used as an inherited congenital hydrocephalic strain and 6-aminonicotinamide (6-AN, a niacinamide antimetabolite)-induced hydrocephalus was studied as an exogenous insult-induced hydrocephalus.

In LEW/Jms rats, aqueduct obstruction was observed on gestational day 17, prior to definite evidence of ventricular enlargement. The form of the aqueductal obstruction was found to be simple stenosis, according to Russell's classification. This finding suggested that aqueductal stenosis was the primary cause of hydrocephalus in the LEW/Jms hydrocephalic strain. This strain might be a model of human sex-linked hydrocephalus.

In 6-AN-induced hydrocephalic rats, dilatation of the whole ventricular system was observed. In this model, evidence of cerebral dysgenesis was suggested by bromodeoxyuridine (BUdR) immunostaining. However, the ventricular dilatation was resulted not only from cerebral dysgenesis, but also from increased intracranial pressure. This model was characteristic in that, in addition to the hydrocephalic state, various central nervous system malformations existed, such as cerebellar dysgenesis, absence of corpus callosum, and so on. These pathological findings suggested that 6-AN-induced hydrocephalus might be a model of human Dandy-Walker syndrome.

Keywords. Congenital hydrocephalus — X-Linked Hydrocephalus — LEW/Jms strain — 6-Aminonicotinamide — Dandy-Walker syndrome

Introduction

The cause of congenital hydrocephalus is various in both human and experimental forms of the condition. However, an important problem, the etiopathogenesis of hydrocephalus in many strains, has been left unsolved.

[1] Department of Neurosurgery, Kobe University, Kobe, 650 Japan
[2] Department of Neurosurgery, Hyogo Medical Center for Adults, Akashi, Hyogo, 673 Japan

We studied two kinds of experimental congenital hydrocephalus in rats, the LEW/Jms strain as an inherited hydrocephalus and 6-aminonicotinamide (6-AN)-induced hydrocephalus as an exogenous insult-induced bydrocephalus. The purpose of this study was to observe the light microscopic pathological findings of congenital hydrocephalus in both these models during the perinatal period and to elucidate the etiology of hydrocephalus in these rats.

Materials and Methods

Inherited Congenital Hydrocephalus

In the LEW/Jms strain, hydrocephalic anomaly was present in about 20% of the animals, as reported by Sasaki et al. (1983). Normal male and female siblings of hydrocephalic rats were mated. After mating, vaginal smears were inspected each morning for signs of sperm. The day copulation was confirmed was designated as day 0 of gestation. Fetuses were collected by uterotomy on gestational days 17, 18, and 20. Newborn pups were also sacrificed. Materials were put in Bouin's solution and embedded in paraffin. In order to investigate and elucidate the morphological changes of the entire CSF pathway, serial sagittal sections, 4 μm thick, were stained with hematoxylin and eosin. Serial coronal sections were also made as the need arose. As it was impossible to distinguish between hydrocephalic and normal embryos from their physical appearance, specimens from all of the siblings were checked. When hydrocephalic rats were included, their morphological changes were compared with those of normal siblings.

Exogenous Insult Hydrocephalus

Male and female Sprague-Dawley (SD-JCL, CLEA Japan) rats were allowed to mate. Vaginal smears were inspected each morning for signs of sperm after mating. The day copulation was confirmed was designated as day 0 of gestation. On the 13th day of gestation, 8 mg/kg of 6-AN was given as a single ip injection; this dosage is known to cause a high frequency of hydrocephalus in fetuses near term (Chamberlain and Nelson 1963). Fetuses were collected by uterotomy 1, 2, 4, and 8 days after injection. Materials were put into Bouin's solution, embedded in paraffin, and cut into 5 μm sections. All fetuses were serially sectioned either sagittally or coronally. Untreated fetuses at the same periods of development were used as controls; all materials were stained with hematoxylin and eosin.

On gestational day 17 (4 days after 6-AN injection), bromodeoxyuridine (BUdR), at a dose of 50 mg, was given as a single ip injection to one pregnant rat 1 h before uterotomy. The fetuses collected from this rat were then put into 70% ethanol and embedded in paraffin, cut into 5 μm sections, and deparaffinized. Specimens were denatured for 30 min in 2N HCl and incubated for 30 min in ethanol with 0.3% H_2O_2 to avoid endogenous peroxidase activity.

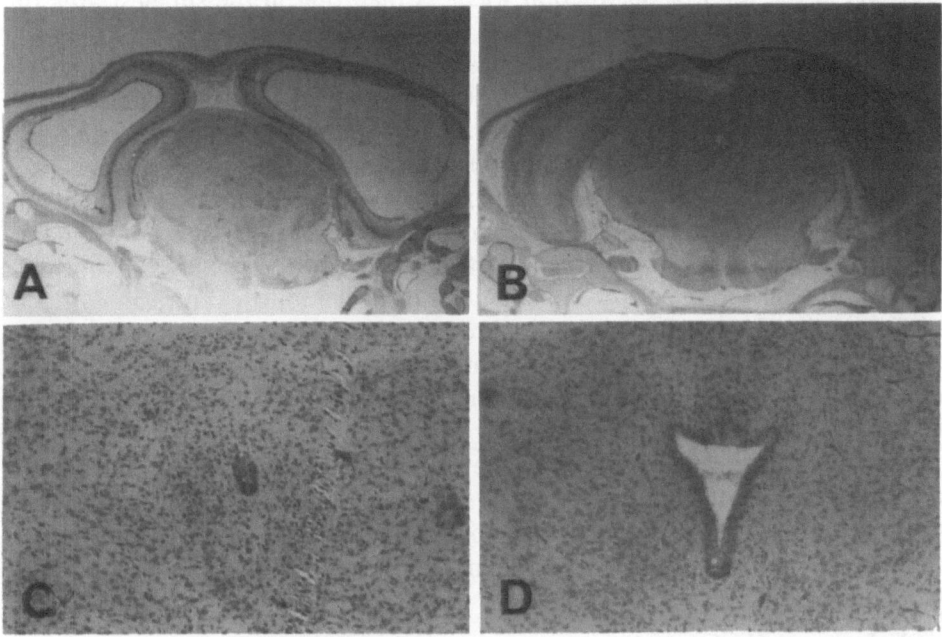

Fig. 1. Newborn rats in coronal section. **A** and **C** show a hydrocephalic and **B** and **D** show a normal rat; **C** and **D** are magnifications of the aqueduct. Complete obstruction of the aqueduct with a simple stenosis is observed in hydrocephalus (**C**), while in the normal rat, the aqueduct is patent with a triangular shaped lumen (**D**) (A.B From H. Yamada et al (1991) Published with permission)

They were then reacted with a 1:30 dilution of purified anti-BUdR monoclonal antibody in phosphate buffer solution (PBS) for 30 min at room temperature. The specimens were then covered with peroxidase-conjugated anti-mouse immunoglobulin G antibody for 30 min and reacted with 5 mg of diaminobenzidine tetrahydrochloride and 4μ 1 of 30% H_2O_2 of Tris buffer for 5 min. Myer hematoxylin was used to counterstain the tissue sections. Untreated fetuses at the same period of development were labeled with BUdR by the same method.

Results

LEW/Jms Strain

Figure 1 shows coronal sections of 1-day-old normal and hydrocephalic rats. In normal rats, the smallest diameter was located at the anterior part of the aqueduct, which was triangular in shape with the base facing the dorsal side. The shape of aqueductal sections varied from the cephalic to the caudal level, as in the human aqueduct (Woollam and Millen 1953). In hydrocephalic rats, the smallest part of the aqueduct was completely obstructed by a collection of oval shaped ependymal cells. The number of ependymal cells lining the aqueduct at the level of obstruction was less than that in the smallest area of the aqueduct in normal rats.

On gestational days 20 and 18, the basic appearance was the same as that of the new-born pups. In hydrocephalus, the lateral and third ven+ricles were dilated and the pineal body was compressed and shifted behind by the enlarged third ventricle. A serial sagittal section also showed that the aqueduct was obstructed. The obstructed site was next to the caudal side of the junction between the third ventricle and the aqueduct. Normal rats showed a patent aqueduct. There was no difference between the hydrocephalic and normal fetuses in the posterior part of the aqueduct or in the fourth ventricle.

On gestational day 17, eight rats were examined; their ventricles were the same size. Only one of these eight rats was found to be occluded at the aqueduct; the other seven rats had patent aqueducts (Fig. 2). The entire ventricular system of each rat was the same size, irrespective of aqueductal form.

Throughout the gestational period, the site of occlusion was the anterior part of the aqueduct, that is, the level of the anterior colliculus. No difference was detected between hydrocephalic and normal rats in the size or form of the subarachnoid space, brain stem, and spinal cord.

6-AN Induced Hydrocephalus

All 6-AN treated fetuses near term showed evidence of hydrocephalus. Head enlargement could be detected from their physical appearance and the size of the body was smaller than that of the head, in contrast with the appearance of control rats.

The cerebral mantle facing the ventricle was examined on gestational day 14 in control and 6-AN treated (24 h after injection) rats. Many mitotic figures were noted in the cerebral mantle in the control, however, no such figures were seen in the 6-AN treated fetus. Cellular rarefaction was also seen in the 6-AN treated rats. These findings suggested that 6-AN had some toxic effects in the developing brain.

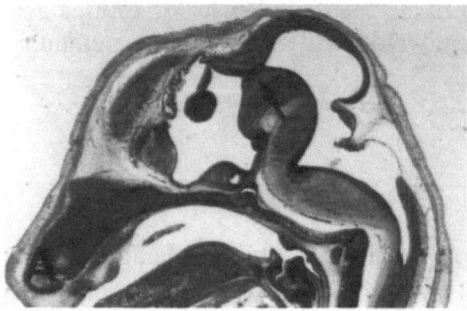 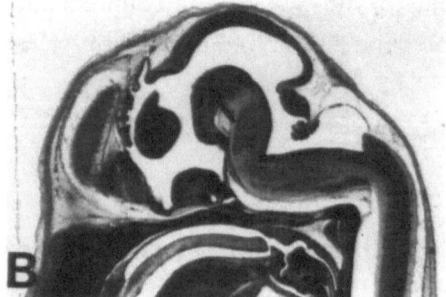

Fig. 2. Midline sagittal section of rat embryo on gestational day 17; **A** showing obstructed aqueduct and **B** showing patent aqueduct. *Arrows* indicate obstructed or patent aqueduct. Ventricles are the same size between A and B. (From H. Yamada et al (1991) Published with permission)

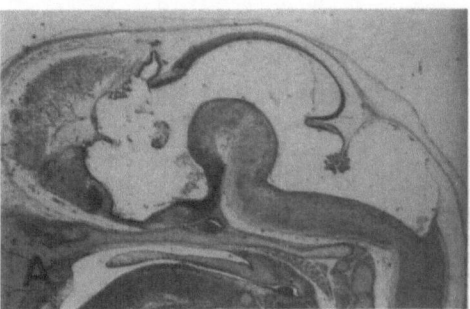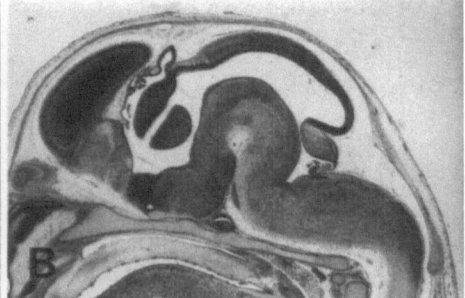

Fig. 3. Midline sag,ittal section of 6-aminonicotinamide (*6-AN*) treated (**A**) and control rat (**B**) embryo on gestational day 17. The 6-AN treated rat showed cystic enlargement (*arrow*) of the fourth ventricle (From H. Yamada et al (1991) Published with permission

On gestational day 17, the 6-AN treated rat showed more severe hypoplasia in all parts of the brain and cellular rarefaction was seen, particularly in the cerebellum. Mild petechial hemorrhage was seen in the tectum of the midbrain. Macrocephalus became clear and ventriculomegaly was confirmed by histological examination. Enlargement of all ventricles, including the aqueduct, was seen, in contrast with findings in the control (Fig. 3). The finding of a thin cortex suggested cerebral hypoplasia. The fourth ventricle was dilated, with cerebellar hypoplasia. In the control, many BUdR positive cells were found in the cerebral mantle around the ventricle. In the 6-AN treated rat, no BUdR positive cells were found in the central nervous system.

On gestational day 21, the finding of macrocephalus became clearer from the physical appearance of the 6-AN treated rats. The skull showed marked distension at the parietal dome. The fact that CSF gushed out when the skull was punctured suggested a high intracranial pressure. The whole ventricular system showed enlargement, including the aqueduct and the fourth ventricle. Agenesis of the corpus callosum was evident on coronal and sagittal sections and normal features characteristic of the cerebellum were not observed (Fig. 4).

Discussion

Many inherited congenital hydrocephalic models have been reported (Berry 1961; Borit and Sidman 1972; D'Amato et al 1986; Green 1970; Higashi et al. 1984; Kohn et al. 1981; Koto et al. 1987; Raimondi et al. 1976); however, few examples of primary aqueductal stenosis have been described. The strain we used, LEW/Jms, was first studied by Sasaki et al. (1983), who reported postnatal developmental changes which they examined histologically. They observed the unbalanced dilatation of both the posterior horn of the lateral ventricle and the upper part of the third ventricle in the postnatal period, and speculated that stenosis of the third ventricle and the anterior part of the

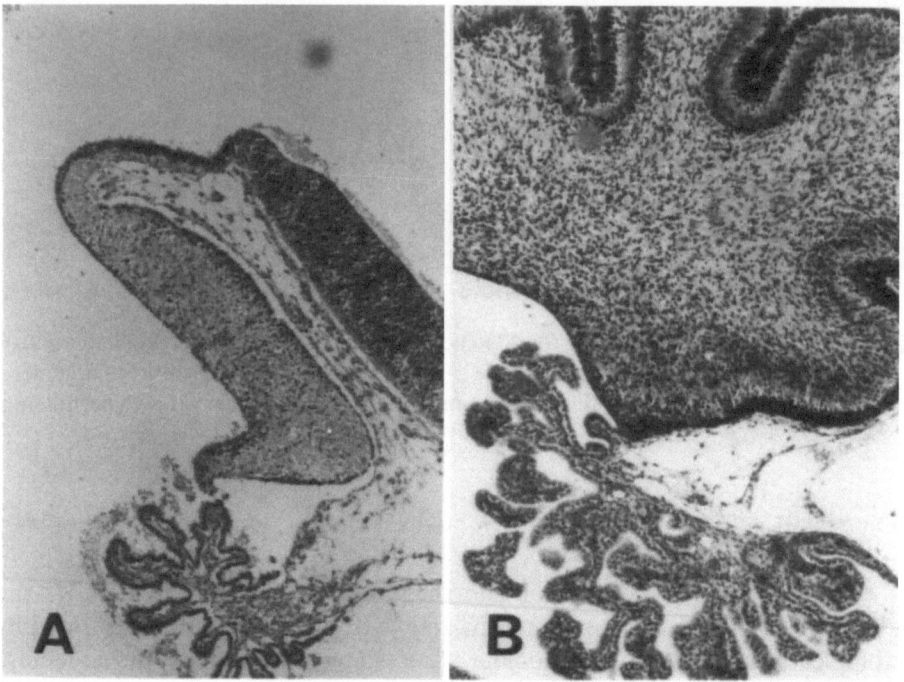

Fig. 4. Cerebellum and choroid plexus in the fourth ventricle of 6-AN treated (**A**) and control rat (**B**) embryo on gestational day 21. No normal features characteristic of the cerebellum were found in the 6-AN treated rat. A hypoplastic choroid plexus is also shown in this rat (From H. Yamada et al (1991) Published with permission)

lateral ventricle in fetal life was a main cause of hydrocephalus. Our study in the fetal period revealed that aqueductal obstruction preceded hydrocephalus and we concluded that aqueductal obstruction in the rats we studied was a primary change and not a secondary phenomenon due to compression by ventricular dilatation. We find support for this thesis in the observation that there was a decrease in the number of ependymal cells lining the aqueduct. Although the entire aqueduct was lined with ependymal cells, the sit of obstruction was the anterior part of the aqueduct.

In humans, there is a form of hydrocephalus with some resemblance to the models presented. In 1949, Bicker and Adams described a family in which all of the sons and four of six brothers of a healthy woman died at birth with hydrocephalus. An autopsy in one case showed evidence of aqueductal stenosis. There have been a number of related reports (Edwards et al. 1961; Holmes et al. 1963) and more information about this sex-linked hydrocephalic disease has been compiled. In the case cited above the entire aqueduct was narrowed; However, there was no septum formation, periaqueductal gliosis, or ependymitis. The narrowest site was reported to be at the rostral portion of the inferior colliculus. As the pathological findings in human hydrocephalus at autopsy are usually those of an advanced stage of hydrocephalus, it is very difficult to conclude whether the aqueductal stenosis described is a primary or a secondary change. In human congenital hydrocephalus, case reports have speculated upon this, but it has yet not been proven that aqueductal stenosis or obstruction are primary changes. In the present study of the hydrocephalic fetal model LEW/Jms rat; we conclude that aqueductal obstruction is a primary change and not a secondary one. The mechanism of aqueductal obstruction in this model is still unclear; however, it is our position that morphological studies in this model will be helpful in resolving the cause of hydrocephalus.

The remarkable pharmacological and toxicological properties of the agent 6-AN have been revealed in experimental animals (Horita et al. 1978; Sasaki 1982). This agent acts not only on the spinal cord, but also on the other sites of the central nervous system (CNS) (Henken et al. 1974; Sasaki 1982). The large amount of 6-phosphogluconate which accumulates in neural tissue in adult rats supports the concept that the primary action of this drug is its inhibition of 6-phosphogluconate dehydrogenase in the pentose phosphate pathway(Henken et al. 1974).

Chamberlain (1970) first reported the morphological changes of 6-AN induced congenital hydrocephalus; however, he showed no histological studies of the models he described. We studied the same model, investigating the developing morphological changes by light microscopic study. This model is very characteristic of with cerebral dysgenesis confirmed by the BUdR immunohistochemical method and various anomalies in the central nervous system. The ventricular dilatation in this model was a result not only of cerebral dysgenesis, but also of increased intracranial pressure, shown by the enlarged head size compared with body size.

Representative human forms of hydrocephalus associated with CNS and systemic anomalies include Dandy-Walker syndrome, Arnold-Chiari malformation, and so on. Several theories relating to the pathogenesis of Dandy-Walker syndrome have been proposed. The most widely accepted view is that the foramina of Luschka and Magendie fail to open, resulting in cystic enlargement of the fourth ventricle with consequent failure of the proper development of the cerebellar vermis (Dandy and Blackfen 1914; Schreiber and Reye 1954; Taggart and Walker 1942). Hart et al. (1972) reported a clinicopathological study on 28 cases of the Dandy-Walker syndrome and concluded that this syndrome was likely to be caused by foraminal atresia. However, none of these proposed mechanisms provide explanations for the many and various associated CNS anomalies. We feel that there is still room for further study. The present model showed cystic enlargement of the fourth ventricle and many CNS anomalies, such as absence of the corpus callosum, cerebellar hypoplasia, maldevelopment of the choroid plexus, and so on, which are associated with hydrocephalus. These findings show that there are interesting similarites between this model and the Dandy-Walker syndrome; the findings indicate that the cause of the Dandy-Walker syndrome is not limited to malfunction in the vicinity of the fourth ventricle, but is due to general systemic metabolic errors, such as niacin deficit in fetal life, as described above. The anomalies seen around the fourth ventricle in the Dandy-Walker syndrome may be one of the features of the systemic disease.

References

Berry RJ (1961) The inheritance and pathogenesis of hydrocephalus-3 in the mouse. J Pathol Bacteriol 81: 157–167

Bicker DS, Adams RD (1949) Hereditary stenosis of the aqueduct of Sylvius as a cause of congenital hydrocephalus. Brain 72: 246–262

Borit A, Sidman RL (1972) New mutant mouse with communicating hydrocephalus and secondary aqueductal stenosis. Acta Neuropathol (Berl) 21: 316–331

Chamberlain JG (1970) Early neurovascular abnormalities underlining 6-aminonicotinamide (6-AN)-induced congenital hydrocephalus in rats. Teratology 3: 377–388

Chamberlain JG, Nelson MM (1963) Multiple congenital anomalies in the rat resulting from acute maternal niacin deficiency during pregnancy. Proc Soc Exp Biol Med 112: 836–840

D'Amato CJ, O'Shea KS, Hicks SP, Glover RA, Annesley TM (1986) Genetic prenatal aqueductal stenosis with hydrocephalus in rat. J Neuropathol Exp Neurol 45: 665–682

Dandy WE, Blackfen KD (1914) Internal hydrocephalus: An experimental, clinical and pathological study. Am J Dis Child 8: 406–482

Edwards JH, Norman RM, Roberts JM (1961) Sex-linked hydrocephalus. Report of a family with 15 affected members. Arch Dis Child 36: 481–485

Green MC (1970) The developmental effects of congenital hydrocephalus (ch) in the mouse. Dev Biol 23: 585–608

Hart MN, Malamud N, Ellis WG (1972) The Dandy-Walker syndrome. A clinico-pathological study based on 28 cases. Neurology 22: 771–780

Herken H, Lange K, Kolbe H, Keller K (1974) Antimetabolic action on the pentose phosphate pathway in the central nervous system induced by 6-aminonicotinamide. In: (Genazzani E, Herken H eds) Central nervous system studies on metabolic regulation and function. Spring, New York, pp 41–54

Higashi K, Asahisa H, Ueda N, Noda Y, Tashiro M (1984) An experimental model of congenital hydrocephalus in the rat (in Japanese). Shoni no Noshinkei 9: 257–264

Holmes LB, Nash A, ZuRhein GM, Levin M, Opitz M (1963) X-linked aqueductal stenosis: Clinical and neuropathological findings in two families. Pediatrics 63: 1104–1110

Horita N, Oyanagi S, Ishii T, Lzumiyama Y (1978) Ultrastructure of 6-aminonicotinamide (6-AN)-induced lesions in the central nervous system of rats. 1. Chromatolysis and other lesions in the cervical cord. Acta Neuropathol (Berl) 44: 111–119

Kohn DF, Chinookoswong N, Chou SM (1981) A new model of congenital hydro-cephalus in the rat. Acta Neuropathol (Berl) 54: 211–218

Koto M, Miwa M, Shimizu A, Tsuji K, Okamato M, Adachi J (1987) Inherited hydrocephalus in Csk Wistar-Imamichi rats Hyd strain: A new disease model for hydrocephalus. Exp Anim 36: 157–162

Raimondi AJ, Clark SJ, McLone DG (1976) Pathogenesis of aqueductal occlusion in congenital murine hydrocephalus. J Neurosurg 5: 66–77

Russel DS (1949) Observations on the pathology of hydrocephalus. Medical Res Council Spec. Rep. Series No 265. HMSO, London

Sasaki S (1982) Brain edema and gliopathy induced by 6-aminonicotinamide intoxication in the central nervous system of rats. Am J Vet Res 143: 1691–1695

Sasaki S, Goto H, Nagano H, Furuya K, Omata Y, Kanazawa K, Suzuki K, Sudo K (1983) Congenital hydrocephalus revealed in the inbred rat LEW/Jms. Neurosurgery 13: 548–554

Schreiber MS, Reye RDK (1954) Posterior fossa cysts due to congenital atresia of the foramen of Luschka and Magendie. Med J Aust 2: 743–748

Taggart JK, Walker AE (1942) Congenital atresia of the foramen of Luschka and Magendie. Arch Neurol Psychiat 48: 583–612

Woollam DHM, Millen JW (1953) Anatomical considerations in the pathology of stenosis of the cerebral aqueduct. Brain 76: 104–112

Yamada H, Oi S, Tamaki N, Matsumoto S, Sudo K (1991) Prenatal aqueductal stenosis as a cause of congenital hydrocephalus in the inbred rat LEW/JMS. Child's Nerv Syst in press

Yamada H, Oi S, Tamaki N, Matsumoto S, Taomoto K (1991) Congenital hydrocephalus mimicking Dandy-Walker syndrome induced by 6-aminonicotinamide injection in pregnant rat. Neurol Med Chir (Tokyo) in press

4 — Postnatal Changes of HRP-Labeled Corticospinal Neurons in Congenital Hydrocephalic Rats (HTX)

Toshio Shirai and Katsuyoshi Ishii[1]

Summary. In the present study we examined the influence of hydrocephalic changes on the growth of corticospinal neurons and the formation of their neuronal connection with the spinal cord in the congenital hydrocephalic rat (HTX) during the postnatal period, using the horseradish peroxidase (HRP)-labeling method.

We injected $0.1-2.0 \, \mu l$ of 20%–50% HRP solution into the cervical cords of HTX rats which had either high or slight dilatation of the lateral ventricles, at postnatal days 1, 7, 14, and 21, and observed the HRP-labeled corticospinal neurons in the cerebral cortex and the structure of the brain stem each day.

At postnatal day 1, HRP-labeled neurons were found in layer V, which was in the dorsal and lateral areas of the cerebral cortex in both types of hydrocephalic rats. From this finding these neurons could be identified as corticospinal neurons and their axons seemed to reach into the spinal cord. By postnatal day 21, HRP-labeled corticospinal neurons were found in the area from the dorsal to the lateral part of the cerebral cortex in the hydrocephalic rats with slight dilatation of the lateral ventricles. However, in the hydrocephalic rats with high dilatation of the lateral ventricles, HRP-labeled corticospinal neurons gradually decreased and a few neurons were found in the lateral part of the cerebral cortex. At postnatal day 21, also, degenerative changes appeared in the corticospinal tract through the pyramis of the medulla oblongata.

These findings indicate that the neuronal connection between the cerebral cortex and the spinal cord, made by the corticospinal axons, gradually disappears when cortical neurons, including corticospinal neurons are destroyed, such destruction being caused by the progresive dilatation of the lateral ventricles and subsequently by the secondary degeneration of the corticospinal axons.

---

[1] Department of Anatomy, Yamagata University School of Medicine, Yamagata, 990-23 Japan

Kohn et al. (1981) reported that, in the congenital hydrocephalic rat (HTX), dilatation of the lateral ventricles appeared at birth and that the thickness of the cerebral cortex gradually decreased, depending on the advancement of lateral ventricular dilatation. These changes seem to influence the differentiation and growth of neurons and neuroglial cells in the cerebral cortex.

Some of the descending projection neurons in the cerebral cortex are corticospinal neurons, which connect the cerebral cortex and the spinal cord. In rats the corticospinal axons are already distributed in the spinal cord at postnatal day 1 (Joosten et al. 1987; Ohtani and Shirai 1988). Moreover, the synaptic formation of the corticospinal neurons advances on their axon terminals in the spinal cord and on their somas through postnatal day 14 (Ohtani et al. 1987; Miyabayashi and Shirai 1988).

In the present study the postnatal development of the corticospinal neurons in the congenital hydrocephalic rat (HTX) was investigated, using the HRP-labeling method, in order to define the effect of hydrocephalic changes on the formation of neuronal connections by cerebral cortical neurons.

Keywords. Congenital hydrocephalic rat — HRP-Labeling method — Corticospinal neurons — Cerebral cortex — Postnatal development.

Materials and Methods

HTX rats with slight and high dilatations of the lateral ventricles at postnatal days 1, 7, 14, and 21 were used. We anesthetized all rats with Nembutal, and immediately injected 0.1–2.0 µl of 20%–50% solution of horseradish peroxidase (HRP) into their cervical cords. One or two days after HRP injection, we perfused them with a fixative consisting of a 1% solution of paraformaldehyde

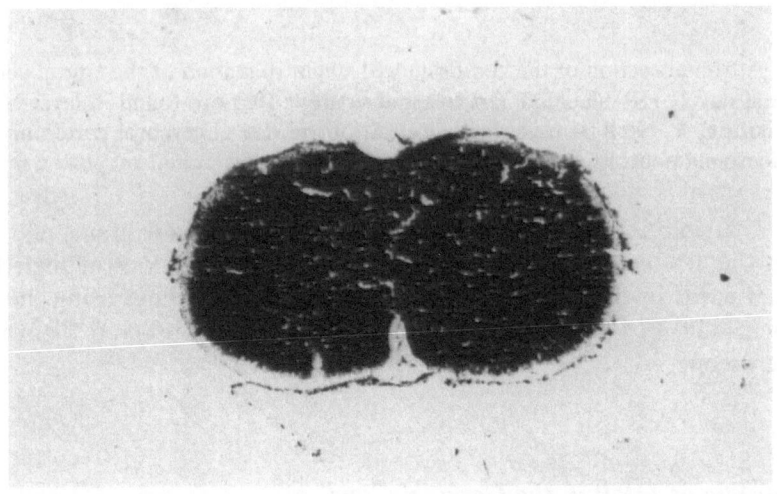

Fig. 1. HRP-injection site in the cervical cord of HTX rat at postnatal day 14. Most area of the spinal cord is stained dark brown with HRP. × 24

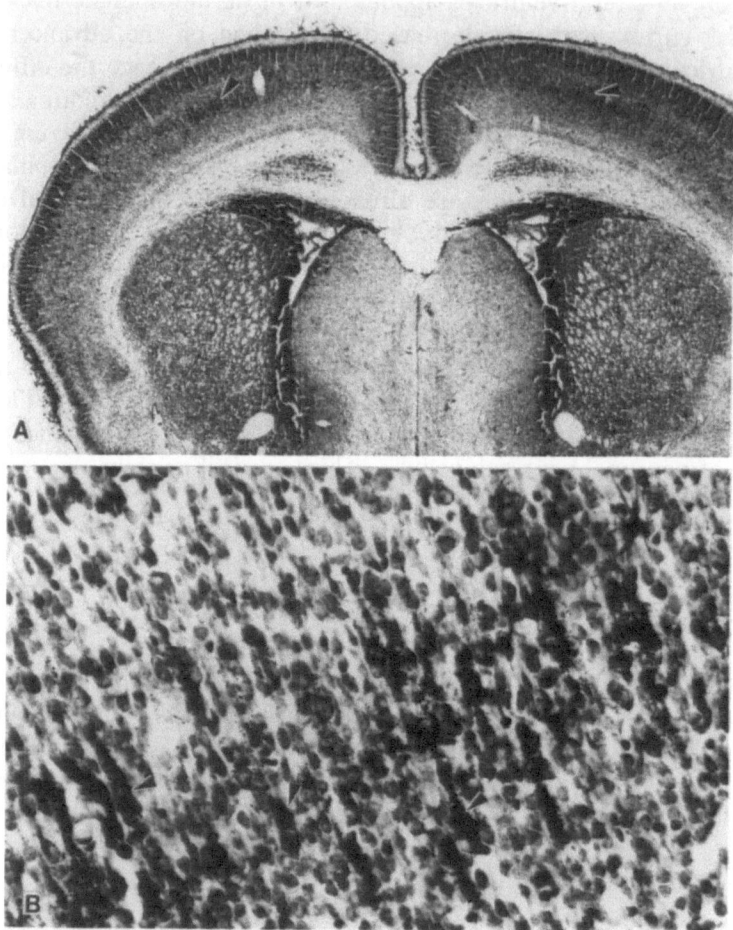

Fig. 2. A A frontal section of the cerebrum with slight dilatation of the lateral ventricles at postnatal day 1. HRP-labeled corticospinal neurons (▶) are found in layer V of the cerebral cortex. × 24. **B** A high magnification of the dorsal cerebral cortex in Fig. 2. The corticospinal neurons (▶) are labeled with HRP. × 380

and a 1.25% solution of glutaraldehyde and immersed their brains and spinal cords into a 20% solution of sucrose. We made serial sections of their brains and spinal cords in thicknesses of 60 or 100 μm, reacted these using the tetra-methylbenzidine (TMB) method (Mesulam 1978), and observed them with a light microscope.

Results

Injection Site of HRP in the Cervical Cord

HRP was injected into almost the whole area of the cervical cord at postnatal days 1, 7, 14, and 21 (Fig. 1).

Distribution of HRP-Labeled corticospinal Neurons in the Cerebral Cortex

At postnatal day 1, the cerebral cortex consisted of the molecular layer, the cortical plate, including many small cells, and layer V, containing large cells with slight and high dilatations of the lateral ventricles. HRP-labeled corticospinal neurons were found in layer V of the dorsal cortex with both slight and high dilatations of the lateral ventricles (Figs. 2a and 3a). In higher magnification the somas and proximal dendrites of the corticospinal neurons were found to be labeled with HRP (Figs. 2b and 3b).

At postnatal day 7, the dorsal area of the cerebral cortex with the high dilatation of the lateral ventricles appeared to have a thinner cerebral wall than the area with the slight dilatation; HRP-labeled neurons were localized in layer V of both cortices.

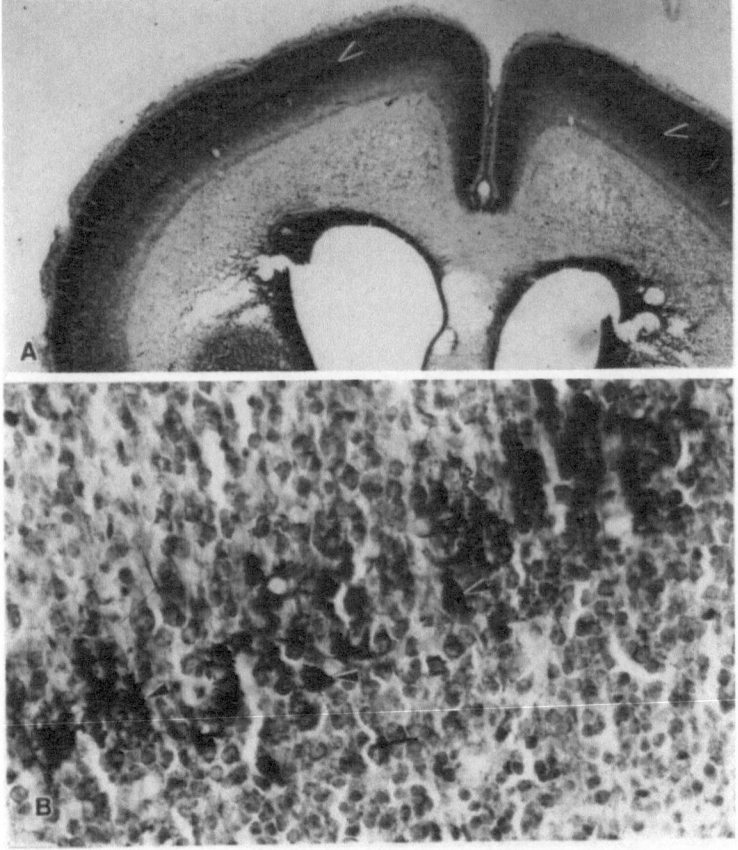

Fig. 3. A A frontal section of the cerebrum with high dilatation of the lateral ventricles at postnatal day 1. HRP-labeled corticospinal neurons (▶) are found in layer V of the dorsal cerebral cortex. × 24. **B** A high magnification of the dorsal cerebral cortex in Fig. 3A. The corticospinal neurons (▶) are labeled with HRP. × 380

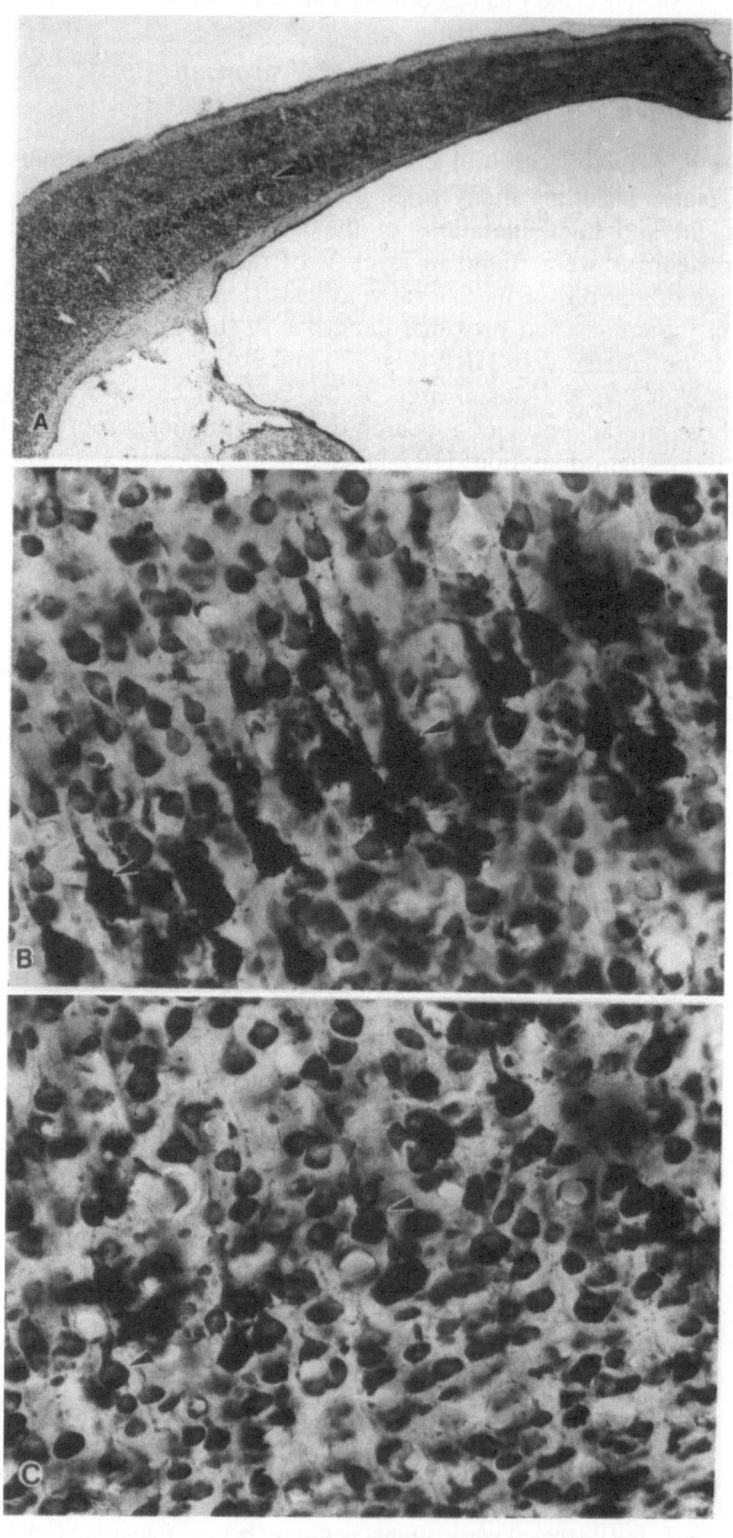

At postnatal day 14, the cerebral cortex with the high dilatation (Fig. 4a) became thinner than that with the slight dilatation (Fig. 5a). The thinnest area appeared in the dorsal area of the cortex with the high dilatation. Many rows of HRP-labeled neurons were found in layer V of the cortex with the slight dilatation (Fig. 5a); however, several rows of these neurons were found in the same layer of the dorso-lateral part of the cortex with the high dilatation (Fig. 4a). The HRP-labeled neurons formed pyramidal cells in the cortex with the slight dilatation and formed such cells in the dorso-lateral part of the cortex with the high dilatation [Figs. 5b and 4b). The same neurons became smaller and flattened in the dorsal part of the cortex with the high dilatation (Fig. 4c).

At postnatal day 21, HRP-labeled neurons were stratified in layer V of the cortex with the slight dilatation, and the growth of their somas increased (Fig. 6a). Only a few HRP-labeled neurons were found in the dorsal part and a few HRP-labeled small neurons were found in the lateral part (Fig. 6b).

Degenerative Changes Appearing in the Pyramis of the Medulla Oblongata of HTX Rats with High Dilatation of the Lateral Ventricles

At postnatal day 21, many macrophages appeared in the pyramis of the lower medulla oblongata and, simultaneously, degeneration of the corticospinal axons was found in this area (Fig. 7).

Discussion

In the normal rat, the corticospinal tract distributed in the posterior horn and the intermediate zone made immature synapses with the developing neurons in these zones at postnatal day 1, and formed a compound synaptic organization, similar to a glomerulus, through postnatal day 14 (Miyabayashi and Shirai 1988).

Also, retrograde labeling studies with HRP have shown that corticospinal neurons were localized in layer V of the cerebral cortex and that their axons reached the cervical cord. By postnatal day 14, their distribution formed an adult pattern and synaptogensis on their somas advanced (Ohtani et al. 1987; Ohtani and Shirai 1988).

In this study we examined the effect of hydrocephalic changes on the postnatal development of corticospinal neurons in the cerebral cortex of the

---

Fig. 4. A A frontal section of the cerebrum with high dilatation of the lateral ventricles at postnatal day 14. Some HRP-labeled corticospinal neurons (▶) are found in the dorso-lateral part of the cerebral cortex. × 24. **B** A high magnification of the dorso-lateral part of the cerebral cortex in Fig. 4A. The somas and the proximal dendrites of the corticospinal neurons (▶) are labeled with HRP. × 380. **C** A high magnification of the dorsal cerebral cortex in Fig. 4A. Several HRP-labeled corticospinal neurons (▶) are found. However, they are smaller than those in the dorso-lateral part and are scattered in layer V. × 380 .

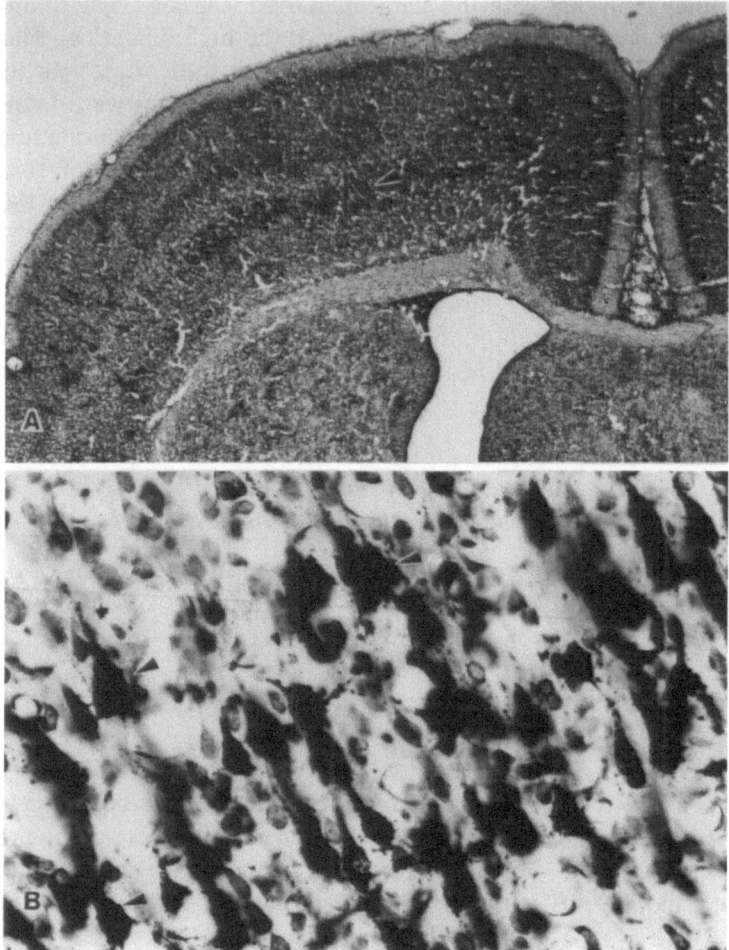

Fig. 5. A A frontal section of the cerebrum with slight dilatation of the lateral ventricles at postnatal day 14. Several rows of HRP-labeled corticospinal neurons (▶) are found in layer V of the dorsal cerebral cortex. × 24. **B** A high magnification of the dorsal cerebral cortex in Fig. 5A. The somas and the proximal dendrites of the corticospinal neurons (▶) are labeled with HRP. × 380

congenital hydrocephalic rat (HTX), compared with corticospinal neurons in the normal rat. At postnatal day 1, HRP-labeled neurons were found in layer V of the cerebral cortex. Therefore, this pattern was the same as that found in the normal rat. Also, it was confirmed that axons of the corticospinal neurons reached the spinal cord not only in the hydrocephalic rat with slight dilatation of the lateral ventricles, but also in the hydrocephalic rat with high dilatation of these ventricles. These findings seemed to show that the outgrowth of axons from the corticospinal neuronal somas to the spinal cord advanced without

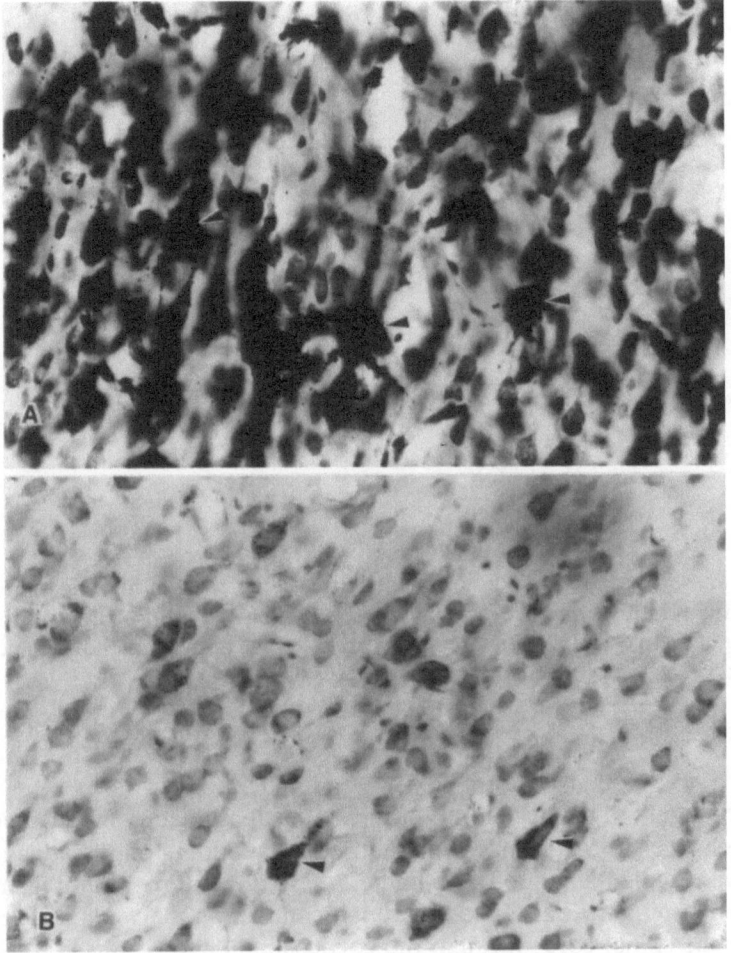

Fig. 6. A HRP-labeled corticospinal neurons (▶) are found in the dorsal cerebral cortex with slight dilatation of the lateral ventricles at postnatal day 21. × 380. **B** A few HRP-labeled corticospinal neurons (▶) are found in the lateral cerebral cortex with high dilatation of the lateral ventricles at postnatal day 21. × 380

being influenced by the progress of lateral ventricular dilatation caused by the birth.

However, as Kohn et al. (1981) have described, the dilatation of the lateral ventricles became remarkable, and subsequently the thickness of the cerebrum reduced during postnatal development. In this process HRP-labeled corticospinal neurons gradually decreased in number. In particular, a few HRP-labeled neurons were scattered in layer V of the lateral part of the cerebral cortex at postnatal day 21. At the same time, axons of the corticospinal neurons appeared to undergo degenerative changes through the pyramis of the

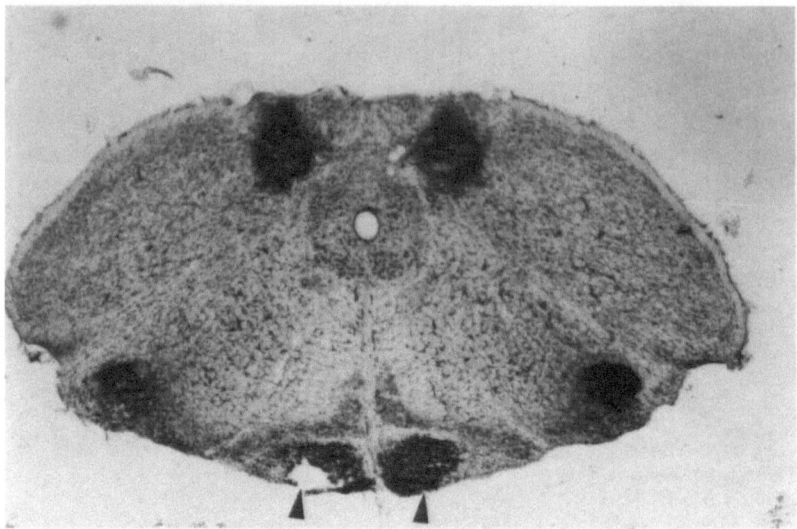

Fig. 7. A transverse section of the lower medulla oblongata with high dilatation of the lateral ventricles in the same hydrocephalic rat as that shown in Fig. 6B at postnatal day 21. The degenerative changes of the corticospinal tract appear in the pyramis of the ventral part. × 24

medulla oblongata. This degeneration in the corticospinal axons seemed to be caused by changes in the corticospinal neurons, depending on the advancement of lateral ventricular dilatation and immediately the anterograde degeneration of the corticospinal axons. The neuronal connection between the cerebral cortex and the spinal cord, through the corticospinal axons, was gradually lost by because of the disappearance of the corticospinal neurons and the degeneration of their axons.

References

Joosten EA, Gribnau AAM, Dederen JWC (1987) An anterograde tracer study of the developing corticospinal tract in the rat: three components. Dev Brain Res 36: 121–130

Kohn DF, Chinookoswong N, Chou SM (1981) A new model of congenital hydrocephalus in the rat. Acta Neuropathol (Berl) 54: 211–218

Mesulam M-M (1978) Tetramethylbenzidine for horseradish peroxidase neurochemistry: a noncarcinogenic blue reaction product with superior sensitivity for visualizing neural afferents and efferents. J Histochem Cytochem 26: 106–117

Miyabayashi T, Shirai T (1988) Synaptic formations of the corticospinal tract in the rat spinal cord. Okajimas Folia Anat Jpn 65:117–140

Ohtani R, Shirai T (1988) The development of corticospinal tract (CST) neurons. Proceedings of the 6th M Singer Symposium pp 473–483

Ohtani R, Shirai T, Kato H (1987) The postnatal distributional changes and synaptogenesis of corticospinal tract neurons in the cerebral cortex of the rat with HRP-labeling method (abstract). Soc Neurosci 13: 1430

5 — Changes in the Cerebral Vascular Bed in Experimental Hydrocephalus: An Angioarchitectural and Histological Study

N. Oka, J. Nakada, T. Nagahori, S. Endo, and A. Takaku[1]

Summary. The angioarchitectural and histological changes of small cerebral blood vessels in experimental hydrocephalus were studied in order to assess changes of the vascular bed in the cerebral mantle.

Changes of the microvasculature assessed from microcorrosion casts by scanning electron microscopy (SEM) and histological changes shown by light and electron microscopy were compared before and after shunting for hydrocephalus. Changes of the regional cerebral blood flow (rCBF) were also evaluated by the hydrogen clearance method.

In hydrocephalus, a reduction in the number and caliber of the capillaries was noted in both the white and gray matter in the SEM study, but the capillaries were preserved and changes were mild and nonspecific in the electron microscopic examination. Shunting resulted in the reversal of all these changes to normal, along with recovery of the rCBF, which had decreased in hydrocephalus.

These observations suggest that changes of the vascular bed participate in the alteration of cerebral mantle width in the hydrocephalic process, and that changes of the microvasculature result not only from damage to the capillaries themselves, but also from changes of the perivascular structures.

Keywords. Hydrocephalus — Ventriculo-peritoneal shunting — Scanning electron microscopy — Electron microscopy — Cerebral blood flow

Introduction

We have previously reported changes of the microvasculature in hydrocephalic rats, as shown by scanning electron microscopy (SEM), in an investigation of the effects of hydrocephalus on the vascular bed in the cerebral mantle (Oka et

[1] Department of Neurosurgery, Toyama Medical and Pharmaceutical University, Toyama, 930-01 Japan

al. 1986). In order to study changes of the microvasculature after cerebrospinal fluid (CSF) shunting, rabbits were used in the present investigation.

Histological changes were assessed using light and electron microscopy and changes of the rCBF were determined by the hydrogen clearance method. All parameters were evaluated before and after shunting to determine changes of the vasculature produced by the relief of hydrocephalus.

Materials and Methods

Hydrocephalus Model and Ventriculo-Peritoneal Shunting

Rabbits weighing 1.5–2.0 kg were used for this experiment. Under intravenous pentobarbital sodium anesthesia (20–25 mg/kg), a 2-cm sterile midline skin incision was made at the occipital region. After exposing and incising the atlanto-occipital membrane, about 1.0–1.5 ml CSF was removed. Then 0.6–0.8 ml of a kaolin suspension (250 mg/ml) was slowly injected into the cisterna magna. To prevent reflux of the kaolin suspension, a piece of muscle with Aron-α was used to cover the incision.

Ventricular size was measured on coronal computed tomography (CT) scans one week, one month, one and a half months, and two months after the kaolin injection. The degree of ventricular dilatation was divided into three categories (mild, moderate, and severe) in accordance with the ratio of the maximum distance between the bilateral anterior horns and the inside diameter of the skull in the same slice (Fig. 1).

In 11 of the 22 rabbits with severe hydrocephalus, ventriculo-peritoneal shunting was performed two months after the kaolin injection.

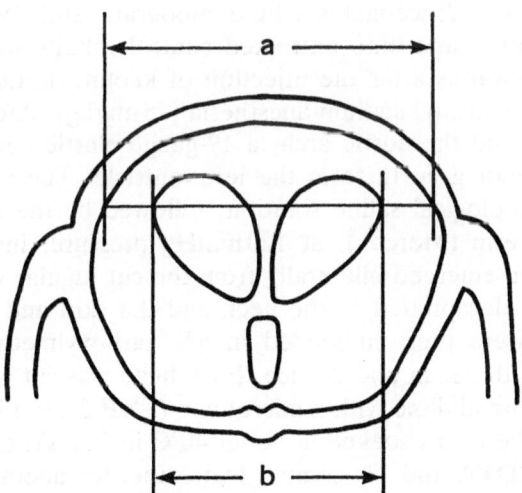

Fig. 1. Classification of hydrocephalus on CT scan. *a*, Inner diameter of the skull; *b*, Maximum width between the anterior horns

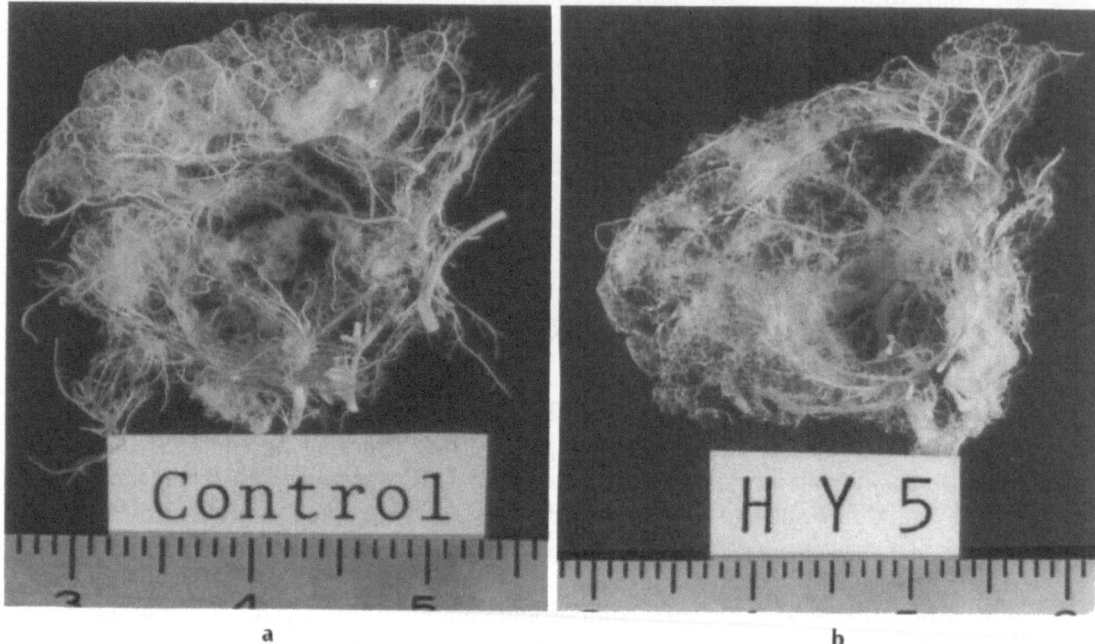

a   b

Fig. 2. a Dense vasculature is seen in a control rabbit. **b** Vasculature becomes sparse and the anterior cerebral artery can be clearly seen in severe hydrocephalus

Scanning Electron Microscopic (SEM) Study

Seven rabbits with hydrocephalus (three moderate and four severe), four rabbits after shunting, and nine untreated control rabbits were used for this experiment. Two months after the injection of kaolin, thoracotomy was performed under pentobarbital sodium anesthesia (25 mg/kg). After ligation of the innominate artery and the aortic arch, a 19-gauge elastic needle was used to cannulate the ascending aorta from the left ventricle. The rabbits were then perfused with physiological saline solution, followed by the slow injection of cooled polyester resin (Mercox), at 120 mmHg pressure, into the ascending aorta until the resin emerged bilaterally from the cut jugular veins.

The heads were decapitated at the neck and the skin and mandibula were removed. Heads were then embedded in 6% carboxylmethyl cellulose and frozen at −70°C with hexan and dry ice. Each head was cut into serial sagittal sections to nearly the midline with a microtome (LKB 2250, PMV450MP). The rest of the hemisphere was soaked at about 40°C in 2% Triton X-100 solution with 25 mM Na$_2$-EDTA and 2 N sodium hydroxide, for about three weeks, to digest the muscle, cranium, and brain tissue. The microvasculature of the gray and white matter in the parietal and frontal areas was then examined by SEM (Hitachi X-650).

Light and Electron Microscopic Study

Eight rabbits with hydrocephalus (four moderate and four severe), four rabbits after shunting, and five untreated control rabbits were used for this study. After thoracotomy under intravenous pentobarbital sodium anesthesia (25 mg/kg), they were perfused via the left ventricular route with 0.5% glutaraldehyde/4% paraformaldehyde in 0.01 M phosphate buffer. The brains were then sectioned coronally into slices of about 3 mm in thickness. For the electron microscopic study, specimens of gray and white matter in the parietal region were soaked in the same fixing fluid for one night, postfixed in buffered 1% osmium tetroxide for 1 hour, dehydrated in ethyl alcohol, and embedded in Epon 812. Ultrathin sections were double-stained with uranyl acetate and lead citrate and examined under an electron microscope (Hitachi H-300). For the light microscopic study, the sections were stained with hematoxylin and eosin (H & E) and periodic acid-methenamine (PAM).

Regional Cerebral Blood Flow (rCBF)

Regional cerebral blood flow was measured in the parietal gray and white matter by the inhalation method in eight rabbits with hydrocephalus (four moderate and four severe), four rabbits after shunting, and five untreated control rabbits.

Results

Scanning Electron Microscopy

Corrosion casts of the rabbits with hydrocephalus showed that the vasculature was sparse; the main trunks of the vessels could be seen more clearly compared with the controls (Fig. 2). In the SEM study, there was an obvious reduction in both the number and the caliber of the capillaries in hydrocephalus, and this change tended to increase in proportion to the severity of the hydrocephalus. The capillaries were about 8–10 μm in diameter in the controls and decreased to a diameter of about 5–8 μm in severe hydrocephalus. The number of capillaries returned to normal and their caliber also recovered to about 6–11 μm after shunting (Figs. 3 and 4, Table 1). These changes were seen almost equally in the gray and white matter.

Table 1. Density and diameter of capillaries

	Control (n = 9)	Hydrocephalus (n = 7)	Post-shunting (n = 4)
Gray matter	Dense 8–10 μm	Sparse 5–7 μm	Dense 7–11 μm
White matter	Dense 8–10 μm	Sparse 5–8 μm	Dense 6–10 μm

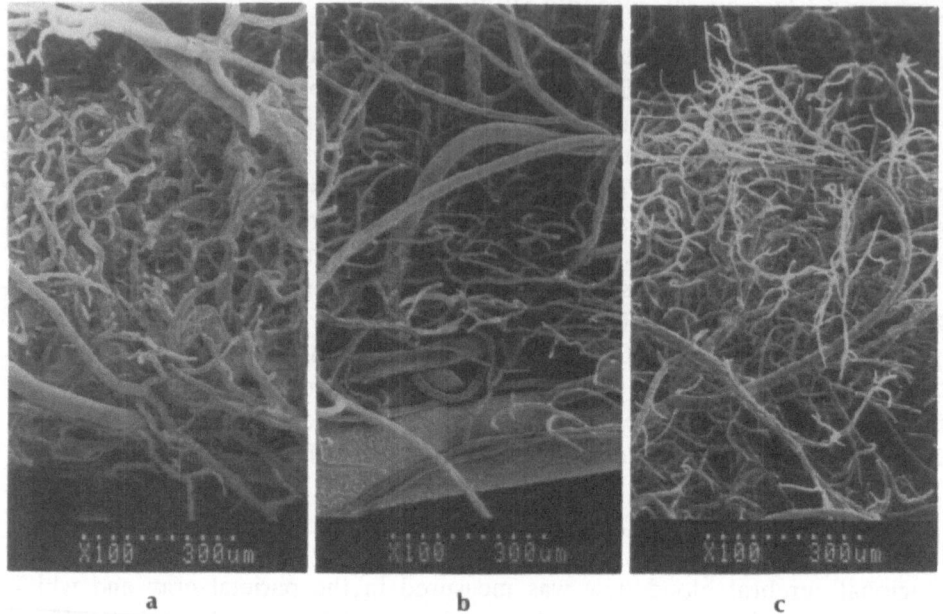

Fig. 3. a Capillaries of the white matter are dense in a control rabbit. **b** Capillaries of the white matter become sparse in severe hydrocephalus. **c** The number of capillaries is increased after shunting

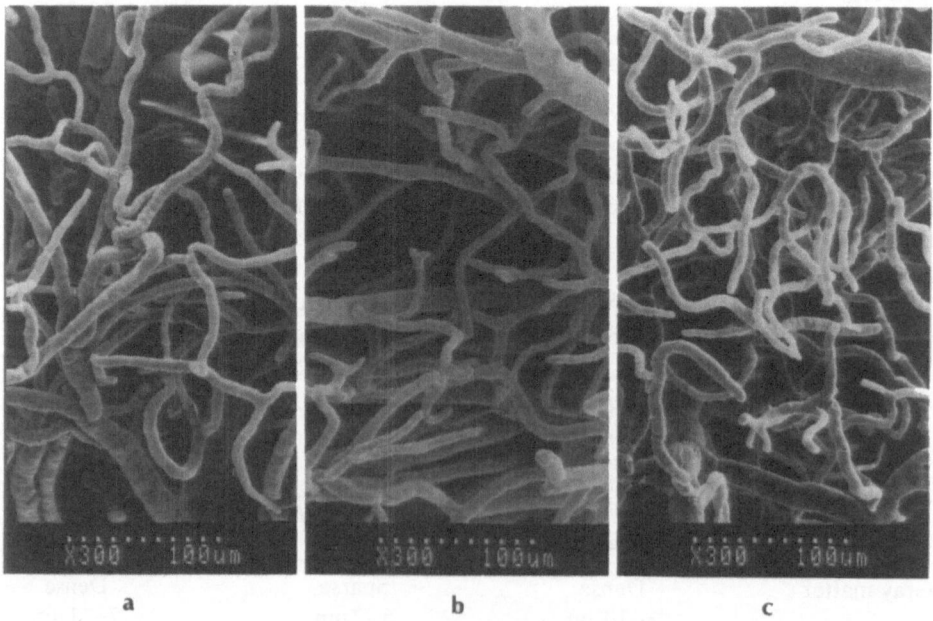

Fig. 4. A Diameters of capillaries are 8–10 μm in a control rabbit. **B** Capillaries narrow to 5–7 μm in severe hydrocephalus. **C** The caliber of capillaries increases to 7–11 μm after shunting

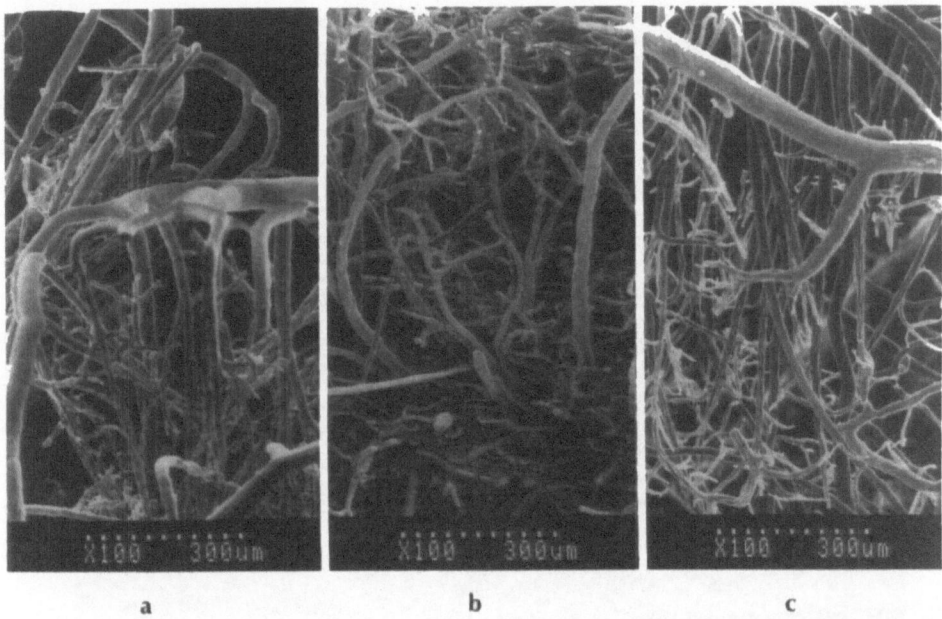

a   b   c

Fig. 5. a Cortical vessels are straight and run parallel, showing a "palisade" pattern, in a control rabbit. **b** The "palisade" pattern disappears in severe hydrocephalus. **c** Cortical vessels become rearranged after shunting

Cortical straight and parallel vessels showing a typical "palisade" pattern were distorted in hydrocephalus and returned to normal after shunting (Fig. 5).

Light and Electron Microscopic Study

The light microscopic study showed that the spongiomatous change which was found in the periventricular white matter in hydrocephalus disappeared after shunting. Pathological vessels could not be found in either the hydrocephalic or the post-shunting groups.

In the electron microscopic study, swelling of astrocytes in the perivascular area was observed in hydrocephalus (Fig. 6). Vacuoles, microvilli, and webs were noted more frequently in the endothelial cells of the capillaries in hydrocephalus as compared to controls (Fig. 7), and these changes were found more frequently in the white matter than in the gray matter. Following shunting, these perivascular and endothelial changes disappeared (Fig. 8). Opening of tight junctions, degeneration and reactive proliferation of endothelial cells, and abnormal vessels indicating neovascularization were not observed in this study.

Regional Cerebral Blood Flow (rCBF)

The rCBF of the gray and the white matter in five normal controls was 34.7 ± 4.5 ml/100 g per min and 17.8 ± 3.3 ml/100 g per min, respectively. Eight

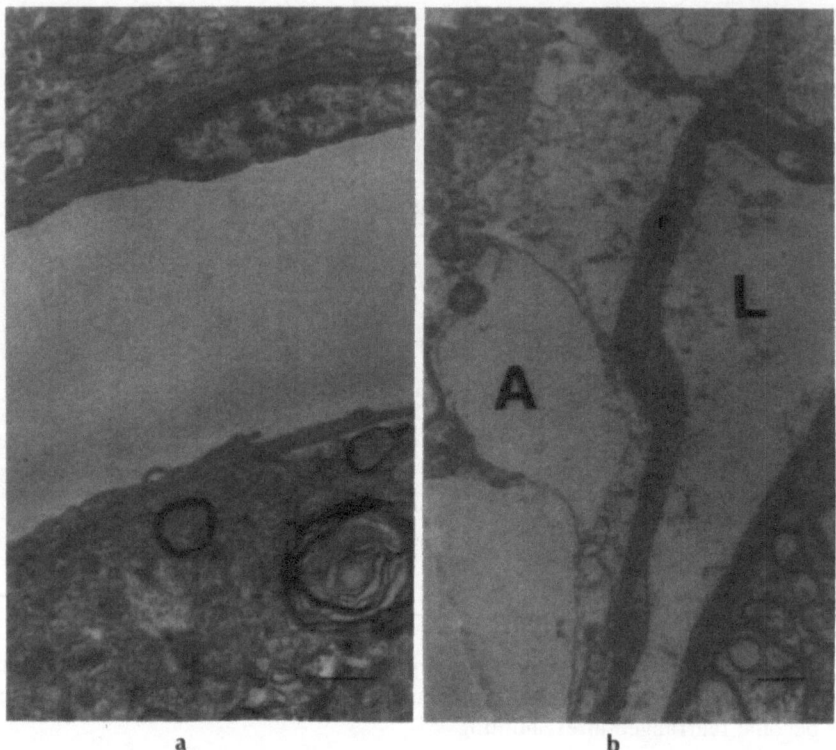

a   b

Fig. 6. a A capillary and its lumen in a control rabbit. *Bar* = 1 μm. × 5000.
b Perivascular astrocytic processes (*A*) are swollen in severe hydrocephalus. L, lumen
of a capillary; *Bar* = 1 μm, × 5000

hydrocephalic rabbits had a rCBF of 24.2 ± 6.7 ml/100 g per min in the gray
matter and 14.8 ± 3.7 ml/100 g per min in the white matter. A decrease in
rCBF was thus noted in both the gray and the white matter, and this change
became more marked in severe hydrocephalus when compared to moderate
hydrocephalus. The rCBF of the gray matter was significantly ($P < 0.05$)
reduced in hydrocephalus compared with that in the normal controls. After
shunting, the rCBF recovered to 37.1 ± 9.7 ml/100 g per min in the gray matter
and to 21.3 ± 4.2 ml/100 g per min in the white matter. These were significant
increases ($P < 0.05$) from the values seen in hydrocephalus (Tables 2 and 3).

Discussion

An early report on the cerebral vasculature in hydrocephalus was made by
Penfield (1929) who performed a macroscopic necropsy study. For the investigation of the cerebral angioarchitecture several methods have been reported,

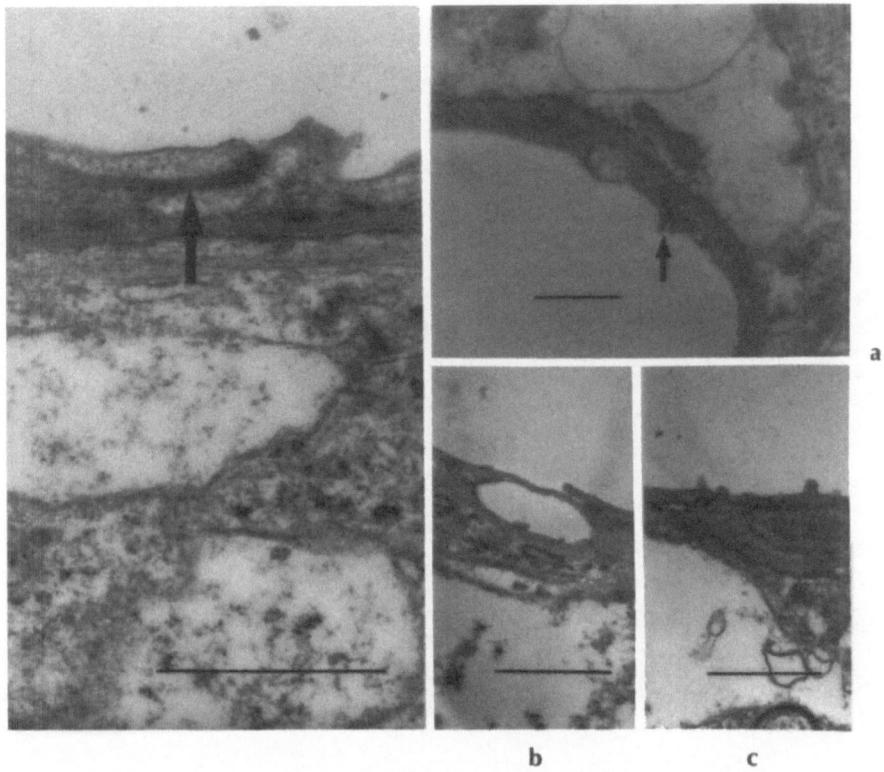

Fig. 7. *Left*, the endothelium of a capillary in a control rabbit. The *arrow* shows a tight junction. *Bar* = 1 µm, × 20 000. *Right*, in hydrocephalic rabbits, web (*a*), inter-endothelial vacuoles (*b*), and microvilli (*c*) are more numerous than in a control rabbit. *Bar* = 3 µm. *a* × 15 000; *b*, × 20 000; *c*, × 20 000

including microradiography (Hassler 1964; Sato et al. 1984; Wozniak et al. 1975), microangiography (Okuyama et al. 1987; Plets 1986; Sato et al. 1984), histological microscopic examination (De 1950; Del Bigio and Bruni 1988), and the use of vascular corrosion casting (Oka et al. 1986).

Table 2. rCBF in hydrocephalic rabbits before and after shunting

	Control (n = 5)	Hydrocephalus (n = 8)	Post-shunting (n = 4)
Gray matter	34.7 ± 4.5	*24.2 ± 6.7	**37.1 ± 9.7
White matter	17.8 ± 3.3	14.8 ± 3.7	**21.3 ± 4.2
		rCBF: ml/100 g per min	

*Mean cortical blood flow in hydrocephalus was significantly reduced compared with normal controls ($P < 0.05$)
**Mean blood flow in both the cortex and the white matter in post-shunting hydrocephalus was significantly increased compared with that in hydrocephalus ($P < 0.05$)
All values are the mean ±SD

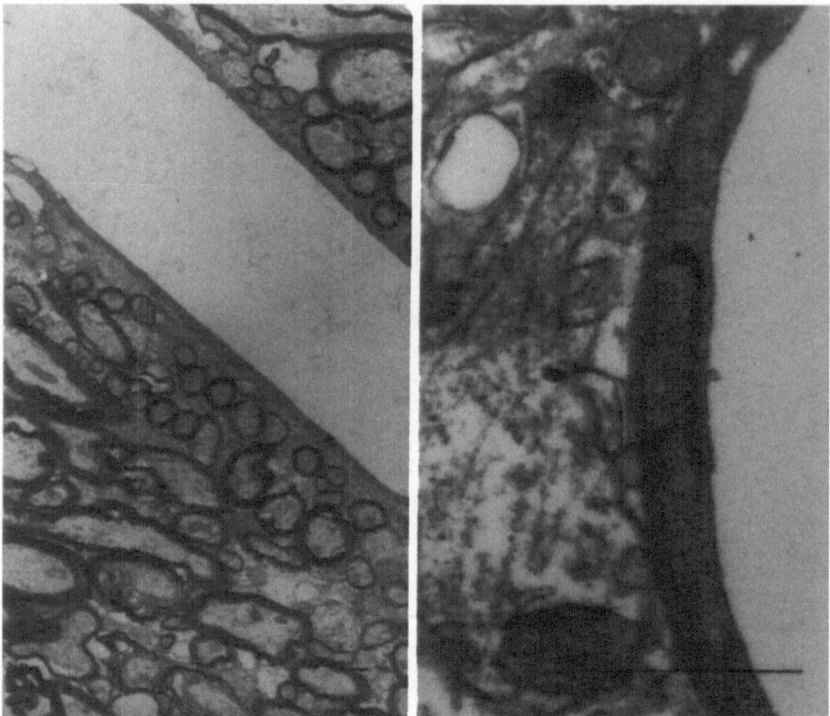

Fig. 8. *Left*, periventricular astrocytic swelling disappears after shunting. *Bar* = 1 μm, × 3000. *Right*, the wall of a capillary normalizes after shunting. *Bar* = 1 μm, × 20 000

Microradiography involves exposing sections of the brain to X-ray films. Although this method produces excellent stereoscopic pictures of the spatial distribution of the vessels, it has several disadvantages: (1) artifacts may be produced during the injection procedure, (2) obstructed vessels cannot be demonstrated, and (3) most of the capillaries and veins do not fill with X-ray contrast medium and are not visualized.

The microangiographic method, which involves observation, under the microscope, of the injection of various dyes into the cerebral vessels, allows the

Table 3. rCBF in rabbits with moderate and severe hydrocephalus

	Moderate (n = 4)	Severe (n = 4)
Gray matter	27.6 ± 8.4	20.9 ± 1.8
White matter	16.5 ± 4.3	13.2 ± 2.3
		rCBF: ml/100 g per min

All values are the mean ±SD

study of smaller vessels than the microradiographic method, but is not so good at showing the spatial distribution of the vessels, because of the thin sections used.

Several histological studies of the angioarchitecture in hydrocephalus have been reported. De (1950) observed the vascular pattern of the smaller vessels using Pickworth's stain. Del Bigio et al. (1988) examined periventricular blood vessels by light microscopy and assessed them by a quantitative method.

Using microvascular corrosion casting, the cerebral vasculature can be observed more stereoscopically and with a better understanding of the successive levels of the vascular tree than is possible by the microradiographic method. Also, the caliber of vessels can be measured more exactly by this method than by microangiography and histological studies, which reveal only sectioned vessels. In addition, this method can demonstrate the capillaries and veins by the injection of polyester resin into the venous system.

Reports on the cerebral angioarchitecture in hydrocephalus have been somewhat varied, probably owing to differences in the methods used and differences in the caliber of the vessels which were observed. Hassler (1964) used microradiography to observe vessels above the precapillary level in experimental hydrocephalus, and described an increase in the number of arteries and veins in the periventricular white matter and in the cortex. Plets (1986) also stated that the arterioles in the subependymal region showed a relative hypervascularization. On the other hand, Wozniak et al. (1975) found a decrease in the number and caliber of the microvessels in advanced hydrocephalus in the congenitally hydrocephalic Hy-3 mouse. There are several other reports that indicate poor visualization of the microvessels in the periventricular region.

As for the capillaries, only a few studies have been published. Hassler (1964) observed the capillaries in the hydrocephalic necropsied brain and in experimental hydrocephalus by the peroxidase staining method, and reported them to seem normal in the atrophic white matter. In contrast, Del Bigio and Bruni (1988) described a significant decrease in the number of capillaries with lamina of $10\,\mu m$ or less in the paraventricular area one week after silicon injection. De (1950) also reported a decrease of the capillaries in hydrocephalus.

After shunting, most studies reported that the microvasculature was restored to normal, although in several studies (Del Bigio and Bruni 1988; Plets 1986) in which CSF shunting was performed in the late stages of hydrocephalus, changes of the microvasculature were irreversible.

The most marked change noted in our study was the reduction in the number and caliber of the capillaries in the white and gray matter in chronic hydrocephalus. This change reversed completely after shunting. However, shunting was performed only two months after the induction of hydrocephalus, so a longer period of observation would be necessary to better assess the reversibility of changes of the cerebral angioarchitecture in hydrocephalus.

Regarding morphological studies of the capillaries using microscopic methods, changes of the capillaries in the hydrocephalic brain seemed to be mild. Nakagawa et al. (1984) found clefts and vacuoles between the tight junctions of the capillaries and postcapillary venules in kaolin-induced hydrocephalus, and suggested that the tight junction acted as a shunt pathway for interstitial edema fluid and cerebrospinal fluid to enter the microvessels. Regarding changes of the tight junctions themselves and changes of the endo-thelial cells in hydrocephalus, Okuyama et al. (1987), from the finding of stenotic or occluded capillaries in the late stage of hydrocephalus, suggested the possible disruption of the blood-brain barrier. In our study, vacuoles, microvilli, and webs, which are thought to be an early and nonspecific response to various stresses, were found in the endothelial cells of the capillaries in hydrocephalus. All these changes reversed after shunting.

The reduction in rCBF in hydrocephalus improved after shunting, which was a similar result to that cited in previous reports (Higashi et al. 1986; Hochwald et al. 1975; Nakamura and Hochwald 1983). The marked decrease in rCBF in the gray matter found in our study, which Murata et al. (1980) also described, contrasted with another report (Sato et al. 1984) of reduced rCBF in the white matter. Aseptic meningitis induced by the injection of kaolin suspension might have been related to the reduction in cortical blood flow.

In hydrocephalus, the vascular bed seemed to decrease with ventricular dilatation and to increase again after shunting. These changes are suggested to participate, not in a small way, in the restoration of cerebral mantle width.

Regarding our results using microcorrosion casting, some questions are raised with regard to the capillaries: (1) Was the sparsity of the vascular cast in hydrocephalus caused by the disappearance of capillaries which actually changed irreversibly? (2) Was this changes caused by the lack of flow of the polyester resin into narrowed capillaries which actually still existed? (3) Was the increase in capillaries after shunting due to the same vessels that were present previously or due to neocapillaries? We also investigated histological changes in order to answer these questions. Our histological studies showed that capillaries were found even in the thinned-out cerebral mantle and that neocapillarization did not occur in the re-expanded mantle after shunting. Therefore, the apparent changes of the capillaries which we observed in hydro-cephalus may not have been caused by changes of the vessels themselves, but may have been secondary to the influence of changes in the periventricular structures. Enlargement of the extracellular space due to interstitial edema and the hypertrophy and accumulation of astrocytes may have caused the capillaries to collapse in hydrocephalus, and these changes were then nor-malized after shunting, leading to capillary re-expansion.

Conclusions

1. A reduction in the number and caliber of the cerebral capillaries was the most marked change seen in hydrocephalus. This change was found in both the gray and the white matter.
2. The number and caliber of the capillaries returned to normal with re-expansion of the cerebral mantle after shunting.

3. Capillary endothelial cells in hydrocephalus showed an increase of vacuoles, microvilli, and webs. These changes were reversed by shunting, and neovascularization was not seen.
4. The rCBF was reduced in hydrocephalus and improved after shunting.
5. These findings suggest that, in the hydrocephalic process, changes of the cerebral vascular bed may participate in the alterations of the cerebral mantle. In addition, the reversal of the changes in the capillaries was apparently brought about not by the vessels themselves, but by changes of the perivascular elements.

References

De SN (1950) A study of the changes in the brain in experimental internal hydrocephalus. J Pathol 112: 197–209

Del Bigio MR, Bruni JE (1988) Changes in periventricular vasculature of rabbit brain following induction of hydrocephalus and after shunting. J Neurosurg 69: 115–120

Hassler O (1964) Angioarchitecture in hydrocephalus. An autopsy and experimental study with the aid of microangiography. Acta Neuropathol (Berl) 4: 65–74

Higashi K, Asahisa H, Ueda N, Kobayashi K, Hara K, Noda Y (1986) Cerebral blood flow and metabolism in experimental hydrocephalus. Neurol Res 8: 169–176

Hochwald GM, Boal RD, Martin AE, Kumer AJ (1975) Changes in regional blood flow and water content of brain and spinal cord in acute and chronic experimental hydrocephalus. Dev Med Child Neurol [Suppl] 17: 42–50

Murata T, Yamagata S, Mori K, Handa H, Nakano Y (1980) Computed tomography in experimental canine hydrocephalus. Part 4: Periventricular lucency (PVL) and regional blood flow in the chronic stage of hydrocephalus (in Japanese). No To Shinkei 32: 219–227

Nakagawa Y, Cervos-Navarro J, Artigas J (1984) A possible paracellular route for the resolution of hydrocephalic edema. Acta Neuropathol (Berl) 64: 122–128

Nakamura S, Hochwald GM (1983) Effect of arterial PCO2 and cerebrospinal fluid volume flow rate changes on choroidal plexus and cerebral blood flow in normal and experimental hydrocephalic cats. J Cereb Blood Flow Metab 3: 369–375

Oka N, Nakada J, Endo S, Takaku A (1986) Angioarchitecture in experimental hydrocephalus. Pediatr Neurosci 12: 294–299

Okuyama T, Hashi K, Sasaki S, Sudo K, Kurokawa Y (1987) Changes in cerebral microvasculature in congenital hydrocephalus of the inbred rat LEW/Jms: light and electron microscopic examination. Surg Neurol 27: 338–342

Penfield W (1929) Cerebral pressure atrophy. In: Penfield W (ed) Proceedings, Association for Research in Nervous and Mental Disease, Vol. 6, Internal pressure in health and disease. Williams and Wilkins, Baltimore, pp 346–361

Plets C (1986) Influence of experimental hydrocephalus on cerebral vascularization. In: Baethmann A, Go KG, Unterberg A (eds) Mechanism of secondary brain damage. Plenum, New York, pp 169–178

Sato O, Ohya M, Nojiri K, Tsugane R (1984) Microcirculatory changes in experimental hydrocephalus: morphological and physiological studies. In: Shapiro K, Marmarou A, Portnoy H (eds) Hydrocephalus. Raven, New York, pp 215–230

Wozniak M, McLone DG, Raimondi AG (1975) Micro- and macrovascular changes as the direct cause of parenchymal destruction in congenital murine hydrocephalus. J Neurosurg 43: 535–545

6 — Impaired Synaptic Plasticity and Dendritic Damage of Hippocampal CA1 Pyramidal Cells in Chronic Hydrocephalus*

Yoichi Katayama, Takashi Tsubokawa, Kosaku Kinoshita, Morimichi Koshinaga, Tatsuro Kawamata, and Shuhei Miyazaki[1]

Summary. The long-term potentiation (LTP) of the Schaffer collateral/CA1 pyramidal cell system of the rat hippocampus was investigated at various periods after induction of hydrocephalus by cisternal kaolin injection. There was a progressive decrease in LTP during the initial 3 weeks, and LTP remained decreased thereafter following the induction of hydrocephalus. Since the intraventricular pressure reached its maximum level within 2 weeks after kaolin injection, the continuous presence of hydrocephalus appeared to be necessary for producing the deficit in LTP induction. Dendritic dysfunction was apparently important for this functional change, since in a previous study by electron microscopy, we revealed a number of swollen dendrites in the CA1 region, while the changes in the axons, synaptic structures, and soma were far less pronounced. In agreement with this interpretation, a swelling of the dendrites of the CA1 pyramidal cells and irregularity of their arrangement was demonstrated by microtubule-associated protein 2-immunohistochemistry to be associated with the decreased LTP. Since LTP is likely to reflect the hippocampal function related to memory retention, functional changes underlying the impaired LTP might be responsible for memory deficit in hydrocephalus.

Keywords. Dendrite — Hippocampus — Hydrocephalus — Long-term potentiation — Synaptic plasticity

Introduction

Deficit in recent memory is one of the major manifestations of chronic hydrocephalus (Fisher 1977). Since several data support a relationship between the hippocampus and recent memory processes (Milner 1970; Bliss 1979),

---

[1] Department of Neurological Surgery, Nihon University School of Medicine, Itabashi-ku, Tokyo, 173 Japan

* This work was presented at the International Symposium on Hydrocephalus, Kobe (1990) under the title "Hippocampal Dendrotoxicity of Hydrocephalus."

hippocampal dysfunction may underlie the memory deficit observed in chronic hydrocephalus. In a previous study by electron microscopy, we revealed a number of swollen dendrites in the hippocampus of hydrocephalic rats (Tsubokawa 1984; Tsubokawa et al. 1988a). In contrast, the changes in the axons and synaptic structures in this region were far less pronounced. No apparent alterations were detected in the soma of the pyramidal cells. The present study was undertaken in order to determine whether or not there were any changes in hippocampal function corresponding to such morphological changes in rats with kaolin-induced hydrocephalus.

For this purpose, alterations in the long-term potentiation (LTP) (Bliss and Lomo 1973; Bliss 1979; Lynch et al. 1983) of synaptic responses in the Schaffer collateral/CA1 pyramidal cell system of the hippocampus were examined. We also investigated the dendritic structure by immunohistochemistry, using microtubule-associated protein 2 (MAP2), a dendrite-specific protein (Vallee 1982; Camilli et al. 1984), in order to confirm whether there was a structural change in dendrites in association with such functional changes. We employed in vivo preparations, since in vitro studies are unavoidably influenced by a transient ischemia-like insult prior to recording and an extracellular environment which is dissimilar to the hydrocephalic condition in vivo. Since hippocampal LTP has been implicated in the mechanism of memory (Bliss 1979), such studies were expected to also provide us with a basis for exploring the mechanisms underlying memory deficit in various disease processes (Landfield et al. 1978; Miyazaki et al. 1989).

Materials and Methods

Male Wistar rats aged 2–3 weeks (250–300 g, $n = 46$) were used for the experiments. In one group of animals, 0.1 ml of kaolin solution (200 mg/ml saline) was injected into the cisterna magna. The animals injected with kaolin were further divided retrospectively into two groups, one of which showed ventricular dilatation (>2 standard deviation (SD); hydrocephalic rats, $n = 19$), while the other showed no significant dilatation of the ventricle (<2SD; non-hydrocephalic rats, $n = 6$). Animals demonstrating severe weight loss or infection were excluded from the study, so that, together with the rats which had died before commencing the experiments, nine rats were excluded from the study. In the other main group of animals, 0.1 ml of saline vehicle was injected into the cisterna magna (sham-operated control rats, $n = 12$). Nine additional rats without any pretreatment were employed as normal controls.

Each group of animals was divided into four subgroups, and each subgroup of animals was subjected to neurophysiological recording at 2–5 weeks after injection. The animals were anesthetized by intraperitoneal injection of Nembutal and occasional supplemental doses were given when required. Local anesthetic (lidocaine) was applied to the wound edges. The animals were placed in a stereotaxic frame and skull holes were drilled at appropriate co-ordinates.

A recording micropipette filled with 3 M NaCl solution and fast green dye (impedance, 5–15 MΩ) was then lowered vertically into the CA1 pyramidal cell layer through a small skull hole (4.0 mm poterior to the bregma, 2.0 mm lateral to the midline). At approximately 2.0–3.3 mm below the brain surface, single unit discharges were encountered. A concentric bipolar electrode (diameter, 100 μm for the inner pole and 250 μm for the outer pole; tip separation, 500 μm) for stimulation was then lowered vertically into the stratum radiatum region containing Schaffer collateral fibers (4.0 mm posterior to the bregma, 3.5 mm lateral to the midline) and the alveus of the hippocampus (4.0–5.0 mm posterior to the bregma, 1.5 mm lateral to the midline). Stimulation electrodes were placed at sites from which typical orthodromic responses can be elicited in CA1 pyramidal cells.

While the anatomical location of the hippocampus is displaced by the development of hydrocephalus (Tsubokawa et al. 1988b), the distinctly laminated anatomical structure of the dorsal hippocampus permits us to make recordings from physiologically will-defined loci. In order to obtain reliable data for quantitative characterization of the functional changes occurring in the CA1 pyramidal cells, the following steps were followed for recording in all experiments. (1) The recording micropipette was initially placed at a depth where spontaneous firings of CA1 pyramidal cells were best recorded. (2) The orthodromic responses to stimulation of the Schaffer collaterals were then recorded. The depth of the stimulation electrode was corrected in relation to the depth of the recording micropipette. The location of the stimulation electrode was then fixed, and remained unchanged thereafter throughout the experiment. The orthodromic responses recorded from the pyramidal cell layer consisted of 3 components (Fig. 1a,c): an initial slow positive wave, a large negative population spike riding on the slow positive wave, and a following large positive wave. Extensive studies have established that these 3 waves comprise a population excitatory postsynaptic potential (EPSP), an orthodromically evoked population spike (PS), and a population inhibitory postsynaptic potential, respectively. (3) The changes in the orthodromic responses were then analyzed by advancing the micropipette in a stepwise fashion at intervals of 0.2-mm. The polarity of the EPSP was reversed when the micropipette was advanced into the dendritic field below the cell layer (Fig. 1a). This information was used to confirm the location of the micropipette. (4) The antidromic response was also recorded as a population spike in response to alveus stimulation from the CA1 pyramidal cell layer. The antidromic spike was confirmed to follow a high frequency stimulation of 300 Hz or more (Fig. 1b). This procedure verified that the recordings had been made from CA1 pyramidal cells. (5) The threshold of PS, as well as the slope of EPSP and the amplitude of PS in response to supramaximal and submaximal (stimulus intensity causing 50% of maximal response) stimulation were determined. The slope of EPSP was expressed as the amplitude of EPSP at 1 ms following the onset of the EPSP. (6) In order to induce LTP, tetanic stimulation was applied to Schaffer collateral fibers. The simulation intensity for observation of the LTP was adjusted to the level which produced 50% amplitude of the maximal

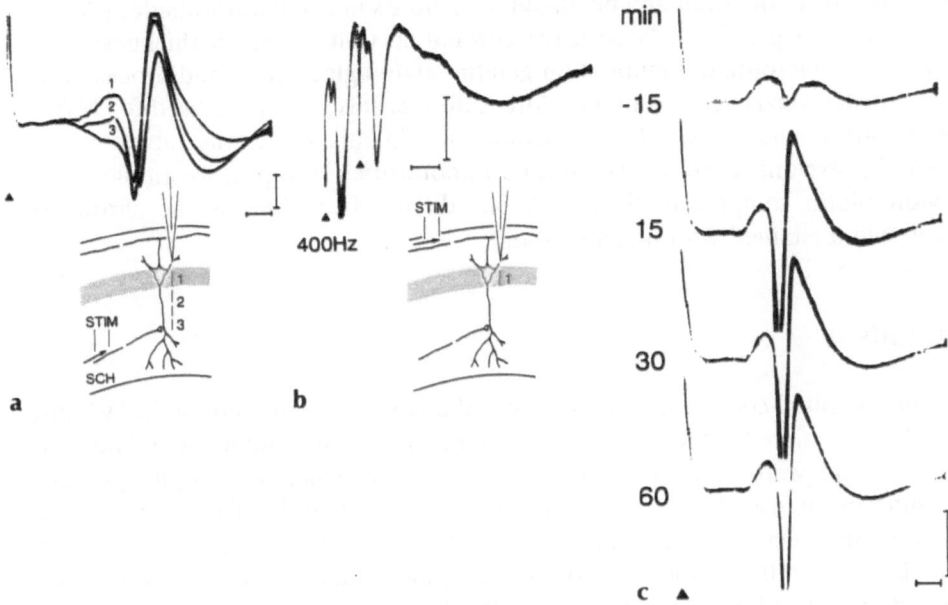

Fig. 1. Representative examples of responses recorded from the CA1 region of the rat hippocampus. Schematic illustrations of the electrode placements are also shown. **a** Orthodromic responses to Schaffer collateral stimulation. There sweeps recorded from different depths (sites 1, 2 and 3) were superimposed, demonstrating that, when the recording micropipette was lowered, the polarity of excitatory post synaptic potential (*EPSP*) was reversed. **b** Antidromic response to alveus stimulation. **c** Long-term potentiation of Schaffer collateral response following tetanic stimulation of the Schaffer collaterals. Three sweeps were superimposed. Time (min) following tetanic stimulation is given at the left side of each record. Note that the amplitudes of EPSP and population spike (*PS*) were potentiated at 15–60 min following tetanic stimulation. STIM, stimulation; SCH, Schaffer collateral; Calibrations, 1 ms and 2 mV. Stimulation is indicated by *solid arrow heads*

PS. The amplitude of PS at 0.3 Hz stimulation was measured at 1, 15, and 30 min after the beginning of tetanic stimulation. The results were expressed as a percentage of the posttetanic amplitude to pretetanic amplitude of PS at 30 min following tetanic stimulation (Fig. 1c).

At the end of the experiment, the intraventricular pressure (IVP) was measured through a needle inserted stereotaxically into the lateral ventricle. The animals were then perfused and processed for histological verification of the electrode placements and the degree of hydrocephalus. The size of the lateral ventricle was measured planimetrically, employing coronal sections at a level 4.0 mm posterior to the bregma.

Three hydrocephalic rats and three sham-operated controls, which were subjected to experimentation at 3 weeks after kaolin-injection, were perfused transcardially with saline followed by 2% paraformaldehyde. The brain was removed from the skull and postfixed for 2 hours in 2% paraformaldehyde, and embedded in paraffin. Consecutive coronal sections, $5\,\mu$m in thickness, were cut with a microtome, mounted on gelatin-coated glass slides and processed for Nissl or Klüver-Barrera staining. Alternate sections were processed for MAP2-immunohistochemistry. The antiserum used in this study was rabbit anti-pig MAP2 polyclonal antibody (Peninsula Laboratories Europe); we employed the avidin-biotin complex method with 3.3'-diaminobenzidine as the chromagen and counterstained with hematoxylin.

Results

Sham-operated control rats did not reveal any substantial increase in IVP after kaolin injection (Table 1). Hydrocephalic rats, which underwent kaolin injection and were later confirmed to display ventricular dilatation, showed a significant increase in IVP at 2 weeks ($P < 0.01$, Table 1). These rats revealed a continued increase in IVP at 3 weeks ($P < 0.01$), 4 weeks ($P < 0.01$), and 5 weeks ($P < 0.05$, Table 1). Non-hydrocephalic rats which underwent kaolin injection but did not develop ventricular dilatation, showed slight increases in IVP at 2 weeks, 3 weeks, and 5 weeks; these increases were always 1 SD level lower than the mean IVP of the hydrocephalic rats.

No apparent differences were observed in the wave-form of the Schaffer collateral responses from the CA1 pyramidal cells, between sham-operated control, hydrocephalic, and non-hydrocephalic rats. The threshold to elicit PS was found to be significantly lowered in hydrocephalic rats. Changes in the threshold of PS and paired pulse facilitation of EPSP have been described in detail elsewhere (Tsubokawa et al. 1988a). Due to the change in threshold, the stimulus intensity that could cause 50% of the maximal response was determined from an intensity-response curve in each animal.

In order to induce LTP, tetanic stimulation was applied to the Schaffer collateral fibers at a stimulation intensity which was adjusted to a level which produced 50% amplitude of maximal PS in each animal (see Methods). Approximately 5 min after tetanic stimulation, we began to see LTP in sham-operated controls. Elevation of the amplitude of PS generally continued for between 5–30 min after tetanic stimulation. The PS then remained at the same

Table 1. Time course of intraventricular pressure after kaolin injection

Group	Before	Time after kaolin injection			
		2 weeks	3 weeks	4 weeks	5 weeks
Sham-operated rats	3.6 ± 0.4 (9)		3.5 ± 0.4 (6)		3.6 ± 0.4 (6)
Hydrocephalic rats		5.8 ± 0.4 (4)**	5.5 ± 0.7 (5)**	5.4 ± 0.8 (6)**	4.9 ± 0.9 (4)*

$* P < 0.05$; $** P < 0.01$
As compared to sham-operated rats before kaolin injection. (n), no. of rats

Table 2. Time course of long-term potentiation after kaolin injection

Group	Before	Time after kaolin injection			
		2 weeks	3 weeks	4 weeks	5 weeks
Sham-operated rats	175.2 ± 28.5 (9)		178.2 ± 28.5 (6)		176.5 ± 26.3 (6)
Hydrocephalic rats		125.8 ± 28.1 (4)*	110.0 ± 6.9 (5)*	108.7 ± 7.5 (6)*	97.8 ± 12.7 (4)*

* $P < 0.01$

As compared to sham-operated rats before kaolin injection. Long-term potentiation was expressed as a percent amplitude of population spike (*PS*) at 30 min following tetanic stimulation as compared to pretetanic amplitude. (*n*), no. of rats

elevated level of amplitude for 3 hours. A significant deficit in LTP induction was observed in hydrocephalic rats (Table 2). While some of the sham-operated controls exhibited a PS in excess of 200% of the pretetanic value of the PS amplitude, such a large LTP was not reached in any of the hydrocephalic rats. Among non-hydrocephalic rats, the LTP was always 2 SD levels greater than the mean LTP of the hydrocephalic rats, when recorded more than 2 weeks after kaolin injection.

Histological examination revealed no significant decrease in the number of CA1 pyramidal cells in any of the hydrocephalic rats from which the above data were collected. The MAP2-immunoreactivity of the CA1 pyramidal cell dendrites did not decrease in hydrocephalic rats as compared to sham-operated controls, both of which were stained simultaneously as a pair (Fig. 2a,c vs b,d). The dendrites of hydrocephalic rats were, however, swollen and their arrangement was somewhat more irregular (Fig. 2b,d) than that of sham-operated controls (Fig. 2a,c). The width of the CA1 region in the dorsoventral direction decreased due, probably, to dilatation of the ventricle (Fig. 2a vs b).

Discussion

The present results demonstrate that the synaptic responses to single-pulse stimulation in the CA1 pyramidal cells of hydrocephalic rats are similar to those of sham-operated control rats, in terms of the wave-forms of the EPSP, the PS, and the inhibitory post-synaptic potential (IPSP). This suggests that axonal conduction and synaptic transmission may not be seriously impaired in the hippocampus of hydrocephalic rats. This inference is consistent with the fact that the central conduction time of the sensory evoked potentials is not prolonged until the terminal stage in the same rat model of hydrocephalus (Tsubokawa 1985).

Significant differences between hydrocephalic rats and sham-operated controls were noted primarily in the induction of LTP. Since a deficit in LTP was not observed in non-hydrocephalic rats which had received kaolin injection but did not develop apparent hydrocephalus and elevated IVP, this type of change

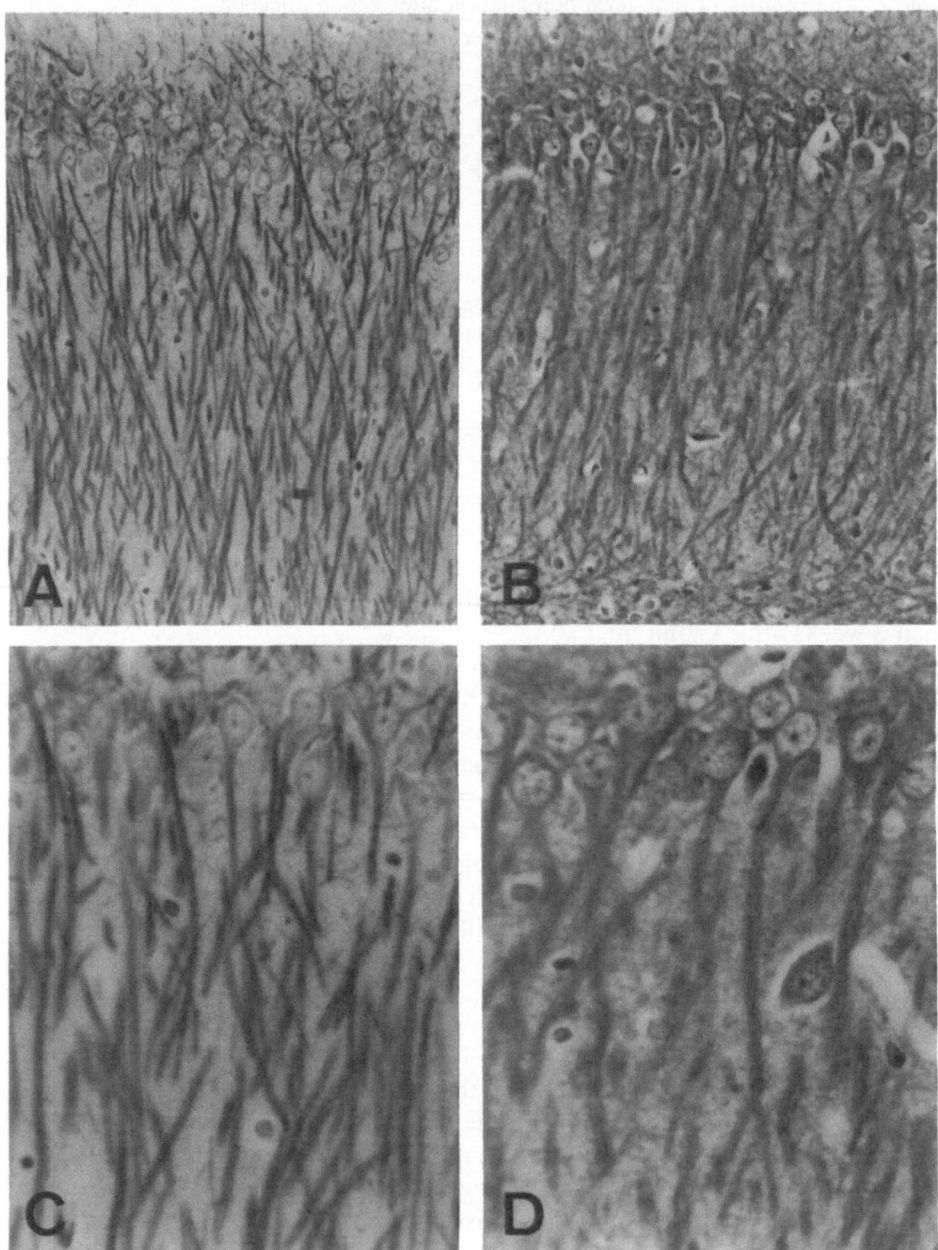

Fig. 2. Representative photomicrographs of microtubule-associated protein 2-immuno-histochemistry of CA1 pyramidal cells. **a** and **c** Sham-operated control rat at 3 weeks after cisternal saline injection; **b** and **d** hydrocephalic rat at 3 weeks after cisternal kaolin injection. Note swollen dendrites and their irregular arrangement in **b** and **d**. The whole width of the CA1 region is decreased in **b**. **a** and **b**, × 200; **c** and **d**, × 400. Counterstained by hematoxylin.

is not considered to be due to the effect of kaolin injection alone, and is therefore related to the existence of chronic hydrocephalus.

Although more research is required to establish the pre- or postsynaptic basis of the deficit for induction of LTP in hydrocephalic rats, there appears to be a reasonable likelihood that the deficit may, at least partially, involve changes in the postsynaptic dendritic processes. Electron microscopic studies on our hydrocephalic rats have revealed a number of swollen dendrites in the CA1 regions, while the changes in the axons and synaptic structures in the same region were far less pronounced (Tsubokawa 1984). In the present study, employing MAP2-immunohistochemistry (Vallee 1982; Camilli et al. 1984), we have also demonstrated that the dendrites of the CA1 pyramidal cells in hydrocephalic rats were swollen and that their arrangement was somewhat more irregular than that of sham-operated controls. While a previous study from our laboratory (Hayashi and Tsubokawa 1991, this volume) has suggested that the MAP2-immunoreactivity of the CA1 region of hydrocephalic rats may decrease, the swelling of the dendrites and the irregularity of their arrangement were more conspicuous in the present study. At least on this point, the present data appear to be consistent with electron microscopic findings indicating the presence of some form of impairment in the dendritic processes rather than in axonal conduction or synaptic transmission in the brain of hydrocephalic rats.

Several lines of biochemical evidence have indicated that the phenomenon of LTP involves postsynaptic intracellular calcium ions (Lynch et al. 1983; Izumi et al. 1987; Melchers et al. 1988). Some electron microscopic observations have also demonstrated that LTP is accompanied by a long-lasting increase in the area of the dendritic spines (Fifkova and Van Harreveld 1977); this has been postulated to cause a facilitation of current spread from the spines to the dendritic branches (Rall and Rinzel 1973). Changes in the intracellular distribution of calcium ions in the CA1 region have been suggested in hydrocephalic rats (Hayashi and Tsubokawa 1991, this volume). Swelling of dendrites in chronic hydrocephalus has been described repeatedly in earlier studies, although it did not draw much comment or attention, in contrast to attention drawn to the interstitial edema within the periventricular structures (Miyagami et al. this volume). It is possible that changes in the mechanisms underlying LTP in hydrocephalic rats have some relation to the pathological processes underlying the dendritic swelling seen in those rats.

The present experiments demonstrated that the impairment in the induction of LTP was progressive during the initial 3 weeks after kaolin injection. In contrast, IVP reached its maximum level within the initial 2 weeks after kaolin injection and remained elevated thereafter. The continuous presence of hydrocephalus thus appears to be necessary for producing progressive dendritic dysfunction. Further studies are required to determine the detailed pathological process which plays an important role in the production of dendritic dysfunction associated with chronic hydrocephalus.

Impaired LTP in the hippocampus of hydrocephalic rats could conceivably influence information processing or storage, and could contribute to the deficits in memory retention seen in rat models of chronic hydrocephalus (Bliss 1979).

Similar changes have been reported in memory-deficient rats in association with aging (Landfield et al. 1978) and concussive brain injury (Miyazaki et al. 1989). In humans, considerable data support a relationship between the hippocampal region and recent memory processes (Milner 1970). Deficits in recent memory represent one of the major synptoms of chronic hydrocephalus in humans (Fisher 1977). Taking all these findings together, there appears to be a strong possibility that impairment of hippocampal function may underlie the deficits in recent memory seen in chronic hydrocephalus in humans as well.

In conclusion, the results of the present study suggest that changes occurring in the hippocampal dendrites, rather than interstitial edema itself or occasional axonal degeneration, are more relevant to the memory deficits encountered in chronic hydrocephalus.

Acknowledgments. This work was supported by a Grant from the Japan Ministry of Health and Welfare. The authors wish to thank Drs. Saburo Nakamura, Nariyuki Hayashi, and Mitsusuke Miyagami of the Department of Neurological Surgery, Nihon University School of Medicine, for their invaluable advice.

References

Bliss TVP (1979) Synaptic plasticity in the hippocampus. TINS 2: 9–12

Bliss TVP, Lomo T (1973) Long-lasting potentiation of synaptic transmission in the dentate area of the anaesthetized rabbit following stimulation of the perforant path. J Physiol (Lond) 232: 331–356

Camilli RD, Miller PE, Theurkauf WE, Vallee RB (1984) Distribution of microtubule-associated protein 2 in the nervous system of the rat studied by immunofluorescence. Neurosciençe 11: 819–846

Fifkova E, Van Harreveld A (1977) Long-lasting morphological changes in dendritic spines of dentate granular cells following stimulation of the entorhinal area. J Neurocytol 6: 211–230

Fisher CM (1977) The clinical picture in occult hydrocephalus. Clin Neurosurg 24: 270–284

Izumi Y, Ito K, Miyakawa H (1987) Requirement of extracellular Ca^{2+} after tetanus for induction of long-term potentiation in guinea pig hippocampal slices. Neurosci Lett 77: 176–180

Landfield PW, McGaugh JL, Lynch G (1978) Impaired synaptic potentiation processes in the hippocampus of aged, memory-deficient rats. Brain Res 150: 85–101

Lynch G, Larson J, Kelso S (1983) Intracellular injections of EGTA block induction of hippocampal long-term potentiation. Nature 305: 719–721

Melchers BPC, Pennartz CMA, Wadmann WJ (1988) Quantitative correlation between tetanus-induced decreases in extracellular calcium and LTP. Brain Res 454: 1–10

Milner B (1970) Memory and the medial temporal regions of the brain. In: Pribram KH, Broadbent ED (eds) Biology of memory, Academic, New York

Miyazaki S, Newlon PG, Goldberg SJ, Katayama Y, Jenkins LW, Hayes RL (1989) Cerebral concussion suppresses hippocampal long-term potentiation (LTP) in rats. In: Hoff JT, Betz A (eds) Intracranial pressure, vol. 7. Springer, Berlin, pp 651–653

Rall W, Rinzel J (1973) Branch input resistance and steady attention for input to one branch of a dendritic neuron model. Biophys J 13: 648–688

Tsubokawa T (1984) Pathogenesis of neurologic deficits in hydrocephalus. Part 1. In: Matsumoto S (ed) Annual report of the Research Committee of Hydrocephalus, Ministry of Health and Welfare of Japan (in Japanese).

Tsubokawa T (1985) Pathogenesis of neurologic deficits in hydrocephalus. Parts 2 and 3. In: Matsumoto S (ed) Annual report of the Research Committee of Hydrocephalus, Ministry of Health and Welfare of Japan (in Japanese).

Tsubokawa T, Katayama Y, Kawamata T (1988a) Impaired hippocampal plasticity in experimental chronic hydrocephalus. Brain Inj 2: 19–30

Tsubokawa T, Katayama Y, Miyazaki S, Ogawa H, Iwasaki M, Sako H (1988b) Brain cell transplantation into the hydrocephalic rat hippocampus. Brain Inj 2: 67–74

Vallee RB (1982) A taxol–dependent procedure for the isolation of microtubule and microtubule-associated proteins (MAPs) J Cell Biol 92: 435–442

7 — Neurotransmitter Changes in Hydrocephalus: Effects of Cerebral Metabolic Activator on Kaolin-Induced Hydrocephalus

Hirohisa Miyake, Patrick Eghwrudjakpor, Takashi Sakamoto, Masahiro Kurisaka, and Koreaki Mori[1]

Summary. We measured the content of monoamine neurotransmitters in kaolin-induced hydrocephalic in rat brain. The effects of neurotransmitter changes in hydrocephalic rat brain after injection of a cerebral metabolic activator (bifemelane hydrochloride) are also discussed.

In this study, norepinephrine (NE), dopamine (DA), and serotonin (5-HT) content were determined in several brain regions including the cerebral cortex, striatum, hippocampus, cerebellum, pons, and medulla oblongata.

Bifemelane hydrochloride (bifemelane) was injected intraperitoneally daily for seven days beginning from the seventh day after kaolin injection and measurement was carried out on 15th day during the subacute phase of hydrocephalus.

As a result of the experimental studies, it was recognized that the content of some monoamines following injection of bifemelane was significantly different from the control values in some brain regions. In particular, differences in the cerebral cortex and striatum were significant.

This study demonstrates the effects of injection of a cerebral metabolic activator (bifemelane) on monoamine neurotransmitters in kaolin-induced hydrocephalus in the rat brain.

Keywords. Hydrocephalus — Monoamine — Neurotransmitter — Cerebral metabolic activator — Bifemelane hydrochloride

Introduction

In the central nervous system, it is generally considered that neurotransmitters play some role in the function of each individual neuron. Numerous reports have recently been made on the relationship between neurotransmitters and neurological disorders. The relationship between hydrocephalus and neurotransmitters has also received much attention in recent times and several reports have been made. (Chovanes et al. 1988; Higashi et al. 1986; Miwa et al. 1982).

---

[1] Department of Neurosurgery, Kochi Medical School, Kochi, 783 Japan

In human hydrocephalus, the concentration of homovanillic acid, the major metabolite of dopamine (DA), is reportedly elevated in ventricular cerebrospinal fluid (CSF) (Andersson and Roos 1965; Del Bigio 1989; Onodera et al. 1988). Norepinephrine (NE) and DA levels have been reported to be decreased in the hydrocephalic rabbit brain (Miwa et al. 1982). In this paper we discuss the effects of cerebral metabolic activator on kaolin-induced hydrocephalus in regard to neurotransmitter changes in hydrocephalic rats. We measured the monoamine neurotransmitter content in rat brains which had kaolin-induced hydrocephalus in the subacute phase. We also examined the effects of injection of a cerebral metabolic activator (bifemelane) on hydrocephalic rats.

Material and Methods

Preparation of Experimental Hydrocephalus

Adult female Wistar rats, 8 weeks-old, weighing 150–160 g, were used in this study. The rats were anesthetized with pentobarbital sodium (50 mg/kg, intraperitoneally) and kaolin (0.1 ml of 200 mg/ml suspension) was injected intracisternally to produce hydrocephalus. During recovery from anesthesia, the rats were placed with their heads slightly lowered to facilitate the flow of kaolin.

Measurement of Monoamines

We measured three monoamines, norepinephrine (NE), dopamine (DA), and serotonin (5-HT), by high-performance liquid chromatography with electrochemical detection.

Preparation of Specimens

Whole brains were cooled on ice immediately after removal and the five following regions were dissected and measured: cerebral cortex, striatum, hippocampus, cerebellum, pons, and medulla oblongata.

Injection of Cerebral Metabolic Activator

The cerebral metabolic activator used in this study was bifemelane hydrochloride. This substance is known to improve neurotransmitter metabolism and cerebral blood flow impairment due to brain ischemia. Clinically, it is administered orally to patients with cerebral infarction and cerebral hemorrhage. Bifemelane was injected intraperitoneally into the kaolin-induced hydrocephalic rats daily for seven days, beginning from the seventh day after kaolin injection. Measurement of monoamines was carried out on the 15th day. As control, bifemelane was injected intraperitoneally into normal rats by the same procedure. The amount of bifemelane injected was 10 mg per kg per day. (Fig. 1)

Results

In the kaolin-induced hydrocephalus, edematous changes of the periventricular layer appeared in the acute phase (Day 3) and ventricular dilatation was noted in the subacute phase (Day 15). Differences in body weight loss, impairment of mobility, and reduction of food and water intake between the bifemelane-injected group and the control group (non bifemelane-injected group) were not significant.

Changes of NE content in hydrocephalic brain are shown in Table 1 in the upper section. After kaolin injection, NE content increased in the striatum, hippocampus, pons and medulla oblongata, while it did not change in the cerebral cortex and cerebellum. The NE content of the bifemelane-injected group tended to show increases as compared to the control group (non-bifemelane-injected group), except in the striatum. In the striatum, there was a decrease in NE content in the bifemelane-injected group, as shown. In particular, the differences in the cerebral cortex and striatum are statistically significant. In the bifemelane-injected group of normal rats, increases of NE content were seen in the cerebral cortex, striatum, and hippocampus.

Changes of DA content in several brain regions are shown in Table 1-middle section. After kaolin injection, the DA content increased in the striatum. No significant changes were seen in other brain regions. There tended to be an increase of DA in the striatum following bifemelane injection, but the difference was not significant. Increase of DA content was seen in the striatum and hippocampus in the bifemelane-injected group of normal rats.

Changes of 5-HT content are shown in Table 1, bottom section. After kaolin injection, 5-HT content decreased in the cerebral cortex and cerebellum and increased in the striatum. In hydrocephalic rats, there tended to be an increase of 5-HT content in all brain regions following bifemelane injection. In particular, the differences in the cerebral cortex and cerebellum were statistically significant. In the bifemelane-injected group of normal rats, increase of 5-HT content was seen in all brain regions.

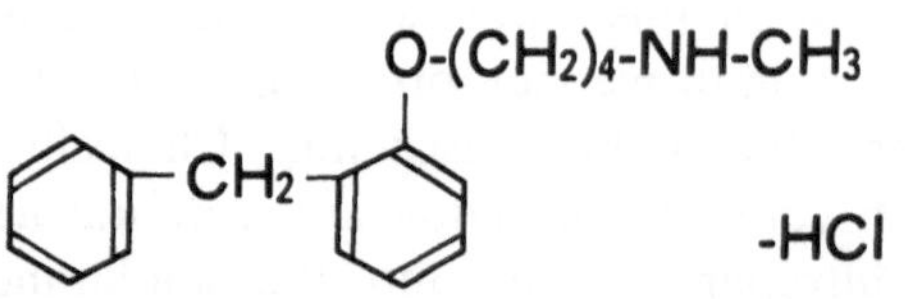

$$O\text{-}(CH_2)_4\text{-}NH\text{-}CH_3$$

CH$_2$

-HCl

4-(o-benzylphenoxy)-N-methylbutylamine hydrochloride (bifemelane hydrochloride)

Fig. 1. Chemical structure of bifemelane hydrochloride

Table 1. Changes in NE, DA, and 5-HT content in kaolin-induced hydrocephalus after injection of bifemelane hydrochloride.

Brain regions	normal	normal rats	hydrocephalic rats in subacute phase	
		bifemelane 10 mg/kg ⊕	bifemelane ⊖	bifemelane 10 mg/kg ⊕
Norepinephrine (ng/g wet tissue)				
Cerebral cortex	217 ± 31	274 ± 35	239 ± 55	319 ± 26 *
Striatum	19 ± 7	88 ± 37	135 ± 48	71 ± 33 *
Hippocampus	229 ± 37	266 ± 42	271 ± 62	321 ± 53
Cerebellum	224 ± 29	233 ± 27	229 ± 27	248 ± 13
Pons + Medulla	481 ± 68	485 ± 63	543 ± 93	581 ± 111
Dopamine (ng/g wet tissue)				
Cerebral cortex	38 ± 11	49 ± 17	44 ± 28	50 ± 28
Striatum	12765 ± 1979	18434 ± 2787	16160 ± 2676	17257 ± 2794
Hippocampus	39 ± 19	107 ± 30	60 ± 18	52 ± 11
Cerebellum	8 ± 3	7 ± 4	8 ± 5	9 ± 5
Pons + Medulla	51 ± 9	51 ± 7	59 ± 6	58 ± 10
Serotonin (ng/g wet tissue)				
Cerebral cortex	452 ± 132	484 ± 52	399 ± 87	500 ± 31 *
Striatum	599 ± 131	716 ± 111	722 ± 120	726 ± 150
Hippocampus	465 ± 50	516 ± 57	470 ± 47	513 ± 67
Cerebellum	130 ± 3	155 ± 21	889 ± 16	123 ± 29 *
Pons + Medulla	953 ± 151	1146 ± 187	961 ± 146	1053 ± 182

Results are given as means ± SEM of four or five rats
* : p < 0.05 significantly different from the control values

Discussion

Intracisternal injection of kaolin suspension is a well known procedure for inducing hydrocephalus and intracranial hypertension, which develop as a result of a sterile meningitis and occlusion of the outflow of the CSF through the fourth ventricle (Gonzalez-Darder et al. 1984; Miwa et al. 1982). In this study, edematous changes of the periventricular layer appeared in the acute phase and ventricular dilatation appeared in the subacute phase, which suggested that hydrocephalus had occurred.

Food and water intake were remarkedly reduced and impairment of locomotion, probably due to akinesia and gait disturbance, was observed during the whole course of hydrocephalus formation.

In hydrocephalus, increased intraventricular pressure and edema of the periventricular layer are generally considered to cause decrease of the cerebral blood flow and impairment of axonal flow. It is considered that changes of monoamine neurotransmitter metabolites correlate with cerebral blood flow (Ogura et al. 1988). Consequently, the possibility that improvement of blood flow and axonal flow could occur as a result of injection of a cerebral metabolic activator should also be considered.

Following intravenous and intraperitoneal injection, bifemelane passes through the blood-brain barrier into several brain regions, especially the cer-

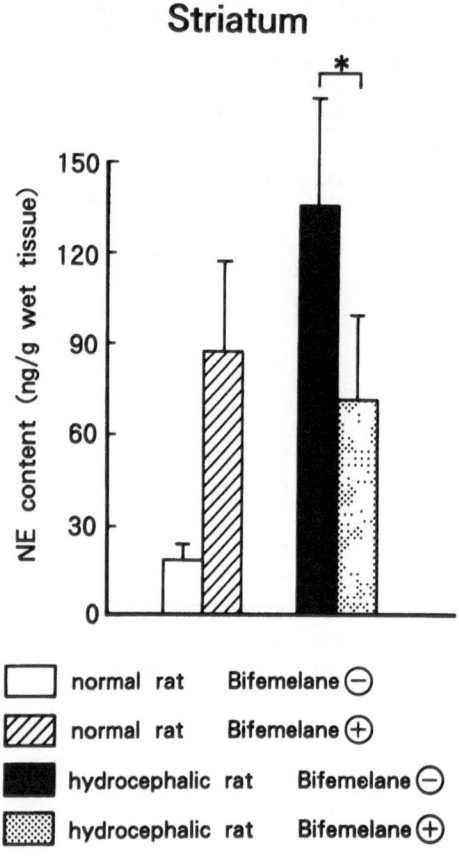

Striatum

Fig. 2. Norepinephrine (*NE*) content in the striatum after injection of bifemelane hydrochloride. *$P > 0.05$: significantly different from the control values

☐ normal rat   Bifemelane ⊖

▨ normal rat   Bifemelane ⊕

■ hydrocephalic rat   Bifemelane ⊖

▨ hydrocephalic rat   Bifemelane ⊕

ebral cortex. This feature is applied clinically to improve neurotransmitter metabolism and impaired cerebral blood flow due to brain ischemia. Clinically, bifemelane is administered orally to patients with cerebral infarction and cerebral hemorrhage (Goto et al. 1988).

Changes of NE content in the striatum are shown in Fig. 2. The NE content in the striatum, which is located on the wall of the lateral ventricles, increased under hypertensive intracranial conditions. This may have been due to the inhibition of the axonal flow of norepinephrinergic nerve fibers passing through the nucleus. After bifemelane injection, the NE content tended to decrease and this may have been due to improvement of the axonal flow of norepinephrinergic nerve fibers.

Changes of 5-HT content in the cerebral cortex are shown in Fig. 3. The 5-HT content decreased after kaolin injection. Since the cerebral cortex includes serotonergic nerve terminals, the decrease of 5-HT content may have been due to inhibition of the axonal flow of serotonergic nerve fibers. In contrast, after bifemelane injection, the content of 5-HT tended to increase. This may have been due to improvement of the axonal flow of serotonergic nerve fibers.

Fig. 3. Serotonin (*5-HT*) content in the cerebral cortex after injection of bifemelane hydrochloride. *P > 0.05: significantly different from the control values

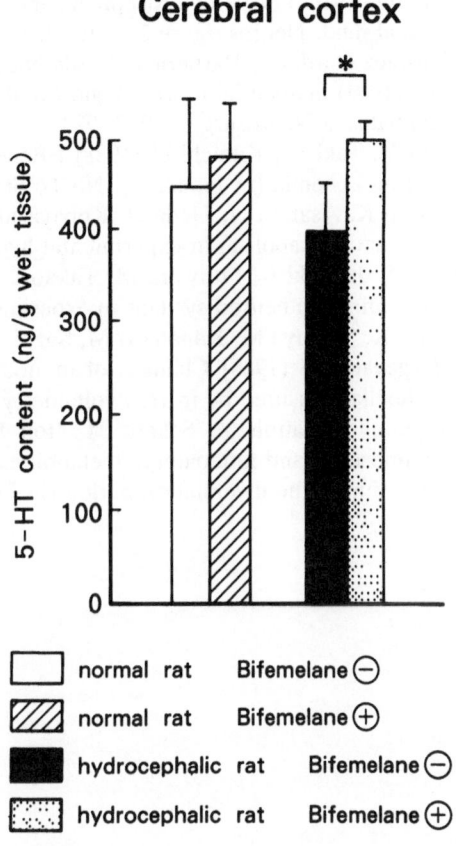

Cerebral cortex

Changes of DA content in all the brain regions after bifemelane injection are, in contrast, not statistically significant.

As a result, this study suggests that monoamines in hydrocephalic rat brains will change after bifemelane injection. In particular, differences in the cerebral cortex and striatum were statistically significant. Changes of NE and 5-HT content after bifemelane injection were observed in some brain regions, but change of DA content was not observed.

Thus, this study demonstrates the effects of a cerebral metabolic activator (bifemelane hydrochloride) on monoamine neurotransmitters in kaolin-induced hydrocephalus in rat brains.

References

Andersson H, Roos BE (1965) Acidic monoamine metabolites in cerebrospinal fluid of children with hydrocephalus. Acta Neurol Scand 41(suppl 13): 149–151

Chovanes GI, McAllister JP II, Lamperti AA, Salotto AG, Truex RC (1988) Monoamine alterations during experimental hydrocephalus in neonatal rats. Neurosurgery 22: 86–91

Del Bigio MR (1989) Hydrocephalus-induced changes in the composition of cerebro-spinal fluid. Neurosurgery 25: 416–423

Gonzalez-Darder J, Barbera J, Cerda-Nicolas M, Segura D, Broseta J, Barcia-Salorio JL (1984) Sequential morphological and functional changes in kaolin-induced hydrocephalus. J Neurosurg 61: 918–924

Goto Y, Taki W, Kikuchi H (1988) Effects of bifemelane on the free fatty acid levels during ischemia (in Japanese). No To Shinkei 40: 1045–1049

Higashi K, Asahisa H, Ueda N, Kobayashi K, Hara K, Noda Y (1986) Cerebral blood flow and metabolism in experimental hydrocephalus. Neurol Res 8: 169–176

Miwa S, Inagaki C, Fujiwara M, Takaori S (1982) The activities of noradrenergic and dopaminergic neuron systems in experimental hydrocephalus. J Neurosurg 57: 67–73

Ogura K, Shibuya M, Kanamori M, Suzuki Y, Ikegaki I, Harada T, Okasa T, Tanoi C, Kageyama N (1988) Changes of monoamine neurotransmitter metabolism in brain ischemia measured by in vivo voltametry (in Japanese). No To Shinkei 40: 87–93

Onodera Y, Saitoh Y, Sakata M, Itoh H, Miwa T (1988) Quantitative fatty acid composition and monoamine metabolites in CSF from congenital hydrocephalic children during the myelination period (in Japanese). Nerv Syst Child 13: 7–13

8 — Changes in the Hypothalamic and Brain Stem Catecholaminergic Systems in Experimental Hydrocephalus: A Histochemical Observation

Kazumasa Ehara[1], *Chikako Tanaka*[2], *Norihiko Tamaki*[1], *and Satoshi Matsumoto*[1]

Summary. Fluorescence histochemical analysis combined with a sensitive assay method using high performance liquid chromatography (HPLC) revealed definite changes in the central catecholaminergic systems in experimental hydrocephalus. Hydrocephalus was induced in rats by injection of kaolin into the cisterna magna. Rats were placed into three groups: control, paired feeding, and hydrocephalic. Then hydrocephalic group was divided into mild and severe subgroups according to the degree of neurological symptoms.

Brain norepinephrine (NE) levels were decreased in the frontal cortex, in the hippocampus, and in the cerebellum. NE levels in the hypothalamus were decreased only in the severe hydrocephalic group. There were no significant differences between the control and the paired feeding groups in brain NE levels. Brain dopamine (DA) concentration was the same in the hydrocephalic and the control groups.

Fluorescent histochemistry revealed the accumulation of NE in the cell body of the locus coeruleus and the subcoeruleus neurons. In contrast, the NE fluorescence of the nerve terminals was reduced in the frontal cortex and the periventricular area of the hypothalamus. Catecholamine histofluorescence was not changed in the striatum and the lower brain stem.

The coerulo-cortical and periventricular pathways of the ascending NE systems were selectively impaired in experimental hydrocephalus.

Keywords. Hydrocephalus — Norepinephrine — Dopamine — rat — Fluorescent histochemistry

Introduction

Hydrocephalus constitutes one of the central issues in clinical neurology and neurosurgery. Not only the symptomatology (Adams et al. 1965; Hakim and Adams 1965), but also the morphological and histopathological changes in

---

[1] Departments of Neurological Surgery and [2] Pharmacology Kobe University School of Medicine, Kobe, 650 Japan

hydrocephalus have been widely investigated in humans and in experimental animals (Penfield and Elvidge 1932; Clark and Milhorat 1970; Milhorat 1972). However, little is known of the related metabolic changes (Moir et al. 1970; Inagawa et al. 1980). This may be due partly to the lack of knowledge of the exact contribution of the neurotransmitter systems to the innervation of structure that may be involved in the mechanism of the metabolic changes. Recent fluorescent histochemical studies have revealed the distribution and precise anatomy of the central monoaminergic systems (Ungerstedt 1971; Lindvall and Björklund 1974) and technological progress has improved the sensitivity of catecholamine assays. Increased catecholamine fluorescence in the locus coeruleus and decreased NE levels in the frontal cortex of the hydrocephalic rat brain have been reported previously by the authors (Ehara et al. 1982). The present study was carried out to assess further changes of entire central monoaminergic pathways, using fluorescent histochemical analysis of serial brain sections, combined with observations of neurological symptoms, and chemical assay of catecholamines by high performance liquid chromatography (HPLC).

Material and Methods

Animal Preparation

Twenty four 6-week-old male Wistar rats were placed into three groups: hydrocephalic, control, and paired-feeding. Hydrocephalus was induced by kaolin injection (Lindauer and Griffith 1938; Matsumoto et al. 1975; Torvik and Stenwig 1977). Rats were anesthetized by 40 mg/kg pentobarbital sodium intraperitoneal injection. After the atlanto-occipital membrane had been exposed through midline suboccipital incision, 0.1 ml of a suspension of kaolin (250 mg of hydrated aluminum silicate in 1 ml of 0.9% saline) was injected through a 27 G needle.

In the control and paired feeding groups, the same amount of physiological saline was injected by the same procedure. Rats were housed in separate cages at 22–24°C under constant day-night rhythm with free access to drinking water and to a commercial diet (Oriental Koubo Industry Co., Tokyo, Japan). Daily food intake, water intake, body weight, and rectal temperature were measured. In the paired feeding group, daily dietary intake was restrict to the mean intake of the hydrocephalic group on each day. All these rats were killed after 4 weeks.

Hydrocephalic rats were divided into a severe group and a mild group according to their neurological symptoms and their degree of body weight loss.

Catecholamine Assay

For chemical assay, brains which had been rapidly removed from decapitated rats were dissected on ice into seven regions: the frontal cortex, occipital cortex, hippocampus, striatum, hypothalamus, cerebellum, and medulla plus pons (Glowinski and Iversen 1966). The samples were homogenized in 5 ml of ice cold 0.4 N perchloric acid containing 5 mg sodium metabisulfite and 20 mg ethylene diamine tetraacetate and then centrifuged for 10 min at 10,000 r.p.m.. Supernatants were assayed for norepinephrine and dopamine, using HPLC with an electrochemical detector (Keller et al. 1976).

Fluorescent Histochemical Preparation

For histochemical demonstration of catecholamine, paraformaldehyde gas treatment combined with glyoxylic acid perfusion was used (Falck et al. 1962; Björklund et al. 1972; Yoshida et al. 1979). Twenty rats were grouped into control and hydrocephalic groups by the procedure outlined under Material and Methods. The rats were anesthetized with pentobarbital sodium (40 mg/kg, i.p.) and the heart was exposed without artificial ventilation. The rats were then perfused through the left ventricles with 600 ml/kg of ice cold 2% glyoxilic acid in phosphate buffered Ringer's solution. Immediately after perfusion, the brains were removed and rapidly frozen in prechilled isopentane with liquid nitrogen. The specimens were freeze-dried at −35°C for 7 days and then exposed to vapor generated from standardized paraformaldehyde at 80°C for 1 h. After this treatment, the specimens were embedded in paraffin in vacuo. Transverse serial sections, each of 100 μ per slice, were prepared. Each 10 μ-thick slice was mounted with a mixture of entellan and xylene. A Zeiss fluorescence microscope with BG 12 and Zeiss # 50 filters was used for analysis.

Results

Neurological Changes

In all rats given kaolin, there was some degree of ventricular dilatation, but the degree of hydrocephalus varied from slight to extensive even after the same amount of kaolin. After 1 week, the rats given kaolin ate less food and exhibited drowsiness and paretic ambulation; after 2 weeks their heads were enlarged and there was a loss of activity; and after 4 weeks their heads were domed. There was a parallel correlation between loss of weight and the neurological symptoms. Two weeks after the operation, the body weight of the control group had increased, but in some rats of the hydrocephalic group (the severe group, $n = 4$), body weight had gradually decreased; however, in the other rats (the mild group, $n = 4$) of the hydrocephalic group, the body weight remained unaltered. Marked decrease of food and water intake was also noted in the severe group and slight decrease of intake was observed in the mild group. The body temperature in the severe group was found to be decreased at 4 weeks, but remained unchanged in the control and the mild group. Also, the skull enlargement and neurological symptoms were remarkable in the severe group.

Assay of Tissue Catecholamine Concentration

The changes in the brain NE concentration in each group are shown in Table 1. In the hydrocephalic rats 4 weeks after operation, brain NE levels were significantly decreased in the cerebral cortex, especially in the frontal cortex, and in the hippocampus and in the cerebellum. In the frontal cortex in particular, the levels of NE were decreased by 67% of the control value. The NE levels in the striatum and in the medulla plus pons remained unaltered. There were no significant changes in NE levels between the control and the paired feeding groups.

As shown in Table 2, there were no statistically significant changes in the DA levels between the control and the hydrocephalic groups. The DA levels in the cerebral cortex were slightly increased in the paired-feeding group.

The NE and DA levels in the hypothalamus of the hydrocephalic group were slightly lower than those in the control group, but were not statistically significant (Table 1). Table 3 indicates the relationship between the degree of hydrocephalus and brain catecholamine levels in the hypothalamus. In the

Table 1. Changes in norepinephrine levels in the hydrocephalic rat brain

	Control	Paired feeding	Hydrocephalus
			(ng/g)
Cerebral cortex	223 ± 14	227 ± 18	146 ± 9**
Frontal cortex	253 ± 18	—	170 ± 9**
Occipital cortex	135 ± 8	—	122 ± 7
Hippocampus	217 ± 9	206 ± 9	172 ± 7*
Striatum	236 ± 44	214 ± 32	316 ± 41
Hypothalamus	1977 ± 14	2013 ± 135	1557 ± 216
Medulla plus Pons	481 ± 27	407 ± 8	507 ± 23
Cerebellum	120 ± 4	105 ± 3	87 ± 8

* $P < 0.01$, ** $P < 0.001$
Each value is the mean ± the standard error of 8 determinations

Table 2. Changes in dopamine levels in the hydrocephalic rat brain

	Control	Paired feeding	Hydrocephalus
			(ng/g)
Cerebral cortex	119 ± 10	172 ± 9*	124 ± 11
Frontal cortex	212 ± 44	—	189 ± 23
Occipital cortex	28 ± 5	—	32 ± 9
Hippocampus	22 ± 3	30 ± 5	21 ± 3
Striatum	9402 ± 831	$10,210 \pm 609$	9939 ± 469
Hypothalamus	669 ± 40	580 ± 85	567 ± 36
Medulla plus Pons	42 ± 3	37 ± 1	42 ± 2
Cerebellum	21 ± 3	18 ± 2	16 ± 2

* $P < 0.01$
Each value is the mean ± the standard error of 8 determinations
Significantly different from each control

Table 3. Relationship between the degree of hydrocephalus and brain norepinephrine and dopaimine levels

		Wet weight (mg)	Norepinephrine (ng/g)	Dopamine (ng/g)
Control	(n = 8)	72 ± 7	1977 ± 141	669 ± 40
Mild hydrocephalus	(n = 5)	72 ± 6	1974 ± 309	564 ± 51
Severe hydrocephalus	(n = 5)	61 ± 6	1117 ± 180*	591 ± 34

* $P < 0.01$
Each value is the mean ± the standard error of 8 determinations
Significantly different from each control

severe cases of hydrocephalus, NE levels in the hypothalamus were markedly decreased by 56% of the control value, but in the mild cases, NE levels were unchanged.

Fluorescent Histochemical Observations

Fluorescent histochemistry revealed changes in the coerulo-cortical NE system. In the hydrocephalic group, fluorescent cell bodies in the locus coeruleus of the midbrain were swollen and catecholamine fluorescent materials had accumulated in the neurons. NE histofluorescence of the dorsal tegmental bundle rostral to the locus coeruleus was also remarkably increased in the brains of the hydrocephalic rats (Fig. 1A,B). In contrast, catecholamine fluorescence in the nerve terminals in the frontal cortex was decreased in the hydrocephalic group (Fig. 1C,D). Fluorescence of the nerve terminals was also slightly decreased in the hippocampus and cerebellum.

In the periventricular NE pathways of the hydrocephalic group, catecholamine fluorescence was decreased in the periventricular and paraventricular nuclei of the hypothalamus (Fig. 2A,B). Even in mild hydrocephalus, catecholamine fluorescence of the nerve terminals was decreased, especially in the periventricular layer of the hypothalamus. However, fluorescence in the lateral portion of the hypothalamus, the medial forebrain bundle, and the supraoptic nucleus was unchanged. Axons of the subcoeruleus, one of the neurons of the periventricular NE pathway, were swollen in hydrocephalus (Fig. 2C,D).

However, there were no significant changes between control and hydrocephalic groups in the histofluorescence of neurons such as A1 (Fig. 3A,B), A2 (Fig. 3C,D), and A3 in the descending NE pathways in the lower brain stem.

Histofluorescence of the dopaminergic nerve terminals in the striatum was unaltered in hydrocephalus (Fig. 4A,B). The fluorescence of dopaminergic neurons in the midbrain, the nucleus of the mesolimbic system (A8), the nucleus of the substantia nigra (A9, Fig. 4C,D), and in the intrapedunclar nucleus (A10) was not changed. DA histofluorescence of the median eminence was reduced in the medial part of the floor of the third ventricle in hydrocephalus (Fig. 5A,B).

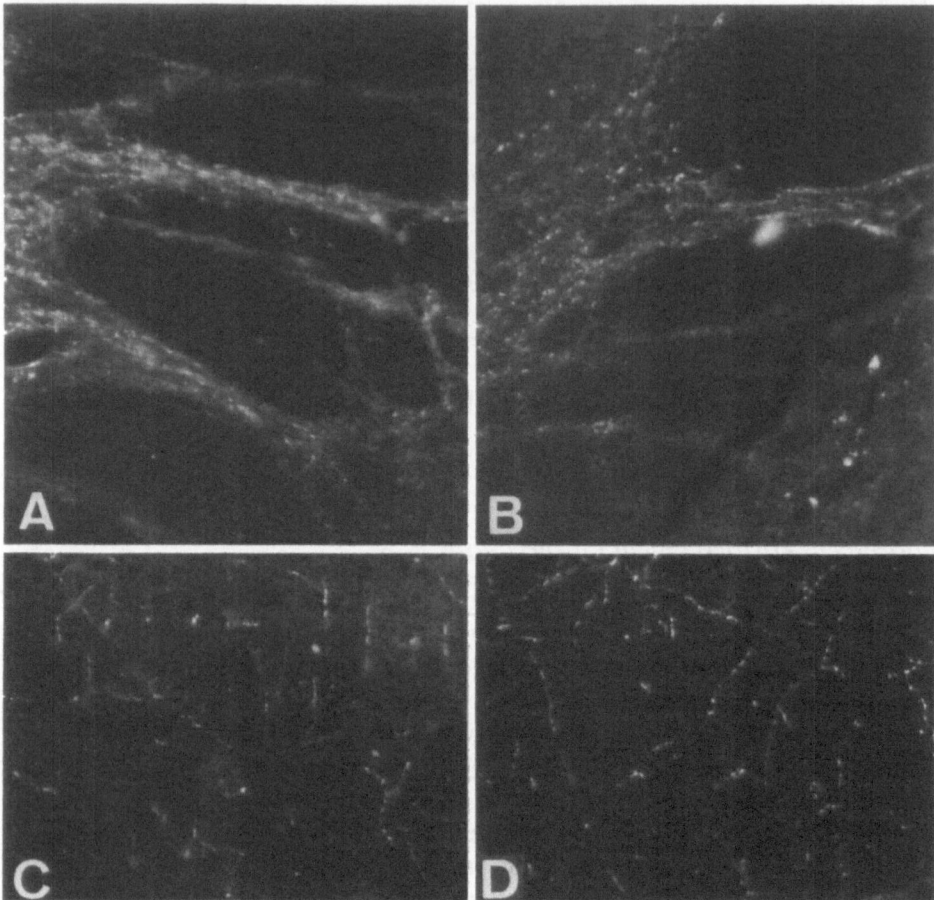

Fig. 1. Norepinephrine fluorescence by combining formaldehyde gas treatment with glyoxylic acid perfusion (× 64). Norepinephrine histofluorescence of the dorsal tegmental bundle rostral to the locus coeruleus in **A** hydrocephalic and **B** control rats. Note that norepinephrine histofluorescence was remarkably increased in hydrocephalus. Catecholamine histofluorescence of the nerve terminals in the frontal cortex in **C** hydrocephalic and **D** control rats. Catecholamine fluorescence was slightly decreased in hydrocephalus

Discussion

The distribution of NE fibers arising from the locus coeruleus has been studied by examining changes in histofluorescence (Dahlström and Fuxe 1964; Ungerstedt 1971; Lindvall and Björklund 1974) and changes in NE content following lesions of the locus coeruleus or related pathways (Kobayashi et al. 1974). These studies have indicated that the major NE innervation to the cerebral cortex, cerebellum, and hippocampus arises from the ipsilateral locus

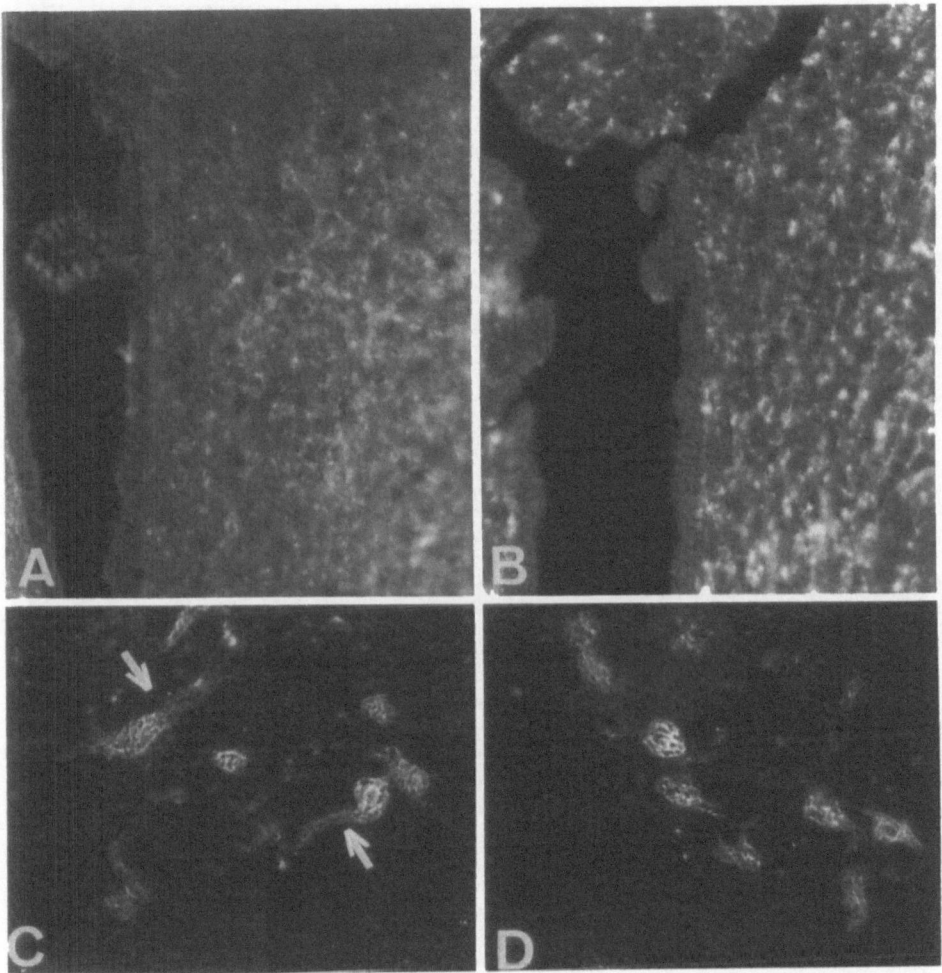

Fig. 2. Coronal section at the level of the paraventricular nucleus in **A** hydrocephalic and **B** control rats. Note the marked reduction of catecholamine fluorescence in the terminals of the periventricular layer of the hypothalamus. The subcoeruleus nucleus in **C** hydrocephalic rats, in which axons of the subcoeruleus were swollen (*arrows*), and **D** control rats

coeruleus, and that the region of the hypothalamus is supplied mainly by axons from NE neurons which emanate from the locus coeruleus and from the subcoeruleus areas.

The reduction of NE in the frontal cortex, the cerebellum, and the hippocampus and the decrease of catecholamine histofluorescence in these brain areas found in the present study, combined with the NE accumulation in nerve cell bodies in the locus coeruleus reported by the authors previously (Ehara et al. 1982), strongly suggest damage to the coerulo-cortical and coerulo-

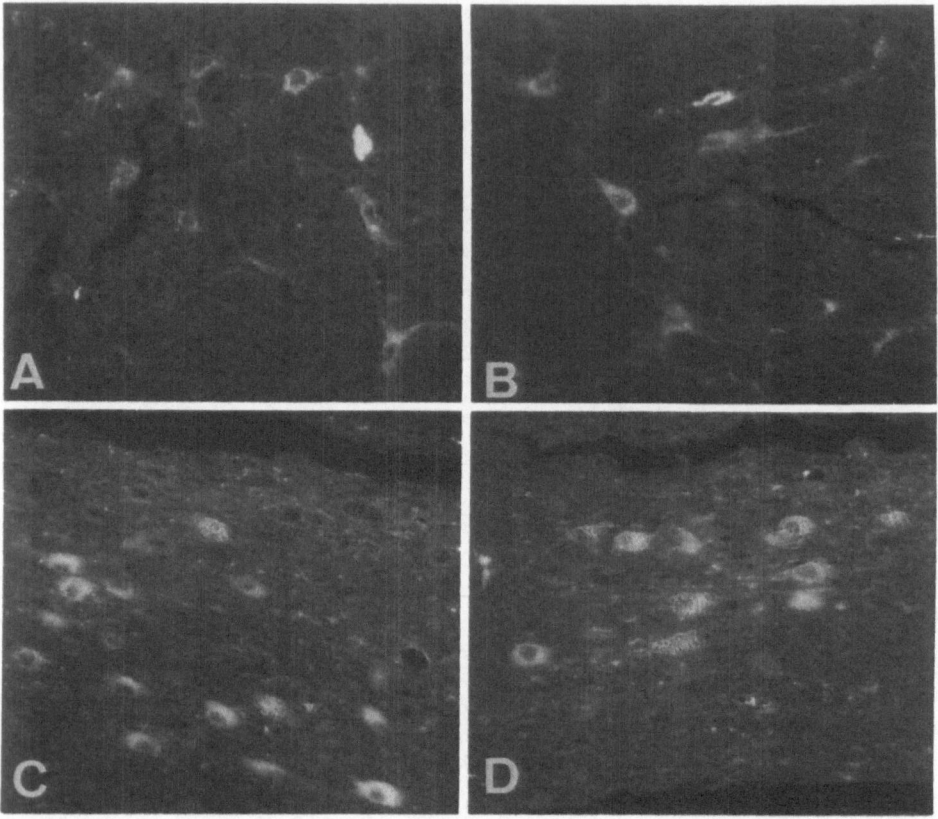

Fig. 3. Norepinephrine fluorescence in the A1 nuclei of the descending pathway in the lateral medulla oblongata in **A** hydrocephalic and **B** control rats. No remarkable change in histofluorescence was observed in either group. Norepinephrine fluorescence in the A2 nuclei of the descending pathway in the dorsal medulla in **C** hydrocephalic and **D** control rats. No remarkable change in histofluorescence was observed in either group

cerebellar NE pathways. According to the fluorescent histochemistry of the serial sections in this study, the coerulo-cortical NE pathway impaired in the area between the medial forebrain bundle in the hypothalamus and the cerebral cortex.

The decrease in hypothalamic NE content found by chemical assay and the decrease in catecholamine histofluorescence in the periventricular hypothalamus, together with the accumulation of NE in the cell bodies of the locus coeruleus and subcoeruleus, indicate damage to the periventricular NE system. These histofluorescence findings closely resemble to axonal injury between cell bodies and nerve terminals (Dahlström and Fuxe 1964).

These histofluorescence findings and the uneven reduction of NE levels in the various cortical regions support this hypothesis. If the neurons of the locus

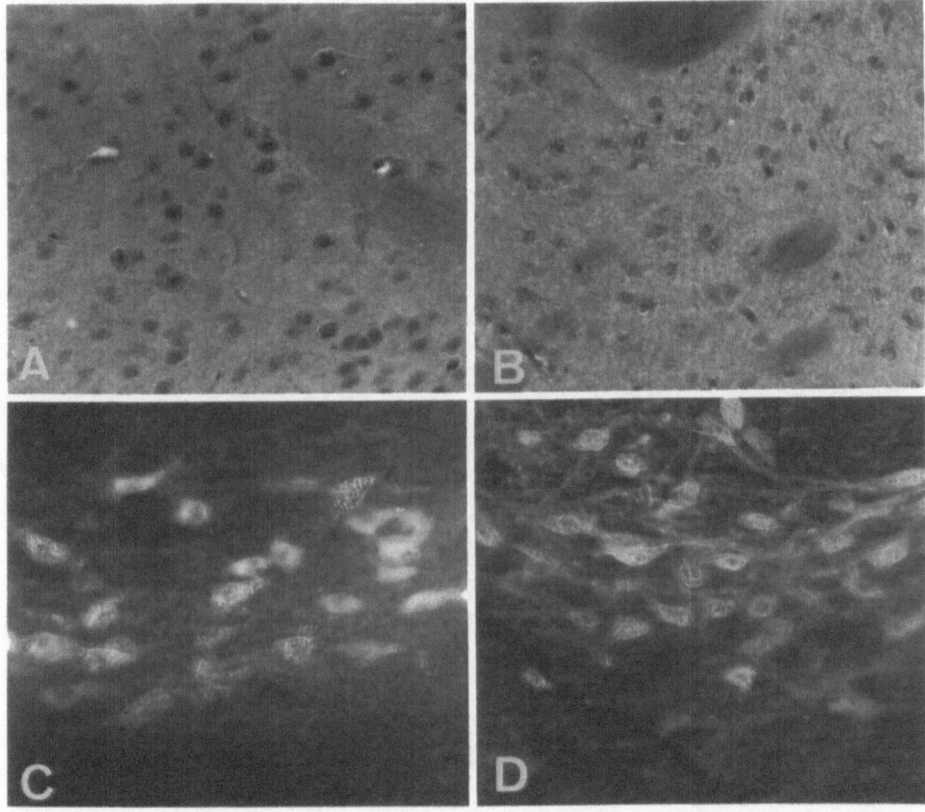

Fig. 4. Dopamine fluorescence in the striatum in **A** hydrocephalic and **B** control rats. No remarkable change in histofluorescence was observed in either group. Dopamine fluorescence of the substantia nigra in **C** hydrocephalic and **D** control rats. No remarkable changes in histofluorescence were observed in either group

coeruleus were highly degenerated, a reduction of NE levels of almost the same amount would be produced in all cortical regions.

This idea is also supported by a physical simulation study using the photoelastic model (Hakim et al. 1976) and by a mathematical simulation using the finite element method (Nagashima et al. 1987), both of which concluded that when the intraventricular pressure was increased, the periventricular white matter was most affected by the physical stress. Histopathological findings for experimental hydrocephalus (Penfield and Elvidge 1932; Clark and Milhorat 1970; Milhorat 1972) have also indicated that edema of the white matter, not the gray matter, was the earliest pathological lesion and that the major atrophic process in hydrocephalus, until the endstage, probably involved the neuroglia and axonal collaterals rather than the neurons, nerve terminals, and the main axonal trunks.

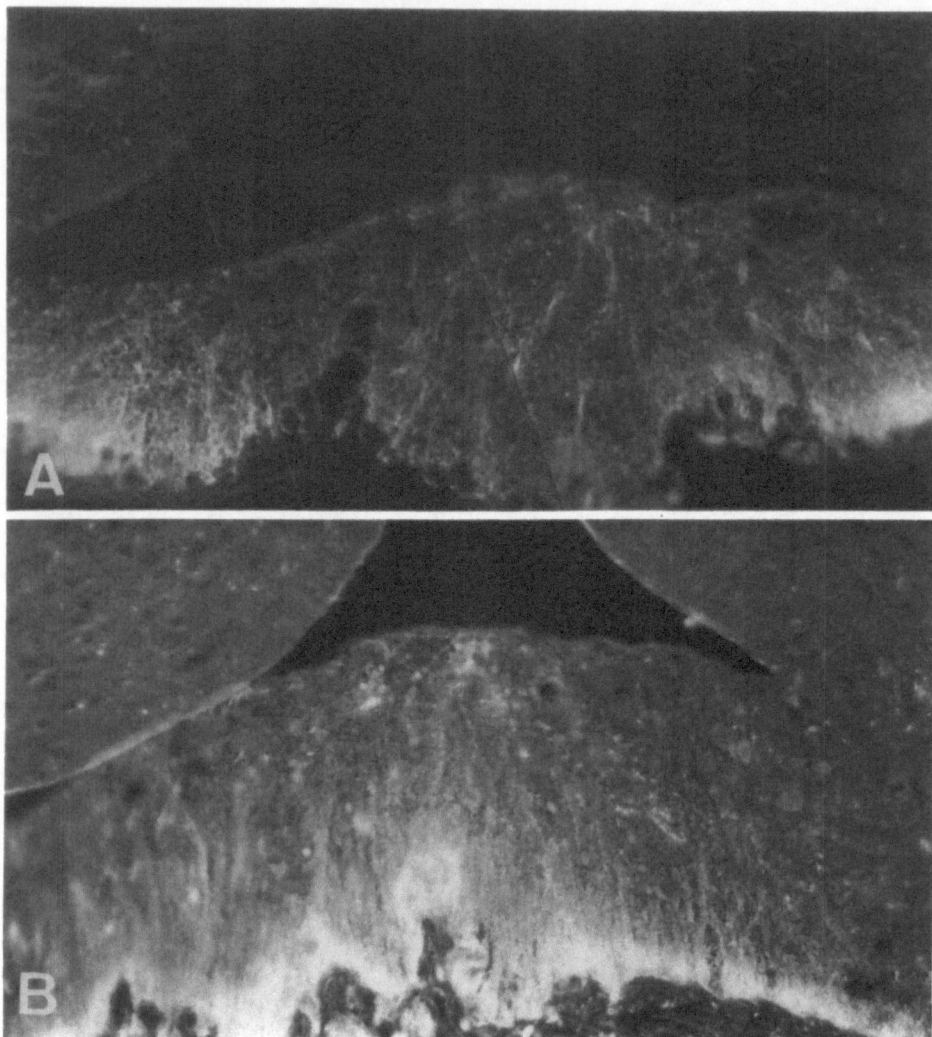

Fig. 5. Dopamine histofluorescence in the median eminence in **A** hydrocephalic and **B** control rats. Note the slight reduction in histofluorescence in the medial part of the floor of the third ventricle at the level of the median eminence

The decrease in NE which occurred in brain tissue when there was an acute increase in intracranial pressure induced by cisternal injection of kaolin suspension in rabbits was first described in 1971 (Owman et al. 1971). Miwa et al. (1982) reported that an NE metabolite, 3-methoxy-phenyl-ethylene-glycol (MHPG), increased in the cerebral cortex in experimental hydrocephalus. The authors, using a HPLC microassay, reported a decrease in NE content in the frontal cortex (Ehara et al. 1982). Decreased NE content in Brodmann's area

4, 17, 22 was also reported recently in kaolin-induced hydrocephalic newborn cats (Lovely et al. 1989). Chemical assay analysis appears to be insufficiently sensitive for the assessment of precise changes in the central monoamine systems because the monoamine fibers run in very complicated pathways in the central nervous system, especially in the brain stem and in the hypothalamus. Therefore we used a combination of histochemistry and microchemical assays for the present study. Our results strongly supported the results of Owman et al. and Lovely et al.

Lovely et al. (1989) also found that early withdrawal of cerebrospinal fluid from the experimental hydrocephalic newborn cats improved the reduction of NE content in Brodmann's area 4 and 22. These data strongly supported the concept that the decrease in NE in the frontal cortex was due to an immediate and reversible effect of disturbance in cerebrospinal fluid dynamics. If the reduction of NE content were related to chronic inflammation or some other mechanism, the levels of NE would not have improved after the withdrawal of ventricular CSF. Paired feeding studies suggest that the reduction of NE content in the various cortical regions was due not to starvation, but to the effect of hydrocephalus induced by kaolin.

The ascending NE pathways are believed to be related to emotion, sleep, and the regulation of appetite, temperature, and urination. The electrical activity of the locus coeruleus is believed to be strongly related to the reticular formation of the brain stem and to be most active in the wakeful state. One of the important roles of the locus coeruleus is believed to involve monitoring of outside stimuli. Wakefulness and learning motivation are also believed to be related to the activity of this nucleus (Aston-Jones and Bloom 1981a,b). Drowsiness, inattentiveness, and loss of spontaneous movement were seen in the chronic stage of experimental hydrocephalus in rats. Psychophysiological analysis of normal pressure hydrocephalus (NPH) has shown decreased cognitive function in normal pressure hydrocephalic patients which suggested that the major mental symptoms of NPH, such as dementia, inattentiveness, and loss of spontaneous activity were related to disturbances in the monitoring of outside environmental stimuli (Katayama et al. 1981). Other reports have also supported the relationship between disturbance of recent memory and the coerulo-cortical NE system. These data strongly supported the relationship between the mental symptoms of hydrocephalus and impairment of the coerulo-cortical NE system.

The periventricular NE system has a close relationship to food intake. Chronic infusion of NE into the ventromedian hypothalamus induced obesity (Shimazu et al. 1986). In experimental hydrocephalus, decrease of NE in the median hypothalamus was observed; this might cause loss of appetite and body weight. The central monoamine system was also believed to be closely related to various autonomic functions such as regulation of body temperature and sexual maturation (Gitler and Barraclough 1987). These results strongly suggest a relationship between the selective impairment of the ascending NE pathway and the various neurological symptomss found in hydrocephalic experimental animals or humans.

References

Adams RD, Fisher CM Hakim S, Ojemann RG, Sweet WH (1965) Symptomatic occult hydrocephalus with "normal" cerebrospinal-fluid pressure. A treatable syndrome. N Engl J Med 273: 117–126

Aston-Jones G, Bloom FE (1981a) Activity of norepinephrine-containing locus coeruleus neurons in behaving rats anticipates fluctuations in the sleep-waking cycle. J Neurosci 1: 876–886

Aston-Jones G, Bloom FE (1981b) Norepinephrine-containing locus coeruleus neurons in behaving rats exhibit pronounced responses to non-noxious environmental stimuli. J Neurosci 1: 887–900

Björklund A, Lindvall O, Svensson LÅ (1972) Mechanisms of fluorophore formation in the histochemical glyoxylic acid method for monoamines. Histochemie 32: 113–131

Clark RG, Milhorat TH (1970) Experimental hydrocephalus, Part 3: Light microscopic findings in acute and subacute obstructive hydrocephalus in the monkey. J Neurosurg 32: 400–413

Dahlström A, Fuxe K (1964) Evidence for the existence of monoamine-containing neurons in the central nervous system. Acta Physiol Scand (Suppl) 62: 232 1–55

Ehara K, Matsumoto S, Yoshida N, Kuno T, Tanaka C (1982) Ascending norepinephrine pathways impaired in experimental hydrocephalus. Jpn J Pharmacol 32: 205–208

Falck B, Hillarp NÅ, Thieme G, Torp A (1962) Fluorescence of catecholamines and related compounds condensed with formaldehyde. J Histochem Cytochem 10: 348–354

Gitler MS, Barraclough CA (1987) Locus coeruleus stimulation arguments LHRH release induced by medial preoptic stimulation. Evidence that the major LC stimulatory component enters contralaterally into the hypothalamus. Brain Res 422: 1–10

Glowinski J, Iversen LL (1966) Regional studies of catecholamines in the rat brain — I. The disposition of [³H]Norepinephrine, [³H]Dopamine and [³H]Dopa in various regions of the brain. J Neurochem 13: 655–659

Hakim S, Adams RD (1965) The special clinical problem of symptomatic with normal cerebrospinal pressure. Obstruction of cerebrospinal fluid dynamics. J Neurol Sci 2: 307–327

Hakim S, Venegas JG, Burton JD (1976) The physics of the cranial cavity, hydrocephalus and normal pressure hydrocephalus. Mechanical interpretation and mathematical model. Surg Neurol 5: 187–210

Inagawa T, Ishikawa S, Uozumi T (1980) Homovanillic acid and 5-hydroxyindoleacetic acid in the ventricular CSF of comatose patients with obstructive hydrocephalus. J Neurosurg 52: 635–641

Katayama Y, Tsubokawa T, Tsukiyama T, Nishimoto H, Moriyasu N (1981) Neurophysiological study on psychiatric symptoms in normal pressure hydrocephalus. Clinical evaluation by contingent negative variation. Neurol Surg (Tokyo) 9: 315–323 (in Japanese)

Keller R, Oke A, Mefford I, Adams RN (1976) Liquid chromatographic analysis of catecholamines, routine assay for regional brain mapping. Life Sci 19: 995–1004

Kobayashi RM, Palkovits M, Kopin IJ, Jacobowitz DM (1974) Biochemical mapping of noradrenergic nerves arising from the rat locus coeruleus. Brain Res 77: 269–279

Lindauer MA, Griffith Jr JQ (1938) Cerebrospinal pressure, hydrocephalus, and blood pressure in the cat following intracisternal injection of colloidal kaolin. Proc Soc Exp Biol Med 39: 547–549

Lindvall O, Björklund A (1974) The organization of the ascending catecholamine neuron systems in the rat brain. Acta Physiol Scand [Suppl] 412: 1–48

Lovely TJ, McAllister II JP, Miller DW, Lamperti AA Wolfson BJ (1989) Effects of hydrocephalus and surgical decompression on cortical norepinephrine levels in neonatal cats. Neurosurgery 24: 43–52

Matsumoto S, Hirayama A, Yamasaki S, Shirataki K, Fujiwara K (1975) Comparative study of various models of experimental hydrocephalus. Childs Brain 1: 236–242

Milhorat TH (1972) Hydrocephalus and the cerebrospinal fluid. Williams and Wilkins, Baltimore, pp 115–118

Miwa A, Inagaki C, Fujiwara M, Takaori S (1982) The activities of noradrenergic and dopaminergic neuron systems in experimental hydrocephalus. J Neurosurg 57: 67–73

Moir ATB, Aschcroft GW, Crawford TBB, Eccleston D, Guldberg HC (1970) Cerebral metabolites in cerebrospinal fluid as a biochemical approach to the brain. Brain 93: 357–368

Nagashima T, Tamaki N, Matsumoto S, Horwitz B, Seguchi Y (1987) Biomechanics of hydrocephalus: A new theoretical model. Neurosurgery 21: 898–904

Owman CH, Rosengren E, West KA (1971) Influence of various intracranial pressure levels on the concentration of certain arylethylamines in rabbit brain. Experientia 27: 1036–1037

Penfield W, Elvidge AR (1932) Hydrocephalus and the atrophy of cerebral compression. In (ed. Penfield W) Cytology and cellular pathology of the nervous system, vol 3. Hafner, New York, pp 1203–1217

Shimazu T, Noma M, Saito M (1986) Chronic infusion of norepinephrine into the ventromedial hypothalamus induces obesity in rats. Brain Res 369: 215–233

Torvik A, Stenwig AE (1977) The pathology of experimental obstructive hydrocephalus, electron microscopic observations. Acta Neuropathol (Berl) 38: 21–26

Ungerstedt U (1971) Stereotaxic mapping of the monoamine pathways in the rat brain. Acta Physiol Scand [Suppl] 367: 1–48

Yoshida N, Taniyama K, Tanaka C (1979) Adrenergic innervation and cyclic adenosine 3'5'-monophosphate levels in response to norepinephrine in stomach of postnatal rats. J Pharmacol Exp Ther 211: 174–180

9 — Regional Changes in Superoxide Free Radicals, Energy Metabolism, and Ca-Calmodulin Binding Protein in the Development of Congenital Hydrocephalus

Nariyuki Hayashi and Takashi Tsubokawa[1]

Summary. Interstitial edema has been proposed as a possible mechanism of neuronal damage in congenital hydrocephalus. Recent studies have demonstrated that oxygen-derived free radicals play an important role in the damage of vascular permeability and cell membrane perturbation in various kinds of edema. Therefore, we studied the regional changes of superoxide free radicals, energy metabolism, and a neuron specific protein, microtubule associated protein 2(MAP2), in the development of congenital hydrocephalus. We present the results in this paper.

Superoxide free radicals increased specifically in the choroid plexus and in periventricular tissue shortly after birth, with degradation of MAP2 in the neural proliferative layer. This specific regional activation of free radicals plays an important role in the development of neural growth and leakage of toxic metabolic substrates from the choroid plexus into the ventricular CSF. In this study, we have demonstrated a free radical trigger mechanism in the development of congenital hydrocephalus.

Key words. Hydrocephalus — Free radicals — Mapping of superoxide anions — Neural proliferative layer — Microtubule associated protein 2(MAP2)

Introduction

The etiology of congenital hydrocephalus remains unclear. A variety of factors, e.g., nutritional deficiencies, heredity, metabolic imbalance, thermal irregularities, and environmental teratogens are implicated in the pathogenesis. A variety of evidence indicates that functional changes in cerebrospinal fluid (CSF) circulation result from failure of movement of ependymal microvilli (Ellington and Margolis 1969; Gilles and Davidson 1971), CSF overproduction by the choroid plexus (Eisenberg et al. 1974), interstitial migration from

[1] Department of Neurological Surgery, Nihon University Medical School, Itabashi-ku, 173 Japan

ependymal tissue (Hopkins et al. 1977), and also, in experimentally induced congenital hydrocephalus rats (Sato 1989), degradation of subependymal tissue and aqueduct stenosis.

Recent studies have demonstrated that oxygen-derived free radicals play an important role in the change of vascular permeability in endothelial vascular damage and tissue degradation with cell membrane perturbation (Chan et al. 1984; Prado et al. 1987; Siesjo et al. 1985; Wei et al. 1985).

One problem is that as free radicals are extremely labile, they are difficult to detect in vivo. We have now developed a new technique for mapping superoxide free radicals, energy metabolism, tissue pH, and vascular permeability, simultaneously, in frozen tissue sections (Hayashi 1990). In this paper, we report on localized changes of superoxide free radicals, energy metabolism, and neuron specific high molecular weight protein (MAP2), which were studied in the progress of congenital hydrocephalus (Koto et al. 1987).

Materials and Methods

Changes in superoxide free radicals, tissue ATP, and MAP2 were studied in experimentally induced congenital hydrocephalus Imamichi rats ($n = 20$) and normal baby Wistar rats ($n = 6$) until 15 days after perturbation (Fig. 1). The brain was frozen in liquid nitrogen suitable for the study of tissue ATP and superoxide free radicals and was fixed in 5% sucrose 95% ethanol mixed solutions for the study of immunohistochemical staining of MAP2. For the mapping of tissue ATP and superoxide free radicals, 15 μ frozen tissue sections were cut by cryostat from the experimental tissue slices.

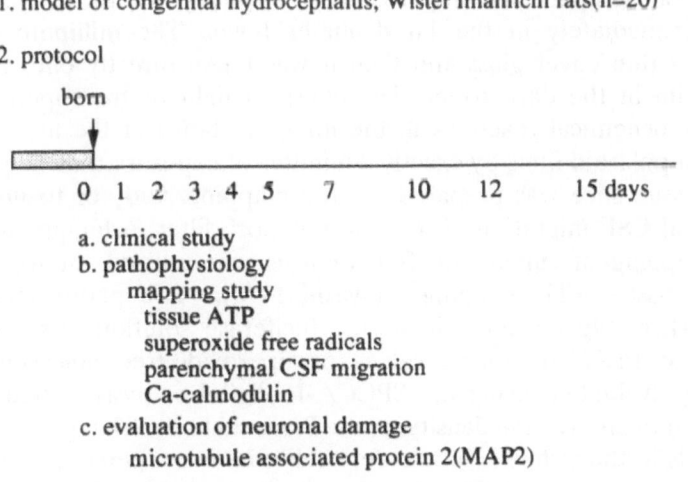

1. model of congenital hydrocephalus; Wister Imamichi rats(n=20)

2. protocol

born

0 1 2 3 4 5   7   10   12   15 days

a. clinical study
b. pathophysiology
    mapping study
      tissue ATP
      superoxide free radicals
      parenchymal CSF migration
      Ca-calmodulin
c. evaluation of neuronal damage
    microtubule associated protein 2(MAP2)

Fig. 1. Experimental protocol

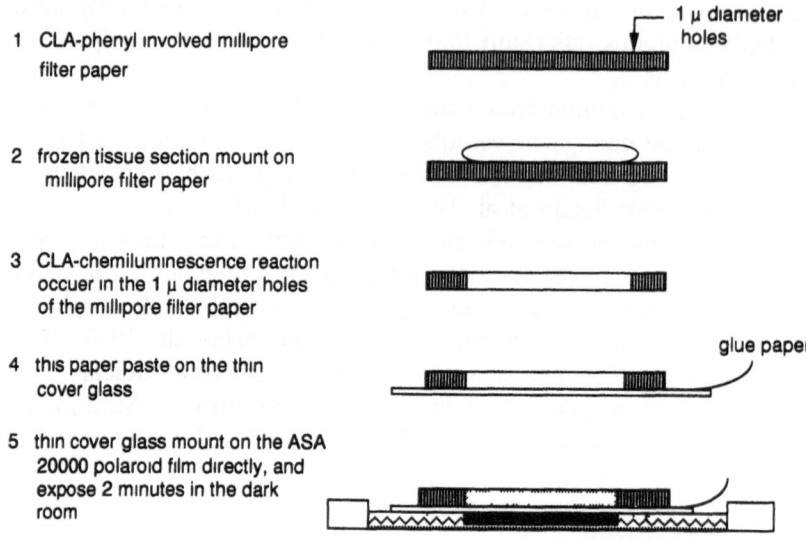

Fig. 2. Mapping technique for superoxide free radicals

Mapping of Superoxide Free Radicals

Determination of the distribution of superoxide anions in the CNS was based on 380 nm chemiluminescence of 2-methyl-6-pheny1-3, 7-dihy-droimidazode-[1,2a]pirazie-3-one(CLA-phenyl) upon reaction with superoxide in the tissue (Nakano et al. 1986). The frozen tissue section was mounted on millipore filter paper (CA 250/0, Schleicher and Schuell Co., Germany) that contained saturated CLA-phenyl solution in the millipore holes. (Tokyo Kasei Kogyo Co., Ltd.). Frozen tissue sections melted and were trapped in the millipore holes at room temperature. Superoxide CLA-phenyl photochemical reactions occurred immediately in the 1μ diameter holes. The millipore paper was pasted on a thin cover glass and then it was taken directly onto ASA-20000 Polaroid film in the dark room. The emission light of the superoxide-CLA-phenyl photochemical reactions in the millipore holes of the filter paper was pictured on polaroid films by exactly 2 minutes of exposure time (Fig. 2). Next, a frozen tissue slice was prepared for the mapping study of tissue ATP and parenchymal CSF migration. The same millipore filter technique as described for the mapping of superoxide free radicals was utilized for topographical, quantative tissue ATP mapping (Hayashi 1990). As a photochemical fluorescent marker, Mg including luciferine fuciferase solution was used (Sigma Chemical Co. FLE-50). Normal values for superoxide free radicals in the brain tissue were evaluated, using the SPCCA-II digital analysis system (Olympus Co., Tokyo) to analyze the density on the Polaroid films. Changes in superoxide free radicals in the ischemic lesion were calibrated as a percent change (%) of normal brain tissue values. The change in brain tissue MAP2 was studied by an immunohistochemical technique using a Vectastain ABC kit.

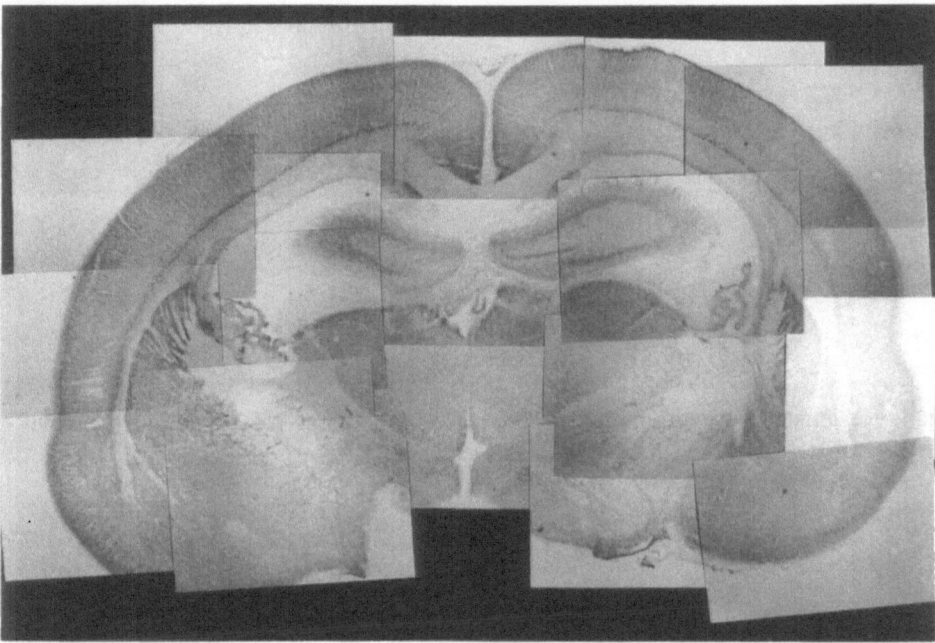

Fig. 3. Immunohistochemical staining of microtubule associated protein 2(MAP2) in the normal baby Wistar rat. The neuron specific protein, MAP2, distributed in especially high density in the neuron proliferative layer

Results

(1) Hormal Wistar rats

Normal Wistar rats showed no progressive ventricular dilatation during the first 2 weeks after birth. Energy metabolism was maintained at 2.8 ± 0.64 m mol tissue ATP; showing no difference from that in adult brain tissue. Superoxide free radicals in brain tissue had a very low density and there was no specific difference between gray and white matter, except in the thalamus.

The distribution of neuron specfic protein (MAP2) was maintained in the whole cortex; in particular, the neuron proliferative layer (subplate layer) showed high density distribution, as shown in Fig. 3.

(2) Wistar Imamichi rats

In Wistar Imamichi rats, ventricular dilatation started shortly after birth and progressed severely for 5–7 days. The ventricular dilatation produced severe brain atrophy in the homogenetic cortex. Damage to the heterogenic cortex that included the hippocampus progressed later than the 5th day after birth. The rate of progression of ventricular dilatation slowed down after this stage and slow destructive hydrocephalus continued to the terminal stage.

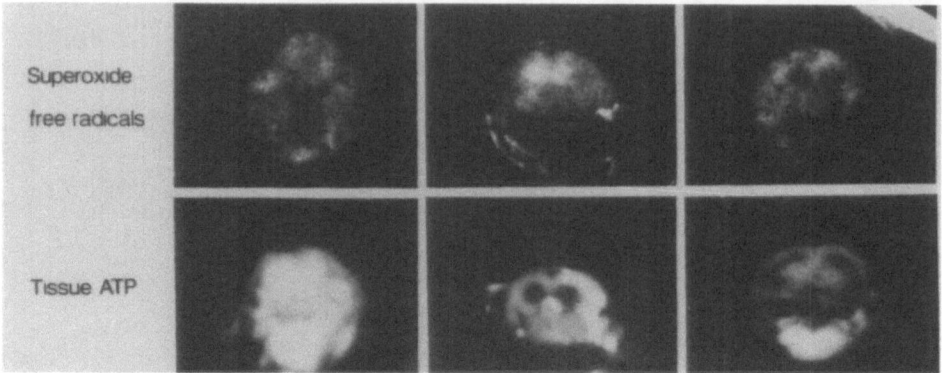

Fig. 4. Regional changes in superoxide free radicals and tissue ATP in various locations in brain tissue in 2-day-old congenital hydrocephalus

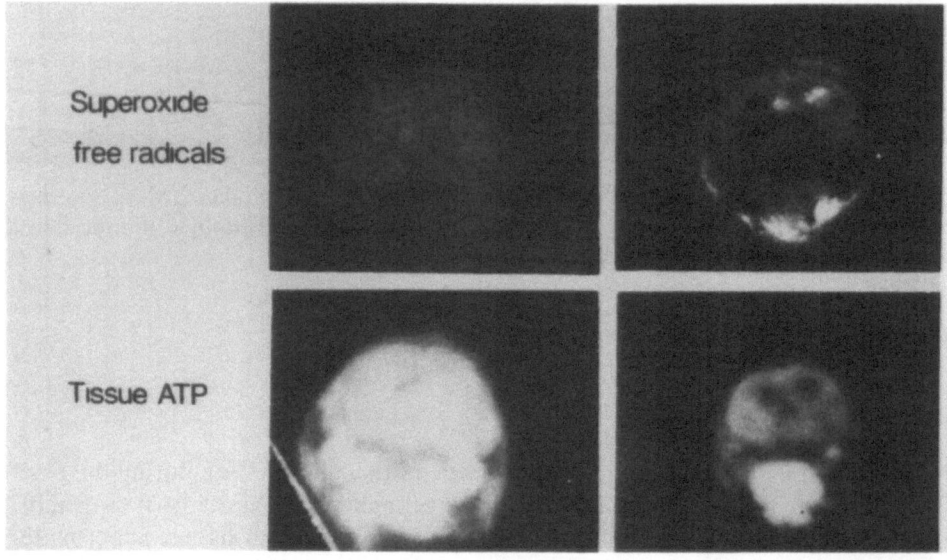

Fig. 5. Regional changes in superoxide free radicals and tissue ATP in the normal Wistar rat and congenital hydrocephalus Wistar Imamichi rat. In congenital hydrocephalus, superoxide free radicals are specifically localized in the choroid plexus

(A) Tissue ATP and Superoxide Free Radicals

Changes of tissue ATP occurred initially in the periventricular tissue, from the second day after birth (Fig. 4). These changes consisted of a maximum of 15% decreasing tissue ATP in the periventricular tissue. Tissue ATP in the congenital hydrocephalus was maintained at a slightly lower level than normal tissue (85%–93%) until the terminal stage, even with severe brain atrophy.

Specific distribution of superoxide free radicals was observed in the Wistar Imamichi rats. On the first day, superoxide free radicals, increased specifically

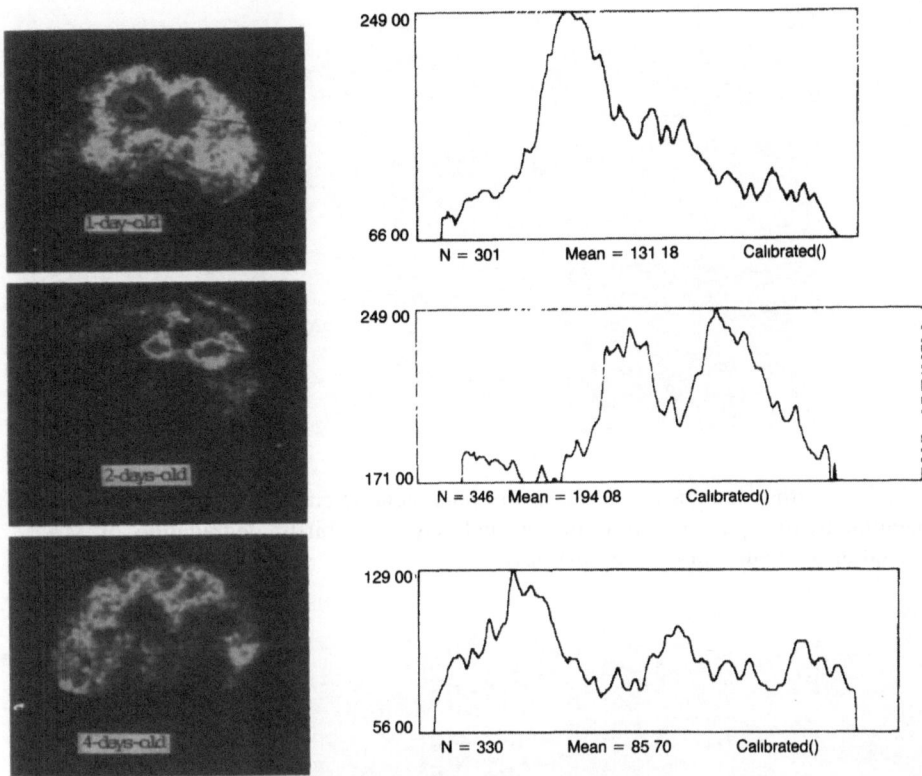

Fig. 6. Sequential changes in regional superoxide free redicals in the development of congenital hydrocephalus. The high density areas in the choroid plexus and periventricular neuronal proliferative layer are limited to shortly after birth

in the choroid plexus, at the foramen of Monro (Fig. 5). The maximum density was 6.8 times higher than normal values and mean values were 5.2 ± 0.82 times higher than those in normal rats. These high density of superoxide specific to the choroid plexus continued at the second day and spread around the periventricular tissue that included the proliferative layer in the homogenetic cortex (Fig. 6). This distribution correlated exactly to the changes of tissue ATP (Fig. 4).

However, the changes in tissue ATP were not severe enough to produce the cell membrane damage seen with cerebral ischemia. The specific activation superoxide free radicals in the choroid plexus was limited to 2 days. This activation in the choroid plexus was followed by severe progression of ventricular dilatation and brain atrophy at between 2–7 days after birth (Fig. 6).

At a later stage of progressive ventricular dilatation, heterogeneous low density superoxide free radicals were observed in the brain mantle. The maximum density was 2.8% higher than that in normal tissue in the parietal area, as shown in Fig. 6. This distribution was not correlated to change in the periventricular CSF migration area.

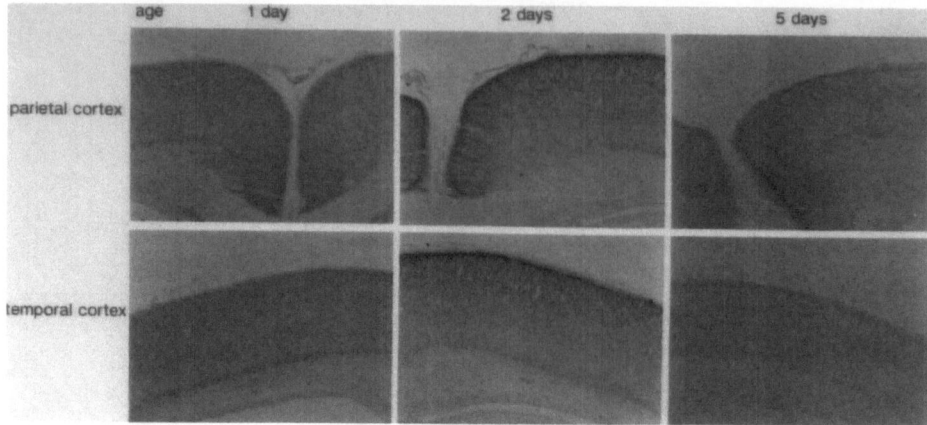

Fig. 7. Sequential changes in MAP2 in the homogenetic cortex in the development of congenital hydrocephalus. From the second day after birth, degradation of MAP2 occurred in the neuronal proliferative layer

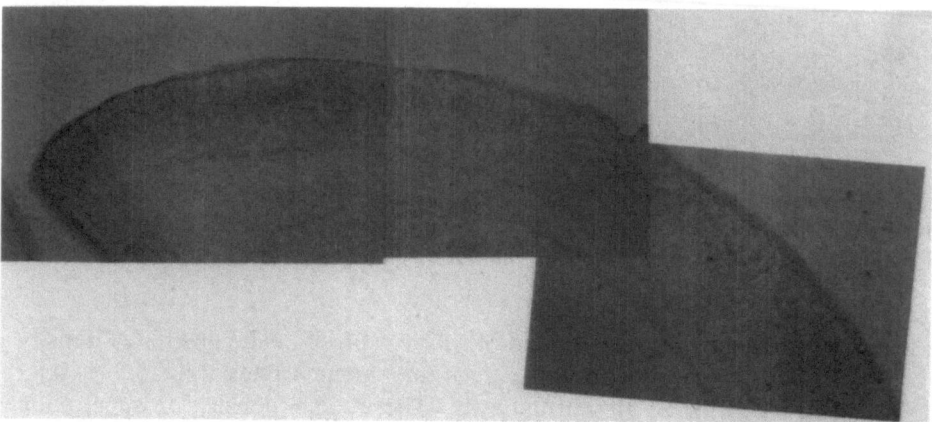

Fig. 8. Changes in MAP2 in the cortex of 5-day-old congenital hydrocephalic rats. Regional changes in MAP2 progressed more severely in the cortex of the watershed zone of the anterior and middle cerebral arteries

In the Wistar Imamichi rats, the role of free radicals in the development of congenital hydrocephalus was limited to the few days after birth.

(B) Changes of Neuron Specific Protein (MAP2)

MAP2 was very sensitive to tissue damage in the progress of hydrocephalus. The distribution of MAP2 was maintained very well in the homogenetic and heterogenetic cortex on the first day. No MAP2 damage in the neuron pro-

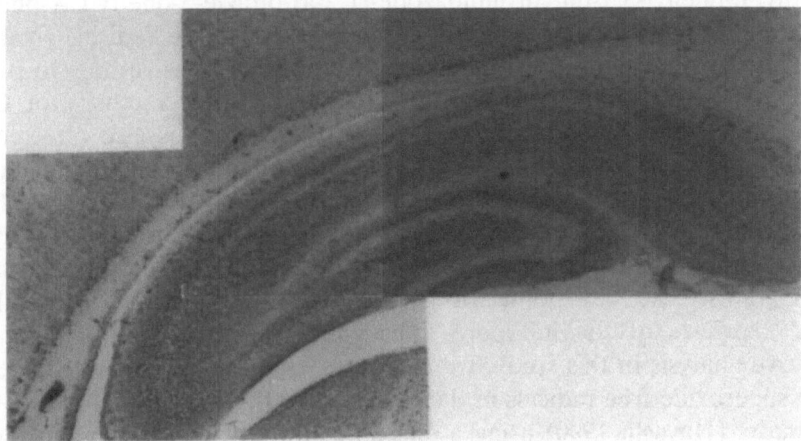

Fig. 9. Regional degradation of MAP2 in the hippocampus CA 1 on the 5th day of hydrocephalus progression

liferative layer was observed. Degradation of MAP2 in the proliferative layer developed on the second day after birth (Fig. 7). The distribution of these changes was observed to correlate with the density of superoxide free radicals and with a low signal of tissue ATP (Fig. 4). At 5–7 days, the peak of progressive ventricular dilatation, degradation of MAP2 progressed in the watershed zone in the brain mantle (Fig. 8) and in the hippocampus CA1 (Fig. 9). These areas are specifically sensitive to disturbances of microcirculation. Therefore, at this stage, the effect of low perfusion pressure caused by increased intracranial pressure added to the damage of MAP2 in the cortex. After 7 days, the changes in MAP2 progressed slowly in layers five and six and then in layers one and two in the homogenetic cortex, until the terminal stage.

Discussion

Interstitial edema has been proposed as a possible mechanism of neuronal damage in congenital hydrocephalus. Recent studies have documented that oxygen derived free radicals such as superoxide anions, hydrogen peroxide, and hydroxy radicals, facilitate the damage of endothelial and parenchymal cell membranes, because of disruption of the structure and damage to enzymatic regulation of ion transport caused by cerebral ischemic insults (Chan et al. 1984; Kollogg et al. 1975; Prado et al. 1987; Siesjo et al. 1985; Wei et al. 1985). Therefore, we have been interested in the role of free radicals, and the tissue damage they cause, in the development of congenital hydrocephalus. Despite this conceptual framework, the location, character, and magnitude of free radical-induced alterations in in vivo lesions is not yet known.

2-Methyl-6-phenyl-3,7-dihydroimidazode-[1,2-a] pirazie-3-one (CLA-phenyl) produces an emission light of 380 nm with superoxide free radicals (Nakano 1986). This emission light is extremely weak, and is responsive only to super-sensitive ASA-20000 film. The quantitative photographic intensity of CLA chemiluminescence upon reaction with superoxide anions is also affected by many factors such as contamination by extra chemiluminescence light during exposure, thickness of the frozen tissue section, sensitivity of the Polaroid film, exposure times, and the concentration of the CLA-phenyl solution. Any of these factors may influence the resultant picture, which may then be unusable for estimations. The key point for getting consistent pictures is exactly 2 minutes' exposure of the millipore filter paper on the Polaroid film. For quantitative analysis in this study, we calibrated changes in the percentages of regional superoxide free radicals in the lesion, compared to normal tissue. Our recent study, (Hayashi 1990) using a photon counting video camera, detected the regional quantitative changes of superoxide free radicals in the tissue.

Basically, hydrocephalus is caused by a disturbance in the CSF circulation. This disturbance is due mainly to disturbances in CSF absorption or to over-production along the CSF pathway, because, in both subacute and chronic hydrocephalus, the rate of formation of CSF continued essentially unchanged (Lorenzo et al. 1990). In congenital hydrocephalus, which comprises most cases of the disease no apparent obstruction in the major pathways can be identified on cisternography (Drayer and Rosenbaum 1978).

The definition of hydrocephalus, therefore, cannot be expressed in such simple terms as non-communicating and communicating hydrocephalus, so common in conventional classifications. Raimondi (1986, 1987) proposed specific classifications that separate intraparenchymal, extraparenchymal, and combined hydrocephalus. Recent reports suggest that aqueduct stenosis is not a primary occlusion but occurs secondary to communicating hydrocephalus (Raimondi et al. 1976; Williams 1973).* CSF circulatory disturbances have been proposed as a mechanism of congenital hydrocephalus. These distur-bances seem to be a more likely mechanism than CSF over production due to such defects as dynein in the microvillis and secondary aqueduct stenosis (Sato 1989).* Because, basically, the choroid plexus has no barrier to the water filtration and no severe morphological changes have been reported.

In this experiment, the specific localized activation of oxygen-derived superoxide free radicals in the choroid plexus has been demonstrated (Figs. 4,5,6). These oxygen-derived free radical reactions increased temporarily specifically in the charoid plexus after sponaneous breathing commenced. Therefore, another mechanism could be nominated for the progress of congen-ital hydrocephalus: The leakage of toxic serum substrate from the chorioidal plexus into the ventricular CSF, could as a consequence, damage microvilli and the CSF circulation. In addition, very toxic free radical reactions in the proliferative layer of the brain mantle influence the development of intra-parenchymal hydrocephalus during and shortly after birth. In kaolin-induced experimental hydrocephalus, ventricular dilatation progresses more severely after serum leakage into the ventricular CSF space. These results strongly

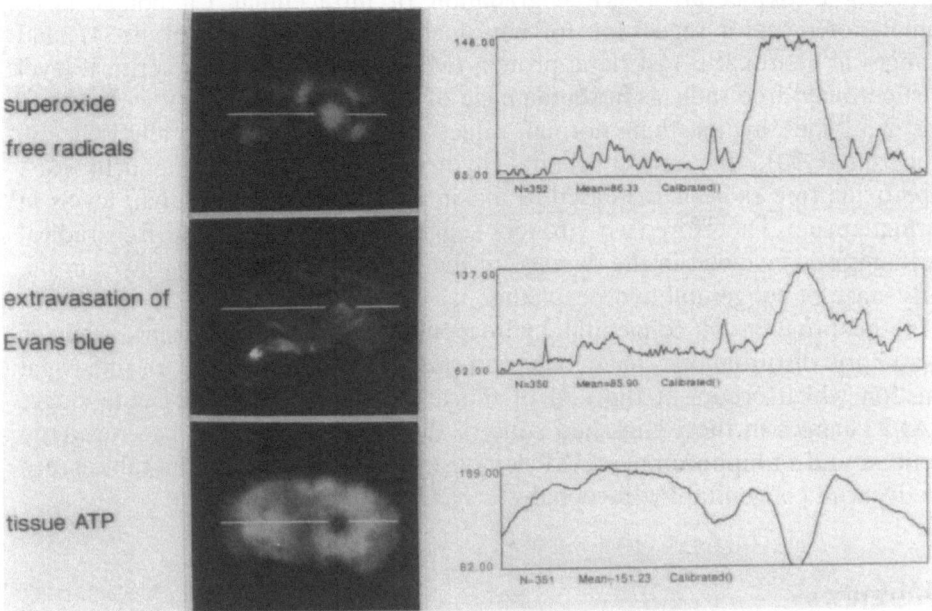

Fig. 10. Simultaneous mapping study of superoxide free radicals, tissue ATP, and vascular permeability in the post ischemic regions. Changes in superoxide free radicals were distributed more severely and widely than changes in tissue ATP and extravasation of Evans bule in the thalamus

suggest that the leakage of toxic substrates into the ventricle and oxygen derived free radicals, play important roles as trigger mechanisms in the progress of congenital hydrocephalus. Various sources of superoxide anions in the biological system have been reported, e.g., oxidization of ubisemiquinone radicals in the respiratory chain (Turrens et al. 1985), prostaglandin synthesis (Kukreja et al. 1986) conversion from available nucleotides (NADPH) (Kukreja et al. 1986), purine degradation with oxidization of xanthine oxidase, conversion of xanthine to urea (Kollogg and Fridovich 1975), and activation of neutrophils (Fantone and Ward 1985). In this study's experimentally induced fore brain ischemia, we have documented superoxide free radical reactions larger than the changes in tissue ATP (Fig. 10). This means that lipid peroxidation with prostaglandin synthesis and activation of neutrophils as sources of superoxide free radicals, play important roles in the functional damage of vascular endothelium and in cell membrane perturbation (Hayashi 1990).* Selective activation of free radicals in the choroid plexus also explains hyperoxygenation on spontaneous breathing with or without inflammatory reaction in the choroid plexus.* The important point is that specific activation of free radicals in the chorioidal plexus was limited to within 2–3 days after birth.

The early changes in MAP2 in the periventricular neuronal proliferative layer are interesting as an initial trigger mechanism for damaging the development of nerve cells (Figs. 7,8). Loss of MAP2 means difficulty of dendrite sprouting (Aoki et al. 1984), degradation of intracellular Ca homeostasis, damage of receptor regulation for neuronal memory (Aoki et al. 1984), and changes in neuronal cytoskeletal protein (Matus et al. 1981). The critical level of superoxide free radicals in the damage of vascular permeability with edema was 2.5 times higher than normal values in 17 minute forebrain ischemia (Hayashi 1990). In our congenital hydrocephalus Wistar Imamichi rats, superoxide free radicals increased to maximum 2.6 times higher than levels in normal tissue. Therefore, we strongly suggest that a superoxide free radical mechanism is involved in the damage of the neuronal proliferative layer in the early stage of congenital hydrocephalus.

In the progress of congenital hydrocephalus, other mechanisms, such as circulatory disturbances, have been proposed for the damage of neuronal function which occurs at the end of the acute stage. After the acute stage, MAP2 changes in the water-shed zone of the homogenetic and heterogenetic cortices, and in hippocampus CA1 demonstrated these to be vulnerable areas in advanced congenital hydrocephalus.

References

Aoki C, Siekevitz P (1984) Plasticity in brain development. Sci Am 259: 34–42

Carcers A, Banker G, Payne M (1984) MAP2 is localized to the dendrites of hippocampal neurons which develop in culture. Dev Brain Res 13: 314–318

Chan PH, Schmidley W, Fishman RA, Longer SM (1984) Brain injury, edema, and vascular permeability induced by oxygen-derived free radicals. Neurology (NY) 34: 315–320

Drayer BP, Rosenbaum AE (1978) Studies of the third circulation: amipaquc CT cisternography and ventriculography. J Neurosurg 48: 946–956

Eisenberg HM, McComb JG, Lorenzo AV (1974) Cerebrospinal fluid overproduction and hydrocephalus associated with choroid plexus papilloma. J Neurosurg 40: 381–385

Ellington E, Margolis G (1969) Block of arachnoid villi by subarachnoid hemorrhage. J Neurosurg 30: 651–657

Fantone C, Ward PA (1985) Polymorphonuclear leucocyte mediated cell and tissue injury. Prog Pathol 16: 973–978

Gilles FH, Davidson RI (1971) Communicating hydrocephalus with deficient dysplastic parasagittal arachnoidal granulations. J Neurosurg 35: 421–426

Hayashi N (1990) Photochemical mapping technique of superoxide free radicals, vascular permeability, and metabolism in the frozen tissue section. Jpn, Laser Med 11(2): 37–44

Hayashi N, Tsubokawa T (to be published) The new mapping study of superoxide free radicals, vascular permeability, and energy metabolism in forebrain ischemic lesions. In: Ito V, Klazo I (eds) Symposium of Maturational Neuronal Death in Cerebral Ischemia

Hayashi N, Prado R, More J, Bunge R, Green BA (1991) Regional changes of free radicals in photochemically induced ischemic injury in the central nervous system. Lasers in the Life Sciences 4: 1–7

Hopkins LN, Bakay L, Kinkel WR, Grand W (1977) Demonstration of transventricular CSF absorption by computerized tomography. Acta Neurochir (Wien) 39: 151–157

Kollogg EW III, Fridovich I (1975) Superoxide, hydrogen peroxide, and singlet oxygen in lipid peroxidation by xanthine oxidase system. J Biol Chem 250: 8812–8817

Koto M, Miwa M, Shimizu A, Tsuji K, Okamoto M, Adachi J (1987) Inherited hydrocephalus in CSsk: Wistar Imamichi rats; Hyd strain: a new disease model of hydrocephalus. Exp Anim 36(2): 157–162

Kukreja RC, Kontos HA, Hess MH, Ellis EF (1986) PGH synthase and lipoxygenase generate superoxide in the presence of NADH or NADPH. Circ Res 59: 612–619

Lorenzo AV, Page LK, Watters GV (1970) Relationship between cerebrospinal fluid formation, absorption and pressure in human hydrocephalus. Brain 93: 679–692

Matus A, Bernhardt R, Hugh-Jones T (1981) High molecular weight microtubule associated protein 2 are preferentially associated with dendritic microtubule in brain. Proc Natl Acad Sci USA 78: 3010–3014

Nakano M, Sugioka K, Ushijima Y, Goto T (1986) Chemiluminescence probe with cypridina luciferin analog, 2-methyl-6-phenyl-3,7-dihydroimidazode (1,2 a) prazin-3-one, for estimating the ability of human granulocytes to generate superoxide. Anal Biochem 159: 363–369

Prado R, Dietrich DW, Watson BD, Ginsberg MD, Green BA (1987) Photochemically induced graded spinal cord infarction. J Neurosurg 67: 745–753

Raimondi AJ (1986) Hydrocephalus: Definition and classification. Presented at the 14th Annual Meeting of the Japanese Society for Pediatric Neurosurgery, Kochi, Japan

Raimondi AJ (1987) Pediatric neurosurgery. Theoretic principles, art of surgical techniques. Springer, New York Berlin Heidelberg

Raimondi AJ, Clark SJ, McLone DG (1976) Pathogenesis of aqueductal occlusion in congenital murine hydrocephalus. J Neurosurg 45: 66–77

Sato K (1989) Mechanisms of genesis in hydrocephalus and movement of microvilli. Annual Report of the Research Committee of "Intractable Hydrocephalus" The Ministry of Health and Welfare of Japan, 1988. pp 138–141

Siesjo Bo K, Bendek G, Koide T, Westerberg E, Wieloch T (1985) Influence of acidosis on lipid peroxidation in brain tissue in vitro. J Cereb Blood Flow Metab 5: 253–258

Turrens F, Alexandre LA, Lehninger AL (1985) Ubisemiquinone is the electron donor for superoxide formation by complex III of heart mitochondria. Arch Biochem Biophys 273: 408–414

Wei EP, Christman CW, Kontos HA, Povlishock JT (1985) Effects of oxygen radicals on cerebral arterioles. Am J Physiol 248: HI57–H162

Williams B (1973) Is aqueduct stenosis a result of hydrocephalus? Brain 96: 399–412

II. Cerebral Hemodynamics and Metabolism

10 — Cerebrovascular Flow and Glucose Transport in the Hydrocephalic Rat

Soon C. Kim, Paul Tompkins, Michael Pollay, Donald D. Horton, and P. Alex Roberts[1]

Summary. This study evaluates regional cerebral perfusion flow and unidirectional glucose transport across the cerebral capillar in hydrocephalic rats. Perfusion flow and glucose influx were measured with ^{99m}Tc-ECD (Dupont Corp.) and ^{14}C-(d)-Glucose, respectively. Perfusion flows for the control and hydrocephalic groups were 1.77 ml/min per g and 1.53 ml/min per g, respectively. The hydrocephalic perfusion flow was significantly lower than the control flow ($P < .05$). Maximal influx of glucose (V_{max}) for the control group was 2.74 µm/min per g. The V_{max} for the hydrocephalic group was 3.19 µm/min per g. Substrate concentration at half maximal transport (Km) was 8.02 mM for the controls and 11.5 mM for the hydrocephalics. There was no substantial difference between control and hydrocephalic groups for these kinetic parameters. These data suggest that reported changes in cerebral metabolism in hydrocephalus are due to derangements in utilization rather than to facilitated diffusion of glucose across the blood brain barrier.

Key words. Hydrocephalus — Glucose transport — Perfusion flow

Introduction

Cerebral glucose utilization in the hydrocephalic rat brain has been shown to be reduced with respect to the non-hydrocephalic brain (Richards et al. 1989; Sogabe et al. 1989). This represents an obvious metabolic deficit with potential pronounced effects on function. These observations do not address the question of whether the primary deficit is in glucose utilization or in glucose delivery/uptake via perfusion flow. We undertook the present study to investigate the parameters of perfusion flow and glucose influx in both the control and the hydrocephalic animal.

---
[1] Division of Neurological Surgery, University of Oklahoma Health Sciences Center, Oklahoma City, OK 73126, USA

Materials and Methods

Adult male Sprague-Dawley rats were used exclusively in this study. Animals for the hydrocephalic group were anesthetized with a 1 ml/kg intraperitoneal injection of ketamine (1 gm), atropine (20 mg), and acepromazine (.54 mg). Following induction of anesthesia, 100 ul of CSF was withdrawn from the cisterna magna and hydrocephalus was induced by means of aseptic cisternal injection of 100 ul of a kaolin suspension (200 mg/ml). Following kaolin injection the wound was closed with a suture and surgically cleansed. After recovery the animals were kept from 7 to 28 days before evaluation of perfusion flow and glucose influx.

The surgical preparation for the measurement of perfusion flow and glucose influx followed that described by Takasato et al. (1984). Animals were placed in a bell jar and anesthesia was induced with 2.5% halothane in oxygen/compressed air (100/900 cc/min) for 20 min. Following induction of anesthesia a tracheostomy was performed and the animals were paralyzed with pancuronium bromide (1 mg/kg) and mechanically ventilated. Adjustments were made to keep blood gases and pH within normal limits. Anesthesia was maintained with 1.5% halothane in the respiratory gas mixture. A catheter was inserted into one femoral artery for the purpose of monitoring systemic blood pressure and sampling blood gases. A neck dissection was performed to expose the carotid arterial system and branches of the external carotid artery were coagulated, as was the pterygopalatine branch of the internal carotid. A PE-50 catheter was inserted into the external carotid as far as the carotid bifurcation. A loose ligature was placed around the common carotid proximal to the bifurcation. Body temperature was maintained at 37°C with a heating pad. The perfusion solution was bicarbonate buffered saline containing the flow marker and ^{14}C-(d)-glucose (in varying concentrations). Perfusion flow was measured using a flow marker (^{99m}Tc-ECD, Neurolite) kindly supplied by the E.I. DuPont Corp. At time zero the common carotid artery was ligated and perfusion solution was infused at a rate of 4 ml/min. This rate of infusion resulted in a perfusion pressure below 160–190 mmHg. Pressures above this level have been shown to damage the blood brain barrier (Hardebo and Nilsson 1981; Rapoport 1976). Acceptable flushing of the cerebral vasculature of the ipsilateral hemisphere was achieved under these conditions with minimal contamination from systemic blood. Perfusion was continued for a total of 15 s (5 s being required for washout of the hemisphere and 10 s allotted for exposure of tissues to the perfusion solution). At time T = 15 s. the animals were killed by decapitation and the brain was rapidly removed. The brain was immediately frozen and mounted for cryostat sectioning at 20 μm. Standards for the perfusion flow marker were prepared from a 2% gelatin solution, also sectioned at 20 μm. ^{14}C standards were purchased commercially from Amersham Corp. in the form of 20 μm strips containing increasing doses of isotope. Brain sections and standards were mounted on glass slides, dried on a warming plate (37°C) and placed in an X-ray film cassette for autoradiography using Kodak XAR-5 film. Exposure for ^{99m}Tc (flow marker) was overnight. Following a decay period of 7

Table 1. Glucose influx, μm/min per gm (± SEM) at varying glucose concentrations

	Mean glucose concentration (mmoles/l)				
	0.12	5	10	20	60
Controls	0.03(0.005)	0.79(0.22)	0.96(0.085)	1.84(0.18)	2.71(0.064)
Hydro.	0.02(0.003)	0.6 (0.049)	1.0 (0.19)	2.42(0.29)	2.68(0.26)

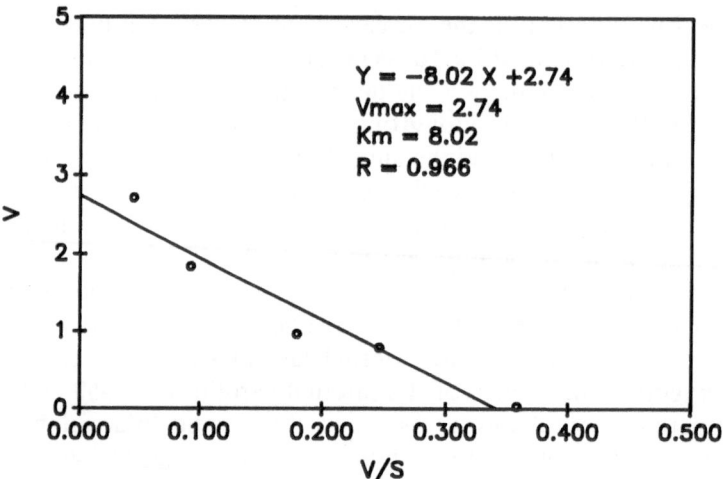

Fig. 1. Hofstee plot for control group

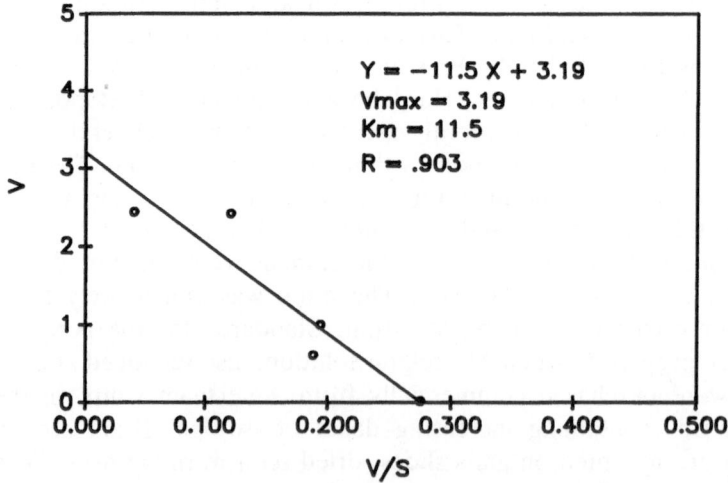

Fig. 2. Hofstee plot for hydrocephalic group

days, the sections were again apposed to film and 2 weeks were allowed for ^{14}C exposure. Each film contained both ^{99m}Tc and ^{14}C standards. Contamination of the overnight image by the ^{14}C isotope was measured by allowing ^{99m}Tc to decay and then placing the sections against film for an overnight exposure. ^{14}C contribution to the overnight image was determined to be less than 5% and was not corrected for in subsequent analyses. Perfusion flow (ml/min per g) and glucose uptake (μmoles/g) were determined from the autoradiography films, using an image analyzer (Imaging Research, Inc., Ontario, Canada). Calibration curves were constructed from the standards on each film and densities in the brain sections were read against these curves. Images were pseudocolored for ease of analysis.

Results

Blood gases and pH were maintained within normal physiological limits. Values for control animals ($n = 31$) were as follows: pH 7.389 (S.D. 0.046), pCO_2 34.68 (S.D. 4.9), and pO_2 176.7 (S.D. 33.1). Corresponding values for hydrocephalic animals ($n = 34$) were: pH 7.41 (S.D. 0.043), pCO_2 34.1 (S.D. 4.08), and pO_2 195.7 (S.D. 21.6). Both groups had similar starting body weights (controls 464 gm S.D. 31.7, hydrocephalics 467 gm S.D. 49.2). After development of kaolin-induced hydrocephalus this group was significantly lower in body weight (419 gm S.D. 74.4, $P < .002$ compared to controls). Mean cortical perfusion flow in the hydrocephalic group was significantly lower than that in the control group (Hydrocephalic 1.53 ml/min per g S.D. 0.057, control 1.77 ml/min per g S.D. 0.058, $P < 0.05$). Table 1 shows glucose influx for the control and hydrocephalic groups at various glucose concentrations in the perfusion solution.

Data from Table 1 were used to construct a Hofstee reciprocal plot of velocity vs velocity/substrate concentration. This procedure linearizes the plot and allows easy determination of the kinetic parameters V_{max} and Km. For the controls, V_{max} was 2.74 μm/min per g and Km was 8.02 mM. These data are shown graphically in Fig. 1. For the hydrocephalics, V_{max} was 3.19 μm/min per g and Km was 11.5 mM. These data are presented graphically in Fig. 2.

Discussion

The autoradiographic technique greatly simplifies the measurement of regional perfusion flow and glucose influx. Regional measurements are difficult to obtain with dissection techniques owing to the contamination of samples with surrounding tissues. If one desires, the cryostat section used for autoradiography may also be stained histologically to determine anatomical landmarks. Prior to kaolin treatment, the hydrocephalic group had the same average body weight as the control group; kaolin-induced hydrocephalus resulted in a significant reduction in body weight in the 28 days of this study. Perfusion flow in the hydrocephalic group was significantly lower than that in the control group, although pH, pCO_2 and pO_2 were the same for both groups. This difference in perfusion flow is probably due to changes in cerebrovascular hemodynamics brought about by the enlarged ventricular system.

Reduced brain utilization of glucose by hydrocephalic animals has been reported by a number of authors (Richards et al. 1989; Sogabe et al. 1989). The present study addresses the role of the glucose transport system in this reduced utilization. The control group in the present study had a V_{max} of 2.74 µm/min per g and a Km of 8.02 mM. These values are in good agreement with literature values for normal animals (Pollay and Stevens 1979). For the hydrocephalic group, V_{max} was 3.19 µm/min per g and Km was 11.5 mM. There was no substantial difference between control and hydrocephalic groups for the kinetic parameters measured in this study.

Previous studies have addressed the question of glucose metabolism in the hydrocephalic rat model without investigating the delivery/influx of glucose into the tissues. Metabolism of glucose in the hydrocephalic rat has been reported as being reduced with respect to the normal animal. Our results suggest that influx of glucose into the cortical region of the hydrocephalic rat brain is essentially normal. This would indicate that reduced utilization of glucose in this hydrocephalic model is predominantly a metabolic disturbance rather than one of delivery.

References

Hardebo JE, Nilsson B (1981) Opening of the blood brain barrier by acute elevation of intracarotid pressure. Acta Physiol Scand 111: 43–49

Pollay M, Stevens A (1979) Simultaneous measurement of regional blood flow and glucose extraction in rat brain. Neurochem Res 4: 109–123

Rapoport SI (1976) Opening of the blood brain barrier by acute hypertension. Exp Neurol 52: 467–479

Richards HK, Bucknall RM, Jones HC, Pickard JD (1989) The uptake of ^{14}C-deoxyglucose into brain of young rats with inherited hydrocephalus. Exp Neurol 103: 194–198

Sogabe T, Matsumae M, Sato O, Miura I (1989) Change in glucose metabolism with time in hydrocephalic rats. Biochem Internat 19(3): 513–518

Takasato Y, Rapoport SI, Smith QR (1984) An in situ brain perfusion technique to study cerebrovascular transport in the rat. (Heart Circ Physiol 16) Am J Physiol 247(2): H484–H493

11 — Effects of Ventricular Enlargement of Experimental Hydrocephalus on the Regional Cerebral Blood Flow, Somatosensory Evoked Potentials, and Biomechanical Factors

Joon Ki Kang, Il Woo Lee, Chun Kun Park, Moon Chan Kim, Dal Soo Kim, Dae Jo Kim, and Chang Rak Choi

Summary. This study was designed to determine the regional cerebral blood flow (rCBF), somatosensory evoked potentials (SEPs), pressure volume index (PVI), and resistance to absorption of cerebrospinal fluid (Ro) in different stages of kaolin-induced hydrocephalus. The experimental animals (cats) were divided into 2 groups; a normal control, and a kaolin-induced hydrocephalic group.

The kaolin-induced hydrocephalic group was divided into 5 subgroups of 10 cats each. These subgroups consisted of cats at 1, 2, 4, 6, and 8 weeks after intracisternal injection of kaolin. Significant decreases in rCBF were revealed both in the frontal cortex and in the periventricular area of kaolin-induced hydrocephalic cats. A reduction of rCBF to 24.7% of control flow (20.4 $\pm$ 2.8 ml per 100 g per min) was detected in the right periventricular area at 2 weeks after kaolin injection. Changes of amplitude and latency in SEPs were more prominent 4 weeks after kaolin injection. The PVI increased significantly from 0.77 $\pm$ 0.02 ml to 1.60 $\pm$ 0.16 ml at 4 weeks after kaolin injection. Ro decreased significantly from 90.6 $\pm$ 1.3 mmHg per ml per min to 36.8 $\pm$ 4.3 mmHg per ml per min at 4 weeks after kaolin injection. It is assumed that some microcirculatory impairment in the brain parenchyma plays an important role which facilitates ventricular expansion with changes of the biomechanical properties of the brain.

Keywords. Biomechanical factors — Regional cerebral blood flow — Somatosensory evoked potentials — Hydrocephalus

Introduction

Traditional views of hydrocephalus unify the varying etiological processes as having in common a defect in the absorption of cerebrospinal fluid (CSF), which creates an imbalance between its formation and absorption. This depic-

[1] Department of Neurosurgery, Kangnam St. Mary's Hospital, Catholic University Medical College, Seoul, Korea

tion of the hydrocephalic process implies that the ventricles will dilate in an extreme way at the expense of the brain as excess CSF is accumulated. However, although this sequence often occurs in the majority of hydrocephalic infants the ventricular enlargement in hydrocephalic infants usually exceeds that found in adults (Shulman and Marmarou 1971; Shapiro et al. 1985a,b).

Based on studies of biomechanical changes in ventricular enlargement, investigators have suggested that a new steady-state balance between neural axis compliance and resistance of CSF absorption occurs in the process of pathological ventricular enlargement (Hochwald et al. 1972a; Guinane 1974; Marmarou et al. 1975; Fried et al. 1987).

The fundamental changes responsible for this ventricular enlargement in hydrocephalus are speculative ones. It is assumed that some microcirculatory impairment in the brain parenchyma plays an important role in ventricular enlargement (Sato et al. 1984).

Laboratory studies of the hydrocephalic process have shown that ventricular size increases progessively after the brain container is altered (Hochwald et al. 1972b; Hochwald et al. 1973).

Most studies have shown that the intact feline hydrocephalic model, using kaolin to incite an inflammatory response, produces moderate enlargement of the ventricle which stabilizes over time (Bering and Sato 1963).

Regarding the pathophysiology of the massive ventricular enlargement associated with CSF circulatory impairment of various causes, it has been suggested that this massive enlargement may result from the inability to establish sufficient transventricular absorption or from a decrease in transventricular absorption of CSF, and also from changes in regional blood flow in brain tissue due to the relatively great effect of pressure on the periventricular areas (Sato et al. 1984; Shapiro et al. 1985a).

We designed this experimental work to examine the relation of ventricular enlargement to regional cerebral blood flow (rCBF) changes, CSF absorption resistance, and somatosensory evoked potentials (SEPs). We also examined the role of altered volume-buffering capacity on progressive ventricular enlargement.

Materials and Methods

Animal Preparation

Fifty-five 8 week-old cats, weighing 900–1300 g, were anesthetized with intra-peritoneal pentobarbital (50 mg/kg) followed by endotracheal intubation; they were then artificially ventilated, through a tracheal tube on an animal pump respirator (Bioscience 815-51190-1, Harbour Estate, Kent, UK), with a 2:1 mixture of nitrous oxide and oxygen and secured in the sphinx position in a stereotactic frame. Indwelling arterial and venous catheters were inserted into the femoral artery and vein for measurement of systemic arterial pressure and for arterial gas determinations. The respirator was adjusted to maintain $PaCO_2$

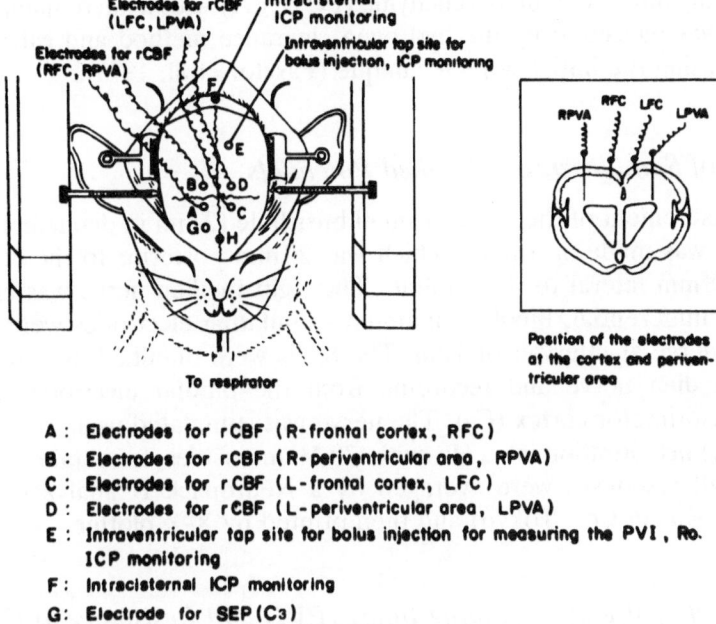

A : Electrodes for rCBF (R-frontal cortex, RFC)

B : Electrodes for rCBF (R-periventricular area, RPVA)

C : Electrodes for rCBF (L-frontal cortex, LFC)

D : Electrodes for rCBF (L-periventricular area, LPVA)

E : Intraventricular tap site for bolus injection for measuring the PVI, Ro.
     ICP monitoring

F : Intracisternal ICP monitoring

G : Electrode for SEP(C3)

H : Reference electrode for SEP(Fz)

Fig. 1. Diagram illustrating the preparation and position of a cat and various equipment. ICP, intracranial pressure

between 35 and 40 torr and PaO_2 greater than 90 torr, and rectal temperature was maintained within the physiological range.

The experimental animals were divided into 2 groups; a normal control group (5 cats), and a kaolin-induced hydrocephalic group (50 cats).

The kaolin-induced hydrocephalic group was divided into 5 subgroups of 10 cats each. These subgroups consisted of cats at 1, 2, 4, 6, and 8 weeks after intracisternal injection of kaolin.

Hydrocephalus was induced in these 50 animals by cisternal kaolin introduction; 1 ml of CSF was withdrawn from the cisterna magna and was replaced with an equal volume of kaolin suspension (250 mg/ml). The animals were placed in the head-down position for 1–2 hours and were allowed to recover.

These animals were re-anesthetized at 1, 2, 4, 6, and 8 weeks after the initiation of hydrocephalus. For the measurement of the regional CSF in these animals four burr holes were made at a point which was 4 mm anterior (frontal cortex, FC) and 2 mm posterior (periventricular area, PVA) to both coronary sutures (Fig. 1).

Measurement of Regional Cerebral Blood Flow

Hydrogen clearance was monitored from the cortex and periventricular area with platinum electrodes of 220 μm diameter; four electrodes were placed stereotactically into the brain parenchyma (FC, PVA) with a micromanipulator. The rCBF was measured by the hydrogen clearance method and calculations were made using the initial-slope technique (Pasztor et al. 1973).

Recording of Somatosensory Evoked Potentials

For the measurement of the SEPs, a small burr hole (2 mm in diameter) on the left parietal was made at a point which was 20 mm posterior to the coronary suture and 8 mm lateral to the midline. The right median nerve was exposed and two circumferential, bipolar, platinum stimulating electrodes were placed around the nerve at intervals of 1 cm. The SEPs were obtained by stimulating the right median nerve and recording from the bipolar electrodes on the opposite sensorimotor cortex (C_3). The nerve was stimulated using rectangular pulses of 0.1 ms duration at 2 Hz with 30-V intensities to obtain a motor response; 128 responses were averaged by a Neuropack II analyzer (MEB-5100; Nihon Koden Co., Tokyo) and then printed by X-Y plotter.

Measurement of Pressure Volume Index (PVI) and Resistance to CSF Absorption (Ro)

A No. 19 scalp vein needle, coupled via saline-filled tubing to a conventional strain-gauge transducer, was inserted into the cisterna magna for the measurement of intracranial pressure (ICP).

For the infusion of the mock CSF into the lateral ventricle, a No. 19 gauge needle was inserted into the lateral ventricle, at a point 15 mm posterior to the coronary suture and 8 mm lateral to the midline.

The output of the strain-gauge transducer was monitored continuously using a conventional strip chart recorder (1 mm/s).

After establishing a steady-state baseline CSF pressure, bolus manipulation of CSF was performed (0.2–0.4 ml). The pressure-volume index (PVI) was calculated from the response of CSF pressure to bolus injection using the equation PVI = ΔV/log (Pp/Po), in which ΔV is the bolus volume, Po is the initial intracranial pressure (ICP) prior to bolus injection and Pp is the peak ICP measured immediately after the bolus injection (Shapiro et al. 1985b).

The resistance to CSF absorption (Ro) was calculated using the formula Ro = Po/PVI × log [Pt/Pp × (Pp − Po)/(Pt − Po)], by extracting, in addition to the Po and Pp, Pt which is the ICP at 1 minute after injection (Marmarou et al. 1975). The animals were reanesthetized 1, 2, 3, 6, and 8 weeks later and placed in the stereotactic frame.

The cisterna magna was recannulated and ventricular fluid pressure was monitored using a No. 25 gauge needle placed stereotactically in the lateral ventricle and connected by saline-filled tubing to a strain-gauge transducer.

Determinations of PVI and CSF absorption resistance were repeated and compared to the values determined for each parameter during the initial experiment (Fig. 2).

Fig. 2. Strip chart record showing the response of intraventricular pressure to bolus injections of the fluid in normal control (*upper*) and 4 week-hydrocephalic animals (*lower*). (△V), Pp is the immediate peak ICP and Pt is the ICP 1 minute after injection. PVI and Ro are calculated from these measurements. The bolus injection sequences show that PVI increased significantly in hydrocephalic cats as compared to normal control cats and that Ro decreased in hydrocephalic cats

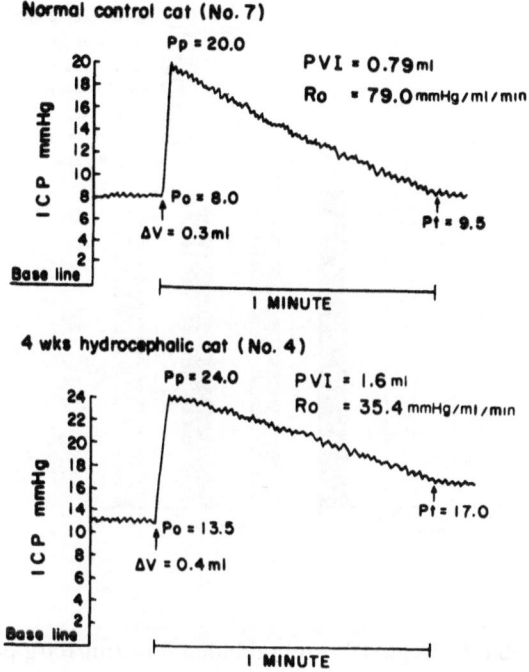

The rCBF and SEPs were measured at each stage, i.e., at 1, 2, 4, 6, and 8 weeks after intracisternal injection of the kaolin.

After completion of these procedures, the animals were sacrificed with intravenous KCl and the brains were removed.

After fixation in formalin, the brains were sectioned in the coronary plane through the foramen of the Monro.

For measurement of the ventricular size, the breadth of the lateral ventricle was determined by the distance from the septum pellucidium (SP) to the head of the caudate nucleus (CN).

Results

Intracranial Pressure

The mean steady-state ICP in the normal control cats was 8.10 ± 0.31 mmHg; the ICP measured in the 2-week-hydrocephalic cats was significantly elevated to 9.6 ± 0.6 mmHg ($P < 0.05$); and the peak value (ICP = 10.2 ± 0.9 mmHg) was obtained in 4-week-hydrocephalic cats ($P < 0.05$), as shown in Fig. 3.

Regional Cerebral Blood Flow

In the normal control cats, the flows were 35.1 ± 2.5 ml/100 g per min in the right frontal cortex, 27.1 ± 3.3 ml/100 g per min in the right periventricular

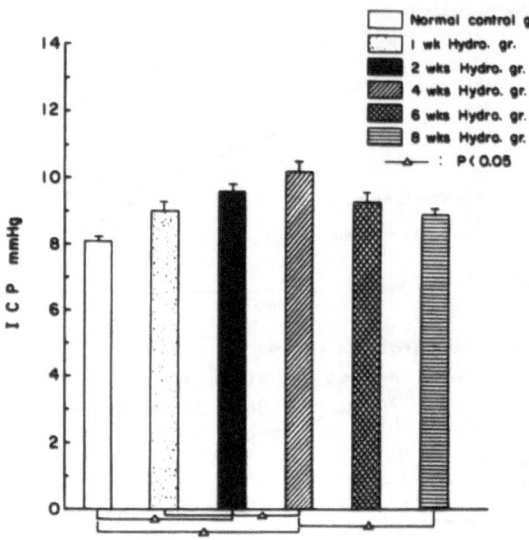

Fig. 3. Steady-state intracranial pressure (*ICP*) in the normal group and in each hydrocephalic group. Hydrocephalic animal groups had statistically different ICPs ($P < 0.05$) compared to the normal control. However there was no significant difference between the ICPs of 6 week-and 8 week-hydrocephalic cats

Table 1. Regional cerebral blood flow (ml/100 g per min, mean ± SD) in the cortex and periventricular area of normal control and hydrocephalic cats

Animal group	No. of animals (n)	RFC	RPVA	LFC	LPVA
Normal control	(5)	35.6	27.1	34.6	26.4
		±2.5	±3.3	±3.4	±3.3
1 week-hydro.	(10)	36.7*	24.9*	36.0	25.3
		±3.6	±2.0	±3.9	±1.9
2 weeks-hydro.	(10)	35.2	20.4*	34.2	19.6*
		±3.6	±2.8	±3.4	±1.2
4 weeks-hydro.	(10)	26.2*	15.9*	27.1*	15.7*
		±2.1	±1.8	±1.4	±1.7
6 weeks-hydro.	(10)	19.5*	10.3*	19.3*	9.9*
		±2.2	±2.4	±1.7	±3.1
8 weeks-hydro.	(10)	18.0*	8.9*	18.2*	8.7*
		±1.6	±1.8	±1.6	±1.5

RFC, right frontal cortex; RPVA, right periventricular area; LFC, left frontal cortex; LPVA, left periventricular area. *$P < 0.05$

area, 34.5 ± 3.4 ml/100 g per min in the left frontal cortex, and 26.4 ± 3.3 ml/100 g per min in the left periventricular area.

Dramatic decreases in rCBF were revealed in both the frontal cortex (FC) and the periventricular area (PVA) in hydrocephalic animals, as shown in Table 1 and Fig. 4. In the 2-week-hydrocephalic cats, a reduction of rCBF to 24.7% of the control flow (20.4 ± 2.8 ml/100 g per min) resulted in the right periventricular area ($P < 0.05$). However, the rCBF of the right frontal cortex

Fig. 4. Regional cerebral blood flow (*rCBF*) in hydrocephalic cats in the RFC and RPVA. Hydrocephalic cat groups had statistically different rCBF compared to normal control animals (*P* < 0.05). Note a significant reduction of flow in the right frontal cortex (*RFC*) in 4 week-hydrocephalic animals and a more advanced reduction of the cerebral blood flow in the right periventricular area (*RPVA*) rather than in the frontal cortex

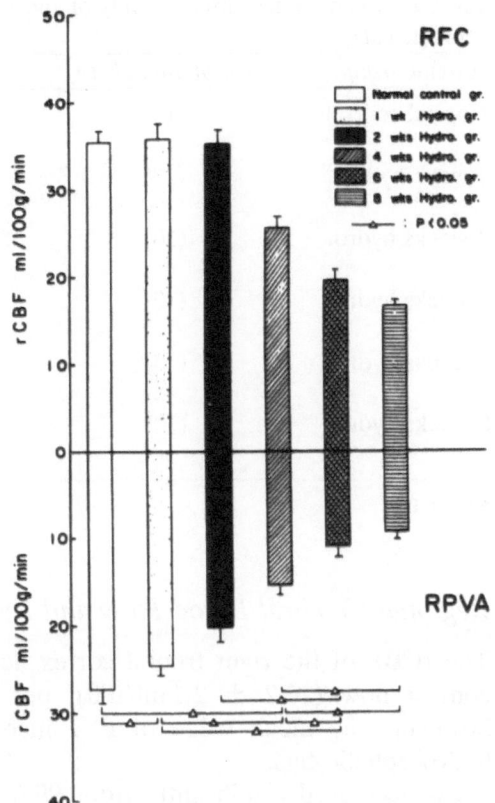

decreased significantly to 26.4% of the control flow (26.2 ± 2.1 ml/100 g per min) in the 4-week-hydrocephalic cats (*P* < 0.05).

The 6-week-hydrocephalic cats demonstrated significant reduction of the rCBF to 45.2% of the control flow (19.5 ± 2.2 ml/100 g per min) in the right frontal cortex and 61.9% of the control flow (10.3 ± 2.4 ml/100 g per min) in the periventricular area (*P* < 0.05).

Pressure-Volume Index (PVI) and Resistance to CSF Absorption (Ro)

The mean value of the PVI was 0.77 ± 0.02 ml and Ro was 90.6 ± 1.3 mmHg per ml per min in normal control cats, as shown in Table 2. The PVI increased significantly from 0.77 ± 0.02 ml to 1.60 ± 0.16 ml at 4 weeks after kaolin injection; this value increased to 2.16 ± 0.34 ml at 6 weeks after kaolin injection (*P* < 0.05).

Ro decreased significantly from 90.6 ± 1.3 mmHg/ml per min to 36.8 ± 4.3 mmHg/ml per min at 4 weeks after kaolin injection and decreased further to 6.2 ± 1.9 mmHg/ml per min at 8 weeks after kaolin injection (*P* < 0.01).

Table 2. Mean values (Mean ± SD) of the PVI and Ro of normal control and hydro-cephalic cats

Animal group	No. of animals (n)	PVI (ml)	Ro (mmHg per ml per min)
Normal control	(5)	0.77 ±0.02	90.6 ±1.3
1 week-hydro.	(10)	0.85 ±0.05	65.6* ±7.2
2 weeks-hydro.	(10)	1.06 ±0.09	59.8* ±5.8
4 weeks-hydro.	(10)	1.60* ±0.16	36.8* ±4.3
6 weeks-hydro.	(10)	2.12* ±0.34	18.5* ±2.7
8 weeks-hydro.	(10)	2.80* ±0.30	6.3* ±1.9

* $P < 0.05$

Regional Cerebral Blood Flow and PVI, Ro

The rCBF of the right frontal cortex decreased significantly to 26.4% of the control flow (26.2 ± 2.1 ml/100 g per min) in 4-week-hydrocephalic cats; however, the mean value of PVI increased to 1.06 ± 0.09 ml in 2-week-hydrocephalic cats.

Ro decreased significantly from 90.6 ± 1.3 mmHg/ml per min to 65.5 ± 7.21 mmHg/ml per min. In the hydrocephalic cats, the reduction of Ro began one week before the reduction of rCBF (FC, PVA); otherwise PVI increased while blood flow reduced in 2-week-hydrocephalic cats. Therefore, a relatively close correlation between rCBF and Ro was found in the hydrocephalic cats.

Somatosensory Evoked Potentials (SEPs) and Ventricular Size

The mean latencies of the wave components in the SEP responses were 6.27 ± 0.12 ms in Po, 8.41 ± 0.25 ms in No, and 12.55 ± 0.36 ms in P1; the mean central conduction time (P1 − Po) was 6.10 ± 0.16 ms in the normal control cats, as shown in Table 3. Changes of amplitude and latency in the SEPs were more prominent 4 weeks after kaolin injection ($P < 0.05$); progressive prolonged latencies of each wave component ($P < 0.05$) and central conduction time resulted 6 and 8 weeks after kaolin injection ($P < 0.05$).

The size of the ventricle (septum pellucidum-caudate nucleus distance) was moderately increased, to 5.19 ± 0.43 mm, in 1-week-hydrocephalic cats and continued to increase up to a maximum size of 9.40 ± 0.7 mm in 4-week-hydrocephalic cats ($P < 0.05$).

However, there was no further enlargement of the ventricle after the 4th week. Changes of the SEPs were related to the ventricular enlargement in 4-week-hydrocephalic cats (Fig. 5).

Table 3. Changes in the amplitude and latency of SEPs in hydrocephalic animals (Mean ± SD)

Component of SEPs	Po		No		P1		CCT[a]
Animal group	Latency (ms)	Amplitude (μV)	Latency (ms)	Amplitude (μV)	Latency (ms)	Amplitude (μV)	(ms)
Normal control	6.27 ±0.12	0.59 ±0.03	8.41 ±0.25	3.31 ±0.26	12.55 ±0.36	7.05 ±0.37	6.10 ±0.16
1 week-hydro.	6.27 ±0.10	0.60 ±0.03	8.37 ±0.19	3.45 ±0.17	12.38 ±0.21	7.04 ±0.42	6.13 ±0.19
2 weeks-hydro.	6.34 ±0.10	0.61 ±0.03	8.41 ±0.17	3.49 ±0.08	12.43 ±0.16	7.09 ±0.41	6.08 ±0.18
4 weeks-hydro.	6.72* ±0.22	0.32* ±0.02	9.14* ±0.15	3.07* ±0.12	13.13* ±0.18	6.29* ±0.18	6.40* ±0.37
6 weeks-hydro.	7.42* ±0.19	0.12* ±0.03	10.34* ±0.07	2.56* ±0.12	15.44* ±0.30	5.67* ±0.26	8.02* ±0.28
8 weeks-hydro.	7.77* ±0.13	0.11* ±0.20	11.43* ±0.07	2.22* ±0.18	16.69* ±0.46	4.90* ±0.05	8.48* ±0.41

* $P < 0.05$

[a] CCT, central conduction time (P1-Po)

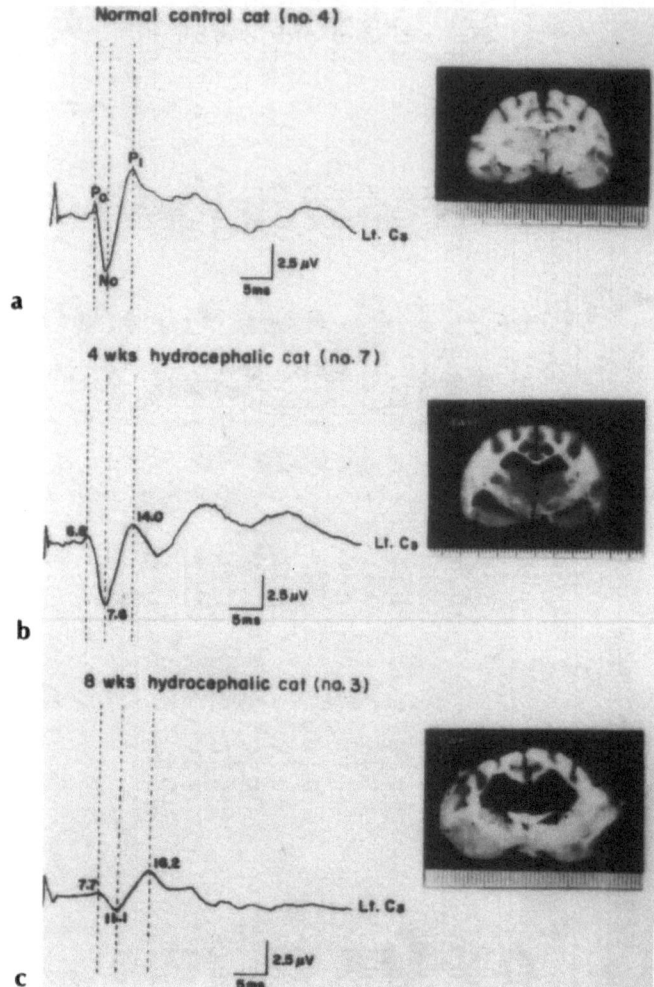

Fig. 5. Changes of SEPs and ventricular enlargements of kaolin-induced hydro-cephalic animals. **a** Wave pattern of SEPs and coronal section of the brain in normal control cat (cat no. 4). **b** Suppressed amplitude and prolonged latency of Po, No, and P_1 components of SEPs 4 weeks after kaolin injection. Note a moderate dilatation of the lateral ventricle 4 weeks after injection (cat no. 7). **c** Marked enlargement of the lateral ventricle corresponded with significant suppressed amplitudes and delayed latencies of Po, No, and P_1 components of SEPs (cat no. 3).

Discussion

The laboratory model of feline kaolin-induced hydrocephalus with alteration of the brain container to augment ventricular size was first used by Hochwald et al. (1972a,b; 1973), to simulate infantile hydrocephalus.

This model was chosen for these laboratory experiments in order to determine whether the demonstrated ventricular enlargement with hydrocephalus could be reproduced in the laboratory setting. Assuming that biomechanical and physiological changes in relation to cerebral circulation in hydrocephalus are substantial, we focused on microcirculatory alterations or changes in both areas of the cortex and deep periventricular area and on the role of biomechanical changes in ventricular enlargement.

Patterns of histological change in hydrocephalus demonstrate that brain-tissue damage occurs in the early stages (Weller and Wisniewski 1969; McLone et al. 1971). Weller and Williams (1975) described major tissue changes in periventricular white matter in hydrocephalus and showed direct evidence of axonal degeneration and myelin breakdown in acute hydrocephalus.

Concurrent with the rapid enlargement of the ventricular system in hydrocephalus, tearing of the ependymal epithelium, particularly at the angle of the lateral ventricle, occurs in association with edematous changes of the white matter; these changes have been well demonstrated by Milhorat et al. (1971).

Furthermore, a significantly reduced cerebral blood flow with raised intracranial pressure has been reported in hydrocephalus (Hochwald et al. 1975), and a similar decrease of regional cerebral blood flow has been disclosed in normal-pressure hydrocephalus (Greitz 1969; Matthew et al. 1975).

Murata et al. (1980) described a marked reduction in rCBF measured in hydrocephalic dogs, in which rather marked decreases in the cortical gray matter flow were found with relatively normal cortical flow, in contrast to findings in the present study.

Changes in ventricular size and cerebral blood flow following kaolin-induced hydrocephalus in dogs have been reported by Sato et al. (1984); they stated that the ventricular system was moderately dilated 7 days after kaolin introduction and that the system continued to increase in size to the 8th week; blood flow was maximally reduced in the first 2 weeks after kaolin injection. They reported that marked decreases in rCBF were revealed in both gray and white matter in hydrocephalic animals, which results were similar to results in our present study. Our study demonstrated that reduction of the rCBF of the deep periventricular area was detected at 2 weeks after kaolin injection, and that the rCBF of the frontal cortex was dramatically decreased at 4 weeks after kaolin injection.

Periventricular lucency (PVL) or periventricular edema was first described by Naidich et al. (1976) and it has been confirmed that PVL is usually encountered in the acute or subacute stages of hypertensive hydrocephalus (Asada et al. 1978; Mori et al. 1980) which result in tearing of the ependymal epithelium, particularly at the angle of the lateral ventricles.

According to our present study, significant abnormal changes in the SEPs were more prominent 4 weeks after kaolin injection and continued progressively to prolong these SEP abnormalities and central conduction time. Therefore, this study suggested that the abnormal SEPs in hydrocephalic animals would result in overstretching of the long paracentral fibers located close to the walls of the lateral ventricles (Yakovlev 1947), in periventricular demyelination

(Weller and Williams 1975), and in poor periventricular blood circulation, and finally, in damage to the parenchyma-presynaptic thalamo-cortical fibers.

One would expect that maneuvers which increase the neural axis volume-buffering capacity would lower CSF pressure. This study demonstrates that the increase in PVI following the introduction of kaolin in hydrocephalic cats should favor the accumulation of volume within the neural axis. The sequential decrease in resistance to CSF absorption following each stage of induced hydrocephalus in the cats facilitated the absorption of CSF and maintained steady-state CSF pressure.

Regarding CSF hydrodynamic studies, Shapiro et al. (1985b), pointed out that if volume was added to the system at a steady state, CSF pressure would change transiently along the pressure-volume curve, but would return to a steady-state pressure, as volume would be absorbed along outflow pathways described by the resistance to CSF absorption parameters; the steady state would be reestablished over time. The present studies demonstrating an increase of the PVI in hydrocephalic cats indicated that enhanced volume-buffering capacity accompanied enlargement of the ventricles.

Although some workers have reported that increased compliance parallels increasing ventricular size (Drapkin and Sahar 1978), other studies have shown that the PVI does not merely reflect ventricular size.

As shown in this report, bolus testing continued to show alteration of the biomechanical properties of the brain with hydrocephalus.

Changes in the white matter of brain tissue, including compression of fiber tracts and loss of myelin, have been described in hydrocephalus (Rubin et al. 1976).

We infer from our present studies that the biomechanical properties of brain parenchyma are altered as these structural changes occur. Guinane (1974) studied the serial changes in CSF absorption resistance and compliance ($\Delta V/\Delta P$) in intact kaolin-induced hydrocephalic cats. He described an acute increase of CSF absorption resistance, which decreased as the ventricle enlarged. His results are similar to those of our present studies. Several investigators have reported enhancement of the absorptive reserve in experimental animals rendered hydrocephalic with kaolin (Löfgren et al. 1973).

Others have found that the central canal of the spinal cord dilates in feline hydrocephalus (Torvik and Murthy 1977) and have suggested that this may be a pathway for accessory absorption (Nakamura et al. 1983).

Takei et al. (1987) reported that, in hydrocephalic animals, the ventricles enlarged rapidly in the first 2–3 weeks and then continued to increase, but at a slower rate. Concomitant with this early increase of ventricular size was a progressive increase in white matter water content both adjacent to and remote from the ventricles. In our present studies, the ventricles enlarged moderately in the 1st week after kaolin injection and then contined to increase to a maximum size in the 4th week after kaolin injection.

From our studies, it is apparent that an absorptive defect is not sufficient to cause progressive ventricular enlargement.

While changes in the biomechanical properties of the brain and microcirculatory alteration in the brain parenchyma facilitate ventricular enlargement, it is unclear whether these factors alone lead to hydrocephalus.

References

Asada M, Tamaki N, Kanazawa Y, Matsumoto S, Matsuo M, Kimura S, Fujii S, Kanada Y (1978) Computer analysis of periventricular lucency on the CT scan. Neuroradiology 16: 207–211

Bering EA Jr, Sato O (1963) Hydrocephalus: changes in formation and absorption of cerebrospinal fluid within the cerebral ventricles. J Neurosurg 20: 1050–1063

Drapkin AJ, Sahar A (1978) Experimental hydrocephalus: cerebrospinal fluid dynamics and ventricular distensibility during early stages. Childs Brain 4: 278–288

Fried A, Shapiro K, Takei F, Kohn I (1987) A laboratory model of shunt-dependent hydrocephalus: development and biomechanical characterization. J Neurosurg 66: 734–740

Greitz T (1969) Effect of brain distension on cerebral circulation. Lancet I: 863–865

Guinane JE (1974) Cerebrospinal fluid resistance and compliance in subacutely hydrocephalic cats. Neurology 24: 138–142

Hochwald GM, Lux WB Jr, Sahar A (1972a) Experimental hydrocephalus: Changes in cerebrospinal fluid dynamics as a function of time. Arch Neurol 26: 120–129

Hochwald GM, Epstein F, Malhan C (1972b) The role of the skull and dura in experimental feline hydrocephalus. Dev Med Child Neurol 14 (Suppl 27): 65–69

Hochwald GM, Epstein F, Malhan C (1973) The relationship of compensated to decompensated hydrocephalus in the cat. J Neurosurg 39: 694–697

Hochwald GM, Boal RD, Marlin AE, Kumar AJ (1975) Changes in regional blood flow and water content of brain and spinal cord in acute and chronic experimental hydrocephalus. Dev Med Child Neurol [Suppl] 17: 42–50

Löfgren J, von Essen C, Zwetnow NN (1973) The pressure-volume curve of the cerebrospinal fluid space in dogs. Acta Neurol Scand 49: 557–574

Marmarou A, Shulman K, MaMorgese J (1975) Compartmental analysis of compliance and outflow resistance of the cerebrospinal fluid system. J Neurosurg 43: 523–535

Matthew NT, Meyer JS, Hartmann A, Ott EO (1975) Abnormal cerebrospinal fluid-blood flow dynamics. Implications in diagnosis, treatment, and prognosis in normal pressure hydrocephalus. Arch Neurol 32: 657–644

McLone DG, Bondareff W, Raimondi AJ (1971) Brain edema in the hydrocephalic hy-3 mouse: Submicroscopic morphology. J Neuropathol Exp Neurol 30: 627–637

Milhorat TM, Clark RG, Hammock MK, McGrath PP (1971) Structual, ultrastructural, and permeability changes in the ependyma and surrounding brain favoring equilibration in progressive hydrocephalus. Arch Neurol 22: 397–407

Mori K, Handa H, Murata T, Nakano Y (1980) Periventricular lucency in computed tomography of hydrocephalus and cerebral atrophy. J Comp Assist Tomogr 4: 204–210

Murata T, Yamagata S, Mori K, Handa H, Nakano Y (1980) Computed tomography in experimental canine hydrocephalus. Part 4: periventricular lucency (PVI) and regional cerebral blood flow in the chronic stage of hydrocephalus. Brain Nerve 32: 219–227

Naidich TP, Epstein F, Lin JP, Kricheff II, Hochwald GM (1976) Evaluation of pediatric hydrocephalus by computed tomography. Radiology 119: 337–345

Nakamura S, Camins MB, Hochwald GM (1983) Pressure absorption responses to the infusion of fluid into the spinal cord central canal of kaolin-hydrocephalic cats. J Neurosurg 58: 198–203

Pasztor E, Symon L, Dorsch NWC (1973) The hydrogen clearance method in assessment of blood flow in cortex, white matter and deep nucleus of baboons. Stroke 4: 556–557

Rubin RC, Hochwald GM, Tiell M (1976) Hydrocephalus: I. Histological and ultrastructural changes in the preshunted cortical mantle. Surg Neurol 5: 109–114

Sato O, Ohya M, Nojiri K, Tsugane R (1984) Microcirculatory changes in experimental hydrocephalus: morphological and physiological studies. In: Shapiro K, Marmarou A, Portnoy HP (eds) Hydrocephalus. Raven, New York, pp 215–230

Shapiro K, Fried A, Marmarou A (1985a) Biomechanical and hydrodynamic characterization of the hydrocephalic infant. J Neurosurg 63: 69–75

Shapiro K, Fried A, Takei F, Kohn I (1985b) Effect of the skull and dura on neural axis pressure-volume relationships and CSF hydrodynamics. J Neurosurg 63: 76–81

Shulman K, Marmarou A (1971) Pressure-volume considerations in infantile hydrocephalus. Dev Med Child Neurol 13 (Suppl 25): 90–95

Takei F, Shapiro K, Kohn I (1987) Influence of the rate of ventricular enlargement on the white matter water content in progressive feline hydrocephalus. J Neurosurg 66: 577–583

Torvik A, Murthy VS (1977) The spinal cord central canal in kaolin-induced hydrocephalus. J Neurosurg 47: 397–402

Weller RO, Williams BN (1975) Cerebral biopsy and assessment of brain damage in hydrocephalus. Arch Dis Child 50: 763–768

Weller RO, Wisniewski H (1969) Histological and ultrastructural changes with experimental hydrocephalus in adult rabbits. Brain 92: 819–828

Yakovlev PI (1947) Paraplegias of hydrocephalics. Am J Ment Defic 51: 561–576

12 — High Energy Phosphate Metabolism in Congenital Hydrocephalic Rats — an in Vivo ^{31}P Magnetic Resonance Spectroscopy Study

Jun Minamikawa, Haruhiko Kikuchi, Masatsune Ishikawa, Kunio Yamamura, and Masaru Kanashiro[2]

Summary. We used phosphorus-31 magnetic resonance spectroscopy (^{31}P-MRS) to obtain in vivo measurements of cerebral energy matabolism and intracellular pH in congenital hydrocephalic rats (HTX). The hydrocephalic group consisted of 20 rats and the non-hydrocephalic group consisted of 15 rats. The rats in the hydrocephalic group were subdivided into three smaller groups according to the degree of hydrocephalus (mild, moderate, and severe). The PCr/Pi ratio was used as the chosen indicator of cellular bioenergetic status.

In the non-hydrocephalic group, the PCr/Pi ratio was 2.99 ± 0.21 (mean $\pm$ SD), and the cerebral intracellular pH was 7.18 ± 0.04 (mean $\pm$ SD). The PCr/Pi ratios in the mild, moderate, and severe hydrocephalic groups were 1.69 ± 0.01, 1.39 ± 0.02, and 0.95 ± 0.09, respectively; these were significantly decreased ($P < 0.01$). The intracellular pHs in the hydrocephalic groups showed no significant differences. In 17 hydrocephalic rats, the correlation between the PCr/Pi ratios and survival days was evaluated to determine the prognosis of these rats from the viewpoint of cerebral energy metabolism. The correlation coefficient between the PCr/Pi ratio and survival time was 0.703. The present study demonstrated the disturbance of cerebral energy metabolism in congenital hydrocephalic rats. It was of particular interest to us that the PCr/Pi ratio seemed to yield data indicative of the prognosis of congenital hydrocephalus.

Keywords: Congenital hydrocephalus — Cerebral energy metabolism — Cerebral intracellular pH — ^{31}P-MRS

Introduction

It is well known that the major pathogenic mechanism of hydrocephalus is disturbance in the cerebrospinal fluid (CSF) circulation. For this reason, many

---

[1] Department of Neurosurgery, Kyoto University, Kyoto, 606 Japan
[2] Nuclear Magnetic Resonance Laboratory, National Cardiovascular Center, Osaka, 565 Japan

studies on hydrocephalus, both experimentally and clinically, have been carried out from the viewpoint of CSF circulation (Schurr et al. 1953). However, so far, few studies have been done in vivo on cerebral energy metabolism in hydrocephalus.

Recent advances in magnetic resonance spectroscopy (MRS) allow non-invasive study of cerebral energy metabolism in vivo. In vivo phosphorus-31 (^{31}P) MRS is a potentially useful tool for noninvasive examination of the physiological and biochemical nature of organs. With this method, it is possible to evaluate not only changes of high-energy phosphate, but also changes of intracellular pH. Therefore this method has been used to study the brain under a variety of experimental conditions such as rest (Chance et al. 1978, 1980), ischemia (Delpy et al. 1982; Thulborn et al. 1982; Andrews et al. 1987), hypoxia (Litt et al. 1986), hypoglycemia (Cox et al. 1983; Behar et al. 1985), cyanide intoxication (Decorps et al. 1984), anesthesia (Litt et al. 1985), and status epilepticus (Petroff et al. 1984). In the present study, ^{31}P MRS was used to investigate cerebral energy metabolic changes in congenital hydrocephalic rats.

Materials and Methods

In this experimental study, congenital hydrocephalic rats of the HTX strain were used; these HTX rats were bred by Kohn et al. in 1981 (Kohn et al. 1981). The average incidence of development of congenital hydrocephalus in newborn HTX rats is more than 40% and the average survival time is about 4 weeks. Within a few days after birth, the hydrocephalic rats show communicating hydrocephalus; this pathologic form changes gradually to the obstructive form (Jones et al. 1987).

Thirty-five HTX rats aged from 20 days to 31 days were anesthetized by intraperitoneal injection of chloral hydrate (3.6 mg/g body weight). The animals were then placed in an in vivo nuclear magnetic resonance (NMR) spectrometer in the supine position, so as to center the cranial cavity on the volume of the homogenous magnetic field of the instrument. Magnetic field homogeneity was maximized by shimming the fields by observation of the proton signal from tissue water. During the experiments, spontaneous respiration continued and body temperature was maintained within 36.0 ± 1.0°C by using specially designed pads.

The animals were divided into two groups depending on the shape of the cranial vault: a hydrocephalic group ($n = 20$) and a non-hydrocephalic group ($n = 15$). The crania of the rats in the hydrocephalic group bulged outwardly; the crania in the non-hydrocephalic group were normal in shape. The rats in the hydrocephalic group were subdivided into three smaller groups according to the degree of cranial vault bulging on inspection: mild ($n = 6$); moderate ($n = 6$); and severe ($n = 8$). The degree of cranial vault bulging corresponded well to the degree of hydrocephalus.

Spectral Measurement of ^{31}P

In vivo NMR spectra were obtained with a JEOL JNM-SMR270 spectrometer (Nihon Denshi Co., Tokyo, Japan; 6.34 Tesla) by means of a 9-mm diameter surface coil in a 70-mm diameter probe with a Fourier transform mode, operating at the phosphorus resonant frequency (109.0MHz). The spectra were collected at the free-induction decays, using quadrature phase detection, and were digitized and processed by computer. The ^{31}P spectra were obtained as 400 times-averaged free-induction decays, using a repetition time of 2.0s. The region of interest giving rise to the ^{31}P spectra was found to be in the forebrain, because the bulk of cerebral cortex and subcortex brain tissue is not so small in this area in hydrocephalic rats. The spectral signals obtained by using this type of surface coil are gained from the brain tissue within a few millimeters depth of the scalp surface. So, even in the hydrocephalic rats whose bulk of cerebral cortex and subcortex is small, the signals of ^{31}P-MRS are thought to be derived from cerebral cortex and subcortex brain tissue. Approximately 13 minutes were required for each ^{31}P spectral measurement.

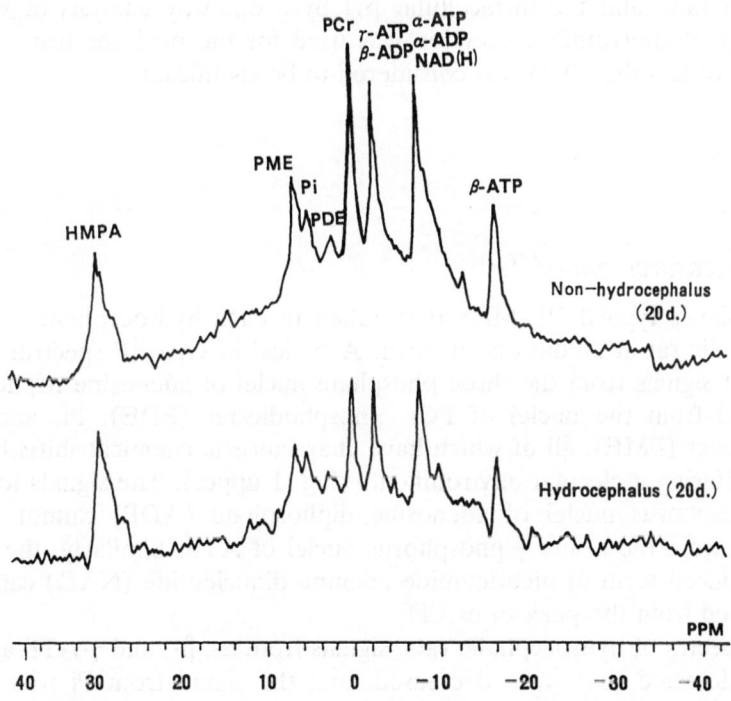

Fig. 1. ^{31}P NMR spectra obtained in a rat 20 days after birth. Non-hydrocephalic rat (*upper*), hydrocephalic rat (*lower*). *ATP*, adenosine triphosphate; *PCr*, phosphocreatin; *Pi*, inorganic phosphate; *ADP*, adenosine diphosphate; *NAD*, nicotinamide adenine dinucleotide; *HMPA*, hexamethyl phosphoramide (external reference) *PME*, phosphomonoester; *PDE*, phosphodiester. Three ATP peaks and the PCr peak are decreased and the Pi peak is slightly increased

Analysis of ^{31}P Spectra

The broad component of the spectra, assigned to relatively immobile phosphate residues in cranial bone (Ackerman et al. 1984; Gonzalez-Mendez et al. 1984) was removed mathematically by using a convolution difference technique (Campbell et al. 1973). Since phosphocreatine (PCr) and inorganic phosphate (Pi) have a similar low relaxation time, their saturation effects are similar and the error in their ratio is only 10% (Chance et al. 1980). Regarding the objective detection of the cellular bioenergetic status, evaluating the signal intensity ratio between PCr and Pi makes shimming differences in individual rats less influential in intensity than evaluating the absolute signal intensity of each peak. Therefore, in previous studies, the PCr/Pi ratio, instead of the absolute signal intensity of β-ATP, has been used as the chosen indicator of cellular bioenergetic status (Chance et al. 1985; Gyulai et al. 1985; Vink et al. 1987). In this study, we too used the PCr/Pi ratio as the chosen indicator of cellular bioenergetic status.

The intracellular pH was calculated from the chemical shift of the Pi resonance peak relative to the PCr resonance peak (Bailey et al. 1981; James 1984). Intergroup statistical analysis was performed by evaluating changes in the PCr/Pi ratio and the intracellular pH by a one-way analysis of variance (ANOVA). Bonferroini's correction was used for the post-hoc test. A probability (P) of less than 0.05 was considered to be significant.

Results

Spectral Measurement of ^{31}P

Figure 1 shows typical ^{31}P MRS data taken in each hydrocephalic and non-hydrocephalic rat at 20 days after birth. A typical in vivo ^{31}P spectrum shows component signals from the three phosphate nuclei of adenosine triphosphate (ATP) and from the nuclei of PCr, phosphodiester (PDE), Pi, and phosphomonoester (PME), all of which have characteristic chemical shifts because of their differing molecular environments (Fig. 1 upper). The signals for the α and γ phosphorus nuclei of adenosine diphosphate (ADP) cannot be distinguished from the α and γ phosphorus nuclei of ATP. Similarly, the signals for the reduced form of nicotinamide adenine dinucleotide (NAD) cannot be distinguished from the peak of α-ATP.

In the spectra of hydrocephalic rats, signals from α-, β-, and γ-ATP and PCr could be detected, but were decreased, and the signal from Pi was slightly increased, in comparison with the signals of non-hydrocephalic rats (Fig. 1 lower).

In the non-hydrocephalic group, the PCr/Pi ratio was 2.99 ± 0.21 (mean ± SD), and the cerebral intracellular pH was 7.18 ± 0.04 (mean ± SD). The PCr/Pi ratios in the mild, moderate, and severe hydrocephalic groups were

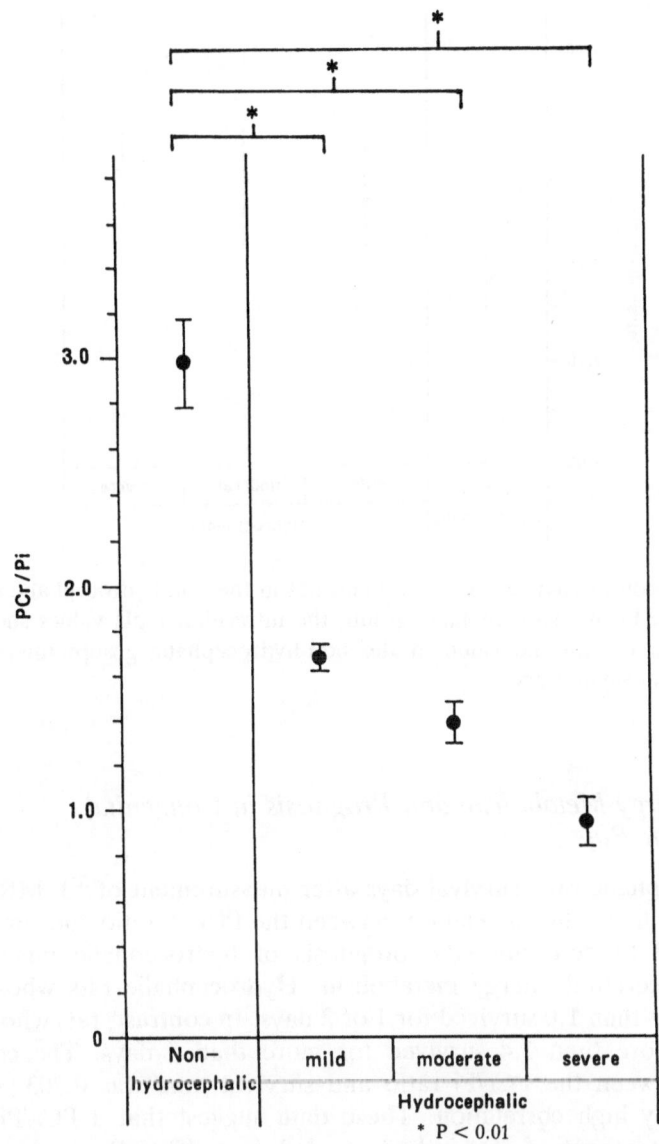

Fig. 2. Comparison of changes in the PCr/Pi ratio in the non-hydrocephalic and hydrocephalic groups. In the hydrocephalic group, the values for the PCr/Pi ratio show a significant decrease compared with the value in the non-hydrocephalic group

1.69 ± 0.01, 1.39 ± 0.02, and 0.95 ± 0.09, respectively. These PCr/Pi ratios in the hydrocephalic groups were significantly decreased; $P < 0.01$ (Fig. 2). On the other hand, the cerebral intracellular pHs were 7.26 ± 0.06, 7.28 ± 0.06, and 7.29 ± 0.06 in the mild, moderate, and severe hydrocephalic groups, respectively. These intracellular pHs showed no significant differences (Fig. 3).

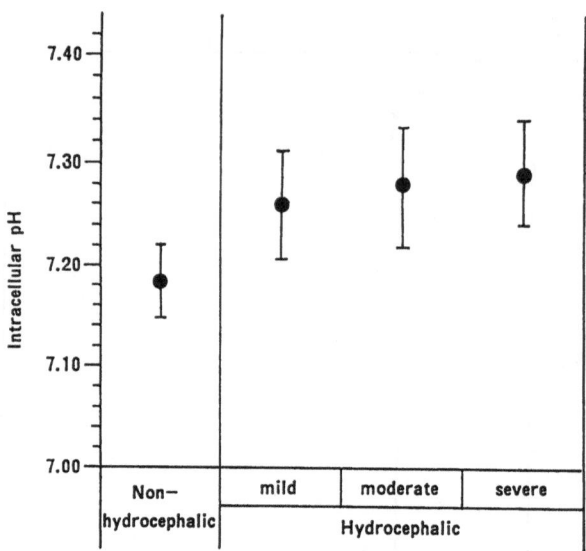

Fig. 3. Comparison of changes of intracellular pH in the non-hydrocephalic and hydro-cephalic groups. In the hydrocephalic group, the intracellular pH values show a slight increase compared with the value in the non-hydrocephalic group; this increase is without statistical significance

Cerebral Energy Metabolism and Prognosis in Congenital Hydrocephalic Rats

In 17 hydrocephalic rats, survival days after measurement of ^{31}P MRS spectra could be identified. The correlation between the PCr/Pi ratio and survival days was evaluated to determine the prognosis of hydrocephalic rats from the viewpoint of cerebral energy metabolism. Hydrocephalic rats whose PCr/Pi ratios were less than 1.0 survived for 1 or 2 days. In contrast, rats whose PCr/Pi ratios were more than 1.4 survived for more than 5 days. The correlation coefficient between the PCr/Pi ratio and survival time was 0.703, which in-dicated a fairly high correlation. These data suggest that a PCr/Pi index is valuable as a prognostic factor in hydrocephalic rats (Fig. 4).

Discussion

Regarding the evaluation of cerebral energy metabolism in vivo, Chance et al. reported the first ^{31}P MR spectroscopic analyses of a whole mouse head in 1978 (Chance et al. 1978). In 1980, Ackerman et al. showed that radio-frequency surface coils allowed selective acquisition of spectra from the brain in the intact rat (Ackerman et al. 1980). Since then, it has been demonstrated that ^{31}P spectroscopy permits rapid and repeated noninvasive in vivo analyses of ATP, PCr, Pi, and intracellular pH in the brain, mainly under experimental condi-tions such as cerebral ischemia and hypoxia (Delpy et al. 1982; Thulborn et al.

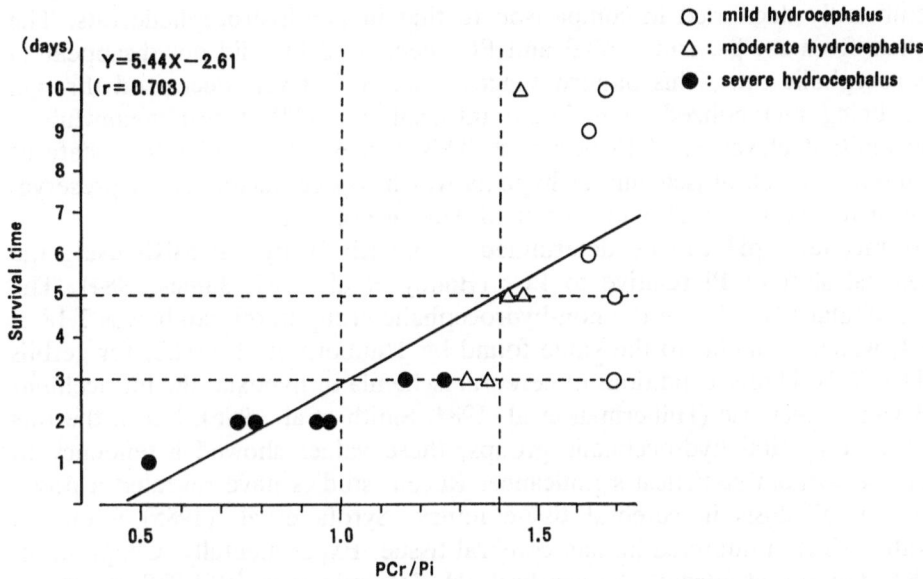

Fig. 4. Correlation between the PCr/Pi ratio and survival time. In the severe hydrocephalic group, the survival time is less than 3 days after examination of cerebral energy metabolism. When the value of the PCr/Pi ratio was less than 1.0, the survival time was 1 or 2 days. The survival time was more than 5 days when the value of the PCr/Pi ratio was more than 1.4. The correlation coefficient (r) was 0.703

1982; Hilberman et al. 1984; Litt et al. 1986; Andrews et al. 1987). However, few ^{31}P-MR spectroscopy studies of hydrocephalus have been carried out. In this present study, we investigated cerebral energy metabolic changes in congenital hydrocephalic rats.

In a general way, as cerebral energy metabolism deteriorates, PCr is metabolized to maintain intracellular ATP stores, Pi increases, and the PCr/Pi ratio decreases as a result (Nilsson et al. 1975). In congenital hydrocephalic rats, these cerebral energy metabolic changes occurr in a way which depends on the degree of hydrocephalus. So in this study, we chose the PCr/Pi ratio as the indicator of cerebral energy metabolic state. The PCr/Pi ratio in the non-hydrocephalic group was 2.99 ± 0.21, which is similar to the values for brain PCr/Pi ratios in rats published previously (Naritomi et al. 1988). In complete generalized ischemia, energy disturbance is rapid and extensive, and PCr and ATP may disappear within several minutes (Ljunggeren et al. 1974). On the other hand, energy disturbance in incomplete generalized ischemia or hypoxia seems to be gradual, showing a stepwise deterioration. In mild ischemia or hypoxia, accumulation of acid metabolites in the tissue at first occurrs without changes in PCr, Pi and ATP and PCr begins to decrease, with a concomitant elevation in Pi as ischemia or hypoxia becomes deeper. Finally, in more extensive ischemia or hypoxia, ATP begins to decrease (Siesjo et al. 1971; Duffy et al. 1972). In congenital hydrocephalic rats, the PCr/Pi ratio was significantly decreased in comparison to that in non-hydrocephalic rats. The signals from α-, β-, and γ-ATP and PCr decreased but did not disappear in hydrocephalic rats. This pattern suggests that PCr levels decreased through PCr being metabolized to maintain intracellular ATP stores; meanwhile a concomitant elevation of Pi occurred. This process was similar to a state of incomplete cerebral ischemia or hypoxia which was characterized by preservation or recovery of ATP and continued decrease of PCr.

Intracellular pH can be determined noninvasively by ^{31}P MRS using the chemical shift of Pi relative to PCr (Bailey et al. 1981; James 1984). The intracellular pH value in the non-hydrocephalic group in this study was 7.18 ± 0.04, which is similar to the value found by Thulborn et al. (1982) for gerbils (pH = 7.2). Under conditions of cerebral ischemia or hypoxia, the intracellular pH values decrease (Hilberman et al. 1984; Smith et al. 1986), but in the rats of the congenital hydrocephalic groups, these values showed a tendency to increase without statistical significance. Recent studies have revealed a possibility of alkalosis in cerebral tissue injury. Syrota et al. (1985) found an alkaline shift in infarcted human cerebral tissue. Experimentally, Chopp et al. (1990) found that intracellular cerebral pH, determined by ^{31}P-MRS, increased significantly 1 week after cerebral ischemia. They suggested that intracellular cerebral alkalosis in the chronic stage of cerebral ischemia might signal severe and irreversible cell damage. With reference to these reports, the increase in intracellular pH in the congenital hydrocephalic rats may indicate cerebral cell damage associated with the development of hydrocephalus.

The PCr/Pi ratio may reflect changes of cerebral blood flow (CBF) or tissue oxygenation. Thulborn et al. (1982) reported that changes in MRS phosphate do not occurr until CBF is less than 20 ml per 100 g per min. Relative to this report, the CBF in the congenital hydrocephalic rats seemed to be rather decreased.

In cerebral ischemia, analysis of the PCr/Pi ratio failed to provide additional prognostic data concerning the reversibility or irreversibility of the metabolic insult (Andrews et al. 1987). In this study, the PCr/Pi ratio seemed to yield data indicative of the prognosis of the congenital hydrocephalic rats. This may be due to differences of disease types or to the differences between ischemia and hydrocephalus in the rapidity of disturbance in cerebral energy metabolism.

The present study has demonstrated the disturbance of cerebral energy metabolism in congenital hydrocephalic rats. It was of particular interest to us that the PCr/Pi ratio seemed to yield data indicative of the prognosis of congenital hydrocephalus.

References

Ackerman JJH, Grove TH, Wong GG, et al. (1980) Mapping of metabolites in whole animals by ^{31}P NMR using surface coils. Nature 283: 167–170

Ackerman JJH, Evelhoch JL, Berkowitz BA, et al. (1984) Selective suppression of the cranial bone resonance from ^{31}P NMR experiments with rat brain in vivo. J Magn Reson 56: 318–321

Andrews BT, Weinstein PR, Keniry M, et al. (1987) Sequential in vivo measurement of cerebral intracellular metabolites with phosphorus-31 magnetic resonance spectroscopy during global cerebral ischemia and reperfusion in rats. Neurosurgery 21: 699–708

Bailey IA, Williams SR, Radda GK, et al. (1981) Activity of phosphorylase in global ischemia in the rat brain. Biochem J 196: 171–178

Behar KL, den Hollander JA, Petroff OAC, et al. (1985) Effect of hypoglycemic encephalopathy upon amino acids, high-energy phosphates, and pH in the rat brain in vivo: deterction by sequential 1-H and 31-P NMR spectroscopy. J Neurochem 44: 1045–1055

Campbell ID, Dobson CM, Williams RJP, et al. (1973) Resolution enhancement of proton NMR spectra using the difference between a broadened and a normal spectrum. J Magn Reson 11: 172–181

Chance B, Nakase Y, Bond M, et al. (1978) Detection of ^{31}P nuclear magnetic resonance signals in brain by in vivo and freeze trapped assays. Proc Natl Acad Sci USA 75: 4925–4929

Chance B, Eleff S, Leigh JS (1980) Noninvasive, nondestructive approach to cell bioenergetics. Proc Natl Acad Sci USA 77: 7430–7434

Chance B, Leigh JS, Clark BJ, et al. (1985) Control of oxidative metabolism and oxygen delivery in human skeletal muscle: a steady-state analysis of the work/energy cost transfer function. Proc Natl Acad Sci USA 82: 8334–8338

Chopp M, Linde AMQV, Chen H, et al. (1990) Chronic cerebral intracellular alkalosis following forebrain ischemic insult in rats. Stroke 21: 463–466

Cox DWG, Morris PG, Feeney J, et al. (1983) ^{31}P-NMR studies on cerebral energy metabolism under conditions of hypoglycemia and hypoxia in vitro. Biochem J 212: 365–370

Decorps M, Lebas JF, Leviel JL, et al. (1984) Analysis of brain metabolism changes induced by acute potassium cyanide intoxication by ^{31}P-NMR in vivo using chronically implanted coils. FEBS Lett 168: 1–6

Delpy DT, Gordon RE, Hope PL, et al. (1982) Noninvasive investigation of cerebral ischemia by phosphorus nuclear magnetic resonance. Pediatrics 70: 310–313

Duffy TE, Nelson SR, Lowry OH (1972) Cerebral carbohydrate metabolism during acute hypoxia and recovery. J Neurochem 19: 959–977

Gonzalez-Mendez R, Litt L, Koretsky AP, et al. (1984) Comparison of ^{31}P-NMR spectra of in vivo rat brain using convolution difference and saturation with a surface coil. Source of the broad component in the brain spectrum. J Magn Reson 57: 526–533

Gyulai L, Roth Z, Leigh JS, et al. (1985) Bioenergetic studies of mitochondrial oxidative phosphorylation using ^{31}Phosphorus NMR. J Biol Chem 260: 3947–3954

Hilberman M, Subramanian VH, Haselgrove JC, et al. (1984) In vivo time-resolved brain phosphorus nuclear magnetic resonance. J Cereb Blood Flow Metab 4: 334–342

James TL (1984) In vivo nuclear magnetic resonance spectroscopy. In: Moss AA, Ring EJ, Higgins CB (eds) NMR, CT and interventional radiology. Department of Radiology, University of California, San Francisco, pp 235–244

Jones HC, Bucknall RM (1987) Changes in cerebrospinal fluid pressure and outflow from the lateral ventricles during development of congenital hydrocephalus in the H-Tx rat. Exp Neurol 98: 573–583

Kohn DF, Chinookoswong N, Chou SM (1981) A new model of congenital hydrocephalus in the rat. Acta Neuropathol (Berl) 54: 211–218

Litt L, Gonzalez-Mendez R, Severinghaus JW, et al. (1985) Cerebral intracellular changes during subercarbia: an in vivo ^{31}P nuclear magnetic resonance study in rats. J Cereb Blood Flow Metab 5: 537–544

Litt L, Gonzalez-Mendez R, Weinstein PR, et al. (1986) An in vivo ^{31}P NMR study of cerebral hypoxia in rats. Magn Reson Med 3: 619–625

Ljunggren B, Schutz H, Siesjo BK (1974) Changes in energy state and acid-base parameters of the rat brain during complete compression ischemia. Brain Res 73: 277–289

Naritomi H, Sasaki M, Kaneshiro M, et al. (1988) Flow thresholds for cerebral energy disturbance and Na$^+$ pump failure as studied by in vivo ^{31}P and ^{23}Na nuclear magnetic resonance spectroscopy. J Cereb Blood Flow Metab 8: 16–23

Nilsson B, Norberg K, Siesjo BK (1975) Biochemical events in general ischemia. Br J Anaesth 47: 751–760

Petroff OAC, Prichard LW, Behar KL, et al. (1984) In vivo phosphorus nuclear magnetic resonance spectroscopy in status epilepticus. Ann Neurol 16: 169–177

Schurr PH, McLaurin RL, Ingraham FD (1953) Experimental studies on the circulation of the cerebrospinal fluid and methods of producing communicating hydrocephalus in the dog. J Neurosurg 10: 515–525

Siesjo BK, Nilsson L (1971) The influence of arterial hypoxemia upon labial phosphate and upon extracellular and intracellular lactate and pyruvate concentrations in the rat brain. Scand J Clin Lab Invest 27: 83–96

Smith ML, von Hanwehr R, Siesjo BK (1986) Changes in extra- and intracellular pH in the brain during and following ischemia in hyperglycemic and in moderately hypoglycemic rats. J Cereb Blood Flow Metab 6: 574–583

Syrota A, Samson Y, Boullais C, et al. (1985) Tomographic mapping of brain intracellular pH and extracellular water space in stroke patients. J Cereb Blood Flow Metab 5: 358–368

Thulborn KR, de Boulay GH, Duchen LW, et al. (1982) A ^{31}P nuclear magnetic resonance in vivo study of cerebral ischemia in gerbil. J Cereb Blood Flow Metab 2: 299–306

Vink R, McIntosh TK, Weeiner MW, et al. (1987) Effects of traumatic brain injury on cerebral high-energy phosphates and pH: A ^{31}P magnetic resonance spectroscopy study. J Cereb Blood Flow Metab 7: 563–571

13 — Cerebral Hemodynamics in Hydrocephalus During Infancy: Experimental and Clinical Studies

Hiromi Sato, Noriko Sato[1], Norihiko Tamaki, and Satoshi Matsumoto[2]

Summary. We carried out a series of experimental and clinical studies in an attempt to clarify the cerebral hemodynamics of hydrocephalus during infancy. Experimental hydrocephalus was induced in SD-JCL rats by the transplacental administration of N-methyl N-nitrosourea (MNU). Postnatal change of cerebral blood flow (CBF) was assessed by the hydrogen clearance method. Angioarchitecture was studied by India ink injection and the resin cast method. Clinically, in 30 infants, the threshold of the cerebral perfusion pressure (CPP) related to the intracranial pressure situation was assessed by computerized analysis. In 34 infants with hydrocephalus, the distribution pattern of CBF was assessed with N-isopropyl-p-[123-I]iodoamphetamine single photon emission computed tomography (CT) before and after shunting. In MNU-induced hydrocephalic rats, during the first postnatal week, CBF was progressively reduced to 27.5% of the control value then later up to 65% of the control values were regained, Angioarchitecture showed the relative increase of precapillary anastomotic channels with a reduction of capillaries. Clinically, the age-related threshold level of CPP which tightened the intracranial cavity was shown. Although in neonatal hydrocephalus, frontally dominant reduction of CBF was more evident that in the controls, after 4 months of age this pattern was detected only in those with rapidly progressive hydrocephalus. These results indicate the critical role of the microcirculaltion in the impaired cerebral hemodynamics of hydrocephalus during infancy.

Keywords. Hydrocephalus — Hemodynamics — CBF — CPP — ICP

Introduction

Although increased intracranial pressure (IICP) causes brain damage through impaired microcirculation, few studies have reported on the cerebrohemodynamics of hydrocephalus during infancy. A series of experi-

[1] Department of Neurosurgery, Shizuoka Children's Hospital, Shizuoka, 420 Japan
[2] Department of Neurosurgery, Kobe University School of Medicine, Kobe, 650 Japan

mental and clinical studies were performed in an attempt to clarify these cerebrohemodynamics.

Materials and Methods

Experimental Production of Congenital Hydrocephalus

Sprague-Dawley (SD-JCL, CLEA Japan Inc., Takatsuki) rats were used. After 2 weeks of acclimation, virgin females aged 10–12 weeks and in proestrus were caged overnight with males. The day when copulation was confirmed by plugs was designated as day 0 of gestation. The rats were maintained under controlled temperature and received tap water ad libitum. Pregnant females were given a single does of 10 mg/kg of MNU intraperitoneally on day 9 of gestation. Naturally delivered pups were sacrificed at the ages of 7, 14, and 21 days. Fifteen hydrocephalic rats in each age group, as well as age-matched controls, were studied.

Morphological Studies

Skull roentogenograms were obtained using a Softex. For light microscopic studies, complete transverse sections from the level of the interventricular foramen to the level of the fastigum of the fourth ventricle were taken and stained with hematoxylin and eosin (H-E) and Klüver-Barrera (K-B).

Observation of Microangioarchitecture

Hydrocephalic rats and their age-matched controls at 1, 2, and 3 weeks of postnatal age were used. For preparing India-ink injection sections, the anesthetized brains were perfused via the heart synchronously with the heart beat, first with cacodylate buffer, then with heparinized cacodylate buffer, and finally with india-ink suspended with Karnovsky's fixative. Freeze-sectioned specimens were cleared with xylene, embedded in gelatin, and observed under light microscope. Corrosion casts of the microvessels were made using polyester resin (Mercox CL2B and its hardening agent; Dai-Nippon Ink Inc., Tokyo) after the perfusion-fixation process described above. After resolving the brain tissue by immersion in NaOH solution for 5 days, the resin cast was washed by ultrasonic washer, then dried at the critical point with CO_2. Microvasculatures at the parietal lobe were observed under SEM (Hitachi-Akashi Mini-SEM, Akashi Manufacturing Inc., Osaka) after coating with gold (Eiko ion-coater, Eiko Inc., Tokyo).

Measurement of Regional Cerebral Blood Flow

Regional cerebral blood flow at the parietal cortex was measured in experimental congenital hydrocephalic rats induced by MNU and in age-matched controls at 1, 2, and 3 weeks of postnatal age. In each age group, 10 hydro-cephalic and 10 control rats were measured by the hydrogen clearance method, using a UH-meter: PHG-201, a recorder: D2R1M, and a data processor: DDU-100 (Unique Medical Inc., Tokyo). Rats were tracheostomied under sodium pentobarbital anesthesia administered by intraperitoneal injection (40 mg/kg·bw), and ventilated by artificial respirator. At measurement, a small amount of hydrogen was mixed through the respiration side tube. Through a burr hole made by dental drill over the anteromedial parietal lobe, a needle-type hydrogen electrode (UHE 100: 0.2 mm in diameter, 2 mm in length, Unique Medical Inc. Tokyo) was introduced and fixed to the skull. A saucer-type indifferent electrode was placed intraperitoneally. After measurement, the appropriate location of the inserted needle was confirmed histologically.

Clinical Subjects and Methods

Thirty hydrocephalic infants underwent ICP analysis. Abnormal cerebrospinal fluid (CSF) dynamics were confirmed by metrizamide CT cisternography. Forty three percent of the infants had congenital hydrocephalus. The analysis was done with a newly invented computerized monitoring system using a micro-computer with a conventional polygraph. Four variables were used: intracranial pressure (ICP), radial arterial pressure (systemic arterial blood pressure: SABP), electrocardiogram (pulse rate: PR), and respiratory waves. Values for these variables were converted to analogue/digital form for data processing on a microcomputer. Real time and online collection, printing and display of raw data, trend graphs of the variables, and calculated data were all processed at the bedside. Simultaneously, analogue data were recorded on a strip chart as waves. Data were collected for 8 h without sedation. ICPs were recorded with a Statham P-50 pressure transducer (Gould Statham Instruments Inc., Puerto Rico) connected to a ventricular catheter introduced into the right anterior horn. The reference point was set at the mid-cranium with the patient in a supine position. As an index of cerebrovascular compromise of ICP circum-stances which reflect intracranial compliance, the transmission ratio of SABP to ICP as defined by Ikeyama was used: {η HB: [pulse pressure (PP) of ICP/PP of SABP} (Ikeyama 1976: Rougemond 1976). Apart from the temporal profile of these variables, correlations between each parameter were calculated. Analogue waves and their patterns recorded on chart strips were correlated with the sequential digital data. Evaluation of psychomotor development was done 6–36 months after shunting.

Qualitative Analysis of Cerebral Blood Flow

In 34 infants with hydrocephalus of various etiologies, the distribution pattern of CBF was assessed with [123-I]iodoamphetamine single photon emission CT ([123]IMP—SPECT) (Kuhl et al. 1981; Lassen et al. 1983). A control study was performed in 22 infants whose complaints consisted of skull deformity and minor head trauma. In each examination, early and delayed patterns of CBF distribution were compared. A total of 98 examinations were analyzed.

The patients were premedicated with $4 mg/kg \cdot bw$ potassium iodide solution for 3 days prior to the study. For imaging, 2–3 mCi of [123]IMP (Nihon Mediphysics, Takarazuka) was injected intravenously. Scanning was started at 30 min and 5 h after injection. The detector employed was a rotating gamma camera, with a large field of view, equipped with a slant-hole collimeter of low energy ($159\% \pm 15\%$ keV) supported by a gantry (ZLC-7500: Siemens, Erlagen). Data acquisition required 64 projections using a 64x64 matrix format during 360° rotation. Data were analyzed by Scintipack 700 (Shimazu, Kyoto) and were processed into axial, coronal, and sagittal sections 6 mm in thickness. The distribution patterns were correlated with the findings of X-ray CT.

Results

Establishment of an Appropriate Induction Method and its Evaluation as a Model of Congenital Hydrocephalus

Experimentally, congenital hydrocephalus was induced in SD-JCL rats by the transplacental administration of N-methyl N-nitrosourea (MNU). Teratological studies demonstrated that a dose 14 mg/kg of MNU administered by intraperitoneal injection on day 9 of gestation induced progressive hydrocephalus in high incidence, that is, 60% of live siblings, thus providing the chance for postnatal study up to 3 weeks of age (Fig. 1).

Observation of Microangioarchitecture in Experimental Hydrocephalus using India-Ink Injection and Resin Cast Methods

Controls showed the regular angioarchitecture of long and perpendicular transcortical branches which mainly supply the white matter and short cortical branches which form the capillary network, as described by Gillian (1971). Hydrocephalus, both in the progressive and in the terminal stage, showed tortuous shortening of the transcerebral branches with a sparse and irregular capillary network. Sections stained with H-E showed engorged subependymal venules. Scanning electron microscopical observations of the resin cast specimens of the microvasculatures showed the relative increase of precapillary and interarteriolar anastomotic channels (Nakai et al. 1981), with the reduction of capillaries (Fig. 2).

Chronological Alteration of the CBF Value in Experimental Congenital Hydrocephalus

Chronological change of the cerebral blood flow value was assessed by the hydrogen clearance method in MNU-induced hydrocephalic rats and their age-

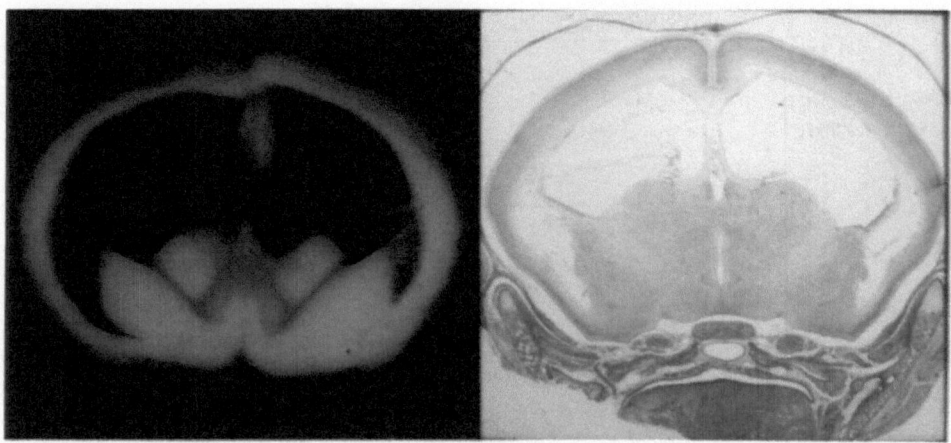

Fig. 1. Macroscopical view of experimental congenital hydrocephalus, induced by Methylnitrosourea (MNU), in rat at 7 days of postnatal age, showing the symmetrical dilatation of ventricles with spongy alteration of the periventricular region

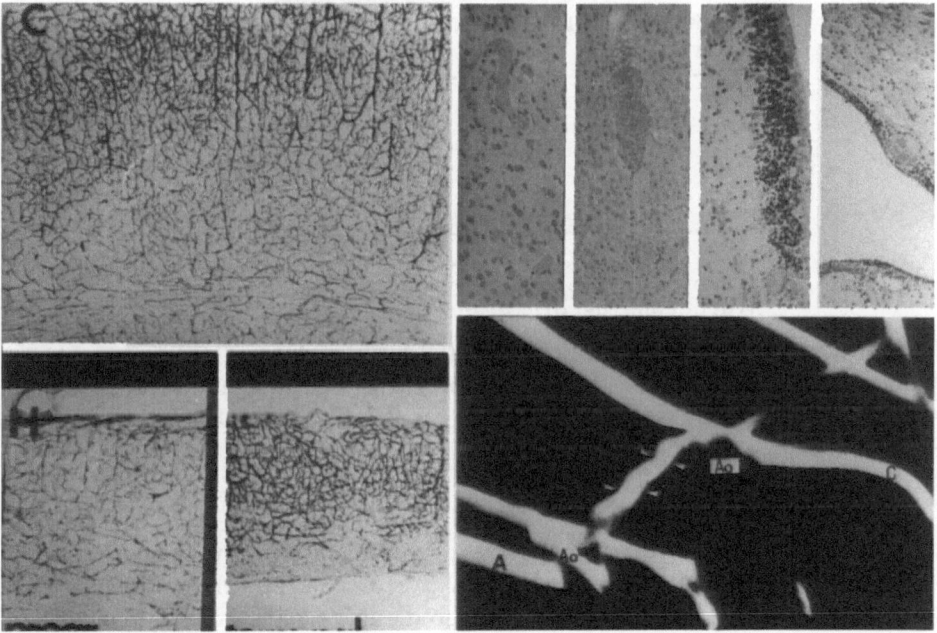

Fig. 2. Representative angioarchitecture studied by India-ink perfusion method (*left*) and resin-cast method (*lower right*). C, control; H, hydrocephalus, progr, progressive stage; terminal, terminal stage. Tortuous shortening of cortical branches with sparse and irregular capillary networks are shown in hydrocephalus. Sections stained with H and E show engorged venules (*upper right*). Relative increase of precapillary shunt through the interarteriolar channels is shown in the resin cast preparations

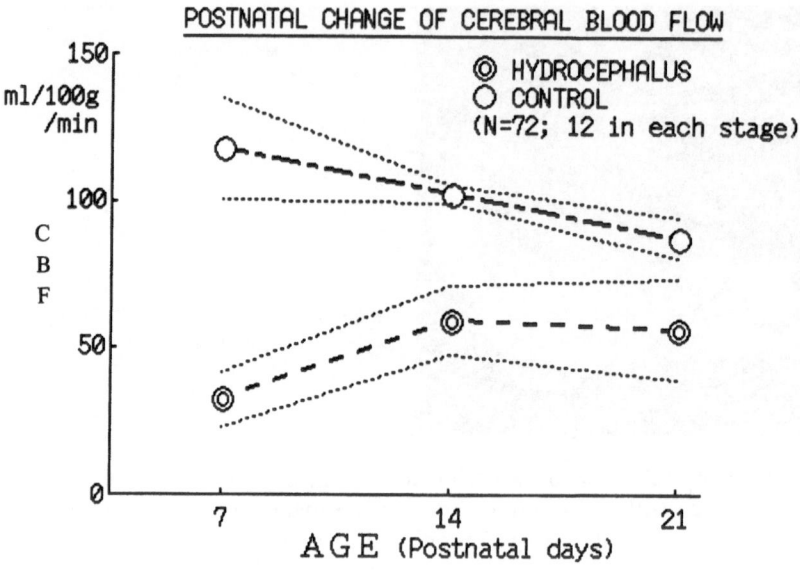

Fig. 3. The chronological change of rCBF in experimental congenital hydrocephalic rats (*lower*) and their normal litter mates (*upper*). The reduction ratio between hydrocephalus and controls is most prominent on day 7, when the progression of hydrocephalus is evident.

matched controls. In hydrocephalic rats, cerebral blood flow values reduced during the first postnatal week, up to 27.5% of control values, then at two weeks of postnatal age, the CBF recovered, up to 65% of the mean CBF control value. The CBF reduction ratio between hydrocephalus and controls was most prominent in the progressive stage of hydrocephalus (Fig. 3).

Clinical Assessment of Intracranial Pressure-Situation in Hydrocephalus During Infancy by Computerized Analysis

There is an age-related threshold level of CPP which tightens the intracranial cavity, even in infants who have an almost open intracranial cavity (Fig. 4). In

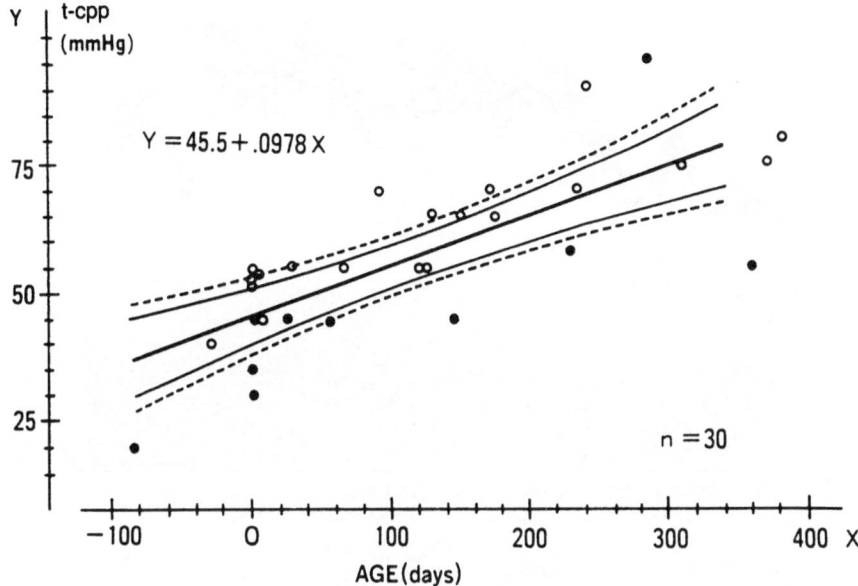

Fig. 4. Age-related change of threshold of cerebral perfusion pressure (*t-cpp*) which is shown in the correlation between CPP and η HB. Patients marked showed poor psychomotor outcome; DQ, IQ ≦ 50 in the follow-up evaluation. η HB, pulse pressure (PP) of ICP/PP of SABP; DQ, developmental quotient; IQ, intelligence quotient

hydrocephalic infants, so-called pressure waves appear (Hayashi et al. 1977; Paraicz 1978) which tighten the intracranial cavity with a reduction of CPP. It is assumed (Kjallquvist et al. 1964; DiRocco et al. 1975) that this critical situation is frequently induced by the suppression of respiration. The lower column in Fig. 5 shows a compiled schema of the chronological changes of physiological parameters of autoregulation, adapting Rosner's cascade theory (Rosner and Becker 1984).

Clinical Evaluation of the CBF Distribution Pattern in Hydrocephalus During Infancy Before and After Shunting

In controls younger than 7 months of age, the frontal lobes showed a relative reduction of CBF (Fig. 6). Most of the controls older than 8 months of age gained an even distribution of CBF. Neonates with congenital hydrocephalus of the so-called simple type showed either frontally dominant CBF reduction or diffuse reduction. In some of these infants, occipitally low CBF was combined with spinal dysraphism. Other infants such as those with postmeningitic hydrocephalus, showed various low-CBF patterns. Most of them showed an increased uptake in the delayed scanning, which suggested a state of reversible ischemia (Creutig et al. 1986).

Follow-up studies at mean 6 months after shunting disclosed sustained low CBF in various locations in 20% of the hydrocephalus cases. Dysgenetic hydrocephalus comprised most of these.

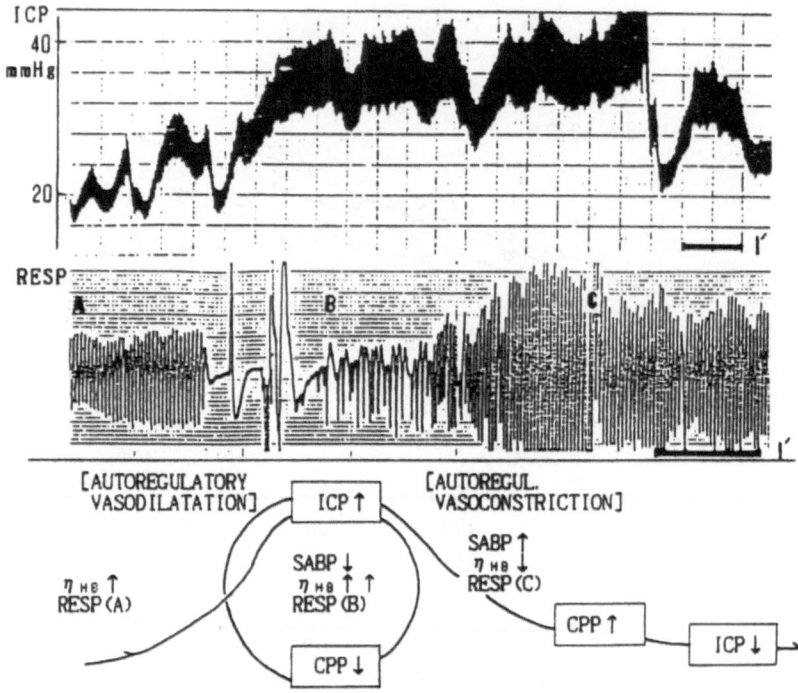

Fig. 5. A representative change of respiratory pattern (*middle and lower graph*) during the appearance of pressure waves (*upper graph*). The *lower figure* is a schematic presentation of the intracranial pressure circumstances related to cerebral perfusion pressure, based on trends of the physiological parameters related to the appearance of pressure waves. Autoregulatory changes were proposed by Rosner (1984). ICP, intracranial pressure; CPP, cerebral perfusion pressure; SABP, systemic arterial blood pressure; η HB, pulse pressure (PP) of ICP/PP of SABP; bar, one minute

In 8 of 11 hydrocephalus cases, ^{123}I-IMP-SPECT detected the frontally reduced CBF which could not be detected by CT. However, in hydrocephalic infants older than 8 months of age, this method disclosed no remarkable alterations, except for progressive and hypertensive hydrocephalus. Figure 6 shows the diffuse reduction with recovery after shunting in a neonate with congenital hydrocephalus.

Discussion

Intracranial hypertension is deleterious when cerebrovascular dynamics are compromised (Portnoy and Chopp 1982) and adverse cerebrohemodynamic effects are emphasized in infants with increased intracranial pressure. Our study further elucidated the factors related to the hemodynamics of hydrocephalus.

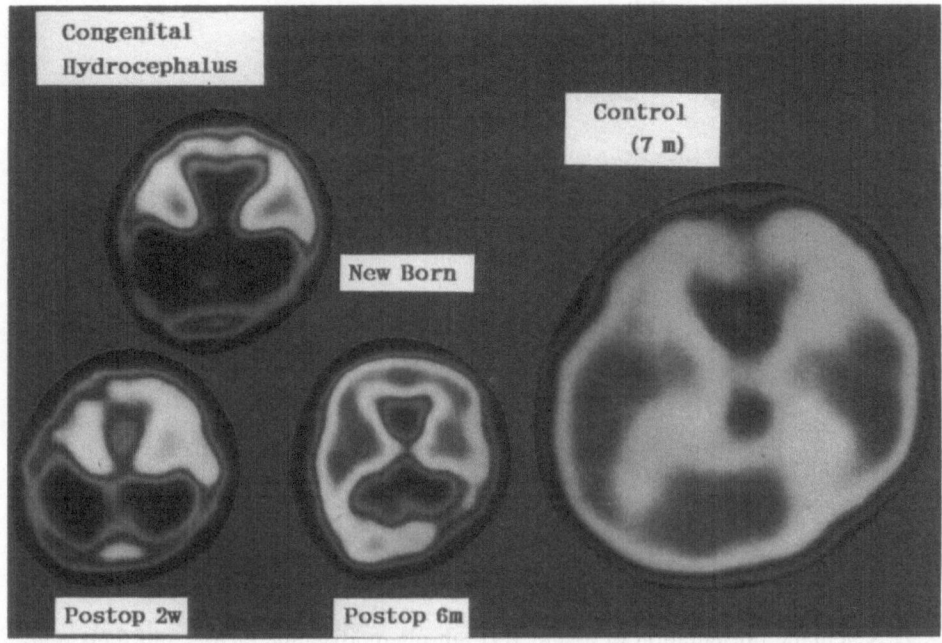

Fig. 6. A sequential change of ^{123}I-IMP SPECT images in a hydrocephalic newborn after shunting, which shows significant recovery of CBF distribution after shunting (*left*). On the *right* is a representative CBF distribution pattern in a 7-month-old control

The induction method of congenital hydrocephalus was originally described by Koyama, Matsumoto, and their colleagues in 1970. Using this model, we reported morphological findings including the pathogenetical sequence of secondary aqueductal stenosis (Sato 1986), and added support to the findings on hy-3 mice (Raimondi and McLone 1976).

Morphological studies have disclosed that the experimental hydrocephalus produced by transplacental MNU is progressive hydrocephalus. Submicroscopical findings lead to the supposition that the pathogenesis of congenital hydrocephalus in this model is based on the immaturity of the germinal cell layer and the rapid maturing of the choroid plexus during the late fetal and early postnatal periods.

Physiologically, the postnatal increase of CBF which is correlated with rapid cortical maturing has been reported both experimentally and clinically (Cross et al. 1976; Denays et al. 1989; Leahy et al. 1979; Rubinstein et al. 1988; Sankaran et al. 1981). Topographically, the increase in frontal lobe is prominent (Ohata et al. 1981).

However, few studies have yet described the pathomechanism of CBF reduction in hydrocephalus during infancy (Hill and Volpe 1982; Wozniak et al. 1975).

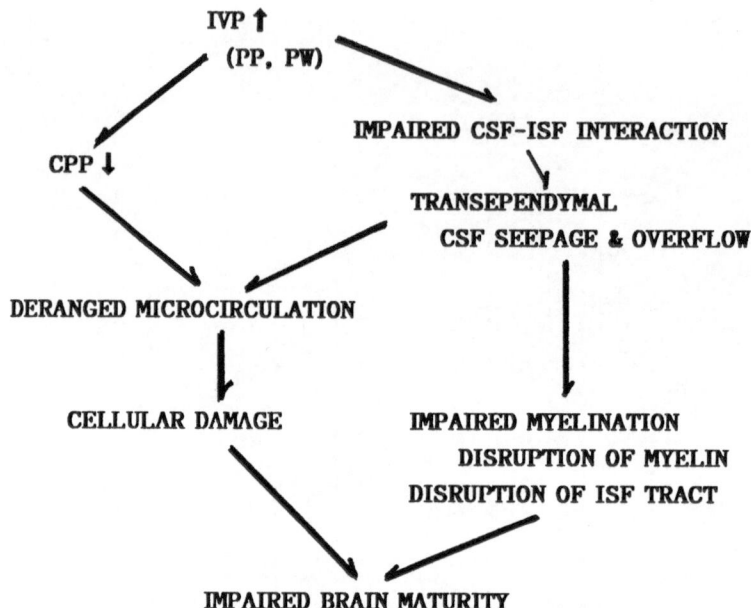

Fig. 7. Schematic presentation of assumed cerebrohemodynamic factors and their relation in hydrocephalus during infancy. Deranged microcirculation is assumed to be related to more complicated factors than the adverse effect of increased intraventricular pressure alone. IVP, intraventricular pressure; CPP, cerebral perfusion pressure; PP, pulse pressure; PW, pressure wave; CSF, cerebrospinal fluid; ISF, interstitial fluid

In human infants, cortical maturation and myelination proceed rapidly together with vascular maturity. In rats, the vascular endothelial cells mature during the third postnatal week and the volume of the vascular bed increases rapidly (Conradi and Sourander 1980; Craigie 1925; Donahue and Pappas 1961; Donahue 1964). Relatively high vaso-reactivity and high $CMRO_2$ are characteristic of immature brains. Many reports have stressed the important role of adequate CBF in brain maturity during the perinatal and infantile periods (Goiten et al. 1983; Lou et al. 1979; Raju et al. 1982; Sankaran et al. 1981; Volpe 1981; Volpe et al. 1983).

On the other hand, pathophysiologically, the microcirculation plays a key role in the maintenance of tissue metabolism. Donahue (1964) claimed that the precapillary blood shunting through the interarteriolar anastmotic channels was the major cause of microcirculatory failure. The low perinatal CBF caused by respiratory distress or hypoxic insults limits the maturation of the brain (Lou et al. 1979).

Regarding the effects of pressure, compression of the vascular bed and reduced intraluminal pressure are assumed to reduce the CBF in normal pressure hydrocephalus in adults (Greitz et al. 1969; Lying-Tunnell et al. 1977). However, it is also known that the reduction of CBF occurs only in the extremely high intracranial pressure range; 450 mmH₂O in adults, if the pressure increased gradually (Kety et al. 1948; Lewis and McLaurin 1971). In an earlier study, we described the intermittent reduction of compliance in infantile hydrocephalus which is related to the supression of the respiratory function (Sato et al. 1988). In hydrocephalus during infancy, we believe that the spong-iness of the periventricular white matter caused by the seepage of CSF pre-disposes to the significant reduction of CBF which is induced by the reduced intracranial compliance which is itself related to the intermittent and acute rise of pressure.

Taking these suppositions into consideration, we compiled our findings on the factors which lead to microcirculatory failure in hydrocephalus. These are presented schematically in Fig. 7. In conclusion, we emphasize the role of micro-circulatory failure in the damage of the developing brain in hydrocephalus.

References

Conradi NG, Sourander P (1980) The early internal vascularization of the rat brain. Acta Neuropathol (Berl) 50: 221–226

Craigie EH (1925) Postnatal change in vascularity in the cerebral cortex of the male albino rat. J Comp Neurol 39: 301–324

Creutig H, Schober O, Gielow R, Friedrich H, Becker H, Dietz H, Hundeshagen H (1986) Cerebral dynamics of N-isopropyl-[^{123}IMP]p-iodoamphetamine. J Nucl Med 27: 178–183

Cross KW, Dear PRF, Warner RM, Walting GB (1976) An attempt to measure cerebral blood-flow in the new-born infant. J Physiol (Lond) 260: 42–43

Denays R, Van Pachterbeke T, Tondeur M, Spehl M, Toppet V, Ham H, Piepsz A, Rubinstein M, Nöel P, Haumont D (1989) Brain single photon emission computed tomography in neonates. J Nucl Med 30: 1337–1341

DiRocco C, McLone DG, Shimoji T, Raimondi AJ (1975) Continuous intraventricular cerebrospinal fluid pressure recording in hydrocephalic children during wakefulness and sleep. J Neurosurg 42: 683–689

Donahue S (1964) A relationship between fine structure and function of blood vessels in the central nervous system of rabbit fetuses. Am J Anat 115: 17–26

Donahue S, Pappas GD (1961) The fine structure of capillaries in the cerebral cortex of the rat at various stages of development. Am J Anat 108: 331–347

Gillian LA (1971) Blood supply to primitive mammalian brains. J Comp Neurol 145: 209–222

Goiten KJ, Amit V, Mussaffi H (1983) Intracranial pressure in central nervous system infections and cerbral ischemia in infancy. Arch Dis Child 58: 184–186

Greitz TVB, Grepe AOL, Kalmer MSF, Lopez J (1969) Pre- and postoperative evalua-tion of cerebral blood flow in low pressure hydrocephalus. J Neurosurg 31: 644–651

Hayashi M, Kobayashi H, Handa Y, Nozaki J, Fujii H, Yamamoto S (1977) A hypoth-esis for the pathogenesis of plateau waves. Neurol Med Chir (Tokyo) 17: 23–29

Hill A, Volpe JJ (1982) Decrease in pulsatile flow in the anterior cerebral arteries in infantile hydrocephalus. Pediatrics 69: 4–7

Ikeyama J, Maeda S, Banno K, Ito A, Nagai H, Kageyama N (1976) Normal intra-cranial circumstances — The theory of "the open and the closed cavities". Brain Nerve 28: 539–547

Kety SS, Shenkin HA, Schmidt CF (1948) The effect of increased intracranial pressure on cerebral circulatory function in man. J Clin Invest 27: 493–499

Kjallquvist A, Lundberg N, Ponten U (1964) Respiratory and cardiovascular changes during rapid spontaneous variations of ventricular fluid pressure in patients with intracranial hypertension. Acta Neurol Scand 40: 291–317

Koyama M, Handa J, Handa H, Matsumoto S (1970) Methylnitrosourea-induced malformations of brain in SD-JCL rats. Arch Neurol 22: 342–347

Kuhl DE, Wu JL, Lin TH, Stein C, Phelps M (1981) Mapping local cerebral blood flow by means of emission computed tomography of N-isopropyl-p[^{123}I]iodoamphetamine (IMP). J Cereb Blood Flow Metab (suppl 1): S25–26

Lassen NA, Henriksen L, Holmes S (1983) Cerebral blood- flow tomography: xenon-133 compared with isopropyl-amphetamine-iodine-123: concise communication. J Nucl Med 24: 17–21

Leahy F, Sankaran K, Cates D, MacCallum M, Rigatto H (1979) Changes in cerebral blood flow (CBF) in preterm infants during inhalation of CO_2 and 100% O_2 (abstract). Pediatr Res 13: 526

Lewis HP, McLaurin RL (1971) Regional cerebral blood flow and increased intracranial pressure produced by stimulated hydrocephalus, mass lesion, and cerebral edema. Surg Forum 22: 424–426

Lou HC, Skov H, Pedersen H (1979) Low cerebral blood flow: a risk factor in neonates. J Pediatr 95: 606–609

Lying-Tunnell V, Lindblad BS, Malmund HO, Persson B (1977) Cerebral blood flow and metabolic rate of oxygen, glucose, lactate, pyruvate, ketone bodies and amino acids in patients with normal pressure hydrocephalus before and after shunting and in normal subjects. Acta Neurol Scand (Suppl) 56: 338–339

Nakai K, Imai H, Kamei I, Itakura T, Komari N, Kimura H, Nagai T, Maeda T (1981) Microangioarchitecture of rat parietal cortex with special reference to vascular "Sphincters" — Scanning electron and dark field microscopic study. Stroke 12: 653–659

Ohata M, Sundaram W, Fredericks MR, London ED, Rapoport SI (1981) Regional cerebral blood flow during development and aging of the rat brain. Brain 104: 319–332

Paraicz E (1978) "A-waves" in infantile and children's hydrocephalus. J Neurosurg Sci 22: 169–171

Portnoy HD, Chopp M (1982) Intracranial fluid dynamics. Interrelationship of CSF and vascular phenomena. In: Raimondi AJ (ed) Concepts in pediatric neurosurgery 3. Karger, Basel, pp 133–142

Raimondi AJ, McLone DG (1976) Pathogenesis of aqueductal stenosis in congenital murine hydrocephalus. J Neurosurg 45: 66–77

Raju TNK, Doschi UV, Vidyasager D (1982) Cerebral perfusion pressure studies in healthy preterm and term newborn infants. J Pediatr 100: 139–142

Rosner MJ, Becker DP (1984) Origin and evolution of plateau waves. Experimental observations and a theoretical model. J Neurosurg 31: 312–324

Rougemond J de, Benabid AL, Chirossel JP, Barge M (1976) The brain vasomotor tone index as a prognostic leader in severe head injuries. In: Becks JWF, Bosch DA, Brock M (eds) intracranial pressure III. Springer, Berlin Heidelberg New York, pp 119–123

Rubinstein M, Denays R, Van Pachterbeke T, et al. (1988) Brain maturation in human newborns: a cerebral blood flow (CBF) study using 123-IMP SPECT (abstract). J Nucl Med 29: 893

Sankaran K, Peters K, Finer N (1981) Estimated cerebral blood flow in term infants with hypoxic-ischemic encephalopathy. Pediatr Res 15: 1415–1418

Sato H (1986) Experimental congenital hydrocephalus — Pathogenetic process in differentiating brain. Neurol Med Chir (Tokyo) 26: 11–18

Sato H, Sato N, Tamaki N, Matsumoto S (1988) Threshold of cerebral perfusion pressure as a prognostic factor in hydrocephalus during infancy. Childs Nerv Syst 4: 274–278

Volpe JJ (1981) Neurology of the newborn. WB Saunders, Philadelphia, pp 141–298

Volpe JJ, Herschowitch P, Perlman JM, et al. (1983) Positron emission tomography in the newborn: extensive impairment of regional cerebral blood flow with intracerebral involvement. Pediatrics 72: 589–601

Wozniak M, McLone DG, Raimondi AJ (1975) Micro- and macrovascular changes as the direct cause of parenchymal destruction in congenital murine hydrocephalus. J Neurosurg 43: 535–545

14 — Cerebral Blood Flow and Oxygen Metabolism in Children with Hydrocephalus

Reizo Shirane, Shinya Sato, Motonobu Kameyama, Akira Ogawa, Takashi Yoshimoto[1], Jun Hatazawa, and Masatoshi Ito[2]

Summary. In this study, we measured regional cerebral blood flow (rCBF) and the cerebral metabolic rate for oxygen (rCMRO$_2$), using positron emission tomography (PET) with O^{15}-radiopharmaceuticals, to clarify the pathophysiology of hydrocephalus in the developing brain. Seven hydrocephalic children without severe neurological deficit were studied. Hypoperfusion and lower rCMRO$_2$ values were observed in the prefrontal, parietal, and visual association cortices which surrounded the dilated anterior or posterior horns of the lateral ventricle. In those cases with markedly enlarged anterior or posterior horns, the surrounding cortices showed relatively lower rCMRO$_2$ values with the fall of rCBF. Hydrocephalus tended to damage various association cortices where functional development occurs later than in other cortical regions.

Keywords. Infant — Hydrocephalus — Cerebral blood flow — Oxygen metabolism — PET

Introduction

Hydrocephalus in children continues to produce long-term brain damage. Although extensive studies have been made on its pathophysiology from the viewpoint of cerebrospinal fluid dynamics, little is known about cerebral circulation and metabolism in this condition. In adults, the value of PET with oxygen-15 (^{15}O) radiopharmaceuticals in the study of regional cerebral blood flow (rCBF), blood volume (rCBV), and the cerebral metabolic rate of oxygen (rCMRO$_2$) is well established.

In this study, we measured cerebral blood flow and oxygen metabolism in seven hydrocephalic children in order to clarify the pathogenesis of ventriculomegaly in the developing brain.

[1] Division of Neurosurgery, Institute of Brain Diseases, and [2] Division of Nuclear Medicine, Cyclotron RI Center, Tohoku University, Sendai, 980 Japan

Table 1. Clinical summary of cases studied

Case	Age (days/months)	Sex	Diagnosis	Symptoms	DQ
1	12d	M	Myelomeningocele (S3–5) Chiari malformation	Increased ICP	—
2	25d	F	Holoprosencephaly (labor type)	Increased ICP	—
3	4m	M	Aqueductal stenosis	Increased ICP	60
4	6m	F	Aqueductal stenosis	Developmental retardation	64
5	6m	F	Post IVH	None	100
6	11m	F	Aqueductal stenosis	Increased ICP	81
7	18m	F	Post IVH	Motor develop. retardation	85

ICP, intracranial pressure

Subjects and Methods

The subjects of this study were seven children with ventricular dilatation under the age of 1½ years. Table 1 shows a clinical summary of the cases. None of these patients had severe neurological deficits. They were operated on (ventriculoperitoneal shunt) after PET study and all of them showed some recovery from their symptoms.

All PET studies were performed in accordance with the policies of the Committee for Clinical PET Study of Tohoku University. Informed consent was obtained from the parents. We used a PT-931 (CTI, Knoxville, Tennessee). (Spinks et al. 1988) The spatial resolution of the image was 8 mm, and the slice thickness was 7 mm. Seven slices were obtained simultaneously. All subjects were scanned at the axial tomographic level from the midbrain to the upper-ventricular level. The PET images were reconstructed using measured attenuation correction. Venous and arterial catheters were inserted in a hand vein and radial artery, respectively, under local anesthesia. Thiopental sodium was administered (3 mg/kg) intravenously 20 minutes prior to the emission scan in order to stabilize the patient during the examination. Measurements of rCBF, oxygen extraction fraction (OEF), rCMRO$_2$ and rCBV were carried out with steady state inhalation of tracer amounts of $C^{15}O_2$, $^{15}O_2$, and inhalation of $C^{15}O$, respectively (Frackowack et al. 1980; Lammertsma et al. 1978). The neonatal brain-blood partition coefficient used in this study was 1.1 ml/g, in accordance with the report of Herscovitch and Raichle (1985). For children older than 1 month, the applied value was 1.0 ml/g. The CO$_2$, O$_2$, and CO content of the inhaled air was approximately 10% of the content used for adults. Arterial blood was drawn for the analysis of blood gases and radioactivity.

Results

In neonates, PET revealed lower rCBF and rCMRO$_2$ values in every region. Among these values, those of the thalamus, brain stem, and sensorimotor

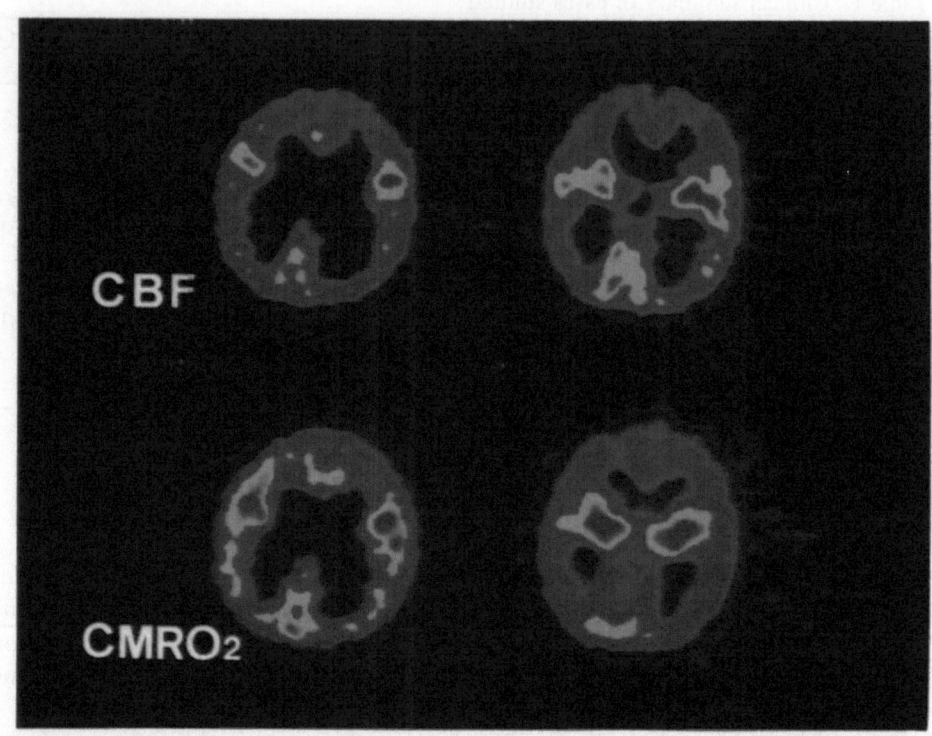

a

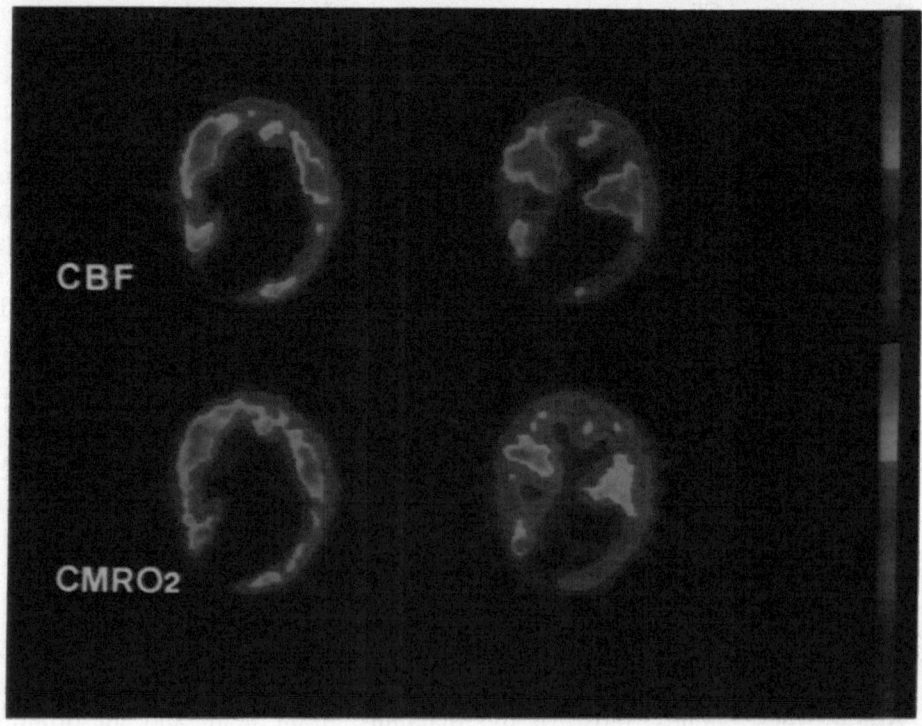

b

cortex showed relatively higher CBF and oxygen metabolism values. (Fig. 1; Table 2)

In infants with aqueductal stenosis, lower rCBF and higher OEF values were observed in the prefrontal, parietal, and visual association cortices. (Table 3; Fig. 2a) Post-operative study revealed a decrease of regional differences in the cerebral cortex. (Fig. 2b) In case 6, which had markedly enlarged anterior horns, the surrounding cortices showed very low rCMRO$_2$ values with the fall of rCBF. (Fig. 3; Table 4)

Table 2. Neonate with Chiari malformation (case 1)

Region	rCBF	rCMRO$_2$	OEF	rCBV
Prefrontal c.	14	0.65	0.20	2.3
Sensorimotor c.	32	0.78	0.17	3.6
Parietal c.	22	0.58	0.14	2.4
Calcarine c.	40	0.62	0.13	6.3
Visual association c.	21	0.53	0.11	2.3
Thalamus	44	1.3	0.16	3.2
Cerebellum	33	0.51	0.10	5.1
Brain stem	66	1.7	0.13	4.2

rCBF: ml/100 per min; rCMRO$_2$: ml/100 g per min; rCBV: ml/100 g

Table 3. Six-month-old girl with aqueductal stenosis (case 4)

Region	rCBF	rCMRO$_2$	OEF	rCBV
Prefrontal c.	30	2.1	0.41	3.2
Sensorimotor c.	39	2.3	0.34	3.4
Parietal c.	34	2.8	0.46	3.8
Calcarine c.	44	2.1	0.26	14.8
Visual association c.	30	2.6	0.50	4.1
Thalamus	66	2.7	0.31	4.0

rCBF: ml/100 g per min; rCMRO$_2$: ml/100 per min; rCBV: ml/100 g

Table 4. Eleven-month-old girl with marked dilatation of anterior horns (case 6)

Region	rCBF	rCMRO$_2$	OEF	rCBV
Prefrontal c.	18	2.8	0.62	5.2
Sensorimotor c.	30	3.8	0.52	4.1
Parietal c.	38	4.5	0.56	4.8
Calcarine c.	57	6.8	0.52	6.1
Visual association c.	34	4.0	0.56	4.3
Thalamus	49	4.7	0.42	3.1

rCBF: ml/100 g per min; rCMRO$_2$: ml/100 per min; rCBV: ml/100 g

Fig. 1. Images of rCBF and rCMRO$_2$ in neonates: **a** Case 1, **b** case 2. Thalamus, sensorimotor cortex and visual cortex show higher blood flow and metabolism

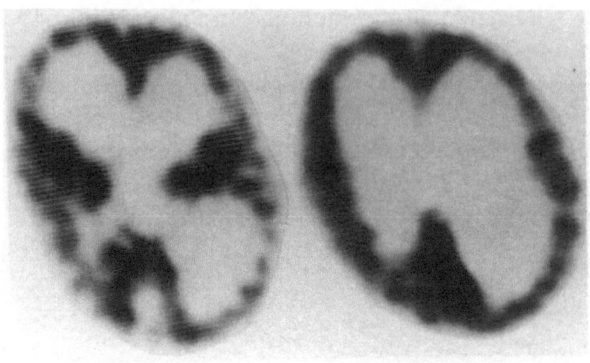

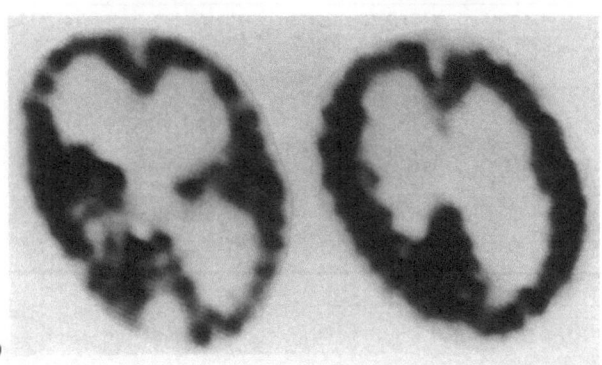

Fig. 2. a Preoperative CBF image in case 4, showing lower perfusion in prefrontal, parietal, and visual association cortices than in thalamus, visual, and sensorimotor cortex. **b** Postoperative study, performed one month after ventriculoperitoneal (*VP*) shunt, showing decreased regional differences

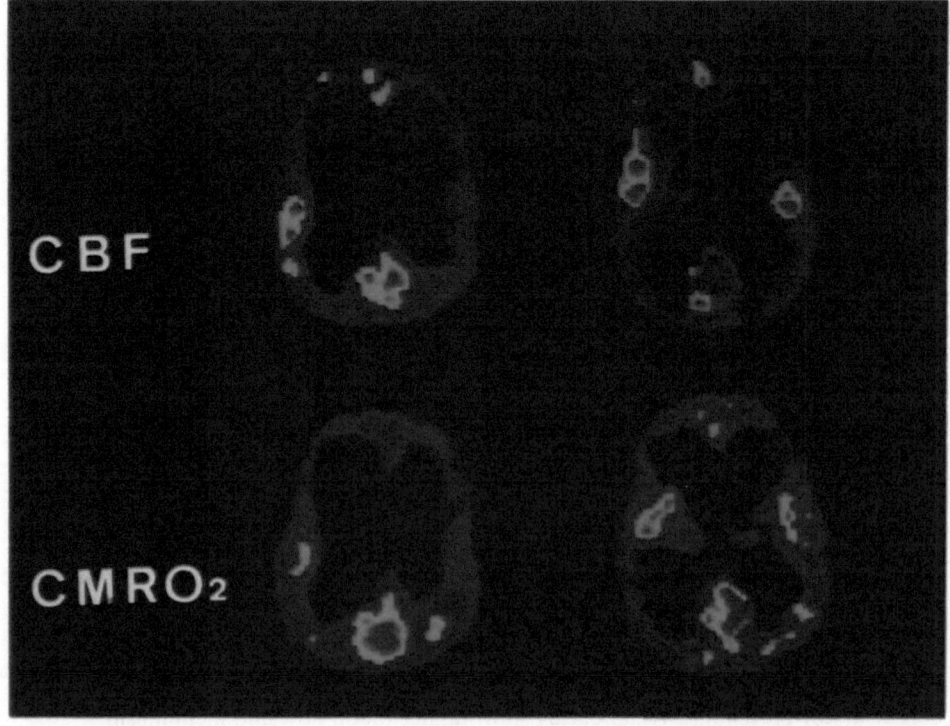

In cases with hydrocephalus after intra-ventricular hemorrhage, marked ventricular dilatation was observed in the posterior horns of the lateral ventricle. No obvious neurological deficit or developmental retardation was observed in this group of patients. PET revealed very low CBF and $CMRO_2$ values in the parietal and visual association cortices. The OEF in those regions was not elevated. (Fig. 4; Table 5)

No particular tendency was observed in the rCBV values in the results of the present study. However, the visual cortex showed higher values than those of the other regions, as reflected in the blood in the venous sinus.

Discussion

In infants, hydrocephalus can present acutely, with symptoms of raised intracranial pressure or, more insidiously, with developmental retardation. The most important pathologic effects include atrophy of the white matter and spongy edema of the brain surrounding the ventricle. These changes have been shown to involve primary destruction of axons, a secondary loss of myelin, and chronic astrogliosis. In contrast, neurons were selectively spared. Weller and Shulman (1972) showed by brain biopsy that the pathologic effects of hydrocephalus were fully reversible on shunting in a 28-day-old infant with white matter edema, while older hydrocephalic infants with associated white matter atrophy and gliosis remained retarded after a shunting operation.

The decision whether or not to shunt an infant with enlarged ventricles and no obvious symptoms of intracranial hypertension depends on an understanding of the damage that is done by ventriculomegaly and the risks inherent in the therapy. Rekate (1984) estimated that when there is less than 2.8 cm of cortical mantle the risk of ventriculomegaly overcomes the risk of a shunting operation. However, the many etiologies of ventriculomegaly make it difficult to predict by conventional neurological or neuroradiological examination whether or not the ventriculomegaly will cause developmental retardation in the infant (Rapin 1976; Young et al. 1973).

In the neonate, PET revealed lower cerebral blood flow and oxygen metabolism; the thalamus, brain stem, and sensorimotor cortex showed relatively higher metabolism. Very low rOEF and $rCMRO_2$ values in preterm infants were also reported by Altman (1989) and the pattern of neonatal cerebral blood flow and metabolism in the present study was similar to the rCMRGlu pattern in the neonatal period reported by Chugani and Phelps (1986) and Chugani et al. (1987). However, it was still unclear whether this metabolic change was brought by hydrocephalus of immaturity of the brain.

In the other older children, lower rCBF and higher rOEF values were observed in the prefrontal, parietal, and visual association cortices which surrounded the dilated anterior or posterior horns of the lateral ventricle. These

◁————————————————————————————————

Fig. 3. Images of rCBF and $rCMRO_2$ in case 6. Lower blood flow and oxygen metabolism are observed in the frontal cortex than in the other cortical regions

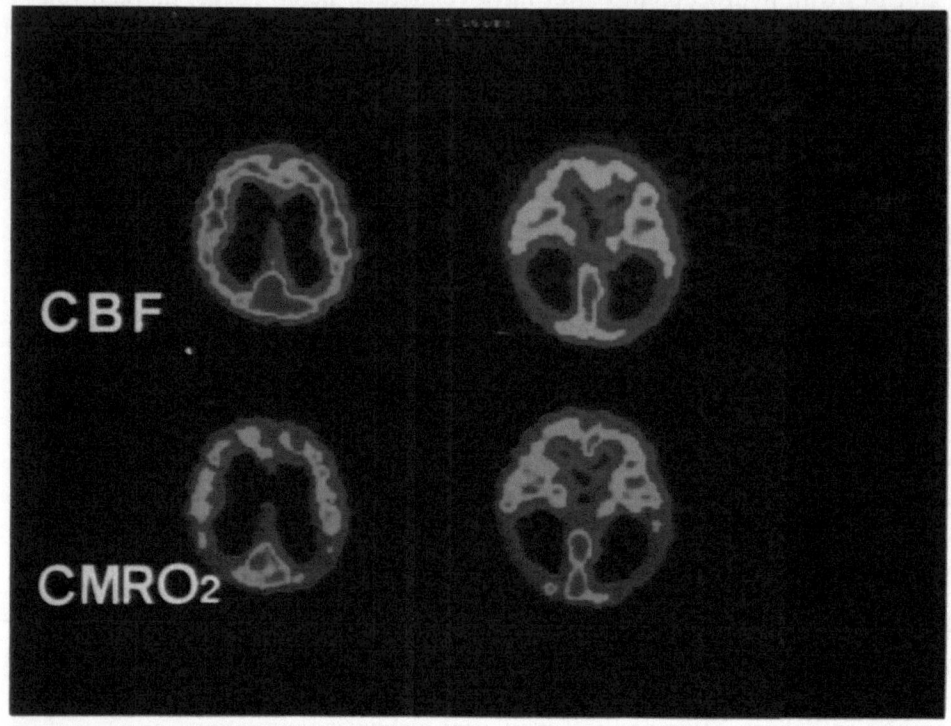

Fig. 4. Images of rCBF and rCMRO₂ in case 5. Parietal and visual association cortices and surrounding posterior horns of lateral ventricle, showing lower blood flow and metabolism in hydrocephalus after intra-ventricular hemorrhage

Table 5. Six-month-old girl with marked dilatation of posterior horns after intra-ventricular hemorrhage (case 5)

Region	rCBF	rCMRO₂	OEF	rCBV
Prefrontal c.	38	1.6	0.47	4.3
Sensorimotor c.	54	2.2	0.38	3.6
Parietal c.	28	1.2	0.33	2.5
Calcarine c.	55	2.5	0.47	5.7
Visual association c.	20	0.6	0.39	2.2
Thalamus	54	2.4	0.44	4.3

rCBF: ml/100 g per min; rCMRO₂: ml/100 per min; rCBV: ml/100 g

regions are "watershed zones" of major cerebral arteries. This regional hypo-perfusion and elevated OEF seemed to be brought about by a combination of brain expansion, interstitial edema, and raised intracranial pressure. The regional differences in rCMRO₂ were not as evident as those observed in rCBF. On the other hand, in the cases with markedly enlarged anterior or posterior horns, the surrounding cortices showed relatively lower rCMRO₂ values with the fall of rCBF. Brooks et al. (1986) reported that a coupled reduction in the rCMRO$_2$ and rCBF of the cerebral cortex was observed in adult patients with long-standing hydrocephalus. When these patients were re-studied after VP shunt, no increases were observed in their rCMRO$_2$ or rCBF levels. This may indicate that irreversible damage such as gliosis existed in the brain.

In the study ·of infants, maturational changes in cerebral blood flow and metabolism should be considered (Ogawa et al. 1989). Chugani et al. (1986, 1987) reported that, in the neonatal period, local cerebral metabolic rate for glucose (lCMRGlc) is highest in the sensorimotor cortex, thalamus, brain stem, and cerebellar vermis. During the 2nd and 3rd months, increases occur in the basal ganglia and in the parietal, temporal, and primary visual cortices. By approximately 8 months, the frontal and various associated cortical regions have also shown a notable increase in lCMRGlc. The anatomical pattern of lCMRGlc typically observed in the young healthy adult is present by the end of the first year of life. Normal maturational changes in the cerebral blood flow and oxygen metabolism of infants have not yet been studied, but it is known that blood flow and oxygen and glucose metabolism show a good correlation with each other in normal subjects. In the present study, lower rCBF and rCMRO$_2$ levels, and the increase or decrease in OEF, were observed mainly in various association cortices in which metabolic maturation is completed after six months. We could not determine whether the low rCBF and rCMRO$_2$ levels in those regions were pathologic or not. However, the disproportion between rCBF and rCMRO$_2$, shown as a change in OEF, might indicate metabolic deterioration produced by hydrocephalus.

One of the technical difficulties of applying this procedure is the stabilization of infants during PET study. Therefore, some anesthetics should be admin-istered; thiopental sodium was used in this study. Barbiturates are known to suppress the cerebral metabolism, therefore, in order to reduce the influence of the substance on cerebral blood flow and metabolism, the dose applied to infants was the minimum one and all studies were performed under the same protocol.

Finally, it should be stressed that hydrocephalus tended to damage the frontal, parietal, and visual association cortices, where functional development occurs later than in other cortical regions (Rapin 1976). Taking this factor into account, the decision whether or not to shunt an infant with enlarged ventricles is difficult, if this decision is based only on neurological examination. The present study indicates that measurement of cerebral blood flow and oxygen metabolism will open a new field in the therapy of hydrocephalus in infants.

References

Altman DI, Volpe JJ, powers WJ (1989) Cerebral oxygen metabolism in newborn infants with positron emission tomography. J Cereb Blood Flow Metab 9 (Suppl 1): s25

Brooks DJ, Beaney RP, Powell M, Leenders KL, Crockard HA (1986) Studies on cerebral oxygen metabolism, blood flow, and blood volume, in patients with hydrocephalus before and after surgical decompression using positron emission tomography. Brain 109: 613–628

Chugani HT, Phelps ME (1986) Maturational changes in cerebral function in infants determined by [18]FDG positron emission tomography. Science 231: 840–843

Chugani HT, Phelps ME, Mazziotta JC (1987) Positron emission tomography study of human brain functional development. Ann Neurol 22: 487–497

Frackowak RS, Lenzi GL, Jones T, Heather JD (1980) Quantitative measurement of regional cerebral blood flow and oxygen metabolism in man using [15]O and positron emission tomography: theory, procedure and normal values. J Comput Assist Tomogr 4: 727–736

Herscovitch P, Raichle ME (1985) What is the correct value for the brain-blood partition coefficient for water? J Cereb Blood Flow Metab 5: 65–69

Lammertsma AA, Wise RJS, Heater JD, Gibbs JM, Leenders KL, Frackowiak RSJ, Rhodes CG, Jones T (1978) Correction for the presence of intravascular oxygen-15 in the steady-state technique for measuring regional oxygen extraction ratio in the brain: 2 results in normal subject and brain tumor and stroke patients. J Cereb Blood Flow Metab 3: 425–431

Ogawa A, Sakurai Y, Kayama T, Yoshimoto T (1989) Regional cerebral blood flow with age: Changes in rCBF in childhood. Neurol Res 11: 173–176

Rapin I (1976) Progressive genetic-metabolic diseases of the central nervous system in children. Pediatr Ann 5: 313–349

Rekate HL (1984) To shunt or not to shunt: hydrocephalus and dysraphism. In: Little JR (ed) Clinical neurosurgery, 32nd edn. Williams and Wilkins, Baltimore, pp 593–607

Spinks TJ, Guzzardi R, Bellina CR (1988) Performance characteristics of a whole body positron tomograph. J Nucl Med 29: 1833–1841

Weller RO, Shulman K (1972) Infantile hydrocephalus: clinical, histological, and ultrastructural study of brain damage. J Neurosurg 36: 255–265

Young HF, Nulsen FE, Weiss MH, Thomas P (1973) The relationship of intelligence and cerebral mantle in treated infantile hydrocephalus: IQ potential in hydrocephalic children. Pediatrics 52: 54–60

15 — Pulsatile Flow in Cerebral Arteries in Neonatal Hydrocephalus

Shigeru Nishimaki[1] and Yasuo Iwasaki[2]

Summary. We studied Pourcelot's index of resistance (RI), which shows cerebral vascular resistance, in the anterior cerebral artery (RI − ACA), and in the basilar artery (RI − BA), and the RI ratio (= RI − ACA/RI − BA) in 13 measurements of hydrocephalus. (1) The mean RI − ACA, RI − BA and RI ratios before treatment were significantly higher than those found after treatment and in normal infants. (2) Before treatment, all RI ratios had increased to 1.00 and more. After treatment and in normal infants, however, all RI ratios had decreased less to than 1.00. We consider that the RI ratio is useful for evaluating the need for or the effect of treatment in hydrocephalus.

Keywords. Pourcelot's index of resistance — Cerebral blood flow velocity — Hydrocephalus

Introduction

Hemodynamic alterations in the cerebral arteries have been evaluated by Doppler sonography in infants using Pourcelot's index of resistance (RI) (Pourcelot 1976). Cerebral blood flow in healthy infants, (Ando et al. 1983; Deeg and Ruprecht 1988; Gray et al. 1983) as well as pathologic blood flow in infants with intraventricular hemorrhage (IVH), (Bada et al. 1979; Perlman and Volpe 1982) asphyxia, (Bada et al. 1979; Deeg et al. 1990) hydrocephalus, (Chadduck et al. 1989; Hill and Volpe 1982) and cardiovascular disease (Lipman et al. 1982; Perlman et al. 1981) have been investigated and published in the literature.

However, these studies have reported only changes of absolute values. To accurately evaluate the need for treatment, we measured RI in both the anterior cerebral arteries (ACAs) and in the basilar artery (BA), and examined the relationship of the two values before and after treatment.

---

[1] Departments of Neonatology, and [2] Neurosurgery, Japanese Red Cross Medical Center, Shibuya-ku, Tokyo, 150 Japan

153

Patients and Methods

Ventriculomegaly was caused by posthemorrhagic hydrocephalus in patients 1, 2, 3, 4, and 5, congenital hydrocephalus in patients 6 and 7, and Arnold-Chiari malformation in patients 8 and 9 (Table 1). Patient 2 had mild progressive hydrocephalus confirmed by computed tomography (CT) scans (Schick and Matson 1961). Nine patients with ventriculomegaly were studied on 13 occasions just before and two hours after treatment. Patent ductus arteriosus (PDA) and other congenital heart diseases were not detected by pediatric cardiologists in any of the patients with hydrocephalus.

Cerebral blood flow velocity was measured through the anterior fontanelle by pulsed Doppler ultrasonograph with a 5-MHz transducer (model RT-5000, Yokogawa Medical Systems, Tokyo). The flow in the ACAs was visualized in front of the third ventricle and the flow in the BA was seen in front of the pons in the sagittal sections. We investigated peak systolic velocity (S) and end diastolic velocity (D). We calculated RI for both ACA(RI − ACA) and BA(RI − BA) from the formula of Pourcelot et al.: RI = (S − D)/S (Fig. 1) (Pourcelot 1976). To study the relationship between RI − ACA and RI − BA, we calculated the RI ratio before and after treatment using the following formula: RI ratio = RI − ACA/RI − BA.

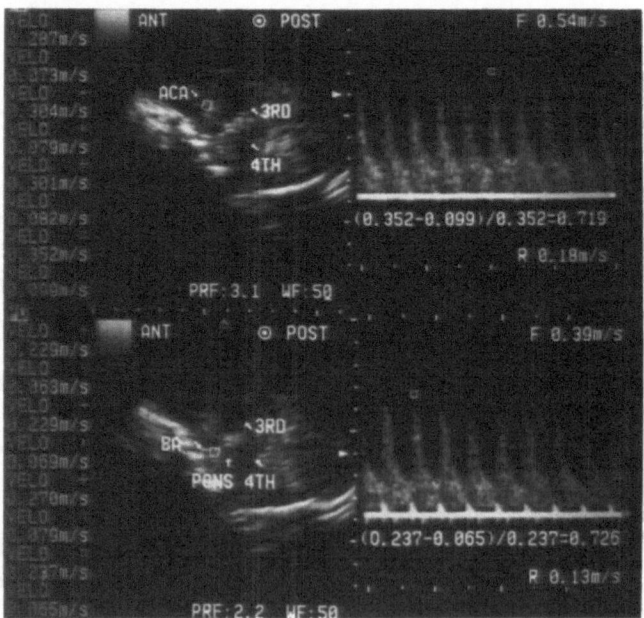

Fig. 1. *Upper left* the flow in the anterior cerebral artery (*ACA*) is visualized in front of the third ventricle (*3RD*). *Upper right* Pourcelot's index (*RI*) in the ACA is calculated from the formula: RI = (S − D)/S. S, peak systolic velocity; D, end-diastolic velocity. *Lower left* the flow in the basilar artery (*BA*) is visualized in front of the pons (*P*). *Lower right* RI in the BA is calculated for RI-BA 4TH, the fourth ventricle

Table 1. RI-ACA, RI-BA, and RI ratio values before and after treatment

Patient no.	Before			Treatment	After		
	RI-ACA	RI-BA	RI ratio		RI-ACA	RI-BA	RI ratio
1	0.845	0.800	1.056	VP shunt	0.739	0.769	0.961
2	0.719	0.698	1.030	VP shunt	0.636	0.648	0.982
3	0.839	0.768	1.092	VP shunt	0.716	0.745	0.961
4	0.880	0.847	1.041	CSF drainage	0.744	0.750	0.992
	0.882	0.847	1.041	CSF drainage	0.761	0.787	0.967
5	0.844	0.788	1.071	VP shunt	0.717	0.755	0.950
	0.982	0.950	1.034	VP shunt	0.705	0.741	0.951
6	0.826	0.815	1.013	VP shunt	0.643	0.682	0.943
	0.742	0.704	1.054	VP shunt	0.535	0.571	0.937
7	0.779	0.768	1.014	VP shunt	0.588	0.629	0.935
8	0.808	0.806	1.002	CSF drainage	0.644	0.706	0.912
	0.899	0.892	1.006	VP shunt	0.632	0.651	0.971
9	0.791	0.777	1.018	VP shunt	0.466	0.476	0.979
Mean	0.834	0.805	1.036		0.656	0.686	0.957
(SD)	(0.069)	(0.069)	(0.027)		(0.088)	(0.089)	(0.027)

The mean RI-ACA, RI-BA, and RI ratios before treatment were significantly higher than after treatment ($P < 0.001$, Figs. 2, 3, and 4). RI, index of resistance; ACA, anterior cerebral artery; BA, basilar artery

At the time of the RI measurements, all patients were in the sleeping state with stable spontaneous respiration. Measurements of blood pressure and hematocrit were within the normal range and stable. Our normal ranges of RI − ACA, RI − BA, and RI ratio were 0.726 ± 0.035 (mean ±SD), 0.753 ± 0.037, and 0.964 ± 0.027, respectively. The data were analyzed using the paired t test.

Results

The results of the measurements of RI − ACA, RI − BA, and RI ratio before and after treatment are shown in Table 1. Measurements of RI − ACA before and after treatment are illustrated in Fig. 2. The RI − ACA values ranged from 0.719 to 0.982 before treatment and from 0.466 to 0.761 after treatment. The mean RI − ACA before treatment (0.834 ± 0.069, ±SD) was significantly higher than that after treatment (0.656 ± 0.088) ($P < 0.001$) and than that in normal infants (0.726 ± 0.035) ($P < 0.001$). The RI − BA values before and after treatment are illustrated in Fig. 3. The RI − BA values ranged from 0.698 to 0.950 before treatment and from 0.476 to 0.787 after treatment. The mean RI − BA value before treatment (0.805 ± 0.069) was significantly higher than that after treatment (0.686 ± 0.089) ($P < 0.001$) and than that in normal infants (0.753 ± 0.037) ($P < 0.05$).

We therefore calculated RI ratios for evaluating the relationship between RI − ACA and RI − BA (Fig. 4). Prior to treatment, the mean RI ratio was 1.036 ± 0.027 (mean ±SD) and ranged from 1.002 to 1.092. All RI ratios in untreated hydrocephalus were 1.000 and more. Following treatment the RI ratios, with a mean of 0.964 ± 0.022 (SD), extended from 0.912 to 0.992. All RI ratios of treated patients were less than 1.000. The mean RI ratio before treatment was significantly higher than that in normal infants (0.964 ± 0.027, mean ±SD) and than that after treatment ($P < 0.001$, respectively).

Discussion

Pulsatile flow measurement using the Doppler technique is useful in infants as it may be carried out at the bedside without disturbing the patient. We studied RI, which shows cerebral vascular resistance, (Pourcelot 1976) in the ACA and BA of hydrocephalic patients. We have two reasons for our choice of the ACAs and BA. First, we can easily detect both the ACAs and the BA in the sagittal section only, therefore there is no need to use different sections for each vessel. Second, we can measure the flow velocities and RI values without angle correction, because the angles between the Doppler flows and the axes of the arteries are almost parallel.

We found marked changes in the values for RI − ACA and RI − BA before and after treatment. The RI ratios presented in this report also demonstrated the need for or the effect of treatment. As previous studies have shown,

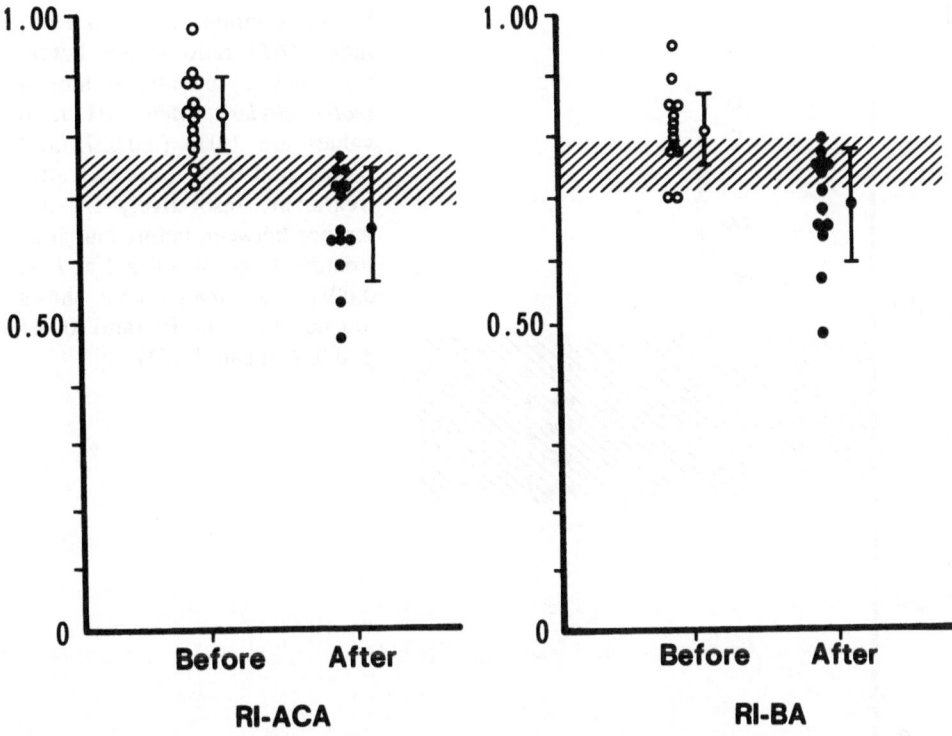

Fig. 2. Relation of Pourcelot's index (*RI*) measurements in the anterior cerebral artery (*RI − ACA*) before (*open circles*) and after treatment (*solid circles*). Mean RI − ACA values are 0.834 (±0.069, SD) before and 0.656 (±0.088) after treatment, respectively. A difference between before and after treatment was significant at $P < 0.001$. The *shaded area* is our normal mean RI − ACA value (0.726 ± 0.035, mean ± SD)

Fig. 3. Relation of Pourcelot's index (*RI*) measurements in the basilar artery (*RI-BA*) before (*open circles*) and after treatment (*solid circles*). Mean RI − BA values are 0.805 (±0.069, SD) before and 0.656 (±0.088) after treatment, respectively. A difference between before and after treatment was significant at $P < 0.001$. The *shaded area* shows our normal mean RI − BA value (0.753 ± 0.037, mean ± SD)

elevated RI measurements decreased after treatment (Chadduck et al. 1989; Hill and Volpe 1982). In our study, after treatment there was, on an average, a 17.8% drop in the RI − ACA value, and only an 11.9% drop in the RI − BA value. The RI − ACA values changed more than the RI − BA values. However, the RI − ACA and RI − BA values in patient 2 (mild progressive hydrocephalus) were within the normal range. With results of the RI values and CT scans, we were undecided whether to treat the patients with a VP shunt operation. On the other hand, there was only a 7.9% drop in the RI ratio; however, all RI ratios before treatment were 1.000 and more, an after treatment they were less than 1.000. The mean RI ratio of untreated hydrocephalic infants (1.036 ± 0.027, ±SD) was significantly higher than that in

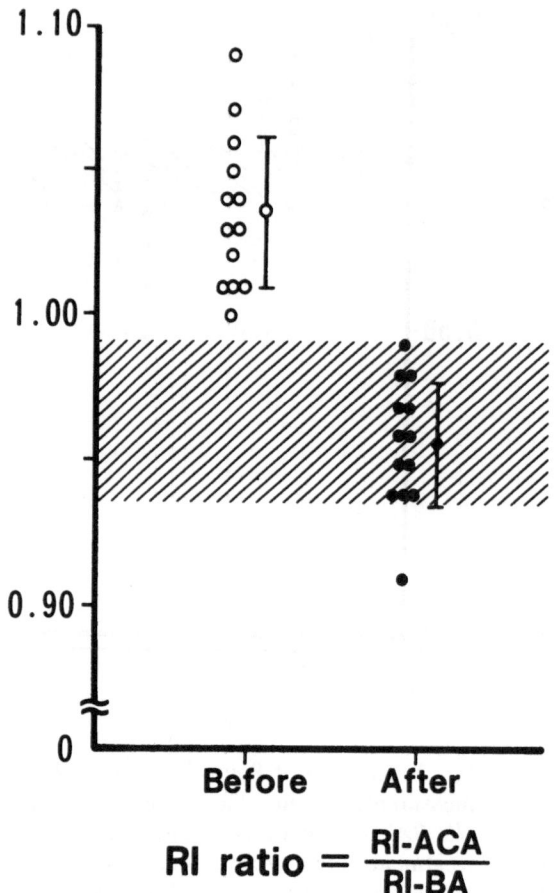

Fig. 4. Relation of Pourcelot's index (*RI*) ratio values before (*open circles*) and after treatment (*solid circles*). Mean RI ratio values are 1.036 (±0.027, SD) before and 0.957 (±0.022) after treatment, respectively. A difference between before and after treatment was significant at $P < 0.001$. The *shaded area* shows our normal mean RI ratio (0.964 ± 0.027, mean ± SD)

normal infants (0.964 ± 0.027) and than that in treated hydrocephalus (0.957 ± 0.022) ($P < 0.001$), respectively. The RI ratio in patient 2 was 1.030 before treatment and 0.982 after treatment. The enlarged ventricles in patient 2 decreased after VP shunt operation. We were therefore able to judge the need of treatment with RI ratios, even in mild progressive hydrocephalus (patient 2 in this study).

The RI values in the ACAs of normal infants were lower than those in the BA. We consider the following to be the reason why the mean RI − ACA value was lower than the mean RI − BA value. In general, the amplitude of the velocity pulse decreases and the waveform develops a rounded shape peripherally (Thompson 1987). RI values therefore decrease with increasing distance from the heart. On the other hand, the RI − ACA values were higher than the RI − BA values in untreated hydrocephalus. In most cases of hydrocephalus, the lateral ventricles enlarge more than the third or fourth ventricles. We consider that the dilated lateral ventricles may compress or stretch the ACAs more than the BA, and thus increase the RI measurements in the ACAs more than in the BA. After treatment, normalized vessels may decrease elevated RI measurements in the ACAs more than those in the BA. Therefore, the mean value of RI − ACA was higher than the value of RI − BA (RI

− ACA > RI − BA) before treatment, and the mean value of RI − ACA was lower than the value of RI − BA (RI − ACA < RI − BA) after treatment.

The results of this study demonstrated that the RI ratios in hydrocephalus were 1.000 and more before treatment, and less than 1.000 after treatment and in normal infants. When RI ratios elevate higher than 1.000, even in mild progressive hydrocephalus, patients not only have enlarged ventricles, but also have an unbalanced cerebral condition. VP shunt operations as well as CSF drainage procedures might be needed in such patients. Besides, we can easily decide how much CSF should be drained in drainage procedures to treat hydrocephalic infants.

We submit that the RI ratio is a useful added tool in evaluating the effect of or the need for treatment in patients with ventriculomegaly. By evaluating hydrocephalus or shunt malfunction at an early stage, we can save the brain from being damaged by ischemia or pressure. Further studies are needed to investigate and estimate cerebral condition in hydrocephalic infants not only immediately after treatment, but also for prolonged periods after treatment.

References

Ando Y, Takahashi S, Takeshita K (1983) Postnatal changes of cerebral blood flow velocity in normal term neonates. Brain Dev 5: 525–528

Bada HS, Hajjar W, Chua C, Sumner DS (1979) Noninvasive diagnosis of neonatal asphyxia and intraventricular hemorrhage by Doppler ultrasound. J Pediatr 95: 775–779

Chadduck WM, Seibert JJ, Adametz J, Glasier CM, Crabtree M, Stansell CA (1989) Cranial Doppler ultrasonography correlates with criteria for ventriculoperitoneal shunting. Surg Neurol 31: 122–128

Deeg KH, Rupprecht T (1988) Pulsed Doppler sonographic measurements of normal values for the flow velocities in the intracranial arteries of healthy newborns. Pediatr Radiol 19: 71–78

Deeg KH, Rupprecht T, Zeilinger G (1990) Doppler sonographic classification of brain edema in infants. Pediatr Radiol 20: 509–514

Gray PH, Griffin EA, Drumm JE, Fitzgerald DE, Duignan NM (1983) Continuous wave Doppler ultrasound in evaluation of cerebral blood flow in neonates. Arch Dis Child 58: 677–681

Hill A, Volpe JJ (1982) Decrease in pulsatile flow in the anterior cerebral arteries in infantile hydrocephalus. Pediatrics 69: 4–7

Lipman B, Serwer GA, Brazy JE (1982) Abnormal cerebral hemodynamics in preterm infants with patent ductus arteriosus. Pediatrics 69: 778–781

Perlman JM, Volpe JJ (1982) Cerebral blood flow velocity in relation to intraventricular hemorrhage in the premature newborn infant. J Pediatr 100: 956–959

Perlman JM, Hill A, Volpe JJ (1981) The effect of patent ductus arteriosus on flow velocity in the anterior cerebral arteries: ductal seal in the premature newborn infant. J Pediatr 99: 767–771

Pourcelot L (1976) Diagnostic ultrasound for cerebral vascular diseases. In : Donald I, Levi S (eds) Present and future of diagnostic ultrasound. Kooyker Rotterdam, pp 141–147

Schick RW, Matson DD (1961) What is arrested hydrocephalus? J Pediatr 58: 791–799

Thompson RS (1987) Blood flow velocity waveforms. Semin Perinatol 11: 300–310

16 — Crossed Cerebellar Diaschisis in Hydrocephalus — Report of Three Cases

Mamoru Abe[1], Hirotoshi Sano, Tetsuo Kanno[2], and Hiroshi Toyama[3]

Summary. Three cases of crossed cerebellar diaschisis (CCD) in hydro-cephalus were studied by single photon emission CT (SPECT) using I-iodoamphetamine (I-123-IMP). In all patients CCD disappeared as a result of effective shunt operations. Abnormal neurological findings were completely normalized in two patients and moderately normalized in the other. One of the three patients had transient brain dysfunction induced in the postoperative course of subarachnoid hemorrhage and the other two patients had local parietal lobe brain damage observed on plain computed tomography (CT). CCD in hydrocephalus has not been reported on so far. As for the mechanism of CCD in these three cases, we speculate that the change of brain tissue press-ure resulting from brain damage may cause abnormal extension of hydrostatic edema, resulting in transneural metabolic depression of the cortico-ponto-cerebellar pathway. It is suggested that neural function is variable in hydro-cephalus with brain damage.

Keywords. Hydrocephalus — Crossed cerebellar diaschisis — I-123-IMP-SPECT

Introduction

The phenomenon of diaschisis as a mechanism of brain dysfunction was first described by Von Monakow in 1941 (Von Monakow 1969). Since then many experimental and clinical studies have entered the literature (Allen and Tsukahara 1974; Baron et al. 1981; Kanaya et al. 1983; Glickstein et al. 1985; Kempinsky 1958; Sasaki et al. 1977). Crossed cerebellar diaschisis (CCD) contralateral to supratentorial infarction was described by Baron et al. (1981), using positron emission tomography (PET) and the steady-state oxygen-15 method.

[1] Department of Neurosurgery, Yachiyo Hospital, Aichi, 470–11 Japan
[2] Departments of Neurosurgery and [3] Radiology, Fujita Health University, School of Medicine, Toyoake, Aichi, 470-11 Japan

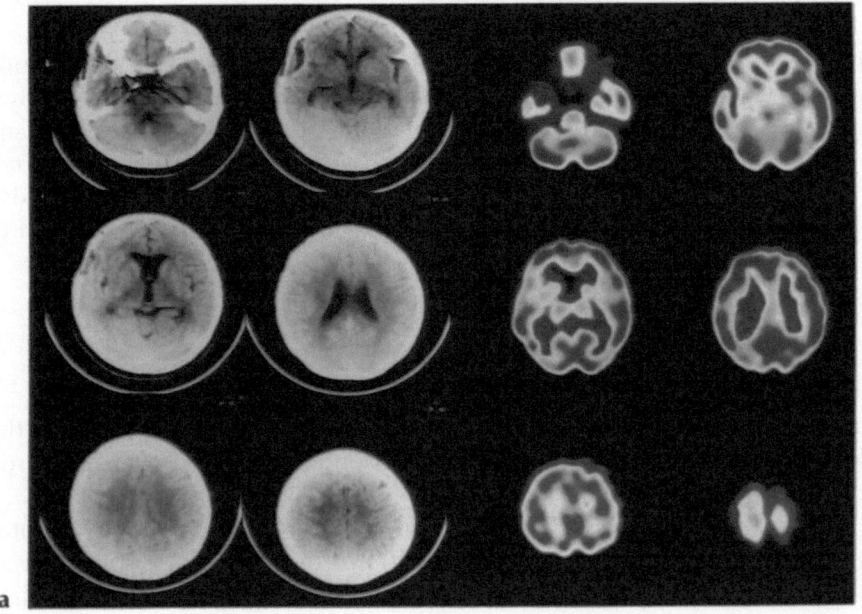

Fig. 1. Case 1: at the time of improved transient aphasia after clipping operation. **a** Plain CT shows ventricle which is only mildly enlarged **b** rCBF image of I-123-IMP-SPECT shows low perfusion in the left temporal lobe.

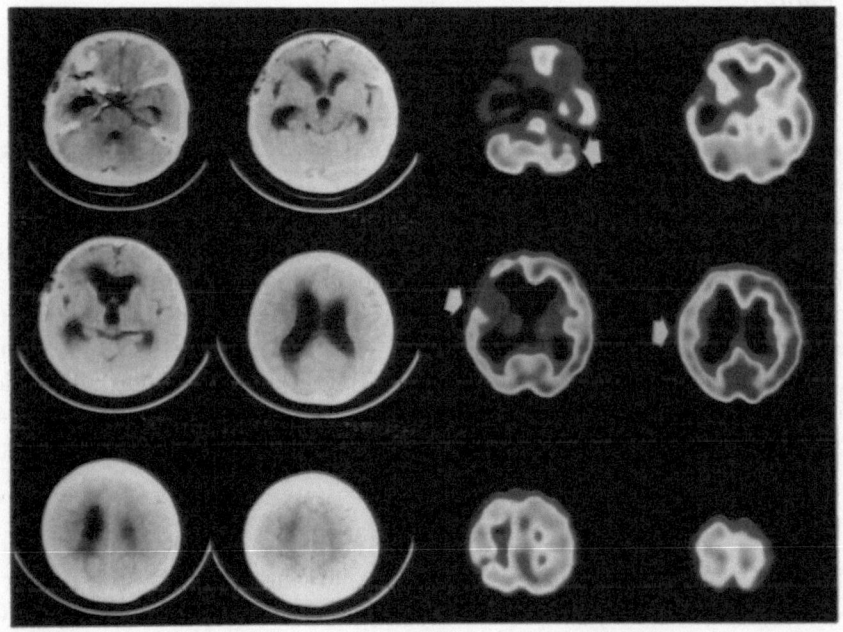

Fig. 2. Case 1: on admission for hydrocephalus. **a** Plain CT shows marked ventricular dilatation with periventricular lucency (*left* > *right*). **b**: I-123-IMP-SPECT shows crossed cerebellar diaschisis, low perfusion of left supratentorial area and contralateral cerebellum (*arrowhead*)

Up to now CCD has not only been reported in relation to cerebral infarction but also in relation to intracranial hemorrhage (Kanaya et al. 1983), moya-moya disease, and arterio-venous malformation (Toshimatsu et al. 1986) and brain tumors (Kusher et al. 1984). However, CCD in hydrocephalus has not been reported on so far. Our findings show that CCD in hydrocephalus disappears as a result of shunt operations. We also looked into the mechanism of CCD in hydrocephalus.

Clinical Materials and Methods

We measured regional cerebral blood flow (rCBF) by I-123-IMP-SPECT in the 3 patients with hydrocephalus; after the shunt operations rCBF was measured in the same way.

We used a ring type SPECT Headtome set-031 (Shimazu Corp., Kyoto, Japan). The full width at half maximum (FWHM) of the spatial resolution was 12.4 mm for high resolution (HR) and 19.8 mm for high sensitivity (HS). Slice thickness was 17.5 mm for HR and 29.0 mm for HS at the center of the field of view. The rCBF study by I-123-IMP was measured on the basis of the microsphere method.

Case Reports

Case 1

A 57-year-old female who had a clipping operation through the left pterion for ruptured aneurysm of the left middle cerebral artery on April 9th 1987. She developed transient postoperative aphasia, but gradually improved. At that time a plain CT showed normal findings (Fig. 1a) and the rCBF image on I-123-IMP-SPECT showed low perfusion in the left temporal lobe (Fig. 1b). Five months after the first operation she developed disorientation. A plain CT showed hydrocephalus (Fig. 2a). The rCBF image on I-123-IMP-SPECT showed CCD (Fig. 2b). A shunt operation was performed which successfully brought about the disappearance of the CCD (Fig. 3a,b) and marked clinical improvement. CCD of this case was also assessed in the r-CBF-study (Fig. 4).

Case 2

A 56-year-old male who had a shunt operation for hydrocephalus after a subarachnoid hemorrhage in 1986. One year following the operation, he developed gait disturbance, dementia and urinary incontinence, which a plain CT showed as hydropcehalus and local brain damage in the right parietal lobe caused by vasospasm (Fig. 5a). The rCBF image on I-123-IMP showed low perfusion of the bi-frontal lobe and CCD (Fig. 5b). We realised that the shunt system was impaired, but fortunately it repaired itself by natural means, and as a result the patient also improved clinically. Plain CT showed an improvement

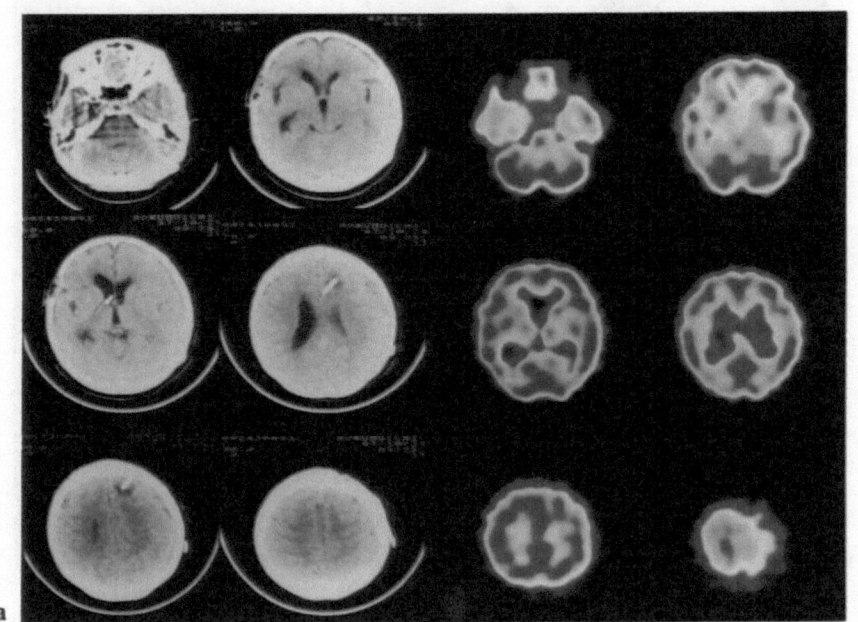

Fig. 3. Case 1: after shunt operation. **a** Plain CT shows reduction of size of ventricule and disappearance of periventricular lucency. **b** I-123-IMP-SPECT shows normal perfusion and disappearance of CCD

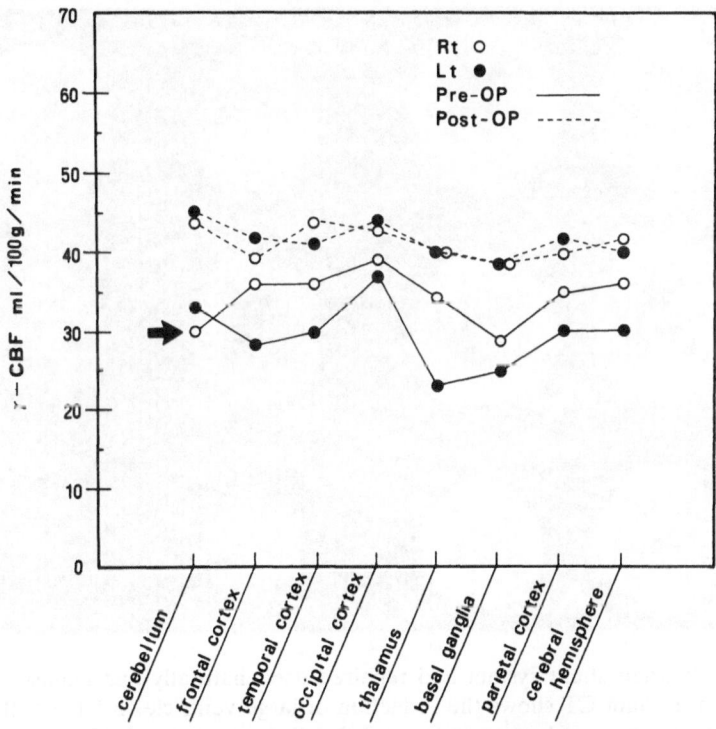

Fig. 4. Case 1: rCBF study on I-123-IMP-SPECT shows the pattern of CCD (*black arrowhead*) and recovery to normal CBF after shunt operation

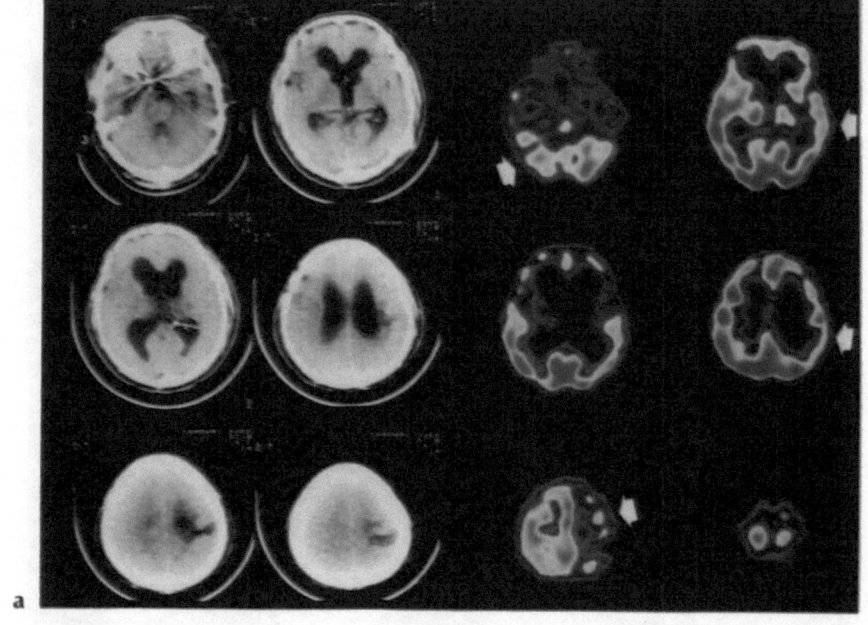

Fig. 5. Case 2: when hydrocephalus developed following shunt malfunction. **a** Plain CT shows hydrocephalus and local brain damage in the right parietal lobe. **b** I-123-IMP-SPECT shows low perfusion of bifrontal lobe and CCD (*white arrowhead*)

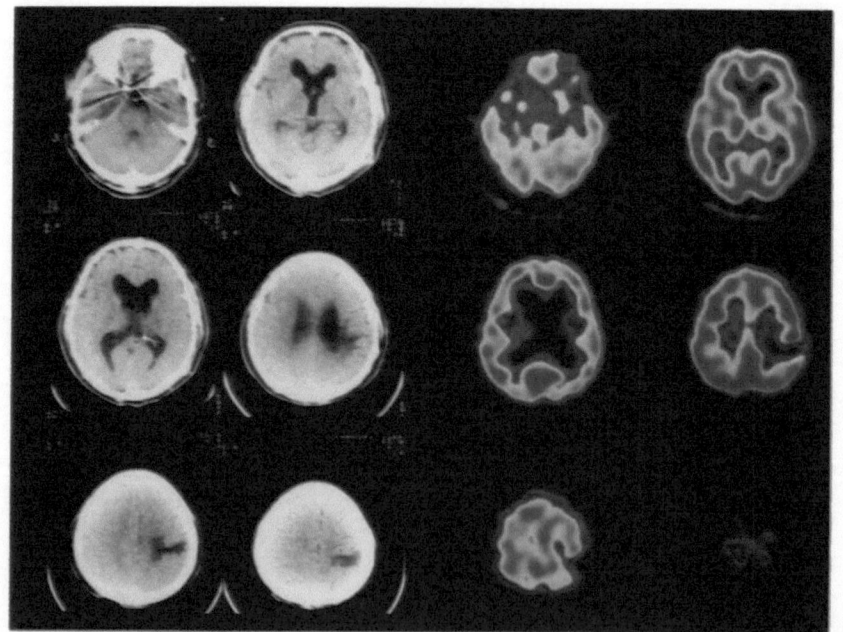

Fig. 6. Case 2: when shunt system had repaired itself naturally and clinical condition had improved. **a** Plain CT shows the reduction of large ventricle. **b** I-123-IMP-SPECT shows the improvement of low perfusion and the disappearance of CCD

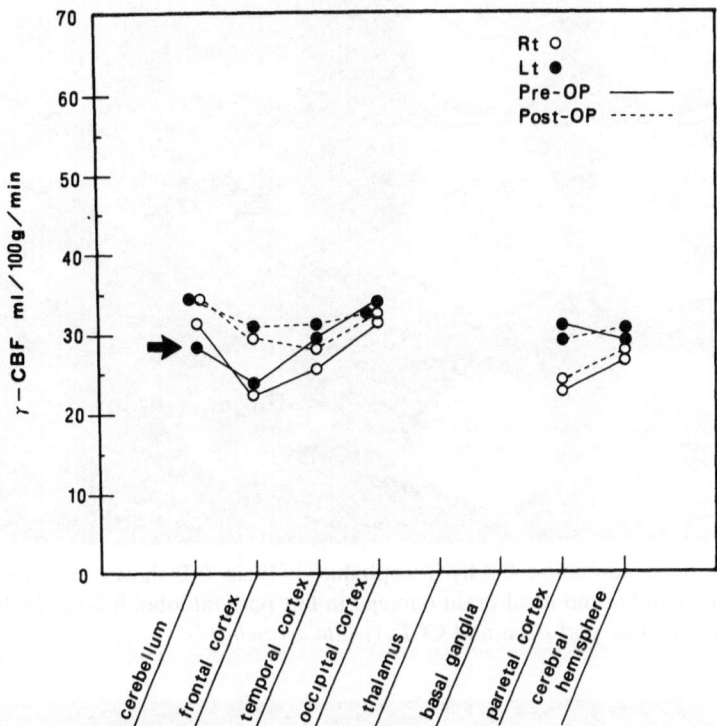

Fig. 7. Case 2: rCBF study (I-123-IMP-SPECT) shows the pattern of CCD (*black arrowhead*) and the improvement after shunt system was repaired

of hydrocephalus (Fig. 6a) and r-CBF image and measurement on I-123-IMP-SPECT showed the disappearance of CCD (Fig. 6b, Fig. 7).

Case 3

A 56-year-old male who was operated for an acute subdural hematoma in the left parietal area in 1986. Hydrocephalus later developed because of meningitis contracted post operatively. He developed dementia, gait disturbance, and urimary incontinence. Plain CT showed hydrocephalus and CCD was shown in the rCBF image on I-123-IMP-SPECT (Fig. 8a,b). A shunt operation resulted in mild clinical improvement and the disappearance of CCD (Figs. 9 and 10).

Discussion

The phenomenon of diaschisis as a mechanism of brain dysfunction was first described by Von Monakow in 1941 (Von Monakow 1969). CCD as one of the diaschisis phenomena was described in supratentorial infarction in a human by Baron et al., using PET, in 1981. Since then CCD has been reported in

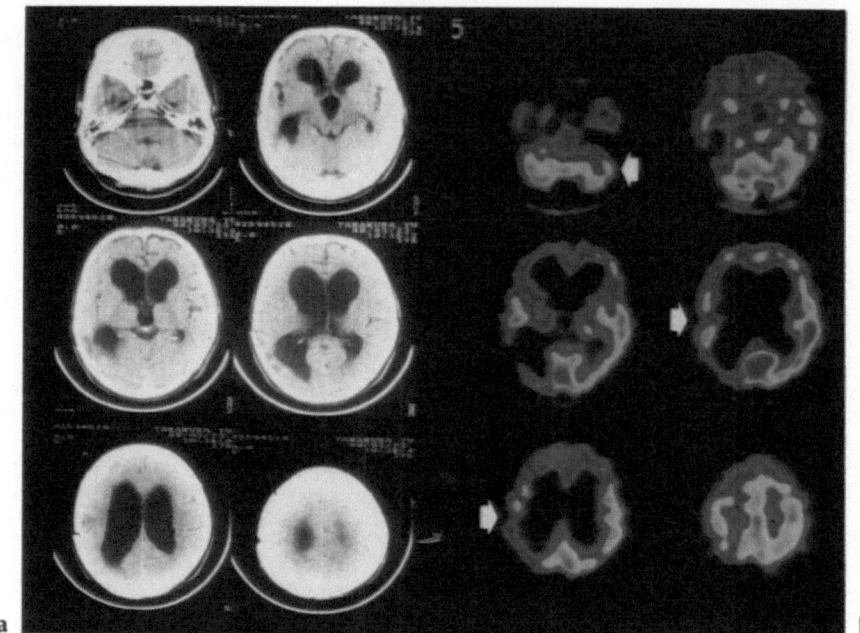

Fig. 8. Case 3: on admission for hydrocephalus. **a** Plain CT shows remarkable large ventricle (*left > right*) and local brain damage in left parietal lobe. **b** I-123-IMP-SPECT shows remarkable low perfusion and CCD (*white arrowhead*)

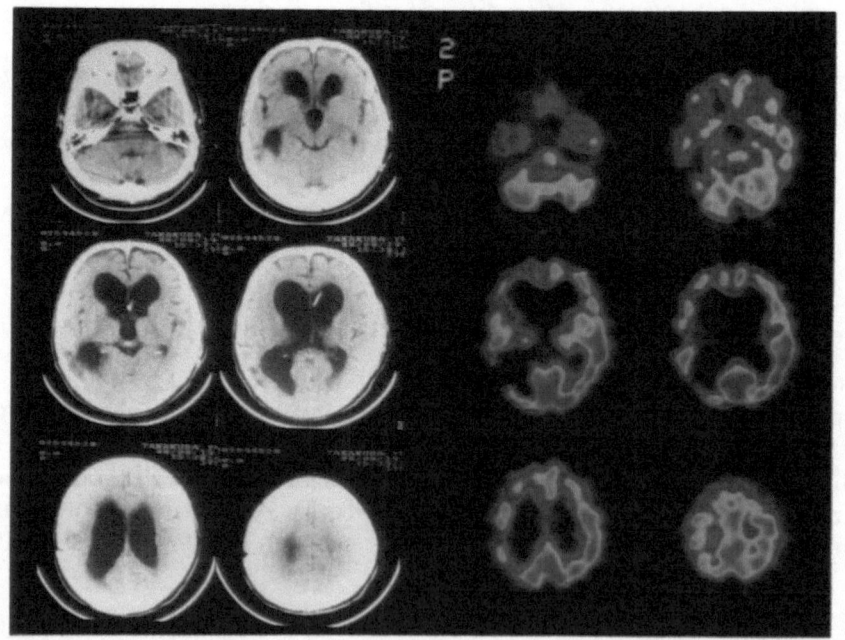

Fig. 9. Case 3: after shunt operation. **a** Plain CT shows minimum reduction of ventricle **b** I-123-IMP-SPECT shows mild improvement of low perfusion and the disappearance of CCD

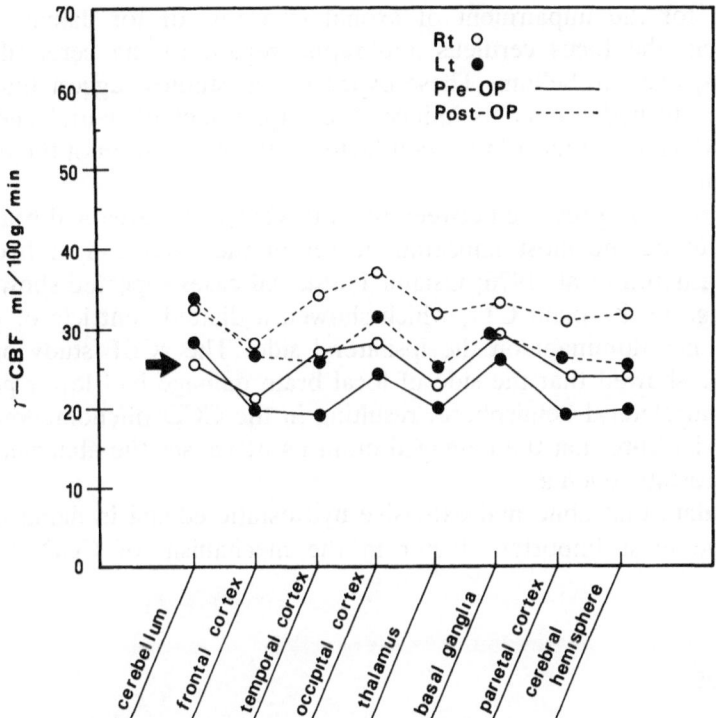

Fig. 10. Case 3: rCBF study (I-123-IMP-SPECT) shows the pattern of CCD and its disappearance and improved rCBF after shunt operation

intracerebral hemorrhage (Kanaya et al. 1983), in moya-moya disease and in arterio-venous malformation (Toshimatsu et al. 1986) and in brain tumors (Kushner et al. 1984).

The mechanism of CCD has been thought to be the most likely cause of transneural metabolic depression through the cerebrocerebellar pathway (Allen and Tsukahara 1974; Brodal 1969, 1978; Glickstein et al. 1985).

Hydrocephalus, namely normal pressure hydrocephalus, was first reported by Hakim and Adams in 1965 as being characterised by three symptoms, dementia, gait disturbance, and urinary incontinence. Shunt operations proved to be remarkably effective in improving these conditions.

The change in intraventricular pressure brought about by cerebrospinal fluid impairment in hydracephalus induces ventricular enlargement and, additionally, hydrostatic edema develops (Marmarou et al. 1976; Osamu 1986). Nariyuki et al. (1987) proved that hydrostatic edema in experimentally induced hydrocephalus resulted in the impairment of cerebral energy metabolism over an extensive area. Also, in hydrocephalus of neonatal rats, George et al. (1988) reported that decreases in norepinephrine, dopamine, and serotonin were observed in the cerebral cortex, neostriatum, and cerebellum. Serotonin and norepinephrine in the brain stem were increased. From the results of these data it is suggested that the alterations of these neurotransmitters may be responsible for the impairment of axonal transport or for damage to projections from the locus ceruleus and raphe region to the cerebral cortex, neostriatum, and cerebellum. These experimental studies suggest that hydrostatic edema in hydrocephalus induces the impairment of neural and axonal transport, which is the most important factor in the mechanism of the diaschisis phenomenon.

The difference in pressure between the intraventricular area and brain tissue is thought to be the most important factor in the extension of hydrostatic edema (Marmarou et al. 1976; Osamu 1986). All cases reported showed local brain damage in the plain CTs, which showed a dilated ventricle or periventricular lucency dominant on the ipsilateral side. The rCBF study on I-123-IMP-SPECT showed that the side of local brain damage had lower perfusion than the contralateral hemisphere, resulting in the CCD phenomenon. These results may indicate that the damaged brain tissue causes the abnormal extension of hydrostatic edema.

We speculate that abnormal extensive hydrostatic edema in damaged brain tissue is the most important factor in the mechanism of CCD in hydrocephalus.

References

Allen GI, Tsukahara N (1974) Cerebrocerebellar communication systems. Physiol Rev 54: 957–1006

Baron JC, Bousser MG, Comar D, Duquesnoy N, Sastre J, Castaigne P (1981) "Crossed Cerebellar Diaschisis" a remote functional depression secondary to supratentorial infarction of man. J Cereb Blood Flow Metab 1 (Suppl 1): S500–501

Brodal A (1969) Neurological anatomy in relation to clinical medicine. Oxford University Press, New York

Brodal A (1978) The corticopontine projection in the rhesus monkey. Origin and principles of organization. Brain 101: 251–283

George I Chovanes, James P McAllister II, Albert A Lamperti, Arnold G Salott, Raymond C Truex (1988) Monoamine alterations during experimental hydrocephalus in neonatal rats. Neurosurgery 22: 86–91

Glickstein M, May JG, Mericier BE (1985) Corticopontine projection in the macaque; the distribution of labelled cortical cells after large injections of horseradish peroxidase in the pontine nuclei. J Comp Neurol 235: 343–359

Hakim S, Adams RD (1965) The special clinical problem of symptomatic hydrocephalus with normal cerebrospinal fluid pressure. Observations on cerebrospinal fluid hydrodynamics. J Neurol Sci 2: 307–327

Nariyuki H, Takashi T, Yasuhide M, Isao K, Tatsuo K (1987) Alteration of cerebral energy metabolism and cytoskeletal protein with intra parenchymal routed CSF migration in the hydrocephalus. Nerv Syst Child 12(1): 11–17

Kanaya H, Endo H, Sugiyama T, et al. (1983) "Crossed Cerebellar Diaschisis" in patients with putaminal hemorrhage. J Cereb Blood Flow Metab 3 (Suppl 1): S27

Kempinsky WH (1958) Experimental study of distal effects of acute focal injury. Arch Neurol Psychiatr 79: 376–389

Kushner M, Alavi A, Reivich M, et al. (1984) Contralateral cerebellar hypometabolism following cerebral insult: A positron emission tomographic study. Ann Neurol 15: 425–434

Marmarou A, Shapiro K, Poll W, Shulman K (1976) Studies of kinetics of fluid movement within brain tissue. In: Beks JWF, Bosch DA, Brock M (eds) Intracranial pressure III. Springer, Berlin Heidelberg New York, pp 1–4

Osamu S (1986) Changes in concept: mechanism of genesis in hydrocephalus. Nerv Syst Child 11(2): 77–83

Sasaki K, Oka H, Kawaguchi S, Jinnnai K, Yasuda T (1977) Mossy fibre and climbing fibre responses produced in the cerebellar cortex by stimulation of the cortex in monkeys. Exp Brain Res 29: 419–428

Toshimatsu M, Noboru K, Junichi N, Kikuo M, Toru O, Kazuhiro T, Toru M, Eiju W, Masahiro I (1986) N-Isoproyl I-123p-iodoamphetamine (I-123IMP) SPECT-crossed cerebellar diaschisis. Jpn J Nucl Med 23(1): 25–34

Von Monakow C (1969) Diaschisis (1914 article translated by G. Harris). Pribram KH (ed) Brain and behavior. I: Mood states and mind. Baltimore, pp 27–36

III. CSF Hydrodynamics

17 — CSF Absorption Rates in Cats with Kaolin-Induced Hydrocephalus — a Study Using Different Kinds of Tracers of Different Molecular Size

Yoshinobu Nakagawa[1], Naomi Fujimoto, and Keizo Matsumoto[2]

Summary. The absorption rate of CSF was studied in experimental hydrocephalus, using three kinds of tracers. Hydrocephalic cats were divided into three groups: (1) acute, (2) subacute, and (3) chronic. Five normal cats were used as controls. Three different kinds of radioisotope — tritiated water (^{3}H), ^{14}C labeled albumin (^{14}C), and NaH_2PO_4 (^{32}P) — were used as tracers. Each tracer, dissolved in artificial CSF (MOS-4; SHIMIZU), was perfused between the lateral ventricles in each group. The perfusion pressure was increased stepwise by $5cmH_2O$ and $15cmH_2O$ before ligation of the spinal cord and was increased to $25cmH_2O$ after ligation. In normal cats the absorption rate of tritiated water was almost twice as much as that of ^{14}C and ^{32}P before and after ligation of the spinal cord. Pressure dependency was noted. In acute hydrocephalus the absorption rate for all tracers was reduced to about 1/3 that in normal cats. In the subacute state, the absorption rate of tritiated water (^{3}H) and electrolyte (^{32}P) gradually recovered. In the chronic state, the absorption rate of ^{14}C-labeled albumin also increased before ligation of the spinal cord. After ligation the absorption rate was reduced but was still perceptible. These findings indicated that there may be different pathways for each tracer.

Keywords. Hydrocephalus — CSF absorption — Blood-brain barrier

Introduction

After the basic study of Bering and Sato (1963), it was widely accepted that transventricular absorption of CSF took place in the hydrocephalic state. However, Eisenberg et al. (1974a) reported that the main absorption route of CSF in experimental cats was the central canal of the spinal cord and there was

[1] Department of Neurosurgery, National Kagawa Children's Hospital, Zentsuji, Kagawa, 765 Japan
[2] Department of Neurosurgery, School of Medicine, University of Tokushima, Tokushima, 770 Japan

negligible absorption of CSF through the ventricular wall. Since then there were no studies which demonstrated the transventricular absorption or existence of minor CSF pathways in experimental hydrocephalus. On the other hand, computed tomography (CT) cisternography has shown transit of contrast medium from the ventricular system to the parenchyma in patients with hydrocephalus. In two earlier studies, we examined paracellular pathways morphologically, using different kinds of tracers and reported that although passage of a large molecular tracer (HRP) was prevented, small molecules such as ionic lanthanum passed through the tight junctions between endothelial cells into the vessel lumens (Nakagawa et al. 1984, 1985). Furthermore, in another study lymphatic pathways were also demonstrated to be a minor CSF pathway in experimental hydrocephalus (Nakagawa et al. 1988). In order to study the transventricular absorption of each component of CSF, we used three different kinds of tracers of different molecular size to investigate CSF absorption rates in cats with kaolin-induced hydrocephalus.

Material and Methods

Experimental hydrocephalus was induced by injection of kaolin suspension into the cisterna magna of 15 adult mongrel cats weighing 3.0–4.0 kg. Hydrocephalic cats were divided into three groups each consisting of five animals: (1) acute (less than 2 weeks), (2) subacute (less than 4 weeks), and (3) chronic state (more than 8 weeks). Five normal cats were used as controls. Three different kinds of radioisotope — tritiated water (^{3}H) as a tracer of water, ^{14}C-labeled albumin as a tracer of protein, and NaH_2PO_4 (^{32}P) as a tracer of electrolyte — were used. The animals were anesthetised by intramuscular injection of ketamin and then intubated. After the insertion of catheters into the femoral artery and vein, the head of the animal was fixed into a stereotactic frame in the sphinx position. Respiration was controlled to maintain: systemic arterial pressure, 100–140 mmHg; pH, 7.30–7.45; $PaCO_2$, 35–45 mmHg; and PaO_2, 80–120 mmHg. After lineal skin incision, two small burr holes were made 3 mm posterior to the coronal suture and 3 mm lateral to the sagittal suture in the bilateral parietal area. Needles (19G) with polyethylene tubes were inserted into each lateral ventricle through the burr holes. The needles were fixed by cranioplasty kit to prevent the leakage of CSF. The ventricular system was then perfused from one lateral ventricle to the other through the needles. Artificial cerebrospinal fluid (Shimizu Mos-4) containing three different kinds of tracers was pumped in at 0.123 ml/min. Before measurement, the ventricular system was perfused for 40–60 min until a stable count of each isotope was obtained. Afterward, CSF flowing out of the ventricle (hydrocephalus) or cistern (control) was collected for 10 min. Six samples were obtained at each perfusion pressure and the mean cerebrospinal absorption was calculated according to the method of Heisey et al. (1962). The perfusion pressure was increased stepwise, by 5cmH$_2$O and by 15cmH$_2$O before ligation of the spinal cord. The baseline was the interaural line. Following ligation,

Table 1. Absorption rate calculated for each tracer at each perfusion pressure before and after spinal cord ligation

tracers	perfusion pressure cmH2O	before ligation		after ligation		
		5	15	5	15	25
control	³H	7.59 ± 2.45	8.62 ± 2.07	7.69 ± 2.02	8.86 ± 2.66	9.87 ± 2.44
	¹⁴C	3.45 ± 1.21	4.66 ± 1.87	3.48 ± 1.57	4.20 ± 1.20	5.60 ± 1.56
	³²P	3.46 ± 1.24	3.98 ± 0.31	3.08 ± 0.60	3.71 ± 0.69	5.75 ± 1.35
acute	³H	2.79 ± 0.60	3.86 ± 0.92	2.69 ± 0.87	2.89 ± 0.75	3.16 ± 0.72
	¹⁴C	1.36 ± 0.33	3.05 ± 1.13	1.60 ± 0.87	1.97 ± 1.06	2.44 ± 1.26
	³²P	0.57 ± 0.15	1.87 ± 0.37	1.00 ± 0.65	1.60 ± 0.74	1.59 ± 0.81
subacute	³H	4.31 ± 1.45	4.76 ± 1.96	2.93 ± 0.95	3.05 ± 0.54	3.55 ± 1.01
	¹⁴C	1.84 ± 0.92	3.31 ± 1.07	1.09 ± 0.64	1.84 ± 0.89	1.91 ± 0.91
	³²P	3.33 ± 1.28	4.15 ± 1.58	2.41 ± 0.91	2.74 ± 0.81	3.11 ± 1.05
chronic	³H	5.89 ± 1.57	7.53 ± 2.42	5.19 ± 0.91	5.16 ± 0.82	5.66 ± 0.83
	¹⁴C	3.56 ± 1.05	5.56 ± 2.46	1.96 ± 0.85	2.13 ± 0.97	2.64 ± 1.02
	³²P	3.71 ± 1.68	5.42 ± 2.12	2.36 ± 0.85	2.87 ± 0.54	3.25 ± 0.75

$\times 10^{-2}$ mℓ/min

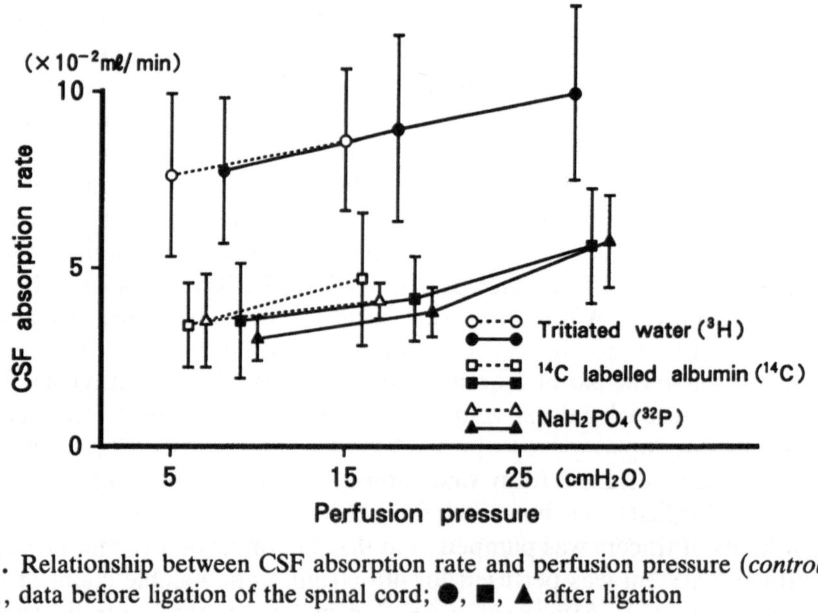

Fig. 1. Relationship between CSF absorption rate and perfusion pressure (*control*). ○, □, △, data before ligation of the spinal cord; ●, ■, ▲ after ligation

the perfusion pressure was increased likewise, by 5cmH₂O and 15cmH₂O to 25cmH₂O. After all the procedures had been carried out, the ventricular system was perfused with Evans-blue and the brain and spinal subarachnoid space were investigated.

Results

In the control animals, the absorption rate of tritiated water was almost twice as much as that of ^{14}C-labeled albumin and electrolyte (^{32}P) (Table 1 and Fig. 1). Before and after ligation of the spinal cord, the absorption rate changed very little and it continued to be dependent on pressure. In the acute state of hydrocephalus, the cerebro-spinal absorption rate for all tracers was reduced to about 1/3 of that in normal cats. At 5cmH$_2$O perfusion pressure, there was no remarkable difference between the absorption rates before and after spinal cord ligation (Fig. 2). In the subacute state, the absorption rate gradually recovered. The absorption rate of tritiated water was more than half that in the controls. Absorption of the electrolyte (^{32}P) increased to the control level. Absorption of ^{14}C-labeled albumin remained at a lower level but showed pressure dependency before spinal cord ligation (Fig. 3). In the chronic state, absorption of tritiated water was still reduced, however, absorption of ^{14}C-labeled albumin and electrolyte (^{32}P) recovered to the normal level. These rates were dependent on the pressure before spinal ligation (Fig. 4). After ligation of the spinal cord, the absorption rates of albumin (^{14}C) and electrolyte (^{32}P) were reduced but were still perceptible, whereas in the study by Eisenberg et al. (a) these absorption rates were found to be zero. The absorption rate of tritiated water showed no remarkable reduction either before or after ligation of the spinal cord. The absorption rate at 5cmH$_2$O perfusion pressure in each state of hydrocephalus is shown in Fig 5. In control and in the acute state there were no remarkable differences between the absorption rate before and after the ligation of the spinal cord. There may be no cerebro-spinal fluid pathways between the ventricular system and the

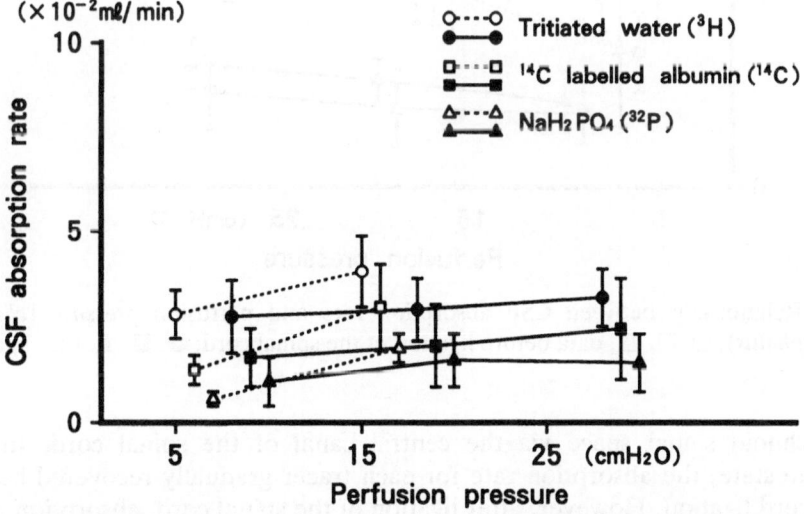

Fig. 2. Relationship between CSF absorption rate and perfusion pressure (*acute hydrocephalus*). ○, □, △, data before ligation of the spinal cord; ●, ■, ▲ after ligation

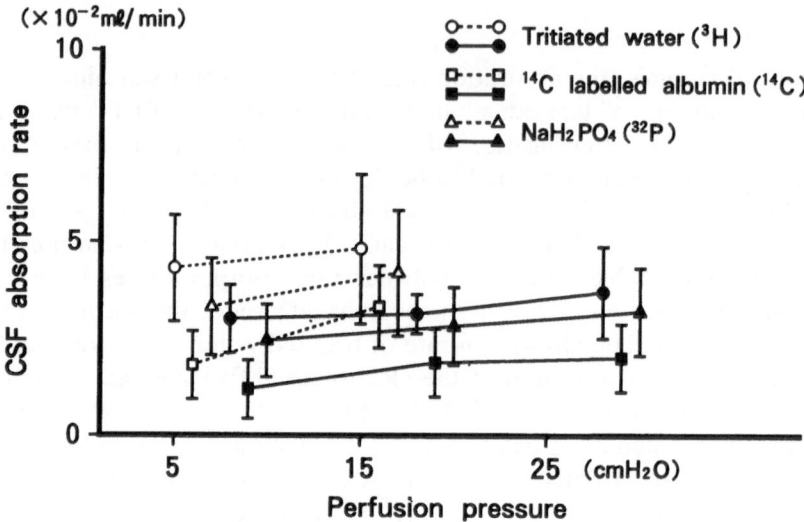

Fig. 3. Relationship between CSF absorption rate and perfusion pressure (*subacute hydrocephalus*). ○, □, △, data before ligation of the spinal cord; ●, ■, ▲ after ligation

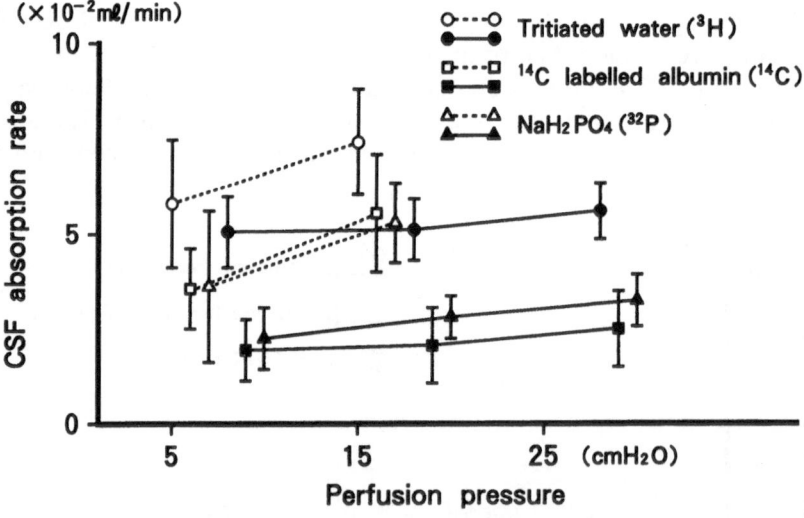

Fig. 4. Relationship between CSF absorption rate and perfusion pressure (*chronic hydrocephalus*). ○, □, △, data before ligation of the spinal cord; ●, ■, ▲ after ligation

subarachnoid spinal space via the central canal of the spinal cord. In the subacute state, the absorption rate for each tracer gradually recovered before spinal cord ligation. However, after ligation of the spinal cord, absorption rates remained lower. In the chronic state, absorption rates recovered to the normal levels. After ligation of the spinal cord, absorption of albumin (^{14}C) and

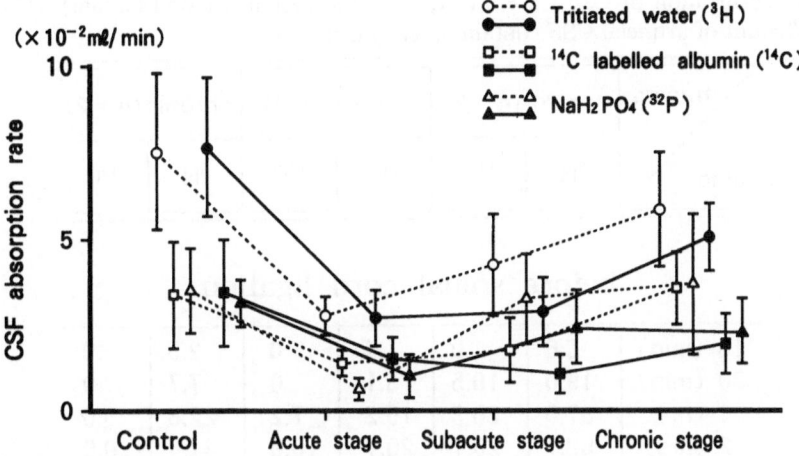

Fig. 5. CSF absorption rates at 5 cmH$_2$O perfusion pressure $\bigcirc$, $\square$, $\triangle$, before ligation and $\bullet$, $\blacksquare$, $\blacktriangle$ after ligation of the spinal cord

electrolyte (^{32}P) was reduced; tritiated water was absorbed at a constant rate before and after spinal cord ligation. These findings indicate that there may be different pathways for the absorption of each tracer in subacute and chronic states of hydrocephalus.

The transit of tracers from the ventricular system of the subarachnoid space into the systemic blood flow was investigated and the energy of each isotope was measured by scintillation counter. Tritium was detected within 5 min after commencing ventricular perfusion. The transit of ^{14}C-labeled albumin was delayed; it was detected 20 min after perfusion (Table 2).

Discussion

Transventricular cerebro-spinal fluid absorption was first proposed by Wislocki and Putnam (1921). Bering and Sato (1963) using the perfusion method, investigated such absorption between a lateral ventricle and the fourth ventricle in experimental hydrocephalic dogs. Their study supported the theory of transventricular absorption and gave an impetus to the idea of parenchymal absorption. Subsequent perfusion studies by Hochwald et al. (1969, 1975), Sahar et al. (1969), and other investigators confirmed the observations of Bering and Sato. Morphologically, however, the cerebrospinal fluid pathways into the parenchymal capillaries were not demonstrated. Eisenberg et al. (1974a,b), using radioisotope-labeled albumin, perfused the ventricular system in kaolin-induced hydrocephalus and investigated the cerebrospinal fluid absorption rate. Their study denied the possibility of transventricular absorption of cerebrospinal fluid. Since then, a few studies have suggested either transventricular absorption or the existence of minor CSF pathways in experimental hydrocephalus. On the other hand, in patients with hydrocephalus

Table 2. Permeation of CSF tracers (^{3}H, ^{14}C) into systemic blood (serum). (Count of serum)/(count of artificial CSF containing each isotope)

tracers / time	control (n = 2)		acute (n = 2)		chronic (n = 2)	
	^{3}H	^{14}C	^{3}H	^{14}C	^{3}H	^{14}C

before spinal cord ligation

15 (min)	5.6	0	1.4	0	2.5	0
30 (min)	19.0	10.5	5.1	0	7.7	0
1 (hr)	37.0	25.3	15.2	7.2	22.8	5.0
2 (hrs)	52.1	20.1	20.1	10.8	31.4	9.9
3	77.2	29.4	23.7	16.4	45.5	14.2
4	102.3	55.0	42.3	19.8	71.6	30.0

spinal cord ligation

5 (hrs)	146.0	64.5	40.2	15.3	63.4	32.1
6	168.4	70.2	50.8	20.2	91.0	50.2
7	179.0	92.3	70.4	34.3	132.1	67.1
8	263.9	142.0	91.5	51.7	164.2	79.5

stop of perfusion

9 (hrs)	54.7	41.4	17.6	12.0	34.2	20.1

$\times 10^{-4}$

computed tomography showed periventricular edema as hypodensity. Furthermore, CT cisternography demonstrated the transit of contrast medium from the ventricular system into the parenchyma of hydrocephalic patients. These findings indicated that interstitial edema fluid may be absorbed into the blood vessels in the parenchyma.

These considerations led us to a morphological study of experimental hydrocephalus. We used three kinds of tracers to look for paracellular pathways in experimental hydrocephalus.

It is well known that large molecular tracers such as horseradish peroxidase pass through the intercellular space between the ependymal cells and into the extracellular space around the neuropil. However, we found that horseradish peroxidase was apparently stopped by tight junctions (Nakagawa et al. 1988). On the other hand, in the same study we demonstrated that ionic lanthanum was present in the entire length of the intercellular space between endothelial cells. We postulated that, in the hydrocephalic state, small molecules may pass through the tight junctions between endothelial cells into the vessel lumens. Furthermore, we also investigated lymphatic pathways as a minor pathway of CSF in experimental hydrocephalus (Nakagawa et al. 1988). We perfused ventricular systems with Evans blue and found that the Evans blue was revealed not only in the spinal subarachnoid space but also in the cervical lymph and deep cervical lymph nodes. We postulated that there may be several pathways for the absorption of CSF in the hydrocephalic state.

In this study, we investigated absorption rates using three different kinds of tracers of different molecular size; we compared the measured rates of absorption in different hydrocephalic states. Tritiated water was used as a tracer for water but tritium can move freely through the membrane of the cell. Therefore, we started the study after a stable concentration of each isotope was obtained. The CSF absorption rate showed remarkable changes after ligation of the spinal cord and revealed pressure-dependent absorption rates. We believe that there are different absorption rates for each state and for each tracer.

According to this and our previous study (Nakagawa et al. 1988), we believe that the main CSF pathway in hydrocephalus is the central canal of the spinal cord. However, there may be other minor pathways for the absorption of CSF; one being the capillaries in the parenchyma and another being the lymphatic system.

References

Bering EA, Sato O (1963) Hydrocephalus: Changes in formation and absorption of cerebrospinal fluid within the cerebral ventricles. J Neurosurg 20: 1050–1063

Eisenberg HM, Mclennar JE, Welch K (1974a) Ventricular perfusion in cats with kaolin-induced hydrocephalus. J Neurosurg 41: 20–28

Eisenberg HM, Mclennar JE, Welch K, Treves S (1974b) Radioisotope ventriculograph in cats with kaolin-induced hydrocephalus. Radiology 110: 399–402

Heisey SR, Held D, Pappenheimer JR (1962) Bulk flow and diffusion in the cerebrospinal fluid system of the goat. Am J Physiol 203: 775–781

Hochwald GM, Sahar A, Sadik AR, Ransohoff J (1969) Cerebrospinal fluid production and histological observations in animals with experimental hydrocephalus. Exp Neurol 25: 190–199

Hochwald GM, Boal RD, Martin AE, Kuman AJ (1975) Changes in regional bloodflow and water content of brain and spinal cord in acute and chronic experimental hydrocephalus. Rev Med Child Neurol 17: 42–50

Nakagawa Y, Cervos-Navarro J, Artigas J (1984) A possible paracellular route for resolution of hydrocephalic edema. Acta Neuropathol (Berl) 64: 122–128

Nakagawa Y, Cervos-Navarro J, Artigas J (1985) Tracer study on a paracellular route in experimental hydrocephalus. Acta Neuropathol (Berl) 65: 247–254

Nakagawa Y, Fujimoto N, Matsumoto K (1988) Minor CSF pathway in experimental hydrocephalus. Nerv Syst Child 13: 463–468

Ogata J, Hochwald GM, Ransohoff J (1972a) Distribution of intraventricular horseradish peroxidase in normal and hydrocephalic cats. J Neuropathol Exp Neurol 31: 154–163

Ogata J, Hochwald GM, Gravito H, Ransohoff J (1972b) Light and electron microscopic studies of experimental hydrocephalus. Acta Neuropathol (Berl) 21: 213–223

Sahar A, Hochwald GM, Ransohoff J (1969) Alternate pathway for cerebrospinal fluid absorption in animals with experimental obstructive hydrocephalus. Exp Neurol 25: 200–206

Wislocki GB, Putnam TJ (1921) Absorption from the ventricles in experimentally produced internal hydrocephalus. Am J Anat 29: 313–320

18 — Subependymal CSF Absorption in Hydrocephalic Edema — Ultrastructural Localization of Horseradish Peroxidase and Brain Tissue Damage

Mitsusuke Miyagami, Tadashi Shibuya, and Takashi Tsubokawa[1]

Summary. The absorption of cerebrospinal fluid (CSF) in hydrocephalic edema was studied in kaolin-induced experimental hydrocephalus in 30 rats by observing the ultrastructural localization of horseradish peroxidase (HRP) as a tracer in relation to neuronal and glial cell brain tissue damage. In the acute stage of hydrocephalus HRP reactive products were diffusely observed in various parts of the deeper brain than in the chronic stage; its reaction products were distributed diffusely in the extracellular spaces and blood vessel walls and some of them were observed in the glial cells and neurons through the routed CSF transport area in both the acute and chronic stage.

In the chronic stage of hydrocephalus, the edema fluid was localized around the ventricle and there were reactive astrocytes with increased glial filaments due to the effects of reactive change caused by intracytoplasmic edema in the glial cells and degenerative changes in some neuronal processes. In blood vessel walls, HRP reactive products were mostly localized in the basement membrane, the increased pinocytotic vesicles of endothelial cells, and in swollen astrocytes in contact with the blood vessels in the subependymal layer. According to these findings, it become clear that hydrocephalic edema in the chronic stage is rapidly absorbed in the limited subependymal layer because of facilitation of CSF absorption caused by increased permeability of the reactive cells of the vessels.

Keywords. Hydrocephalus — CSF absorption — Horseradish peroxidase — Enzymehistochemistry — Hydrocephalic edema

Introduction

Previous studies have suggested that transventricular absorption of cerebrospinal fluid can occur when normal CSF circulation is obstructed and the fluid is prevented from reaching its normal absorption sites (Sahar et al. 1969, 1971).

[1] Department of Neurological Surgery, Nihon University School of Medicine, Itabashi-ku Tokyo, 173 Japan

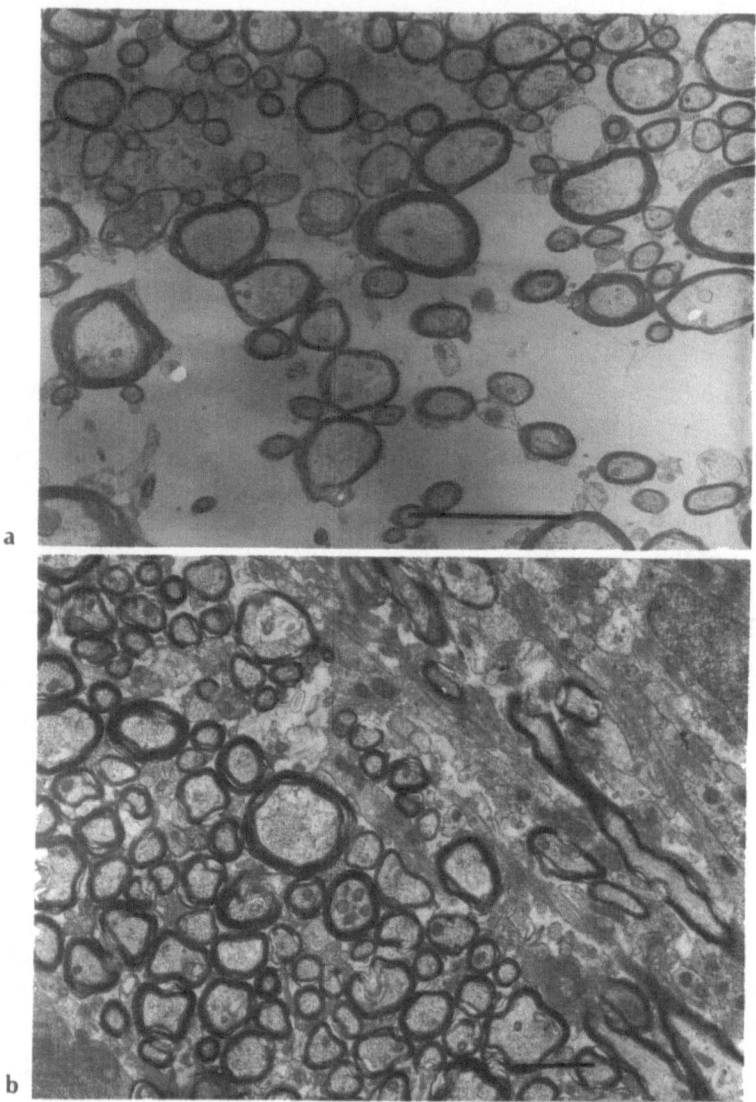

Fig. 1. Electronmicrographs ot **a** acute hydrocephalus 7 days after kaolin injection note marked extracellular spaces in subependymal tissues. **b** Chronic hydrocephalus 7 weeks after kaolin injection note slight enlargement of extracellular spaces and intracellular edema in the neuronal processes of the subependymal tissues. *Bar* = 1 µm

However, the mechanism and routes by which CSF returns to the blood are not entirely clear. Brain tissue damage may be more or less developed in the paraventricular area of hydrocephalus when CSF circulatory disturbance continues.

In this study, subependymal CSF absorption through the cerebral ventricular wall was examined by observing the ultrastructural localization of horseradish

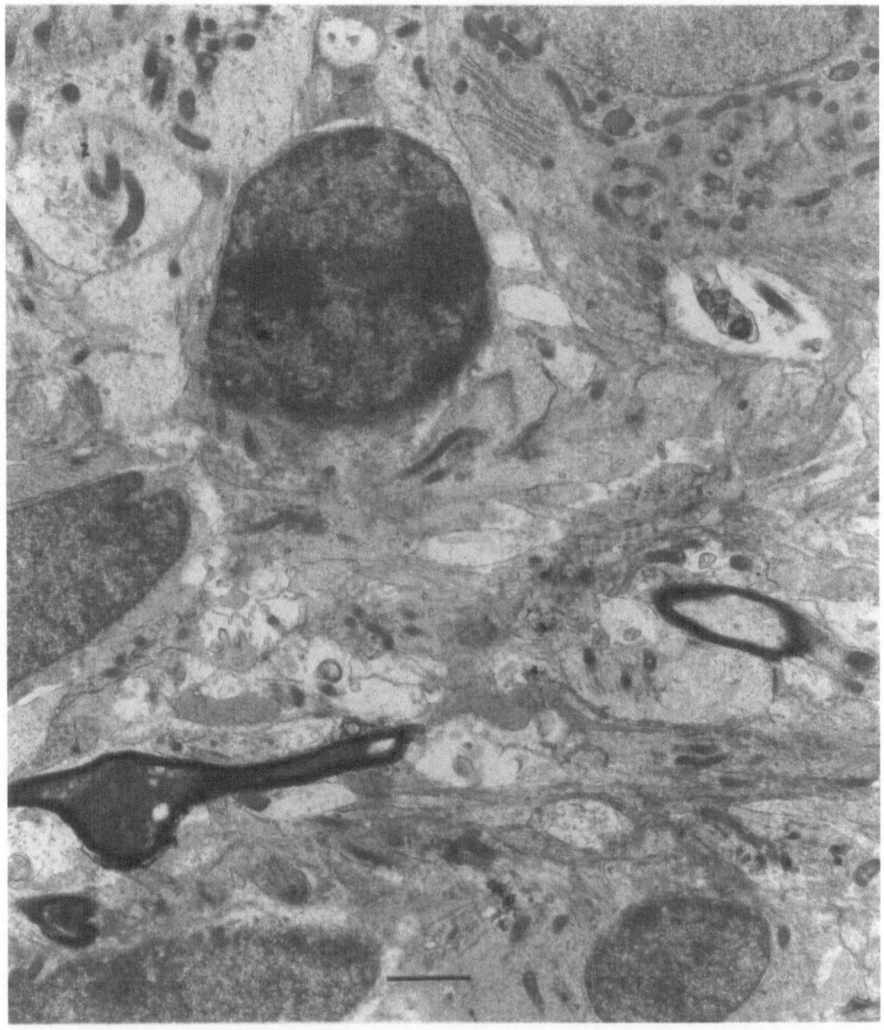

Fig. 2. Vacuole formation in the glial cells and degenerative findings demonstrating extensive increase of electron density and abnormal multi-lamellar bodies in neuronal processes, with intracellular edema in the subependymal tissues, 4 weeks after kaolin injection. *Bar* = 1 μm

peroxidase (HRP) as a tracer in relation to brain tissue damage in kaolin-induced experimental hydrocephalus.

Methods

Experimental hydrocephalus was induced by injecting kaolin 20 mg/0.1 ml into the cisterna magna of 46 rats. One, 2, 3, 4, 7, and 10 weeks after this injection

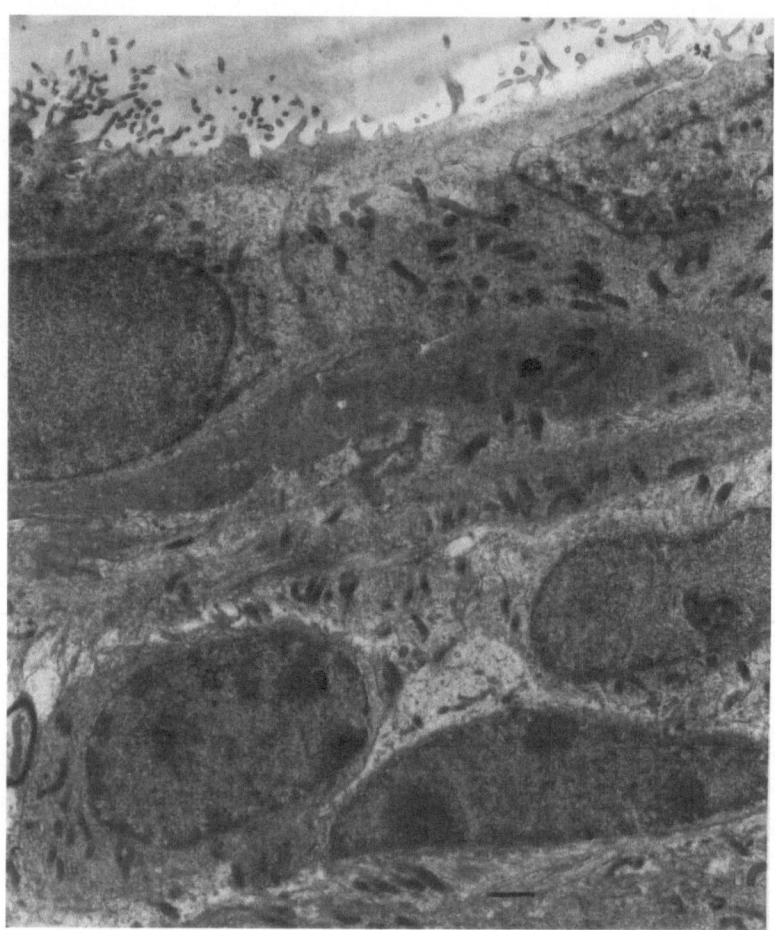

Fig. 3. Increase of glial filaments in the glial cells in the subependymal tissues 7 weeks after kaolin injection. *Bar* = 1 μm

had been carried out the morphological changes in the hydrocephalic rats were studied by light and electron microscope. Hydrocephalus was classified as acute when it occurred 1–3 weeks after kaolin injection and as chronic when it occurred more than 4 weeks after kaolin injection.

In 30 of these hydrocephalic rats, horseradish peroxidase (type II, Sigma) 10 mg per 0.1 ml per 10 min was injected stereotactically into the right lateral ventricle through a burr hole located 1 mm posterior from the bregma and 2 mm lateral from the sagittal suture in the right frontoparietal area. At 1 h after injection of horseradish peroxidase, all hydrocephalic rats were perfused through the cardiac route with 50% Karnovsky fixative. Immediately after the brains were evacuated they were fixed again with 50% Karnovsky solution for 1 h and non-frozen 30–40 μm-thick sections were made with a microslicer,

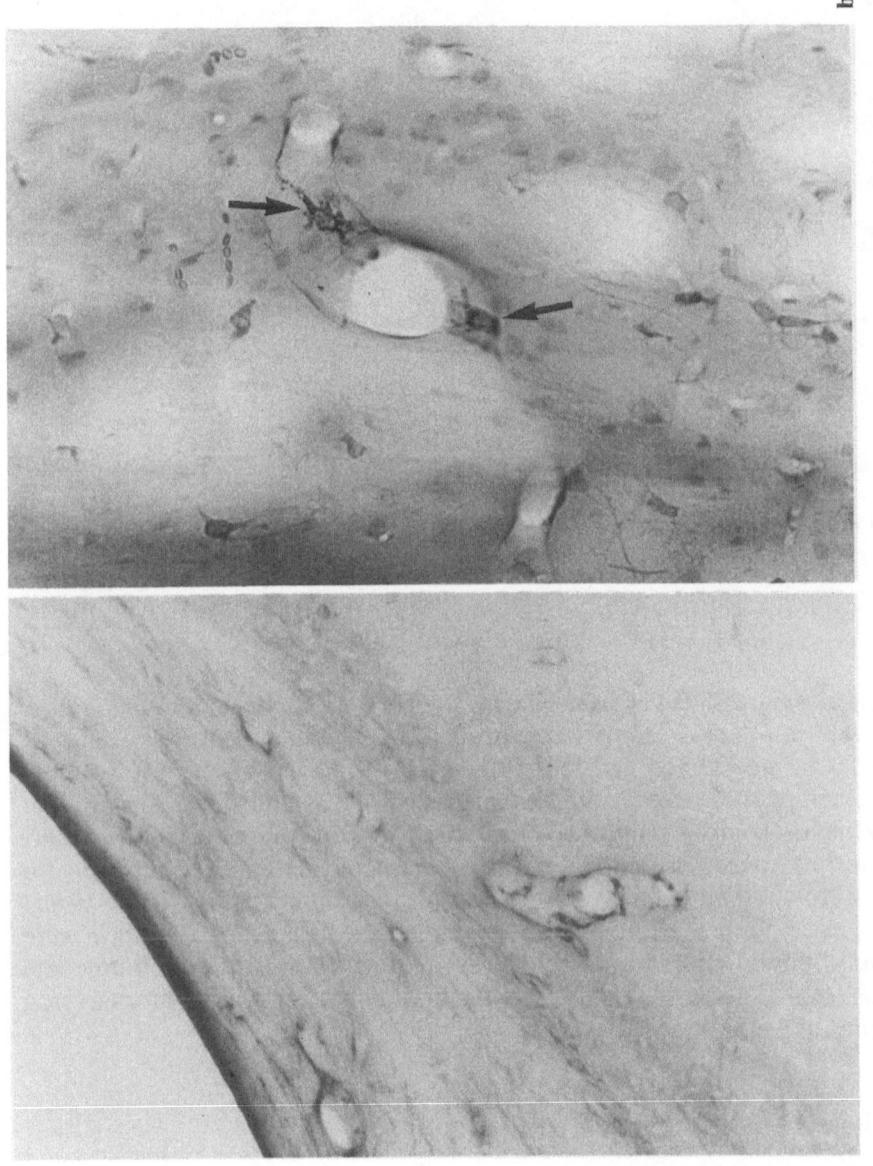

Fig. 4. a Acute hydrocephalus 7 days after kaolin injection. Note dense horseradish peroxidase reaction products from the ependymal surface to the deep brain in periventricular tissues and particularly, in blood vessels and glial cells in contact with them. **b** At high magnification dense dark horseradish peroxidase reaction products are seen in blood vessels and glial cells in contact with them in periventricular tissues (*arrows*)

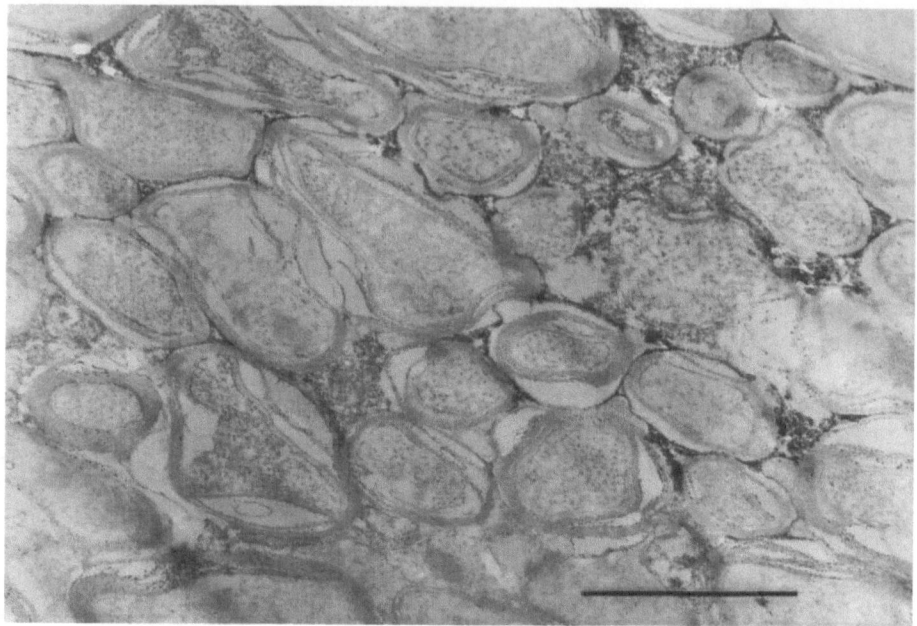

Fig. 5. On electron micrograph dark horseradish peroxidase reaction products are seen in the extracellular spaces around the neuropil and between myelin multilayers. *Bar =* 1 µm

following rinsing with 0.1 M cacodylate buffer (Ph 7.2). For light microscopical study 20–30 µm-thick sections were incubated in Graham-Karnovsky solution (DAB-4HCl 5 mg, 0.05 M Tris-HCl (Ph 7.6) 10 ml, 1% H_2O_2 0.1 ml) for 3 min at room temperature and counterstained with H.E. following rinsing. For electron microscopical study 40–50 µm-thick sections were incubated, using the same procedure as for light microscopical study, after preincubation for 15 min at room temperature with a solution containing DAB 4HCl 10 mg, distilled water 5 ml, 0.2 M phosphate buffer saline (Ph 6.5–7.0). They were then rinsed three times with 0.1 M cacodylate buffer for 10 min each time and were postfixed, dehydrated, and embedded in the manner standard for electron microscopical procedures.

Results

1. Brain Tissue Damage Resulting from Kaolin-Induced Experimental Hydrocephalus

About 1 week after kaolin injection into the cisterna magna, rats exhibited slow movement and gait disturbance together with appetite and weight loss.

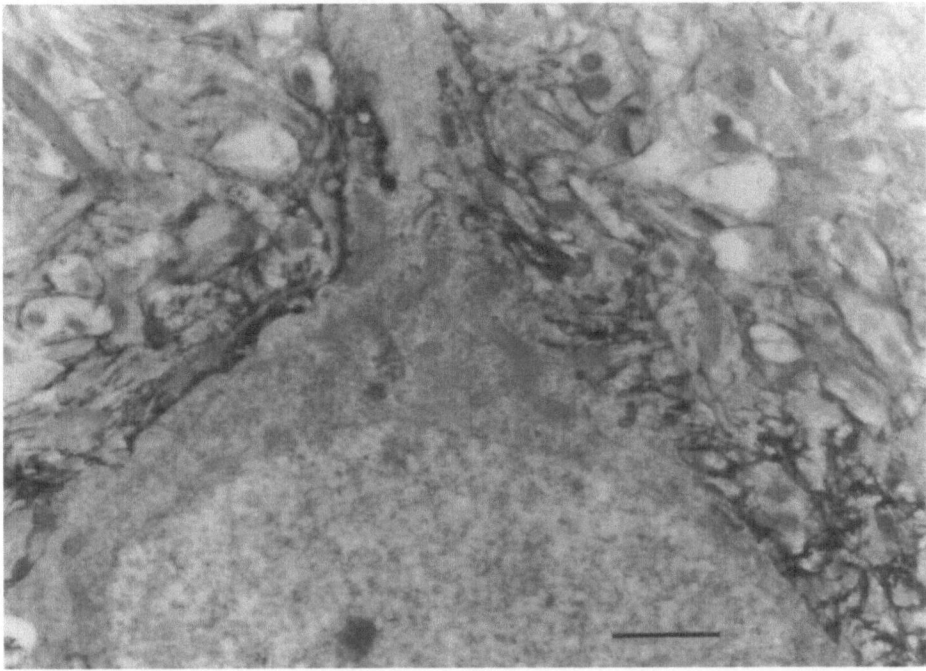

Fig. 6. Horseradish peroxidase observed in some vacuoles and organelles in the cytoplasm of nerve cells and also ın the intercellular spaces between the neuronal processes in the chronic stage, 4 weeks after kaolin injection. *Bar* = 1 μm

Ventricular size enlarged slightly 1–3 weeks after kaolin injection. Four weeks after that, ventricular size enlarged moderately or markedly in 70% of the 46 hydrocephalic rats. Acute hydrocephalus 1–3 weeks after kaolin injection appeared diffuse and spongy, a state caused by hydrocephalic edema; this state was more remarkable in the white matter of the paraventricular area in acute hydrocephalus than in chronic hydrocephalus occurring 4–10 weeks later. Hydrocephalic edema was more apparent in the paraventricular tissues around the lateral ventricle than around the 3rd or 4th ventricles. In chronic hydrocephalus ependymal cells became flat in shape and their cilia decreased in number. Sometimes there were increased macrophages on the ependymal surface and deficit of parts of the ependymal lining. However, the proliferation of glial cells or blood vessels in the subependymal tissues of chronic hydrocephalus did not appear on histological H.E. findings.

Electron microscopical observation of acute hydrocephalus showed marked enlargement of extracellular spaces in the glial cell layer and in the myelinated neuronal process layer of the subependymal tissues, whereas intracellular edema in these tissues was not marked. The neuronal processes and glial cells in these tissues had no degenerative changes. In addition, abnormal changes of organelles were demonstrated in the ependymal cells.

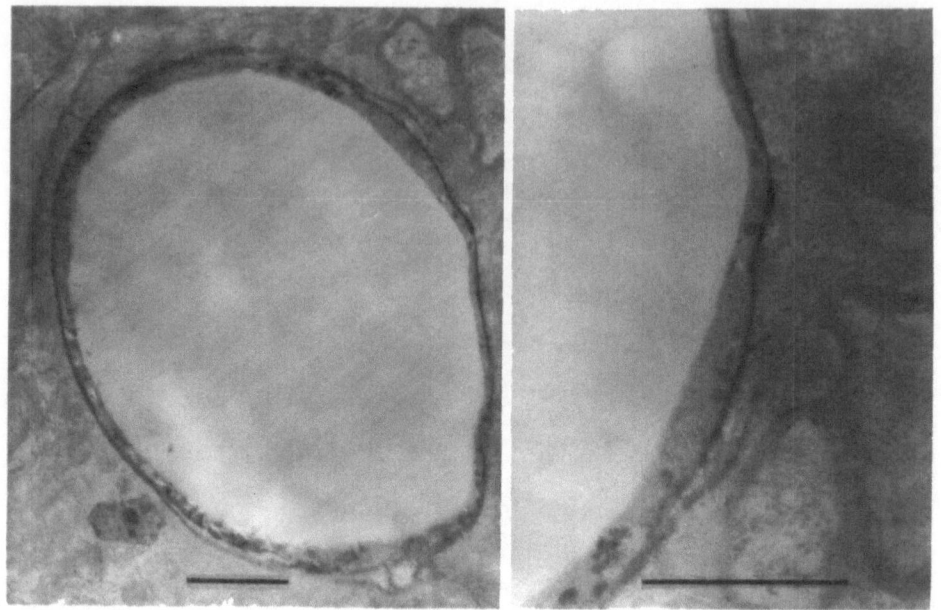

Fig. 7. a Dense horseradish peroxidase reaction products appear in the basement membrane and endothelial cell cytoplasm of a capillary. **b** At high magnification horseradish peroxidase appear in the basement membranes and increased pinocytotic vesicles in the endothelial cell cytoplasm, but not in the tight junction of endothelial clefts.

In chronic hydrocephalus, occurring 4–10 weeks after kaolin injection, ultrastructural findings demonstrated remarkably abnormal changes in the subependymal tissues 50–100 μm from the ependymal surface. Most of the ultrastructural changes in these tissues consisted of decreased electron density and/or swelling of cells due to the intracellular edema of neuronal processes and glial cells, whereas the extracellular spaces in these layers were not extensively enlarged when compared with conditions in acute hydrocephalus. Vacuole formation and obscuring of the neurotubulus in the dendrites and axons were frequently observed. In some dendrites and axons degenerative changes such as the formation of abnormal lamellar structures and extensive increase of electron density were observed; such changes may be a kind of dying back phenomenon of neurons. Some glial cells in the subependymal tissues of chronic hydrocephalus exhibited vacuole formation and cell membrane damage. The frequent appearance of glial cells with increased glial filaments in subependymal tissues may have indicated reactive astrocytosis. Also, glial cells around the capillary were swollen by intracellular edema; however, endothelial cells were not damaged and endothelial clefts were normal.

Deep white matter more than 100 μm from the ventricular surface demonstrated slight intracellular neuronal process and glial cell edema and some

Fig. 8. a Dense horseradish peroxidase reaction products in the cytoplasm of a glial cell around a capillary. **b** Some glial cells in subependymal tissues with dense reaction products in their cytoplasm.

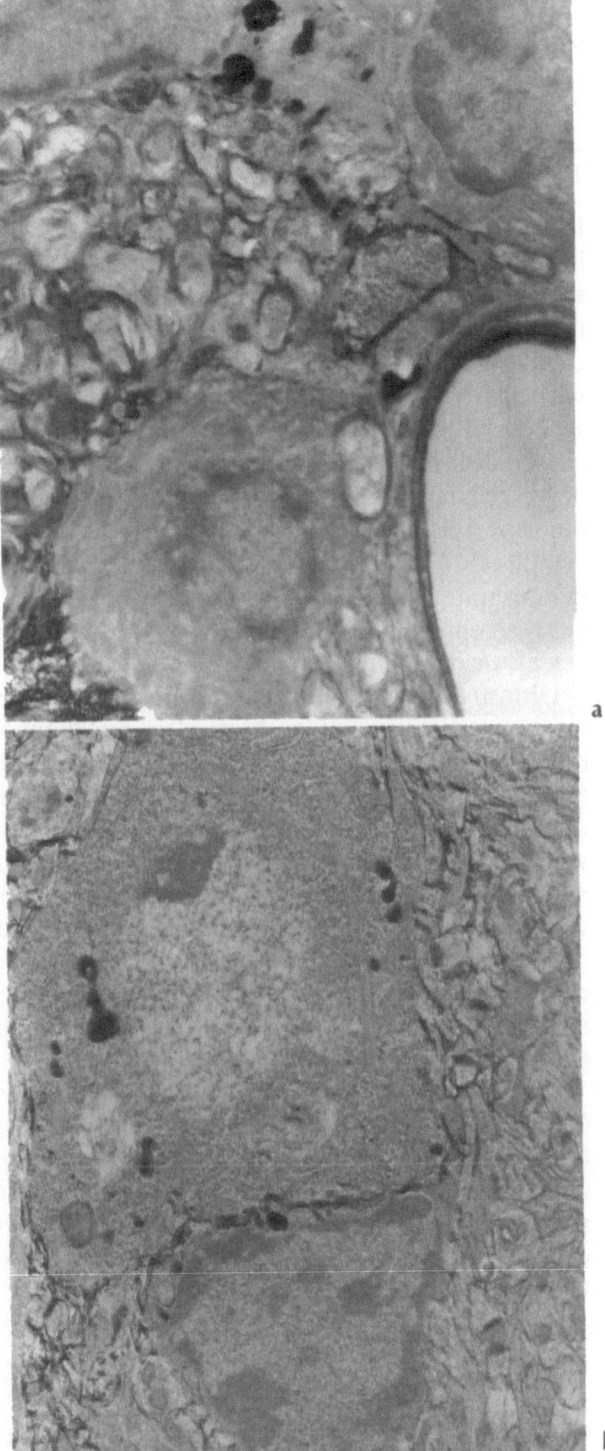

vacuole formation. Gray matter of the cerebral cortex and basal ganglia did not show abnormal changes in the ultrastructure of neuronal processes and glial cells.

2. Light and Electron Microscopical Localization of Horseradish Peroxidase in Experimental Hydrocephalus

In acute hydrocephalus showing a marked spongy state, horseradish peroxidase introduced into the right lateral ventricle appeared more deep and extensive from the ventricular surface than in chronic hydrocephalus. Horseradish peroxidase was distributed at a definite distance from the surface of the ventricular wall (but near the surface) in both acute and chronic hydrocephalus, particularly demonstrating much dark horseradish peroxidase staining in the several layers close to the ventricular surface. The dense reaction products of horseradish peroxidase appeared to be localized in blood vessels and in some nerve cells and glial cells. Some glial cells with cell processes in contact with blood vessels in periventricular tissues showed horseradish peroxidase in their cytoplasm. That finding was clearly observed in the deeper brain tissues which demonstrated decreasing horseradish peroxidase staining. It could be that at least cerebrospinal fluid high molecule proteins were absorbed into blood vessels through their contact with glial cells.

Ultrastructural localization of horseradish peroxidase was observed with non-stained sections. One hour after injection of horseradish peroxidase into the lateral ventricle the dark reaction products of horseradish peroxidase were localized mainly in the intercellular spaces between ependymal cells, glial cells, neuronal processes, and nerve cells and in the perivascular spaces. In the blood vessel walls of experimental hydrocephalus horseradish peroxidase clearly appeared, mainly in the basement membrane and in the increased pinocytotic vesicles of endothelial cell cytoplasm. However, the dense reaction products of horseradish peroxidase were not seen in the tight junctions of endothelial clefts. These findings suggested that horseradish peroxidase was absorbed into blood vessels by endothelial transport through the pinocytotic vesicles in endothelial cells.

Horseradish peroxidase was observed in the intracytoplasmic vacuoles and organelles of some glial cells in contact with blood vessels. This ultrastructural finding was consistent with the light microscopical finding of horseradish peroxidase localization in glial cells with glial processes in contact with blood vessels. In the subependymal layer of experimental hydrocephalus the cytoplasm of some nerve and glial cells had dense reaction products in some vacuoles, endoplasmic reticulum and ribosomes.

Discussion

Evidence for transventricular absorption of CSF as an alternate pathway in experimental hydrocephalus was provided by Wislocki and Putnam (1921). Bering and Sato (1963) showed the transventricular absorption pathway in normal and hydrocephalic dogs at the chronic stage. These workers determined that the CSF absorption rate was in direct proportion to the pressure gradient between the intraventricular pressure and the vein pressure of the superior sagittal sinus, using the perfusion method of Pappenheimer et al. (1962). Brightman and Reese (1969) suggested that both the concentration and the movement of HRP in brain tissues were primarily determined by diffusion. Studies by Sahar et al. (1969, 1971) have also shown that the difference in uptake of radiolabeled albumin in the periventricular white matter of both normal and hydrocephalic cats is dependent on the perfusion time and not on the perfusion pressure and that CSF absorption probably takes place within 2.5–3 mm from the ventricular surface. Lux et al. (1970) using more refined techniques based on the water content of brain slices brought absorption sites to within 600 μm from the ventricular surface. Nakagawa et al. (1985) reported that there were no obvious differences in the peroxidase staining spread from the ependymal surface into brain tissue at time intervals of 1, 2, and 4 weeks after kaolin injection. However, in our study the diffuse spread of horseradish peroxidase was distributed more deeply from the ependymal surface in the acute stage, 1–3 weeks after kaolin injection. It may be suggested that experimental hydrocephalus in the chronic stage has an increased absorption of CSF compared with that in the acute stage. We deduce this from the fact that there was not so much spongy state periventricular brain tissue in the chronic stage of hydrocephalus as in the acute stage and on the basis of the distribution of horseradish peroxidase in each stage.

In hydrocephalic patients periventricular edema has been shown as periventricular hypodensity on CT (Hopkins et al. 1977; Mori et al. 1980). It has been suggested that development of periventricular hypodensity in experimental hydrocephalic dogs is due to an increased transit of CSF from the ventricles into the white matter (Hiratsuka et al. 1982). However, the mechanism of the resolution of CSF or interstitial edema fluid is still disputed. On the basis of morphological and physiologic data gained by using high molecular weight, water-soluble compounds, it seemed likely that periventricular edema fluid in experimental hydrocephalus might be absorbed into blood vessels in the white matter (Bering and Sato 1963; Hochwald et al. 1969; Nakagawa et al. 1985; Ogata et al. 1972). Bowsher (1957) in an autoradiographic study reported that ^{35}S labeled serum protein injected into the ventricle of a normal cat penetrated into the capillaries in the brain tissues through the ependymal.

In this study, light microscopical examination showed that horseradish peroxidase injected into the ventricle distributed from the ependymal surface to various parts of the deep brain by diffusion and localized mainly in blood vessels and in some nerve and glial cells. On glial cells in contact with blood vessels frequently showed horseradish peroxidase in their cytoplasm. Ultrastructural localization of horseradish peroxidase was demonstrated mainly in the blood vessel walls and in the extracellular spaces between neuronal processes, nerve cells and glial cells in the periventricular tissues in both the acute and the chronic stages of hydrocephalus. In the capillaries, horseradish peroxidase localized mainly in the basement membrane and in the increased pinocytotic vesicles of endothelial cells, but not in the tight junctions of endothelial clefts. It is suggested that CSF absorption into the blood vessels was shown by the transendothelial transport through the pinocytotic vesicles of endothelial cells. In previous reports horseradish peroxidase (molecular weight 43 000), microperoxidase (2000), and ferritin (8 000 000) of high molecular weight used as tracers in experimental hydrocephalus penetrated into the extracellular spaces, but not into the tight junctions of endothelial clefts (Brightman 1965a,b; Milhorat et al. 1970; Ogata et al. 1972). However, Nakagawa et al. (1985), Simpson et al. (1977), and Bundgaard (1982) observed that lanthanum of low molecular weight (139.0) passed through the tight junctions of interendothelial clefts. From the present study most of the high molecular weight CSF components were absorbed mainly into the blood vessels directly through the extracellular spaces from the ependymal surface. However, it seemed from our horseradish peroxidase distribution data that some high molecular CSF components penetrated into some glial and nerve cells through the extracellular spaces at first and were then absorbed into the blood vessels by transendothelial transport.

Weller and Wisniewski (1969) and Ogata et al. (1972) found that in experimental hydrocephalic brain tissue damage the enlargement of extracellular spaces between ependymal cells and in the subependymal tissues appeared, on electron microscopical study, to be due to the transfer of CSF from the ventricle into the brain tissue. They called this finding "CSF edema", due to the enlargement of the extracellular spaces. Also, Fishman (1975) called it "hydrocephalic edema" which is consistent with the spongy appearance in the periventricular area that we noted on light microscopical examination of experimental hydrocephalus in this study. In the present study acute hydrocephalus 1–3 weeks after kaolin injection appeared diffuse and spongy, a state caused by hydrocephalic edema; this state was more remarkable in the white matter of the paraventricular area in acute hydrocephalus than in chronic hydrocephalus occurring 4–10 weeks later. On electron microscopical observation, acute hydrocephalus showed marked enlargement of extracellular spaces in the subependymal tissues which correlated with the spongy state seen on light microscopical examination. However, in chronic hydrocephalus the enlargement of extracellular spaces diminished. Most of the ultrastructural changes in the chronic stage demonstrated intracellular edema of neuronal processes and glial cells, with slight enlargement of the extracellular spaces in the white matter of the subependymal tissues. Some neuronal processes and glial cells had degenerative changes such as increased electron density and the formation of vacuoles and abnormal lamellar structures. These ultrastructural changes were observed in the subependymal tissues apparently $100 \mu m$ from the ependymal surface. Previous studies (Clark and Milhorat 1970; Gopinath et al. 1979; Hochwald et al. 1969; Milhorat et al. 1970; Miyagami et al. 1976; Ogata et al. 1972; Rubin et al. 1976; Weller and Wisniewski 1969) have reported brain tissue damage consisting of primary axonal damage and reactive astrocytosis with the enlargement of extracellular spaces in the white matter of subependymal tissues.

In contrast, Torvik et al. (1976) and Torvik and Stenwing (1977), in their light and electron microscopical study, found only hydrocephalic edema, but no neuron and glial cell brain tissue damage in experimental hydrocephalus.

In the present study of chronic hydrocephalus increased glial filaments in the glial cells, which might be due to the reactive changes of intracytoplasmic edema in those cells, were observed in the subependymal tissues. These findings were consistent with the ultrastructural localization of horseradish peroxidase seen in the cytoplasm of some glial cells in the subependymal tissues through the ependymal surface. This reactive astrocytosis was more conspicuous in the chronic hydrocephalus of 7–10 weeks than 4 weeks after kaolin injection and sometimes intracytoplasmic vacuoles and broken cell membranes with intracytoplasmic edema were seen in glial cells, as Gopinath et al. (1979) demonstrated on electron microscopical study of kaolin-induced hydrocephalus in rabbits.

Takei et al. (1987) studied two groups of cats by opening either the calvaria or the calvaria and the dura mater before injecting kaolin into the cisterna magna. In both groups they found large numbers of glial fibrils and reactive astrocytes filled with abnormal organelles of glycogen particles and mitochondria.

References

Bering EA Jr, Sato O (1963) Hydrocephalus: Changes in formation and absorption of cerebrospinal fluid within the cerebral ventricles. J Neurosurg 20: 1050–1063

Bowsher D (1957) Pathway of absorption of protein from the cerebrospinal fluid: An autoradiographic study in the cat. Anat Rec 128: 23–39

Brightman MW (1965a) The distribution within the brain of ferritin injected into cerebrospinal fluid compartments. I. Ependymal distribution. J Cell Biol 26: 99–122

Brightman MW (1965b) The distribution within the brain of ferritin injected into cerebrospinal fluid compartments. II. Parenchymal distribution. Am J Anat 117: 193–2201

Brightman MW, Rees TS (1969) Junctions between intimately apposed cell membranes in the vertebrate brain. J Cell Biol 40: 648–677

Bundgaard M (1982) Ultrastructure of frog cerebral and pial microvessels and their impermeability to lanthanum ions. Brain Res 241: 57–65

Clark RG, Milhorat TH (1970) Experimental hydrocephalus. Part 3. Light microscopic findings in acute and subacute obstructive hydrocephalus in the monkey. J Neurosurg 32: 400–413

Fishman RA (1975) Brain edema. N Engl J Med 293: 706–711

Gopinath G, Bhatia R, Gopinath PG (1979) Ultrastructural observations in experimental hydrocephalus in rabbits. J Neurol Sci 43: 333–344

Lux WE Jr, Hochwald GM, Sahar A, Ransohoff J (1970) Periventricular water content: Effect of pressure in experimental chronic hydrocephalus. Arch Neurol 23: 475

Hiratsuka H, Tabata H, Tsuruoka S, Aoyagi M, Okada K, Inaba Y (1982) Evaluation of periventricular hypodensity in experimental hydrocephalus by metrizamide CT ventriculography. J Neurosurg 56: 235–340

Hochwald GM, Sahar A, Sadik R, Ransohoff J (1969) Cerebrospinal fluid production and histological observations in animals with experimental obstructive hydrocephalus. Exp Neurol 25: 190–199

Hopkins LN, Bakay L, Kinkel WR, Grand W (1977) Demonstration of transventricular CSF absorption by computerized tomography. Acta Neurochir (Wien) 39: 151–157

Milhorat TH, Clark RG, Hammock MK, McGrath PP (1970) Structural, ultrastructural, and permeability changes in the ependymal and surrounding brain favoring equilibration in progressive hydrocephalus. Arch Neurol 22: 397–407

Miyagami M, Nakamura S, Murakami T, Koga N, Moriyasyu (1976) Electron microscopic study of ventricular wall and choroid plexus in experimentally induced hydrocephalic dogs. Neurol Med Chir (Tokyo) 16: 15–21

Mori K, Handa H, Murata T, Nakano Y (1980) Periventricular lucency in computed tomography of hydrocephalus and cerebral atrophy. J Comput Assist Tomogr 4: 204–209

Nakagawa Y, Cervós-Navarro J, Artigas J (1985) Tracer study on a paracellular route in experimental hydrocephalus. Acta Neuropath (Berl) 65: 247–254

Ogata J, Hochwald GM, Clavioto H, Ransohoff J (1972) Distribution of intraventricular horseradish peroxidase in normal and hydrocephalic cats. J Neuropathol Exp Neurol 31: 154–163

Pappennheimer JR, Heisey SR, Jordan EF, Downer JdeC (1962) Perfusion of the cerebral ventricular system in unanesthetized goats. Am J Physiol 203: 763–774

Rubin RC, Hochwald GM, Tiell M, Mizutani H, Ghatak N (1976) I. Histological and ultrastructural changes in the pre-shunted cortical mantle. Surg Neurol 5: 109–114

Sahar A, Hochwald GM, Sadik AR, Ransohoff J (1969) Cerebrospinal fluid absorption in animals with experimental obstructive hydrocephalus. Arch Neurol 21: 638

Sahar A, Hochwald GM, Ransohoff J (1971) Cerebrospinal fluid turnover in experimental hydrocephalic dogs. Neurology (NY) 21: 218

Simpson I, Rose B, Loewenstein WR (1977) Size limit of molecules permeating the junctional membrane channels. Science 195: 294–296

Takei F, Shapiro K, Hirano A, Kohn I (1987) Influence of the rate of ventricular enlargement on ultrastructural morphology of the white matter in experimental hydrocephalus. Neurosurgery 21: 645–650

Torvik A, Stenwing AE (1977) Pathology of the experimental obstructive hydrocephalus — Electron microscopic observation. Acta Neuropathol (Berl) 38: 21–26

Torvik AR, Bhatia R, Nyberg-Hansen (1976) The pathology of experimental obstructive hydrocephalus. Neuropathol appl Neurobiol 2: 42–52

Weller RO, Wisniewski H (1969) Histological and ultrastructural change with experimental hydrocephalus in adult rabbits. Brain 92: 819–823

Weller RO, Wisniewski H, Shulman K, Terry RD (1971) Experimental hydrocephalus in young dogs. J Neuropathol Exp Neurol 30: 613–626

Wislocki GB, Putnam TJ (1921) Absorption from the ventricles in experimentally produced internal hydrocephalus. Am J Anat 29: 313–326

19 — CSF Flow Dynamics in External Ventricular Drains

James M. Drake[1], *Christian Sainte-Rose*[2], *Marcia DaSilva*[1], *and Jean-François Hirsch*[2]

Summary. Fifty-five children had 64 external ventricular drains (EVD) placed predominantly (95%) for cerebrospinal fluid (CSF) shunt infection. In 9 children, a computer monitoring system measured the CSF output each second continuously for up to 24 hours. The monitoring was repeated daily for up to 9 days. The state of arousal of the patients was recorded simultaneously. In all children, daily EVD outputs were related to age, sex, weight, method of establishing the EVD, height of the drip chamber, time since insertion, and type of infecting organism. Computer monitoring revealed wide fluctuations in flow rate, with peak rates frequently greater than 20 cc/h, and periods of flow arrest. These changes were usually associated with increased arousal, but also occurred with sleep. The mean EVD flow rate of all children was 6.3 cc/h. EVD output increased with age and weight and decreased with gram negative or multiple organism infections, and with elevation of the drip chamber. Resolution of the infection, sex of the patient, and method of establishing the EVD had no effect on output. These results predict that — CSF production increases with brain growth in humans; CSF production is depressed by gram negative and multiple organism infections; implanted CSF shunts with standard valves flow at equivalent rates to an EVD in the supine position; and the CSF drainage requirements in this group are approximately equal to their EVD output.

Keywords. Hydrocephalus — Cerebrospinal fluid shunts — Cerebrospinal fluid production — External ventricular drainage

Introduction

External ventricular drainage is used most commonly in children as an interim measure in the treatment of CSF shunt infection (Bayston et al. 1987; Gardner

[1] Division of Neurosurgery, Hospital For Sick Children, University of Toronto, Toronto, Ontario M5G 1X8 Canada[2]

[2] Department of Neurosurgery, Hôpital Enfants Malade, Paris, 75730 France

et al. 1985; McLaurin and Frame 1987; Shapiro and Shulman 1982; Walters et al. 1984). It is less often used in patients with head injury and raised intracranial pressure who have an indwelling ventricular catheter which also serves as a pressure monitor (Shapiro and Marmarou 1983). It is now rarely used in the treatment of intraventricular hemorrhage in premature infants or as a temporary CSF diversion method for hydrocephalus secondary to posterior fossa tumors.

While it is a familiar treatment to all neurosurgeons, the very simple EVD can provide very important information on CSF production and absorption, the in vivo performance of CSF shunts, the CSF drainage requirements of hydrocephalic patients, and finally, design criteria for new CSF shunt designs. The measurement of the minute to minute, or dynamic changes in EVD flow, required the development of a computer monitoring system, on which the patient's activity level could also be recorded. The factors that affected the background, or steady state EVD flow, upon which the dynamic changes were superimposed, required the analysis of the 24-h EVD outputs of a large group of patients by means of a chart review.

Methods

External ventricular drains were established by either the externalization of the distal portion of a CSF shunt system, or by the removal of the shunt system and the insertion of a new ventricular catheter. The ventricular CSF was collected into a closed sterile system, typically a drip chamber and collecting bag (Codman External Drainage System, Codman Corporation, Randolph, Mass. or Cordis External Ventricular Drainage Set, Cordis Corporation, Miami, Flo.). The drip chamber was placed at a specified height above the middle of the head. The patients were confined to bed except for brief intervals at which time the collecting tube was occluded. The fluid in the collecting system was sampled daily for evidence of infection. The patency of the system was determined frequently by examining the drip chamber.

Dynamic EVD Flow — Computer Monitoring System

To measure the dynamic changes in EVD flow, a computer monitoring system was developed (Fig. 1). The drip chamber and collecting bag were suspended from the weighing hook of a digital balance (Mettler PJ3000, Mettler Instrument Corporation, Hightstown, N.J.). The balance was attached to a platform which could be raised and lowered so that the drip chamber was at the appropriate height. The balance was equipped with bidirectional interface and connected to an IBM compatible computer (Compaq Deskpro 286, Compaq Computer Corporation, Houston, Tex.) by means of an RS232 port.

The weight of the collecting system plus the accumulated CSF was measured every s to the nearest 0.01 g. A mean weight for each minute was determined. Flow rates were calculated from the difference in mean weights in consecutive minutes.

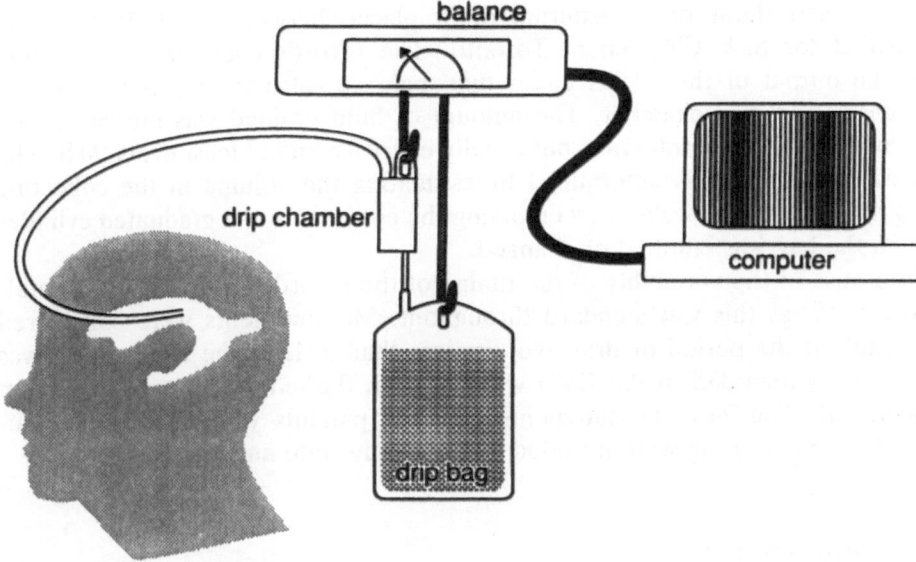

Fig. 1. Schematic of the computerized monitoring system. The drip chamber and collecting bag are suspended from a balance that records the weight each s and transmits the data to the computer. Interactive display allows the entry of patient functional status as well as displaying current flow rate and previous 12-h outputs

So that the relationship between level of arousal and flow rate could be determined, an interactive display on the computer system was developed. Arousal was graded from low to high among four categories, namely, "asleep", "awake", "crying", and "nursing care". The medical staff could enter a change in functional status by simply pressing one of four corresponding function keys. The functional status was displayed and was assumed to be unchanged unless a different status was entered.

The EVD flow data was displayed on the computer screen. In addition to the functional status, it included the weight of the CSF, the calculated flow rate for each min, the weight and flow rates for the previous 15 min, and the hourly output for the previous 12 h. This helped in determining whether the EVD was patent and also with recording the EVD output in the hospital chart. The program could be paused if the collecting system was manipulated and the reason for the pause recorded with the data. The data was stored on the hard disk for subsequent analysis. Four patients from the Hopital Enfants Malades in Paris and five from the Hospital for Sick Children in Toronto were monitored in this fashion.

Steady State EVD Flow — Hospital Record Review

To determine what factors influenced EVD output in the steady state we reviewed retrospectively the hospital records of all children who had either an externalised shunt or an external drain placed between 1984–1988 at the Hospital for Sick Children in Toronto. The records contained information on the output of the EVDs under fluid balance calculations, as well as the height of the drip chamber. The amount of fluid drained was measured and recorded at variable intervals, but usually every 8 h and at least every 24 h. The measured output was determined by estimating the volume in the collecting bag according to its scale or by emptying the contents into a graduated cylinder when the bag was emptied or changed.

Because of the variability of the timing of the recorded outflows, 24-h totals were used, as this was standard throughout. Measurements were considered unusable if the period of drainage was less than 24 h, if the information was improperly recorded, if the EVD was clamped, flushed, or thought to be non functional. The 24-h measurements in the 9 patients who underwent computerized monitoring were included in the steady-state analysis.

Statistical Analysis

The effect of individual variables on steady state EVD output was tested with either linear regression or analysis of variance. The model of steady state EVD output was constructed by multiple linear regression analysis. Those variables having no significant effect on the model were excluded.

Results

Nine patients underwent computerized monitoring. Forty-six patients had undergone external drainage during the period 1984–1988. Of this group, five patients had two periods of external drainage and two had had three periods of drainage, all for repeat shunt infections. This produced a total of 64 periods of external drainage for study. Each period of drainage was treated as an independent measurement for data analysis.

Hydrocephalus in association with myelomeningocele was by far the commonest etiology at 34.5%. Sixty-one of the 64 periods of external drainage were for infected shunts. One EVD was placed following intraventricular rupture of an abscess prior to placing a ventriculoperitoneal (VP) shunt; one was placed following a failed attempt to place a VP shunt with subcutaneous emphysema; one was placed for hydrocephalus associated with presumed Tuberculous meningitis. The commonest infecting organisms were gram positive. *Staphylococcus epidermidis* was the most frequent, accounting for 40.9% of the organisms identified. Fifteen patients were infected with more than one organism. The patients were treated with a variety of antibiotic regimens according to the identity and sensitivity of the infecting organisms.

Twenty-five patients had external ventricular drains. Thirty-four patients had the peritoneal end of their shunt externalised. One patient with bilateral VP shunts had both peritoneal catheters externalised. Two patients had one of two

Table 1. External ventricular drainage

	Mean	SE	n[a]	Median	Range
Age (years)	4.51	±0.7	55	2.61	0.04–18.4
Sex Male	32				
Female	23				
Weight (kg)	15.4	±1.8	64	10.95	2.3–65.7
Duration EVD (days)	16.4	±1.2	62	13.5	4–44
# Usable 24-h measurements per patient	11.2	±0.9	64	8.5	1–39
Height of EVD (cm above middle of head)	3.9	±0.22	637	5	−10–20
24-h Output (cc)	152	±4.2	717	122	2–533
(cc/h)	6.33	±0.173	717	5.08	0.08–22.2

[a] Number of patients

VP shunts externalised. In one patient the method of establishing external drainage was not recorded.

The median age of the patients was 2.61 years, ranging from a few days of age to 18 years (Table 1). There were 32 boys and 23 girls. The median duration for the EVD to be in place was 13.5 days with a minimum of four and a maximum of 44 days. The median number of usable 24-h measurements per patient was 8.5. The average height of the EVD was 3.9 cm but ranged from −10 to 20 cm. The average 24-h rate for all patients was 6.33 ccs per hour. The maximum flow rate in any 24-h period for all patients was 22.2 ccs an hour.

Dynamic Characteristics of EVD Flow

The nine children underwent an average of 5.7 days of computer monitoring (range 2–9). The monitoring system worked extremely well. The nursing staff found this a convenient way to evaluate EVD function and record EVD output. The requirement to record the functional status of the patient was not an undue burden. Care had to be insured that the balance was not disturbed and that the drip chamber and collecting system hung free. These patients were monitored closely by the medical personnel, but changes in functional status could have occurred and not have been recorded on the computer.

Examples of the min to min variation in flow rate, obtained by computerized monitoring, are shown in Fig. 2. In this patient, a 1-year-old child with an EVD inserted for abdominal wound dehiscence, there was periodic variation in the flow rate while asleep. These variations occurred every 60 min, lasted approximately 20 min, and had peak values in the 70 cc/h range. The total amount of CSF vented during these episodes was approximately 10 cc. The period of increased flow was followed by a period of flow arrest. These variations may have occurred in association with REM sleep in which case the increased flow would be in response to vasodilatation, and the flow arrest would occur as CSF production accounted for the vented CSF. This pattern was not seen in the other 8 children.

In the other children, peak flow rates tended to occur in response to wakefulness, crying, or when they were being manipulated for nursing care. Some-

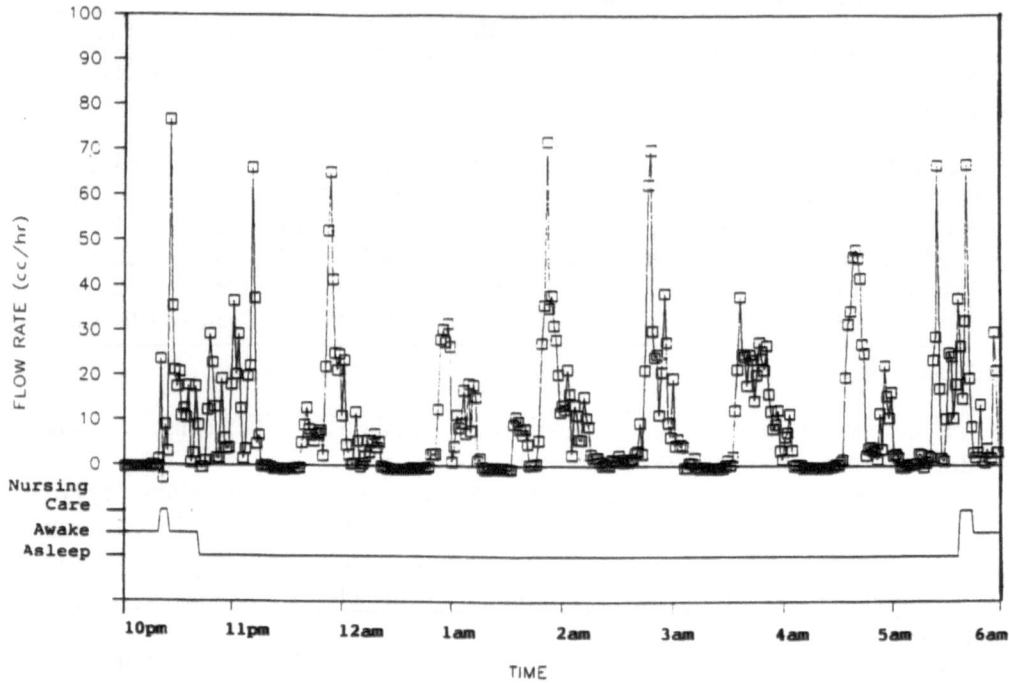

Fig. 2. Min to min variation in flow rate in 1-year-old child with EVD for abdominal wound dehiscence. The average flow rate for this 8-h period is 10 cc/h. The height of the EVD is 10 cm. There are periodic increases in flow rate to approximately 70 cc/h. These occur during sleep and last approximately 20 min. They are followed by arrest of flow for approximately an equal time period

times the pattern was chaotic, particularly in a restless child. The striking finding was the variability of the flow rate.

Effects on Steady State EVD Flow

The relationship between age and average daily flow rates is shown in Fig. 3. The increase with age follows a logarithmic profile with a correlation coefficient of 0.6755. The flow rates in children less than 1 year of age are quite low, less than 4 ccs per h. In older children the values are higher, although quite variable. As age and weight are highly correlated, a similar type of profile occurred with weight vs flow rate, with a similar correlation coefficient.

Other factors which might be expected to influence the steady state flow rates include height of the EVD, type of infecting organism, time elapsed since insertion, type of EVD, and sex. Using multiple regression analysis a model was fitted to 24-h flow data, using these factors as well as age and weight.

There was no significant effect due to time elapsed since insertion, type of EVD, or sex. Age and weight had a significant effect. The height of the EVD

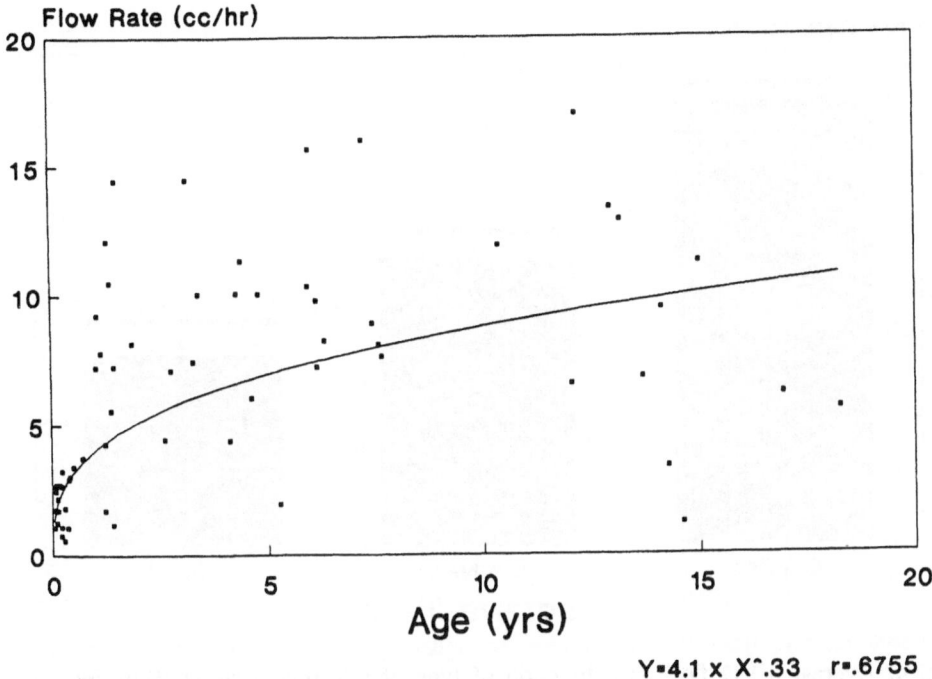

Y=4.1 x X^.33   r=.6755

Fig. 3. Average EVD flow for each patient over entire drainage period as a function of age

had a significant negative effect on output. This same effect seen in the group as a whole was also seen in individual patients when the EVD level was altered during the drainage period. Finally, the type of infecting bacteria had a significant effect. Flow rates were highest in patients with gram positive infections and lowest in patients with gram negative and mixed infections (Fig. 4). There was no significant difference in age, weight, or height of the reservoir, between patients infected with gram positive, gram negative, or mixed infections.

Discussion

An EVD consists of a ventricular catheter, a connecting tube to a drip chamber, and a collecting bag. There may be an integral one way valve, or if the shunt is externalized, a proximal shunt valve. The height of the drip chamber acts as a hydrostatic valve analogous to the opening pressure of standard shunt valves. The total opening pressure of the system is the sum of the height of the drip chamber plus any intervening valves. An EVD, like a standard shunt valve, has very little resistance to flow once open and similarly has a closing pressure at which it closes passively.

In this configuration, the EVD drains CSF at a rate equal to the CSF production minus the CSF absorption. If the total pressure of the EVD is less

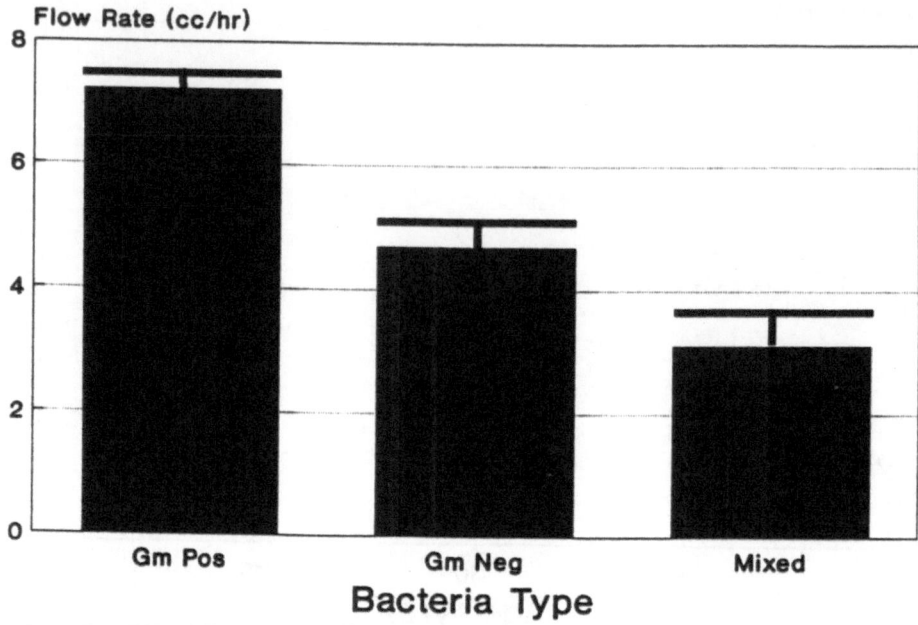

Fig. 4. Average EVD flow as a function of type of infecting bacteria. Bars indicate standard error. Average EVD flow is significantly lower with gram negative or mixed infections, $P < 0.001$

than the pressure in the superior sagittal sinus, then the EVD flow rate should equal the CSF production rate.

As an EVD has a proximal ventricular catheter and a hydrostatic valve, the main difference between the mechanics of an EVD and an implanted shunt lie with the distal end. The drip chamber is always at atmospheric pressure. Although measurement of the intraperitoneal pressure in infants with hydrocephalus has shown it to be near atmospheric pressure at rest, 0–50 mm H_2O (Yamada et al. 1975), there are large increases in intraabdominal pressure which accompany crying, coughing, and straining. These are associated with the corresponding increases in intracranial pressure occurring with the same events.

The absence of this distal increase in intraperitoneal pressure leads to venting of the CSF with these activities with an EVD. This was quite evident in the patients undergoing computerized monitoring where flow rates in excess of 20 cc/h were common and flow rates as high as 100 cc/h occurred for a few minutes with increased activity. While one would expect venting to be less with an implanted shunt, in fact increased flow, as measured by radioisotope injection, has been reported with these activities (Harbert et al. 1974).

Other differences between a patient with an EVD and a shunt include the constant recumbent position and initial CSF infection. The EVD flow in a patient lying quietly at rest would therefore be expected to be the same as in a patient with a shunt of equal pressure characteristics. This level of activity, while proportionally much higher in infants, would still occupy approximately 25% of the time in adults.

The average EVD flow rate we observed in 55 children, median age 2.61 years, with the drip chamber at an average height of 3.9 cm was 6.33 cc/h. EVD flow increased logarithmically with increasing age and weight, being very low in infants. As some CSF absorption may have taken place with the EVD in place, no comments regarding the absolute EVD output and CSF production can be made. However the relationship between age and output indicates that CSF production is a function of age or, more probably, brain weight. This concept is also supported by animal studies where CSF production is a function of size of the species studied; 0.02 cc/h in the mouse; 0.6 cc/h in rabbits; and 9.2 cc/h in the goat Davson (1984).

To date, there have been few studies on the CSF production in man and previously there has been no suggestion that the CSF production in children might be different from that in adults. A group of older children and adults undergoing CSF perfusion chemotherapy for central nervous system neoplasms had a CSF production rate of 0.37 cc/min (22.2 cc/h) (Rubin et al. 1976). There was no obvious difference between children and adults in this study. Cutler et al. (1968) studied 12 children, ages 5–13, also undergoing cerebrospinal fluid perfusion chemotherapy and found production rates of 0.35 cc/min (21 cc/h). Page et al. (1973) studied 8 children with hydrocephalus, ages 1 month–8 years, and found a CSF production rate of 0.25 cc/min (15 cc/h).

CSF absorption, although impaired in hydrocephalus, remains pressure dependent (Marmarou et al. 1983). One would expect absorption to increase and EVD flow to fall with increasing height of the drip chamber. This was observed both as an overall effect on the model and in individual patients. Casey and Vries (1989) also observed this negative effect of increasing height in EVD output. In fact, neurosurgeons make use of this effect all the time when adjusting the height of the EVD to control output or by selecting a higher pressure valve to attempt to reduce the effects of over drainage.

The effect of infection on CSF production has not been studied in man, to our knowledge. A decrease in CSF production in the presence of gram negative ventriculitis in infants undergoing external drainage, however, was reported as an "observation" by McComb (Breeze et al. 1989) There is animal model evidence for the effects of infection on CSF production. Breeze et al. (1989) produced E. coli ventriculitis in the rabbit and noted a 50% reduction in CSF output in the infected animals. They speculated that this reduction was due to either a reduction of choroid plexus blood flow, or to a reduction in ionic transport caused by enterotoxins. Similarly, Scheld et al. (1980) found that the most pronounced reduction of CSF production in experimental meningitis in the rabbit occurred with E. coli. Cooper et al. (1968) failed to find a reduction in CSF production in a model of Streptococcus pneumoniae meningitis in the dog.

Our data on the effects of infection on EVD flow supports these experimental results and is the first evidence for this in man. Gram negative infections had lower EVD flow rates. Mixed infections also produced lower rates. While some of these included gram negative organisms, they may have also indicated a more severe infection. Perhaps the most interesting effect of an infection was the failure of the flow rates to increase with resolution of the infection. The average duration of the EVD in this study was 16.4 days, with a maximum of 44 days. How long the flow levels would remain at this level is unknown, but gram negative infections may produce changes in the choroid plexus, such as destruction or scarring, which are long lasting.

The limited circumstances under which EVD flow is equivalent to shunt flow have been discussed. There was no change of EVD flow rate with time during the drainage period, and these children were in a state of equilibrium in terms of CSF drainage. One would therefore expect shunts implanted immediately following the EVD to perform in the same way, in the recumbent position, providing the opening pressure of the valve and the height of the drip chamber were the same. The average drip chamber height of 3.9 cm corresponds to a low pressure valve. The average EVD flow rate was 6.3 cc/h. This gives some indication of the probable shunt flow rates and CSF drainage requirements in this group of children, at least in the immediate post EVD period.

In vivo shunt flow rates have been comparable to the values we measured with the EVD. Measurement by means of an implanted electrolysis unit showed a wide variation in flow rates anywhere between 0.6 and 116 cc/h (Hara et al. 1983; Numoto et al. 1984). The average flow rate in 2 patients was approximately 15 cc/h. (Hara et al. 1983). Using magnetic resonance imaging (MRI) phase imaging in 5 teenagers and young adults we found flow rates between 3 and 19 cc/h (Martin et al. 1989). Using injection of radioisotope and an external detector which had to be calibrated for each type of reservoir (Harbert et al. 1974) gave values similarly over a wide range from <1 cc/h to greater than 20 cc/h (Brendel et al. 1983; Chervu et al. 1984; Harbert et al. 1974; Matsumae et al. 1989). With the computer monitoring system we measured flow rates anywhere from 0 to greater than 100 cc/h. The average flow over a 24-h period had a mean of 6.33 cc/h with a range between 0.08 and 22.2 cc/h.

The dynamic fluctuations in EVD flow rate were predominantly related to increased level of arousal. Similar fluctuations may occur in implanted shunts. The fluctuations which occurred during sleep in one child (Fig. 2) could certainly occur in implanted shunts. Hara et al. (1983) also noted an increase in shunt flow at night, lasting several h, and suggested the possibility of a circadian rhythm. The fluctuations in our patient occurred much more rapidly. The particular pattern we observed may be related to REM sleep. Hydrocephalic infants have been found to have periodic increases in intracranial pressure, associated with increased intracerebral blood volume, occurring with REM sleep (Barritault et al. 1980). These occurred approximately every h and lasted about 20 min. Transient increases in intracerebral blood volume occurring with REM sleep in a patient with an EVD would be expected to produce the type of flow pattern shown in Fig. 2.

Important differences between EVD flow and in vivo shunt flow occur with patients in the erect posture. We noted increased EVD flow with decreasing drip chamber height and when the drip chamber was dropped well below head level the EVD rapidly vented. An increase in shunt flow (Brendel et al. 1983; Matsumae et al. 1989) and remarkably high negative intracranial pressures have been measured in the sitting position in patients with implanted shunts (McCullough and Fox 1974). One can surmise from these two observations that, in patients with standard valves and without anti-siphon devices, there is similarly an initial venting in the erect posture, followed by an average CSF flow rate equal to the CSF production.

The data from EVD flow measurement can be used to predict the performance of currently implanted valves and new valve designs. However, the average rate and range of flow rates required to optimize the treatment of hydrocephalus are unknown. It is very unlikely that these flow rates are the same for all causes of hydrocephalus or for all patients at every stage of development. Perhaps in the future, with improved knowledge of the pathogenesis of hydrocephalus, and more sophisticated valve design, each patient will have a shunt tailored to their specific needs.

References

Barritault L, Rimbert JN, Hirsch JF, Pierre-Kahn A, Lacombe J, Zouaoui A, Mises J, Gabersek V (1980) Vasomotor origin of intracranial pressure waves in hydrocephalic infants. Eur J Nucl Med 5: 511–514

Bayston R, Hart CA, Barnicoat M (1987) Intraventricular vancomycin in the treatment of ventriculitis associated with cerebrospinal fluid shunting and drainage. J Neurol Neurosurg Psychiatry 50: 1419–23

Breeze RE, McComb JG, Hyman S, Gilles FH (1989) CSF production in acute ventriculitis. J Neurosurg 70: 619–622

Brendel AJ, Wynchank S, Caster JP, Barat JL, Leccia F, Ducassou D (1983) Cerebrospinal fluid shunt flow in adults: radionuclide quantitation with emphasis on patient position. Radiology 149: 815–818

Casey KF, Vries JK (1989) Cerebral fluid over-production in the absence of tumor or hypertrophy of the choroid plexus. Nerv Syst Child 5: 332–334

Chervu S, Chervu LR, Vallabhajosyula B, Milstein DM, Shapiro KM, Shulman K, Blaufox MD (1984) Quantitative evaluation of cerebrospinal fluid shunt flow. J Nucl Med 25: 91–95

Cooper AJ, Beaty HN, Oppenheimer SI, Goodner CJ, Petersdorf RG (1968) Studies on the pathogenesis of meningitis, VII. Glucose transport and spinal fluid production in experimental pneumococcal meningitis. J Lab Clin Med 71: 473–483

Cutler RWP, Page L, Galicich J, Watters GV (1968) Formation and absorption of cerebrospinal fluid in man. Brain 91: 707–720

Davson H (1984) Formation and drainage of the cerebrospinal fluid. In: Shapiro K, Marmarou A, Portnoy H (eds) Hydrocephalus. Raven, New York, pp 3–41

Gardner P, Leipzig T, Phillips P (1985) Infections of central nervous system shunts. Med Clin North Am 69: 297–314

Hara M, Kadowaki C, Konishi Y, Ogashiwa M, Numoto M, Takeuchi K (1983) A new method for measuring cerebrospinal fluid flow in shunts. J Neurosurg 58: 557–561

Harbert J, Haddad D, McCullough D (1974) Quantitation of cerebrospinal fluid shunt flow. Radiology 112: 379–387

Marmarou A, Ward JD, Wilson JT, Maset AL, Becker DP (1983) Biomechanics of hydrocephalus: Application of pressure volume dynamics to test CSF absorption in hydrocephalic infants. In: Ishii (ed) Hydrocephalus: Proceedings of the International Symposium on Hydrocephalus, Tokyo, Japan. Excerpta Medica, Tokyo, pp 31–38

Martin AJ, Drake JM, Lemaire C, Henkelman RM (1989) MR measurement of CSF shunt flow. Radiology 173: 243–247

Matsumae M, Sato O, Itoh K, Fukuda T, Suzuki Y (1989) Quantification of cerebrospinal fluid shunt flow rates. Nerv Syst Child 5: 356–360

McCullough DC, Fox JC (1974) Negative intracranial pressure hydrocephalus with shunts and its relationship to the production of subdural hematoma. J Neurosurg 40: 372–375

McLaurin RL, Frame PT (1987) Treatment of infections of cerebrospinal fluid shunts. Rev Infect Dis 9: 595–603

Numoto M, Hara M, Tatsuo S, Kadowaki C, Takeuchi K (1984) A noninvasive CSF flowmeter. J Med Eng Technol 8: 218–220

Page LK, Bresnam MJ, Lorenzo AV (1973) Cerebrospinal fluid perfusion studies in childhood hydrocephalus. Surg Neurol 1: 317–320

Rubin RC, Henderson ES, Ommaya AK, Walker M, Rall DP (1976) The production of cerebrospinal fluid in man and its modification by acetazolamide. J Neurosurg 44: 735–739

Shapiro K, Marmarou A (1983) Mechanism and treatment of intracranial hypertension in the head injured child. In: Shapiro K (ed) Pediatric head trauma. Future, New York, pp 45–69

Shapiro K, Shulman K (1982) Shunt infections: A protocol for effective treatment Monogr Neural Sci 8: 69–71

Scheld WM, Dacey RG, Winn HR, Welsh JE, Jane JA, Merle AS (1980) Cerebrospinal fluid outflow resistance in rabbits with experimental meningitis. J Clin Invest 66: 243–253

Walters BC, Hoffman HJ, Hendrick EB, Humphreys RP (1984) Cerebrospinal fluid shunt infection influences on initial management and subsequent outcome. J Neurosurg 60: 1014–1021

Yamada H, Tajima M, Nagaya M (1975) Effect of respiratory movement on cerebrospinal fluid dynamics in hydrocephalic infants with shunts. J Neurosurg 42: 194–200

20 — Evidence of CSF Flow in Rostral Direction Through Central Canal of Spinal Cord in Rats

Thomas H. Milhorat, Richard W. Johnson, and Walter D. Johnson

Summary. The movement of Evans blue dye (EBD) through the central canal of the spinal cord was investigated in rats. Following injection into the dorsal columns at T_{5-6}, the marker moved centripedally into the central canal and drained rostrally, to exit through the outlets of the fourth ventricle within 90 min. A similar pattern of clearance was produced by freeze-lesioning the dorsal columns and injecting EBD intravascularly. When the marker was injected into the lateral ventricles, the cisterna magna, or the lumbar subarachnoid space, it failed to enter the central canal. Taken together, these findings are consistent with an intraluminal flow of fluid that moves in a rostral direction through the central canal of the spinal cord in rats.

Keywords. Central canal of the spinal cord — CSF circulation — Hydromyelia — syringomyelia

Introduction

The central canal of the spinal cord is a simple epithelial tubule that is derived in common with the cerebral ventricles from the lumen of the neural tube. At its rostral end, it is anatomically continuous with the fourth ventricle through a well-defined aperture, and it extends the length of the spinal cord to end as the slightly expanded terminal ventricle of the conus medullaris. Although the central canal contains cerebrospinal fluid (CSF), and is lined like the cerebral ventricles by ciliated ependyma, CSF flow through its lumen has not been demonstrated under normal conditions.

There is indirect evidence that the central canal of the spinal cord drains CSF in a caudal direction under certain pathological conditions. In syringomyelia, it is postulated that obstruction of the outlets of the fourth ventricle produces

---

Departments of Neurosurgery, State University of New York, Health Science Center at Brooklyn, and Kings County Hospital Center, Brooklyn, NY 11203, USA

tubular cavitation of the spinal cord by directing the CSF pulse wave caudally (Gardner and Goodall 1950; Gardner and McMurry 1976), or by creating a dissociation of pressure between the fourth ventricle and the spinal sub-arachnoid space sufficient to draw fluid into the central canal (Williams 1980; Williams and Bentley 1980). These and other hydrodynamic theories are sup-ported by the frequent finding of hydromyelia or syringomyelia in association with lesions at the level of the cervical-medullary junction (Aboulker 1979; Ball and Dayan 1972; duBoulay et al. 1974; Gardner and Goodall 1950; Gardner and McMurry 1976; Williams 1980; Williams and Bentley 1980), and by experimental evidence that kaolin-induced basilar arachnoiditis will produce hydromyelia in association with communicating hydrocephalus (Becker et al. 1972; Eisenberg et al. 1974; Hochwald et al. 1975; Williams and Bentley 1980). In severe examples of experimental hydromyelia, the pathological findings may include disruption of the ependymal epithelium, edema of the white matter especially in the region of the dorsal columns, and fistula formation between the terminal ventricle and the subarachnoid space (Becker et al. 1972; Eisen-berg et al. 1974; Hochwald et al. 1975). The changes are thought to be due to the caudal flow of CSF through the central canal (Hochwald et al. 1975) and to constitute an alternative pathway for absorption in hydrocephalus (Eisenberg et al. 1974).

In this study, the movement of Evans blue dye (EBD) through the central canal of the spinal cord was examined in rats. Three sets of experiments were carried out: (1) stereotactic injection of EBD into the dorsal columns of the thoracic spinal cord (T_{5-6}); (2) intravascular injection of EBD in animals with freeze lesions in the same location; and (3) injection of EBD into the lateral ventricles, the cisterna magna, or the lumbar subarachnoid space.

Materials and Methods

Following review and approval by an Institutional Animal Care Committee, adult Sprague-Dawley rats weighing 300–350 g were anesthetized briefly with a mixture of 1% halothane, 70% nitrous oxide, and 30% oxygen.

Parenchymal Injection Experiments

In one set of experiments, the spinal cord was exposed through a small laminotomy at T_{5-6}. The dura was opened and 0.1 microliters (ul) of 2% EBD was injected slowly into the dorsal columns to a depth of 0.1 mm using a 30-gauge needle mounted on a Kopf stereotactic frame. The animals were sacrificed at various intervals with a lethal dose of pentobarbital and perfused through the heart with 10% buffered formalin solution. The brain and spinal cord were removed as a single specimen and were serially sectioned with a fine blade.

Freeze Lesion Experiments

In a second set of experiments, the spinal cord was exposed as described above. The dorsal columns were lesioned by applying a $-70°$ cold probe to the dura for 5 s. Immediately prior to lesioning, 0.5 cc of 2% EBD was injected intravascularly. The animals were sacrificed at various intervals and the brains and spinal cords were prepared as described for parenchymal injection experiments.

CSF Experiments

In a final set of experiments, 1.0 ul of 2% EBD was injected into one of the following CSF spaces: the right lateral ventricle, the cisterna magna, or the lumbar subarachnoid space. Intraventricular injections were made over an interval of 30 s using a 30-gauge needle mounted on a Kopf stereotactic frame with coordinate settings of 1.0 mm posterior to bregma, 1.5 mm lateral to the sagittal suture, and 3.2 mm deep to dura. Cisternal injections were made percutaneously through the atlantooccipital membrane using a 30-gauge needle. For lumbar injections, the dura was exposed through a small laminotomy at L_{4-5} and punctures were made under magnification using a 27-gauge needle. The animals were sacrificed at various intervals and the brains and spinal cords were prepared as described for parenchymal injection experiments.

Results

Parenchymal Injection Experiments

Following stereotactic injection of EBD into the dorsal columns at T_{5-6}, the marker was observed to move centripedally through the parenchyma of the spinal cord and to enter the central canal within 1–5 min. Thereafter, the marker moved rostrally to produce intense staining of the ependyma to the level of the obex within 90 min (Fig. 1). Staining of the fourth ventricle, including the choroid plexus and the foraminal outlets, was present in some cases but not in others, reflecting perhaps the small volume of dye injected. The marker was not observed to move caudally through the central canal except when the injection was excessively forceful or when it was made directly into the lumen. There was usually some local staining of the leptomeninges around the lesion site, but this did not extend more than 1 cm above or below the level of T_{5-6} at 90 min.

Freeze Lesion Experiments

The movement of EBD from freeze lesion sites in the dorsal columns at T_{5-6} was found to occur in a pattern similar to that observed following stereotactic injection. In particular, the marker moved centripedally into the central canal

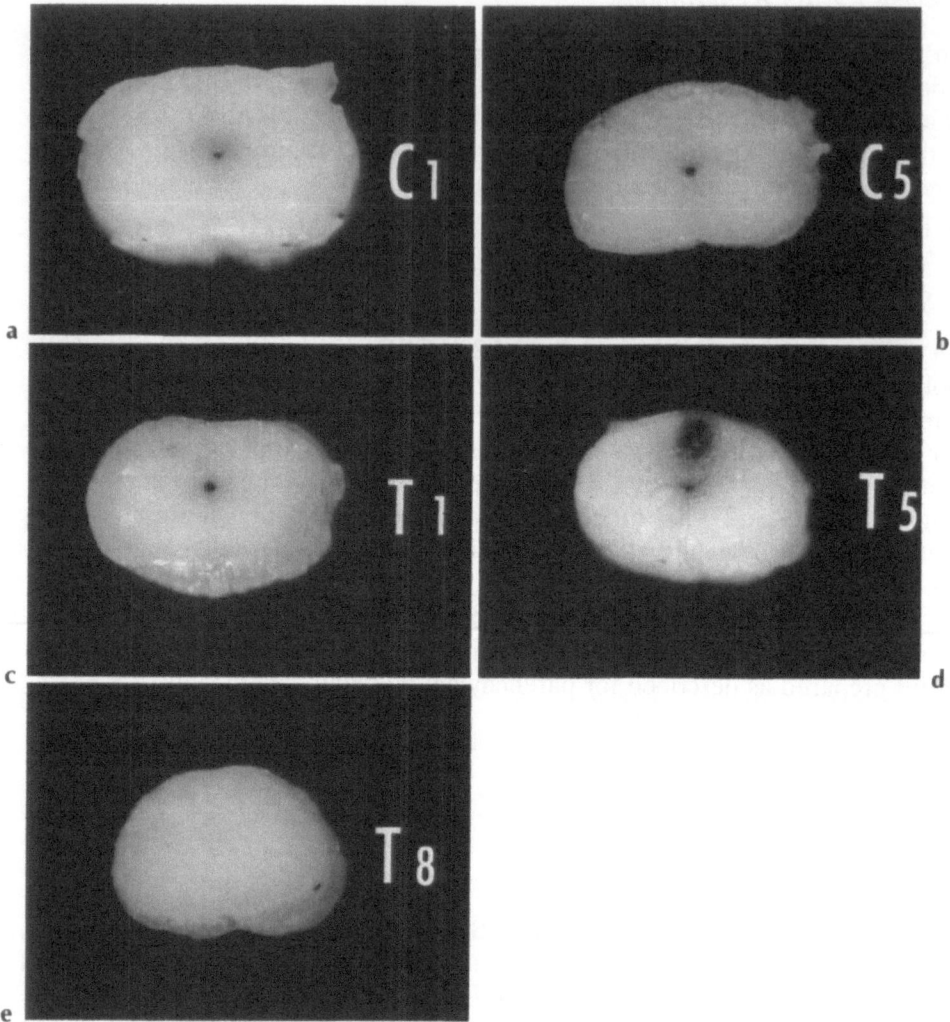

Fig. 1a–e. Distribution of EBD 90 min after stereotactic injection into dorsal columns of thoracic spinal cord. There is staining of the central canal at all levels rostral to the injection site but not below it

within 1–5 min and drained rostrally, to reach the fourth ventricle and its foraminal outlets within 90 min (Figs. 2 and 3). As with the parenchymal injection experiments, there was some local staining of the leptomeninges around the lesion site which did not extend more than 1 cm above or below the level of T_{5-6} at 90 min.

CSF Experiments

Following stereotactic injection of EBD into the lateral ventricles, the marker was observed to pass promptly into the fourth ventricle and to exit into the

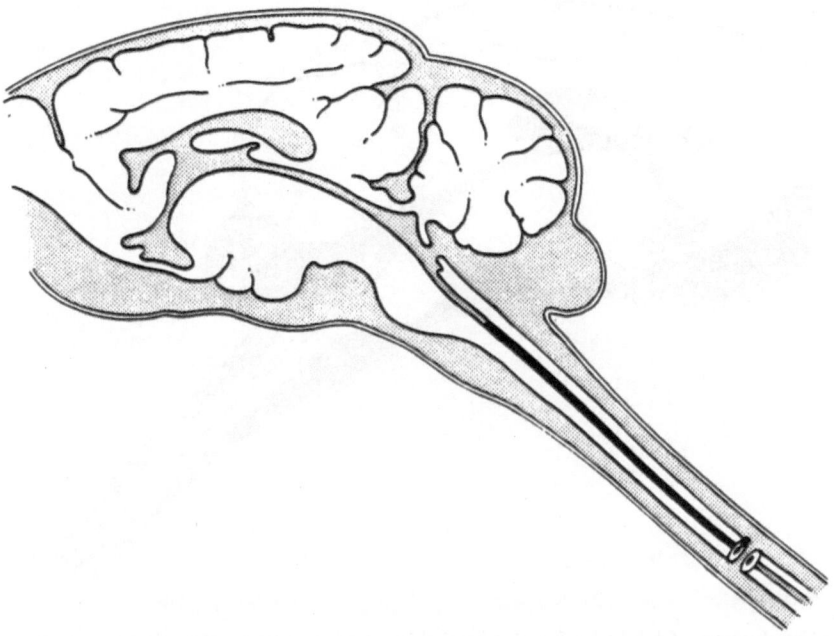

Fig. 2. Movement of EBD (*solid shading*) from freeze lesion site in dorsal columns of thoracic spinal cord, 45 min after intravascular injection

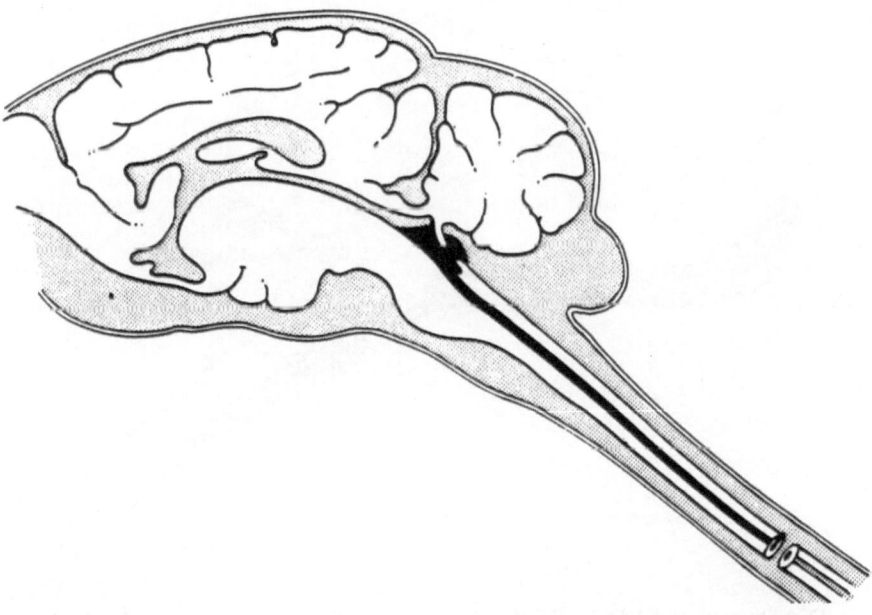

Fig. 3. Movement of EBD (*solid shading*) from freeze lesion site in dorsal columns of thoracic spinal cord, 90 min after intravascular injection

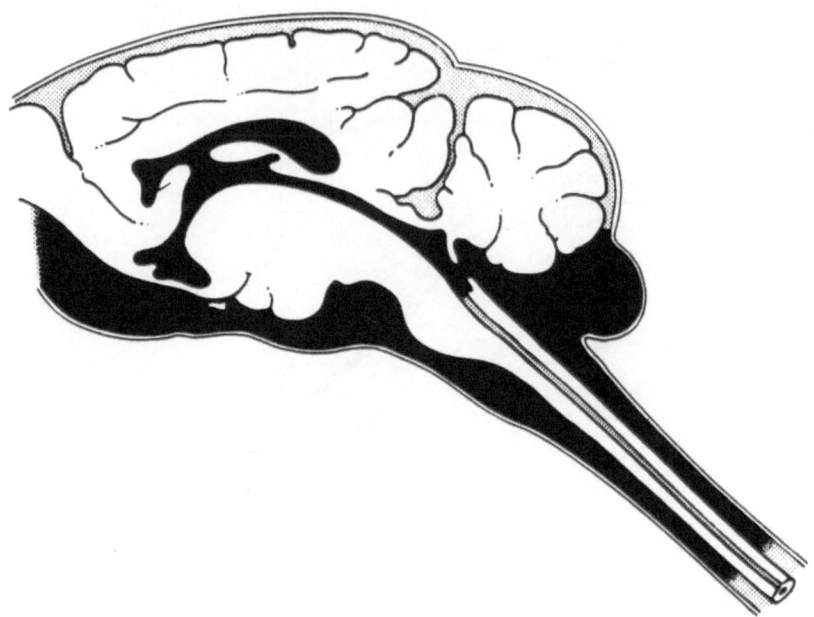

Fig. 4. Distribution of EBD (*solid shading*) 90 min after intraventricular injection

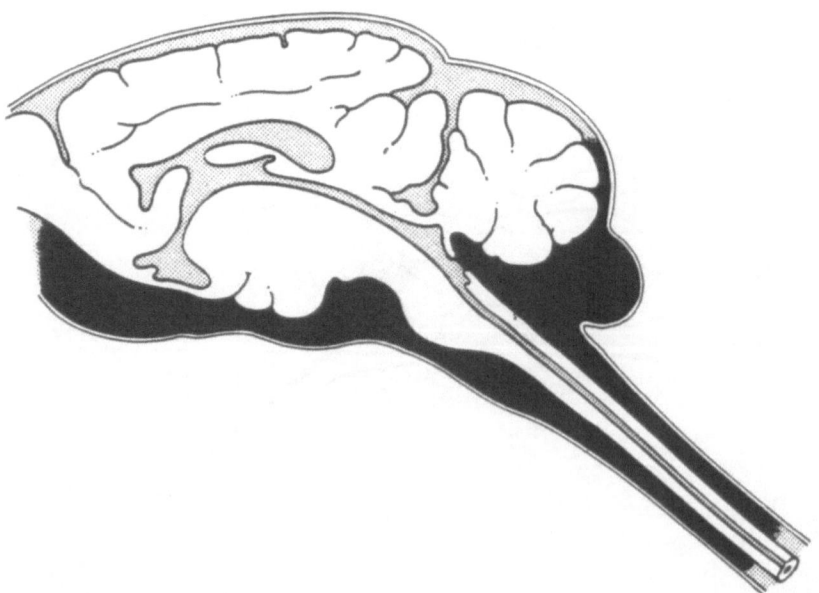

Fig. 5. Distribution of EBD (*solid shading*) 90 min after intracisternal injection

subarachnoid space through the paired lateral foramina of Lushka and the midline foramen of Magendie. Dye passing into the basilar cisterns moved rostrally through the interpeduncular and chiasmatic cisterns to stain the leptomeninges of the olfactory bulb within 45 min. Dye passing into the cisterna magna descended into the spinal subarachnoid space to the level of C_{6-7} at 45 min and T_{3-4} at 90 min, but did not enter the central canal during the interval of this study (Fig. 4).

When EBD was injected into the cisterna magna, the marker ascended through premedullary, prepontine, interpeduncular, and chiasmatic cisterns to reach the level of the olfactory bulb within 45 min. Simultaneously, the marker descended into the spinal subarachnoid space to stain the leptomeninges to the level of T_{1-2} at 45 minutes and T_{5-6} at 90 min. There was no staining of the central canal during the interval of this study (Fig. 5).

Finally, when EBD was injected into the lumbar subarachnoid space, the marker spread locally throughout the sacral sac and moved rostrally to stain the leptomeninges to the level of C_{3-4} at 45 min, and to the level of the premedullary cisterns at 90 min. There was intense staining of the leptomeninges in the lumbar area where the dye penetrated the pial surface of the lumbar and lower thoracic spinal cord to stain white matter to a depth of 1–2 mm at 90 min. Dye within the parenchyma moved centripedally toward the central canal, but did not reach the lumen during the interval of this study (Fig. 6).

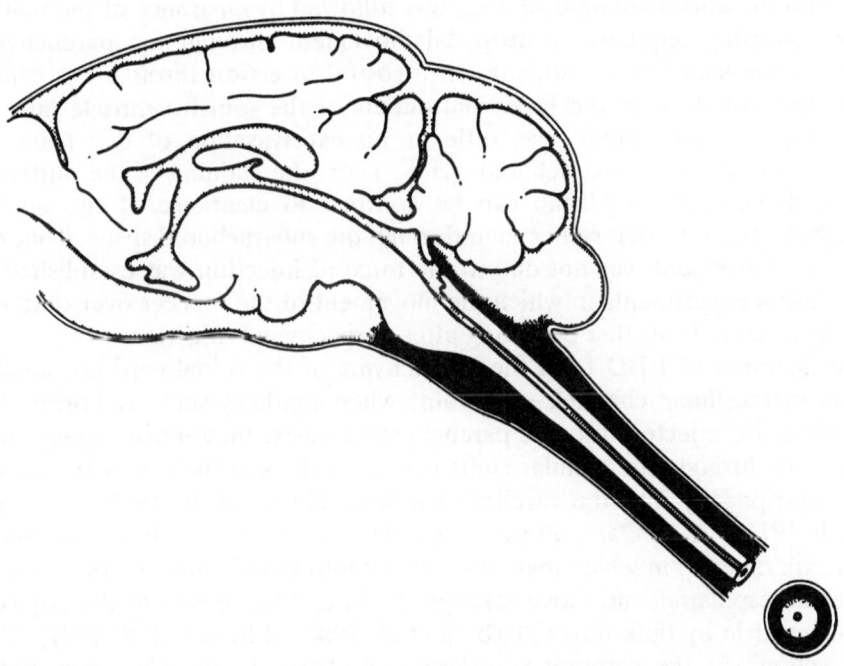

Fig. 6. Distribution of EBD (*solid shading*) 90 min after lumbar injection. *Inset* shows parenchymal staining (*stipple*) of lower thoracic spinal cord

Discussion

The injection of vital dyes into the macroscopic CSF cavities is a reliable means for examining bulk flow patterns (Cserr and Ostrach 1974; Milhorat 1975) and has been used clinically to distinguish obstructive and communicating types of hydrocephalus (Bering 1956; Milhorat and Clark 1970). When vital dyes are injected into blood, they are bound promptly to plasma proteins (Tschingi 1950) so that their distribution in tissue reflects the movement of dye-protein complexes rather than water soluble molecules. In the current experiments, the injection of EBD into the lateral ventricles, the cisterna magna, and the lumbar subarachnoid space did not result in any discernible staining of the central canal over an interval of 90 min. This finding is in agreement with the movement of dyes, radioisotopes, and other tracers injected into the CSF cavities of man, the rhesus monkey, dog, cat, rat, mouse, guinea pig, and sea lamprey (Bradbury and Lathem 1965; DiChiro 1964; Milhorat and Clark 1970). In rabbits, the central canal of the spinal cord stains brilliantly following the intraventricular injection of vital dyes (Bradbury and Lathem 1965), but this finding appears to be species specific (Davson 1970).

Although parenchymal injection experiments and freeze lesion techniques have been used for years to examine bulk flow patterns within the brain interspaces (Blasberg et al. 1980; Cserr et al. 1977; Cserr and Ostrach 1974; Klatzo I 1967), such methodology has not been applied to the study of fluid movement within the spinal cord. In the current experiments, the injection of EBD into the dorsal columns at T_{5-6} was followed by clearance of the marker in the following sequence: centripedal movement through the parenchymal tissues of the spinal cord, drainage in a rostral direction through the central canal, and exit through the foraminal outlets of the fourth ventricle into the subarachnoid space. There was little or no extravasation of dye from the injection site into the subarachnoid space. Thus, the staining of the outlets of the fourth ventricle at 90 min can be ascribed to clearance of the marker through the central canal rather than through the subarachnoid space. That this pattern of movement was not due to the force of injection was established by freeze lesion experiments in which the movement of the marker over time was indistinguishable from that occurring after parenchymal injection.

The clearance of EBD from the parenchyma of the spinal cord presumably follows extracellular channels. In brain, when markers such as horseradish peroxidase are injected into the parenchymal tissues, they move rapidly, predominantly through intercellular clefts between cells and their fiber tracts, and drain centripedally into the cerebral ventricles (Cserr et al. 1977; Cserr and Ostrach 1974). A similar pattern of movement can be produced by freeze lesion experiments, in which markers injected into blood enter the brain across permeable capillaries and move through the interstitial spaces to the adjacent lateral ventricle by bulk flow (Blasberg et al. 1980; Milhorat et al. 1989). This "sink action" of the cerebral ventricles contributes to the clearance of the brain interspaces and is an important mechanism for removing solutes by net transport from brain to CSF (Cserr 1971; Davson 1970; Milhorat 1975).

In the current experiments, the clearance of EBD from the parenchyma of the spinal cord was found to occur in a centripedal direction toward the central canal. This was comparable in rate and direction to the clearance of markers from the parenchyma of the brain, and raises the possibility that the central canal functions as a sink for the interstitial spaces of the spinal cord. From a clinical standpoint, it is well known that computed tomography (CT) myelography will often demonstrate delayed filling of syrinx cavities. Filling can occur whether or not the contrast medium reaches the fourth ventricle and sometimes produces a "target sign" which is caused by opacification of the syrinx concurrent with decreasing opacification of the subarachnoid space. While this finding has been attributed to diffusion of the contrast medium through the parenchymal interspaces (Ikata et al. 1988), such a reversal of concentrations cannot be explained solely by molecular equilibration, and raises the possibility that "sink action" of the central canal may play a role.

The rate of clearance of EBD through the central canal was found to be equivalent to its rate of clearance from the spinal subarachnoid space. For example, when the marker was injected into the dorsal columns at T_{5-6} it ascended to the level of C_{3-4} within 45 min and to the level of the fourth ventricle within 90 min (see Fig. 3). This rate of ascent was approximately the same as that observed following lumbar injection of the marker (see Fig. 6). Since the movement of CSF through the spinal subarachnoid space is known to occur by bulk flow and constitutes a true circulatory current that is influenced by the venous pulse and other physiological variations (DeChiro 1964; Milhorat 1972), it is possible that the movement of EBD through the central canal reflects a similar mechanism.

The arrangement of an ascending flow of fluid through the central canal and a descending flow of fluid through the cerebral ventricles is consistent with the embryologic development of these spaces. Both are derived from the lumen of the neural tube and each develops, respectively, from the caudal and rostral luminal poles to form a continuous cavity that is sealed at either end and lined by ciliated ependymal cells. Following segmentation, the middle third of the neural tube develops three distinct foraminal openings at the level of the emerging fourth ventricle (Arey 1954). These foramina are the only direct communications between the internal cavity and the developing subarachnoid space and they create an outflow pathway for the CSF. Since the ends of the neural tube are closed, it is possible to infer that the movement of fluid, and possibly of cilia, is directed from the rostral and caudal poles toward the foraminal outlets of the fourth ventricle (Fig. 7).

References

Aboulker J (1979) La syringomyelie et les liquides intra-rachidiens. Neurochirurgie 25 (Suppl 1): 1–144

Arey LB (1954) Developmental anatomy. WB Saunders, Philadelphia, pp 465–500

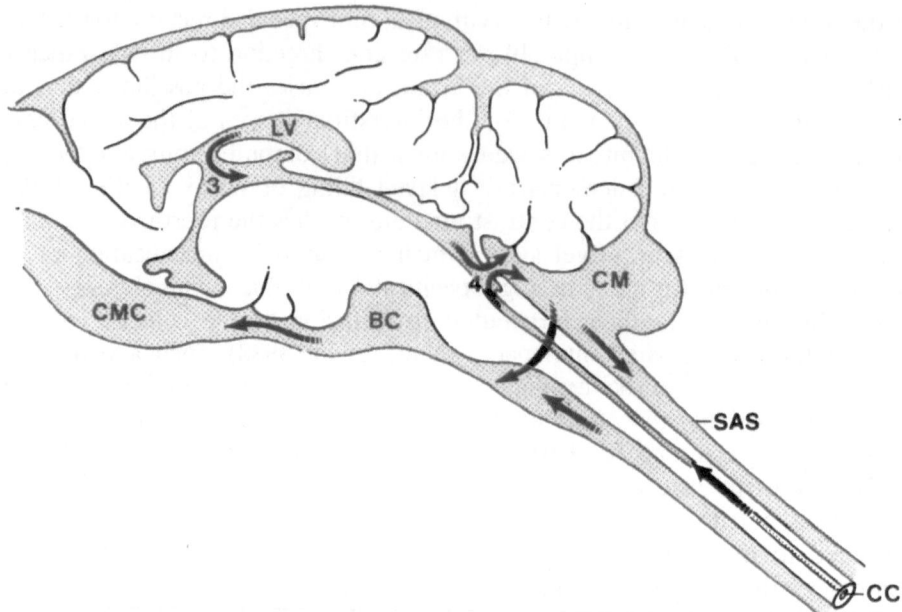

Fig. 7. Major pathways of CSF flow in the rat. LV, lateral ventricle; 3, third ventricle; 4, fourth ventricle; CM, cisterna magna; BC, basilar cisterns; CMC, chiasmatic cisterns; SAS, subarachnoid space; CC, central canal

Ball MJ, Dayan AD (1972) Pathogenesis of syringomyelia. Lancet II: 799–801

Becker DP, Wilson JA, Watson GW (1972) The spinal cord central canal-response to experimental hydrocephalus and canal occlusion. J Neurosurg 36: 416–424

Bering EA Jr (1956) The use of phenosulfonphthalein in the clinical evaluation of hydrocephalus. J Neurosurg 13: 587–595

Blasberg RG, Gazendem J, Patlak CS, et al. (1980) Quantitative autoradiographic studies of brain edema and a comparison of multi-isotope autoradiographic techniques. In: Cervos-Navaro P, Ferszt R (eds) Brain edema. Raven, New York, pp 255–269

Bradbury MWB, Lathem W (1965) A flow of cerebrospinal fluid along the central canal of the spinal cord of the rabbit and communications between this canal and the sacral subarachnoid space. J Physiol 181: 785–800

Cserr HF (1971) Physiology of the choroid plexus. *Physiol Rev* 51: 273–311

Cserr HF, Cooper DN, Milhorat TH (1977) Flow of cerebral interstitial fluid as indicated by the removal of extracellular markers from rat caudate nucleus. Exp Eye Res 25: 461–473

Cserr HF, Ostrach LH (1974) Bulk flow of interstitial fluid following intracranial injection of Blue Dextran 2000. Exp Neurol 45: 50–60

Davson H (1970) *Physiology of the cerebrospinal fluid.* Churchill, London, pp 157–158

DiChiro G (1964) Movement of the cerebrospinal fluid in human beings. Nature 204: 290–291

duBoulay G, Shah SS, Currie JC, et al. (1974) The mechanism of hydromyelia in Chiari Type I malformations. Br J Radiol 47: 579–587

Eisenberg HM, McLennan JE, Welch K (1974) Ventricular perfusion in cats with kaolin induced hydrocephalus. J Neurosurg 41: 20–28

Gardner WJ, Goodall RJ (1950) The surgical treatment of Arnold-Chiari malformation in adults. An explanation of its mechanism and importance of encephalography in diagnosis. J Neurosurg 7: 199–206

Gardner WJ, McMurry FG (1976) "Non-communicating" syringomyelia: a non-existent entity. Surg Neurol 6: 251–256

Hochwald GM, Boal RD, Marlin AE, et al. (1975) Changes in regional blood-flow and water content of brain and spinal cord in acute and chronic experimental hydrocephalus. Dev Med Child Neurol 17 (Suppl 35): 42–50

Ikata T, Masaki K, Kashiwaguchi S (1988) Clinical experimental studies on permeability of tracers in normal spinal cord and syringomyelia. Spine 13: 737–741

Klatzo I (1967) Neuropathological aspects of brain edema. J Neuropathol Exp Neurol 26: 1–14

Milhorat TH (1972) *Hydrocephalus and cerebrospinal fluid.* Williams and Wilkins, Baltimore, pp 24–30

Milhorat TH (1975) The third circulation revisited. J Neurosurg 42: 628–645

Milhorat TH, Clark RG (1970) Some observations on the circulation of phenolsulfonphthalein in cerebrospinal fluid: Normal flow and flow in hydrocephalus. J Neurosurg 32: 522–528

Milhorat TH, Johnson WD, Dow-Edwards, DL (1989) Relationship between edema, blood pressure, and blood flow following local brain injury. Neurol Res 11: 29–32

Tschingi RD (1950) Protein complexes and the impermeability of the blood-brain barrier to dyes. Am J Physiol 163: 756

Williams B (1980) On the pathogenesis of syringomyelia: a review. JR Soc Med 73: 798–806

Williams B, Bentley J (1980) Experimental communicating syringomyelia in dogs after cisternal kaolin injection. Part I Morphology. J Neurol Sci 48: 93–107

21 — Pathogenesis of Syringomyelia with Description of Non-Communicating Type That Arises Immediately Caudal to Obstructive Lesions

Thomas H. Milhorat, Richard W. Johnson, and Walter D. Johnson

Introduction

The pathogenesis of syringomyelia is incompletely understood. Since the condition is known to occur in association with hindbrain malformations and a variety of other lesions that occur at the level of the foramen magnum, attempts have been made to explain its development hydrodynamically. According to Gardner (Gardner et al. 1957; Gardner and Goodall 1950; Gardner and McMurry 1976), syringomyelia is caused by mechanical obstruction of the outlets of the fourth ventricle which results in a redirection of the cerebrospinal fluid (CSF) pulse wave into the central canal. The caudal focusing of the pulse wave presumably distends the central canal and leads to a net accumulation of fluid that may be confined to the lumen of the canal (hydromyelia) or may dissect into the paracentral tissues if the ependymal lining ruptures (syringohydromyelia).

Williams (1978, 1980, 1986) has offered the alternative explanation that obstructions at the level of the cervical-medullary junction produce a dissociation of pressure between the cranial and spinal subarachnoid spaces that draws fluid from the fourth ventricle into the central canal as a consequence of the relatively lower CSF pressure caudal to the block. This pressure gradient has been shown to be sensitive to postural influences and appears to be accentuated during sudden Valsalva maneuvers such as coughing, straining, and sneezing (Williams 1981). Other authors, while agreeing that a pressure gradient contributes to syrinx formation, have provided evidence that CSF within the spinal subarachnoid space is forced under increased pressure (Park et al. 1989) through enlarged Virchow-Robin spaces (Ball and Dayan 1972) or the dorsal roots (Aboulker 1979) into the central canal.

On the basis of the foregoing hypotheses, a number of operative approaches have been proposed as treatment for syringomyelia. The classical procedures

Departments of Neurosurgery, State University of New York, Health Science Center at Brooklyn, and Kings County Hospital Center, Brooklyn, NY 11203, USA

include terminal myelotomy (Gardner et al. 1977), decompression of the foramen magnum with plugging of the obex (Gardner and McMurry 1976; Levy et al. 1983; Logue and Edwards 1981; McLean et al. 1973), and decompression of the posterior fossa with one or more of the following steps: lysis of arachnoidal adhesions, fenestration or drainage of the outlets of the fourth ventricle, amputation of the tips of the cerebellar tonsils, and duraplasty (Batzdorf 1988; Bertrand 1973; Oakes 1985; Rhoton 1976; Williams 1986). No one procedure has been uniformly successful and additional strategies have been advocated, such as ventricular shunting (Krayenbuhl and Benini 1971), syringosubarachnoid shunting (Tator et al. 1982; Vaquero et al. 1987), syringoperitoneal shunting (Barbaro et al. 1984; Lesoin et al. 1986; Phillips and Kindt 1981), and lumboperitoneal shunting following drainage of the syrinx (Park 1989).

The proposition that syringomyelia is caused by a caudally directed flow of CSF through the central canal has not been supported by recent experience with magnetic resonance (MR) imaging. With the widespread availability of this new technology, syrinx cavities can be demonstrated that do not communicate with the fourth ventricle, and occur in the absence of an obvious lesion or in association with lesions such as cervical spondylosis (Dorhmann and Rubin 1986; Yu and Moseley 1987) that are located caudal to the foramen magnum. Even with lesions that obstruct the cervical-medullary junction, the intramedullary cavity usually is found at some distance from the fourth ventricle and is separated from it by a long segment of syrinx-free spinal cord. Thus, in a series of reports (Kokmen et al. 1985; Lee et al. 1985; Park et al. 1989; Pojunas et al. 1984; Samuelsson et al. 1987; Sherman et al. 1986) summarizing MR findings in 127 patients with hydromyelia and syringomyelia, a direct communication between the fourth ventricle and the intramedullary cavity was present in only 4 (3%), including 1 of 13 patients with the Chiari II malformation (Park et al. 1989).

The purpose of the current study was to review the neurologic, neuroradiologic, and surgical findings in patients with MR-documented syringomyelia. Evidence is provided that extramedullary obstruction is a common cause of non-communicating syringomyelia, whereas obstruction of the CSF pathways distal to the outlets of the fourth ventricle tends to produce a communicating type of syringomyelia (hydromyelia) in association with hydrocephalus. Both types of syringomyelia have distinctive neuroradiologic findings and both appear to have different treatment requirements.

Keyword. Syringomyelia — Cerebrospinal fluid — Hydrocephalus

Clinical Material and Methods

Fifty-one patients with MR-demonstrated syringomyelia were the subjects of this study. Excluded from consideration were patients with intramedullary tumors, since syrinx formation in such cases can involve many variables including cystic degeneration of the tumor, peritumoral edema, and transudation of protein rostral or caudal to the lesion. There were 7 children and 44 adults ranging in age from 2 to 76 years, with a mean age of 41.6 years. All patients exhibited varying degrees of weakness or spasticity of the extremities. Additional findings in some patients included: neck or back pain, radicular pain, dissociated sensory loss, paresthesias in the upper extremities, muscular atrophy of the hands, impaired position sense in the lower extremities, urinary incontinence, scoliosis or kyphosis, spina bifida, torticollis, dysphagia, headaches, and macrocephaly.

MR images were obtained on the following scanning units: (1) 0.5 Tesla Magnetom; (2) 0.6 Tesla Teslacon II; and (3) 1.5 Tesla General Electric Sigma. Sagittal and axial T1-weighted spin echo images utilized a repetition time (TR) of 500–700 ms, and an echo time (TE) of 13–20 ms for the Sigma and Magnetom units and 28–32 ms for the Teslacon II unit. Additional information was obtained by plain spine roentgenography, computed tomography (CT) scanning, metrizamide myelography or ventriculography, delayed CT myelography, and gadolinium-enhanced MR imaging.

Twenty-seven patients underwent one or more of the following surgical procedures: (1) ventriculoperitoneal (VP) shunting (12 cases); (2) suboccipital craniotomy and upper cervical laminectomy with lysis of arachnoidal adhesions and duraplasty (3 cases); (3) anterior cervical discectomy and fusion (6 cases); (4) syringosubarachnoid shunting to the lateral medullary cisterna or cisterna magna (5 cases); (5) posterior laminectomy for excision of extramedullary cyst or tumor (2 cases); and (6) posterior cervical fusion (1 case).

Results

Based on neuroradiological criteria, syrinx cavities were divided into 3 general types: (1) communicating syrinxes, that were anatomically continuous with the fourth ventricle; (2) non-communicating syrinxes, that were separated from the fourth ventricle by an intervening segment of syrinx-free spinal cord; and (3) atrophic syrinxes.

Communicating Syringomyelia (Hydromyelia)

A direct communication between the syrinx cavity and the fourth ventricle was present in 9 of 51 patients (18%). An associated finding in all cases was hydrocephalus. The aperture of the syrinx was visualized best on midsagittal MR images and patency was confirmed in some cases by metrizamide ventriculography. There was considerable variation in the size of the syrinx opening, which was found along the floor of the ventricle near its caudal apex at the level of the obex. Since this is the location of the normal opening of the central canal, the term hydromyelia can probably be used to describe these syrinxes.

Treatment consisted of a VP shunt in 7 patients. There was one revision for shunt failure but no other complications over a follow-up period of 2 months to 5 years. Symptoms were improved or relieved in all patients within a few weeks of operation and postoperative MR scans revealed a reduction in ventricular size in 6 of 7 patients and a reduction in syrinx size in 7 of 7 patients.

Non-communicating Syrinxes, Obstructive Type

Extramedullary lesions causing chronic compression of the spinal cord were associated with syrinx formation in 25 of 51 patients (49%). In each case, the lumen of the syrinx appeared to arise immediately caudal to the lower border of the compressive lesion and did not extend rostral to this level. Cavity lengths varied from a mean of 3 levels to those of 6 levels or more which were typically found in younger patients. The obstructing lesions included: (1) cerebellar hernias associated with the Chiari I or Chiari II malformations (14 cases); (2) cervical discs (4 cases); (3) extramedullary cysts or tumors (4 cases); (4) basilar impression (2 cases); and (5) gibbus deformity (1 case).

Sixteen patients underwent operative treatment. Symptomatic improvement and a collapse in syrinx size was achieved in 5 of 5 patients with the Chiari II malformation, myelomeningocele, and hydrocephalus by UP shunting. In 2 of 3 patients with the Chiari I malformation, suboccipital decompression with lysis of arachnoidal adhesions and duraplasty proved to be effective treatment. There was no symptomatic improvement or change in syrinx size in the third patient, and a syringosubarachnoid shunt from the rostral end of the syrinx to the lateral medullary cistern was subsequently performed. In this patient and in 3 additional patients with Chiari I malformations in whom a syringo-subarachnoid shunt was performed as a primary procedure, the results were good over a follow-up interval of 1–6 months.

In 2 of 3 patients with cervical discs, anterior discectomy and fusion resulted in symptomatic relief with complete resolution of the syrinx on follow-up MR scans. However, in both of these cases, the syrinxes were narrow cavities, and in a third patient with a large cervical syrinx, there was no reduction in syrinx size following operative removal of the disc. Effective treatment in this case was achieved by a syringosubarachnoid shunt from the rostral end of the syrinx to the cisterna magna.

A reduction in syrinx size was observed in 2 patients following the removal of extramedullary masses. In a 63-year-old male with a 20 year history of progressive spastic paraparesis, excision of an arachnoid cyst at T_{6-7} produced a significant improvement in symptoms and a marked reduction in the size of the syrinx caudal to the block. Similar results were achieved by excision of a C_7 schwannoma in a 25-year-old male with a syrinx extending from C_7-T_4.

Non-communicating Syringomyelia, Atrophic Type

Non-communicating syrinxes occurring in association with spinal cord atrophy were present in 14 of 51 patients (27%). In typical cases, the syrinx was confined to a focal segment of myelomalacia and appeared as a non-distended cleft that was central in location and flattened in transverse diameter on axial images. In some cases, the lumen of the cavity appeared to extend into the dorsal quadrant of the spinal cord. The causes of spinal cord atrophy included: (1) cervical spondylosis (9 cases); (2) fracture dislocations (2 cases); (3) myelotomy for excision of tumor (2 cases); and (4) spinal cord infarction following cardiac arrest (1 case).

Operative treatment was limited to anterior discectomy and fusion in 3 patients with cervical discs. There was some improvement in symptoms, especially in 2 patients with prominent radicular complaints, but little or no improvement in long tract signs. Postoperative MR scans revealed no change in syrinx size.

Unclassified Syrinxes

Three patients in this series had non-communicating syrinxes that were not associated with extramedullary compression and were not due to spinal cord atrophy.

Case 49

A 48-year-old female with a 10 year history of neck pain that occasionally radiated into one or both shoulders experienced progressive weakness and spasticity in the lower extremities of approximately 6 months duration. There was a past history of multiple injuries to the neck, including one severe whiplash injury 2 years earlier. Neurological examination revealed mild spastic paraparesis, impaired position sense in the lower extremities, and atrophy of the intrinsic muscles of both hands. On MR scanning, there was evidence of a syrinx cavity from C_{2-7} associated with degenerative osteoarthritis and a swan neck deformity. Treatment consisted of a syringo-subarachnoid shunt to the lateral medullary cistern, which resulted in a marked reduction in the size of the syrinx and a significant but incomplete recovery of neurological deficits over a follow-up interval of 3 years.

Case 50

A 47-year-old male who had been paraplegic since a motor vehicle accident 17 years earlier complained of progressive weakness in the upper extremities and occasional difficulty swallowing of 2 months duration. Neurologic examination revealed complete paraplegia with patchy loss of sensation below T_4, slight weakness of the upper extremities, generalized hyperreflexia, and no significant cranial nerve findings. X-rays of the cervical spine were unremarkable except for narrowing of the C_{5-6} disc interspace and evidence of a posterior cervical fusion that had been performed at the time of the original injury. CT myelography and MR imaging revealed a long syrinx cavity that extended from L_{1-2} to the level of the lower medulla.

Case 51

A 37-year-old female with a 10 year history of multiple sclerosis complained of slowly progressive spastic quadriparesis over an interval of several months. MR scans demonstrated multiple white mattter lesions consistent with gliotic plaques surrounding the lateral and fourth ventricles. In the caudal half of the medulla, there was a concentration of plaques that extended to the level of C_1, associated with a narrow syrinx that distended the spinal cord from C_1 to C_7.

Discussion

The diagnosis of syringomyelia has been greatly facilitated in recent years by the advent of MR imaging which provides unique information about the location, extent, and anatomical relationships of intramedullary cavities. As experience has grown, it has become evident that syrinx formation is far more common than previously supposed, and that it can occur in association with a wide variety of lesions that arise at some distance from the cervical-medullary junction (Dohrmann and Rubin 1986; Kokmen et al. 1985; Lee et al. 1985; Pojunas et al. 1984; Sherman et al. 1986; Yu et al. 1987). Perhaps the most unexpected finding is that most syrinx cavities do not communicate directly with the fourth ventricle (Park et al. 1989). This has cast doubt on the traditional hypothesis that CSF flows caudally through the central canal, and has revived interest in the proposition of Ball and Dayan (1972), and subsequently Aboulker (1979), that CSF within the spinal subarachnoid space moves under increased pressure (Park et al. 1989) into the central canal through enlarged parenchymal interspaces.

The findings in the current study confirm previously published data that most syrinx cavities do not communicate with the fourth ventricle. Anatomically continuous syrinxes (communicating syringomyelia, hydromyelia) were found in association with hydrocephalus, and were present in only 9 of 51 patients (18%). The most important findings concerned non-communicating syrinxes. In 25 of 28 cases that were not due to spinal cord atrophy, the intramedullary cavity was found immediately caudal to an extramedullary compressive lesion. The rostral end of these cavities appeared to arise at the lower border of the compressed segment of spinal cord and was separated from the fourth ventricle by a syrinx-free segment that varied in length from a few centimeters in the case of Chiari I malformations, to greater than 40 cm in the case of an extramedullary arachnoid cyst. This relationship is similar to that described by Blaylock (1981), and appears to be evident, in retrospect, on previously published MR images demonstrating syrinx formation in association with the

Chiari I malformation (Batzdorf 1988; Park et al. 1989; Rhoton 1988; Vaquero et al. 1990) and basilar impression (Kohno et al. 1990). It is appropriate to point out that although syrinx formation was not observed to occur rostral to compressive lesions in this study, Quencer et al. (1986) have reported 1 convincing case in which a 56-year-old woman with a cervical schwannoma exhibited syrinx formation above and below the tumor. However, in this case, the patient had suffered a severe neck injury 5 years earlier that may have been a contributing factor.

The finding of syrinx formation caudal to compressive lesions requires a review of prevailing hydrodynamic theories. Given this anatomical relationship, it is unlikely that the formation of non-communicating syrinxes can be attributed to a caudally directed flow of CSF from the fourth ventricle into the central canal, either as the consequence of a redirected CSF pulse wave (Gardner and McMurry 1976), or by the establishment of a pressure gradient between the cranial and spinal subarachnoid spaces (Williams 1980). Likewise, it is unlikely that raised intraspinal pressure (Park et al. 1989) plays a significant role in syrinx formation, since CSF pressure below extramedullary lesions tends to be normal or reduced, depending on the completeness of the block.

A fundamental assumption of prevailing hydrodynamic theories is that the fluid which accumulates within syrinx cavities is derived from the cerebral ventricles and enters the central canal through the fourth ventricle (Gardner and McMurry 1976; Williams 1980) or the spinal subarachnoid space (Aboulker 1979; Ball and Dayan 1972). This has not been firmly established, and in a recent experimental study (Milhorat et al., this volume) evidence has been presented that the central canal of the spinal cord may have an intrinsic circulation that drains CSF in a rostral direction toward the fourth ventricle. Obstruction of this circulatory pathway is a possible explanation for the development of certain non-communicating syrinxes that arise caudal to compressive lesions. Obviously, if mechanical compression of the central canal is a causal factor, it would follow that removal of the obstructing lesion, or decompression of the constricted segment of spinal cord, should improve symptoms and reduce syrinx size in some cases. This was observed in 6 of 8 patients in the current series, and comparable results have been reported following the removal of extramedullary tumors (Blaylock 1981; Quencer et al. 1986), transoral resection of the odontoid process for basilar impression (Kohno 1990), and decompression of the foramen magnum for the Chiari I malformation (Batzdorf 1988; Vaquero 1990).

Although the surgical management of communicating syringomyelia (hydromyelia) has been based on the assumption that CSF flows caudally from the fourth ventricle into the central canal (Batzdorf 1988; Gardner 1976; Williams 1980), experience has shown that plugging of the obex is not effective treatment (Batzdorf 1988; Levy et al. 1983; Williams 1980). Batzorf (1988) has suggested that the occasional success of Gardner's original operation (Gardner 1976) may occur when sealing of the obex is incomplete. On the basis of evidence that the central canal of the spinal cord drains fluid in a rostral direction (Milhorat et al., this volume), it is possible to speculate that obstruction of the CSF pathways distal to the outlets of the fourth ventricle impedes both the ascending flow of CSF through the central canal and the descending flow of CSF through the cerebral ventricles, producing dilatation of the cavities proximal to the block. This explanation would be consistent with the pathological findings in communicating hydrocephalus/hydromyelia and would account for the fact that effective treatment of the condition can often be achieved by either a VP (Krayenbuhl and Berini 1971) or a syringoperitoneal shunt (Barbaro et al. 1984; Lesoin et al. 1986; Phillips and Kindt 1986). In this series, VP shunting tended to produce a uniform reduction in the size of the cerebral ventricles and hydromyelic cavity, except in patients with myelomeningocele and the Chiari II malformation in whom the caudal end of the syrinx often remained distended.

There was a considerable variation in the rostrocaudal length of syrinx cavities. Cervical syrinxes tended to be found in adult patients, whereas longer cavities, especially those extending the length of the spinal cord (holocord enlargement), were more often seen in younger patients or adults with congenital obstructions. In man, the lumbar and thoracic segments of the central canal are frequently obliterated during the middle years of adult life by a proliferation of glial and ependymal cells (Netsky 1953). This is unique to the human and its significance is unknown. However, caudal stenosis of the central canal may explain why syrinx formation, especially of the acquired variety, in adults is frequently confined to the rostral segment of the spinal cord.

In the current series, atrophic syrinxes (syringomyelia ex vacuo) were present in 14 of 51 patients (27%). These were quite characteristic and usually could be distinguished easily from other types of syringomyelia by MR imaging. In typical cases, the syrinx cavity was confined to an atrophic segment of spinal cord and appeared as a narrow cleft that was flattened or collapsed in transverse diameter on axial images. Since the principle etiologic factors were ischemia and trauma the probable cause of cavity formation in these cases was myelomalacia secondary to cell loss and myelinolysis.

Non-communicating syrinxes that were not due to compression or atrophy were present in 3 of 51 patients (7%). In 1 patient with multiple sclerosis, a cervical syrinx was found immediately caudal to a cluster of intramedullary plaques. It could not be established with certainty whether these lesions produced an intrinsic obstruction of the central canal. However, in the absence of any other explanation, occlusion of the central canal secondary to gliosis or scarring is a possible mechanism for syrinx formation in this case and in 2 cases of post-traumatic syringomyelia. The extension of one post–traumatic syrinx (case 50) from the injury site at C_{5-6} to the level of the medulla was presumably the result of rostral dissection through the paracentral tissues. This phenomenon was not seen with syrinxes associated with extramedullary compression, possibly because of the resistance imposed by the compressed segment of spinal cord.

Overall, the findings in the current study are consistent with separately reported experimental evidence that the central canal of the spinal cord drains fluid in a rostral direction (Milhorat et al., this volume), and suggest that obstruction of this circulatory pathway, either proximal or distal to the obex, produces different types of syrinx cavities. The diagnostic distinction between communicating and non-communicating syringomyelia can usually be made by MR imaging, which is also helpful in excluding intramedullary tumors. Findings of importance in the differential diagnosis of syringomyelia are hydrocephalus, myelomalacia, and compression of the spinal cord rostral to the syrinx.

Although it is beyond the scope of this report to discuss specific treatment strategies, several general comments can be made. First, in patients with hydrocephalus and communicating syrinxes (hydromyelia), the treatment of choice appears to be a VP shunt. Plugging of the obex can not be recommended and is probably contraindicated on the basis of evidence reported here. Second, in the treatment of non-communicating syrinxes, a distinction should be made between atrophic and obstructed cavities. Atrophic syringomyelia is not likely to be helped by treatment, although surgery may be warranted to treat the causal lesion or to halt progression of the atrophic process.

The treatment of obstructive syringomyelia is much less certain. In some cases, removal of the obstructing lesion or surgical decompression of the spinal cord may be the treatment of choice. However, direct operations may fail to relieve certain obstructions just as they do in the treatment of non-communicating hydrocephalus. In patients whose syrinxes persist following direct operations, and in those with non-communicating syrinxes not due to extramedullary compression, a syringosubarachnoid shunt may be considered. The principle of treatment should be to divert the syrinx fluid into the subarachnoid space rostral to obstructing lesions. In patients with the Chiari I malformation, we have found it desirable to position the distal end of the catheter in the lateral medullary cistern rather than the upper cervical theca. The value of syringosubarachnoid shunting as a primary treatment for non-communicating syringomyelia is currently under investigation.

Acknowledgment. The authors are indebted to the following colleagues who contributed cases to this study: Richard M. Bergland, M.D., Mark Eastham, M.D., and David Liu, M.D. Robert H. Milhorat provided invaluable assistance in the collection, analysis, and tabulation of data.

References

Aboulker J (1979) La syringomyelie et les liquides intra-rachidiens. Neurochirurgie 25 (Suppl 1): 1–144

Ball MJ, Dayan AD (1972) Pathogenesis of syringomyelia. Lancet II: 799–801

Barbaro NM, Wilson CB, Gutin PH, et al. (1984) Surgical treatment of syringomyelia. Favorable results with syringoperitoneal shunting. J Neurosurg 61: 531–538

Batzdorf U (1988) Chiari 1 malformation with syringomyelia. Evaluation of surgical therapy by magnetic resonance imaging. J Neurosurg 68: 726–730

Bertrand G (1973) Dynamic factors in the evolution of syringomyelia and syringobulbia. Clin Neurosurg 20: 322–333

Blaylock RL (1981) Hydrosyringomyelia of the conus medullaris associated with a thoracic meningioma. J Neurosurg 54: 833–835

Dohrmann GJ, Rubin JM (1986) Cervical spondylosis and syringomyelia: suboptimal results, incomplete treatment, and the role of intraoperative ultrasound. Clin Neurosurg 34: 378–388

Gardner WJ, Goodall RJ (1950) The surgical treatment of Arnold-Chiari malformation in adults. An explanation of its mechanism and importance of encephalography in diagnosis. J Neurosurg 7: 199–206

Gardner WJ, McMurry FG (1976) "Non-communicating" syringomyelia: a non-existent entity. Surg Neurol 6: 251–256

Gardner WJ, Abdullah AF, McCormack LJ (1957) The varying expressions of embryonal atresia of the fourth ventricle in adults. Arnold-Chiari malformation, Dandy-Walker syndrome, "arachnoid" cyst of the cerebellum, and syringomyelia. J Neurosurg 14: 591–607

Gardner WJ, Bell HS, Poolos PN, et al. (1977) Terminal ventriculostomy for syringomyelia. J Neurosurg 46: 609–617

Kokmen E, Marsh WR, Baker HL Jr (1985) Magnetic resonance imaging in syringomyelia. Neurosurgery 17: 267–270

Kohno K, Sakaki S, Shiraishi T, et al. (1990) Successful treatment of adult Arnold-Chiari malformation associated with basilar impression and syringomyelia by the transoral anterior approach. Surg Neurol 33: 284–287

Krayenbuhl H, Benini A (1971) A new surgical approach in the treatment of hydromyelia and syringomyelia. The embryological basis and the first results. J R Coll Surg Edinb 16: 147–161

Lee BCP, Zimmerman RD, Manning JJ, et al. (1985) MR imaging of syringomyelia and hydromyelia. AJR 144: 1149–1156

Lesoin F, Petit H, Thomas CE III, et al. (1986) Use of the syringoperitoneal shunt in the treatment of syringomyelia. Surg Neurol 25: 131–136, 1986

Levy WJ, Mason L, Hahn JF (1983) Chiari malformation presenting in adults: a surgical experience in 127 cases. Neurosurgery 12: 377–390

Logue V, Edwards MR (1981) Syringomyelia and its surgical treatment — an analysis of 75 patients. J Neurol Neurosurg Psychiatry 44: 273–284

McLean DR, Miller JDR, Allen PBR, et al. (1973) Posttraumatic syringomyelia. J Neurosurg 39: 485–492

Oakes WJ (1985) Chiari malformations, hydromyelia, syringomyelia. In: Wilkins RH, Rengachary SS (eds) Neurosurgery, vol. 3. McGraw Hill, New York, pp 2102–2124

Netsky MG (1953) Syringomyelia — a clinicopathologic study. Arch Neurol Psychiat 70: 741–777

Park TS, Cail WS, Broaddus WC, et al. (1989) Lumboperitoneal shunt combined with myelotomy for treatment of syringohydromyelia. J Neurosurg 70: 721–727

Phillips TW, Kindt GW (1986) Syringoperitoneal shunt for syringomyelia: a preliminary report. Surg Neurol 16: 462–466

Pojunas K, Williams AL, Daniels DL, et al. (1984) Syringomyelia and hydromyelia: magnetic resonance evaluation. Radiology 153: 679–683

Quencer RM, Gammal TE, Cohen G (1986) Syringomyelia associated with intradural extramedullary masses of the spinal canal. AJNR 7: 143–148

Rhoton AL Jr (1976) Microsurgery of Arnold-Chiari malformation in adults with and without hydromyelia. J Neurosurg 45: 473–483

Rhoton AL Jr (1988) Microsurgery of syringomyelia and syringomyelic cord syndrome. In: Schmidek HH, Sweet WH (eds) Operative Neurosurgical Techniques. WB Saunders, Philadelphia, pp 1307–1326

Samuelsson L, Bergstrom K, Thuomas K, et al. (1987) MR imaging of syringo-hydromyelia and Chiari malformations in myelomeningocele patients with scoliosis. AJNR 8: 539–546

Sherman JL, Barkovich AJ, Citrin CM (1986) The MR appearance of syringomyelia: new observations. AJNR 7: 985–995

Tator CH, Meguro K, Rowed DW (1982) Favorable results with syringosubarachnoid shunts for treatment of syringomyelia. J Neurosurg 56: 517–523

Vaquero J, Martinez R, Salazar J, et al. (1987) Syringosubarachnoid shunt for treatment of syringomyelia. Acta Neurochir (Wien) 84: 105–109, 1987

Vaquero J, Martinez R, Arias A (1990) Syringomyelia-Chiari complex: magnetic resonance imaging and clinical evaluation of surgical treatment. J Neurosurg 73: 64–68

Williams B (1978) A critical appraisal of posterior fossa surgery for communicating syringomyelia. Brain 101: 223–250

Williams B (1980) On the pathogenesis of syringomyelia: a review. J R Soc Med 73: 798–806

Williams B (1981) Simultaneous cerebral and spinal fluid pressure recordings. 2. Cerebrospinal dissociation with lesions at the foramen magnum. Acta Neurochir (Wien) 59: 123–142

Williams B (1986) Progress in syringomyelia. Neurol Res 8: 139–145

Yu YL, Moseley IF (1987) Syringomyelia and cervical spondylosis: a clinicoradiological investigation. Neuroradiology 29: 143–151

22 — Potential Difference Records from Human Cerebrospinal Fluid

Peter S. Baxter and Robert A. Minns[1]

Summary. The electrical potential difference (PD) between ventricular cerebrospinal fluid (CSF) and blood was recorded simultaneously with intraventricular pressure in children with shunted hydrocephalus. The mean basal value was +4.1 mV. The ECG and small amplitude PD changes which matched the respiratory trace were seen in all patients. More prolonged wave-like PD changes, lasting about ten minutes, preceded A, or plateau, wave changes on the pressure trace, and were followed by a small positive change which lasted throughout the plateau wave. Similar briefer PD waves preceded individual B waves in the pressure trace. During episodes of recurrent B wave activity the overall PD showed more prolonged wave-like changes lasting up to an hour. In one patient a negative PD change was also associated with an episode of increased pulse pressure without an overall rise in pressure. The PD changes suggest that A and B pressure waves in the ventricular CSF are triggered by active secretion.

Keywords. Electrical potential difference — Intraventricular pressure — Plateau wave — B waves

Introduction

Hydrocephalus is caused by obstruction to the flow or absorption of cerebrospinal fluid (CSF), but the origin of pathological pressure changes such as A, B, and C waves remains uncertain. Hemodynamic factors are a generally postulated cause (Rosner and Becker 1984). It is now recognised that two thirds of the CSF is actively secreted by the choroid plexus, which has the ultrastructural characteristics of a secretory epithelium (Carr 1975). Other secretory epithelia such as the intestinal and airway mucosa and sweat glands characteristically have a transmucosal electrical potential difference (PD)

[1] Department of Paediatric Neurology, Royal Hospital for Sick Children, Edinburgh, EH9 1LF, Scotland, UK

which reflects their ion transporting activities and which changes when secretion is stimulated by a regulatory agent such as those acting through intracellular cyclic AMP (Armstrong 1987). A similar PD has been demonstrated between the spinal CSF and blood in man (Sorensen et al. 1978) and animals (Davies et al. 1984). We report the existence of a PD between ventricular CSF and blood in children with shunted hydrocephalus and demonstrate changes that correlate with physiological and pathological changes in pressure.

Patients and Methods

In three children (aged 3 years 4 months–11 years 7 months) with shunted hydrocephalus who had symptoms of shunt dysfunction, the ventricular pressure and PD was recorded through a separate frontal Rickham reservoir before and during sleep. Access was obtained by a 25G short butterfly inserted percutaneously into the reservoir cap which was connected to a non-displacement pressure transducer and a 1M KCl agar bridge after air had been expelled from the system. The other end of the KCl bridge was placed in a calomel half cell and the PD between this and a saline-filled intravenous cannula, which acted as the reference electrode, connected by an identical bridge to a second calomel half cell (back to back PD less than 2 mV, checked before and after each study) was measured by a high impedance battery-operated electrometer (Keithley 602, Keithley Instruments Ltd., Ohio) and recorded simultaneously with the output from the pressure transducer, via an isolated amplifier onto a

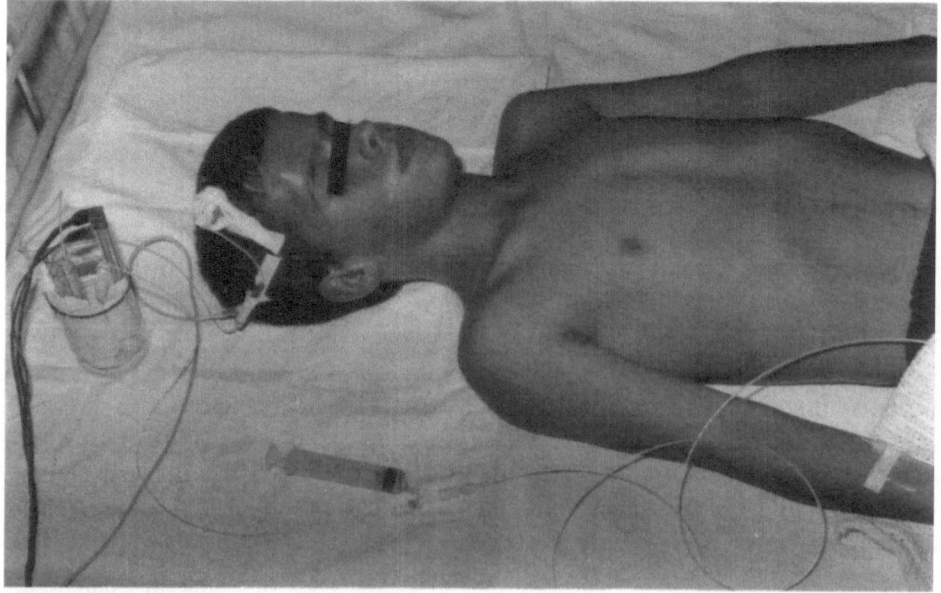

Fig. 1. Patient with P.D. and ICP being recorded through a common ventricular access device. The reference P.D. electrode is from an I.V. cannula

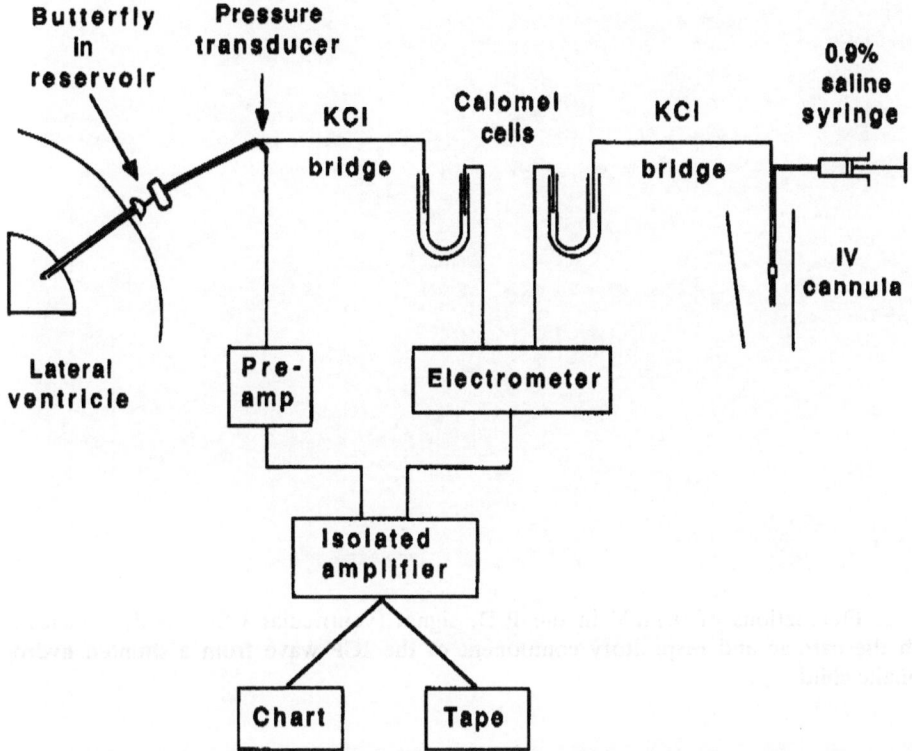

Fig. 2. Schematic diagram of methodology for recording P.D. of ventricular CSF with respect to the extracellular fluid

Table 1. Results

Patients Names	Offset Potential (back-back)		Basal PD	Corrected basal PD (allow +3.1 mV for saline-blood junction potential
AD	Start	+0.8	+0.9	
	End	−1.6	+0.9	
	Mean	−0.8	+0.9	+4.8 mV
IS	Start	+0.9	+0.45	
	End	+1.2	+0.45	
	Mean	+1.05	+0.45	+2.5 mV
SS	Start	−0.1	+1.5	
	End	−0.4	+1.5	
	Mean	−0.25	+1.5	+4.9 mV

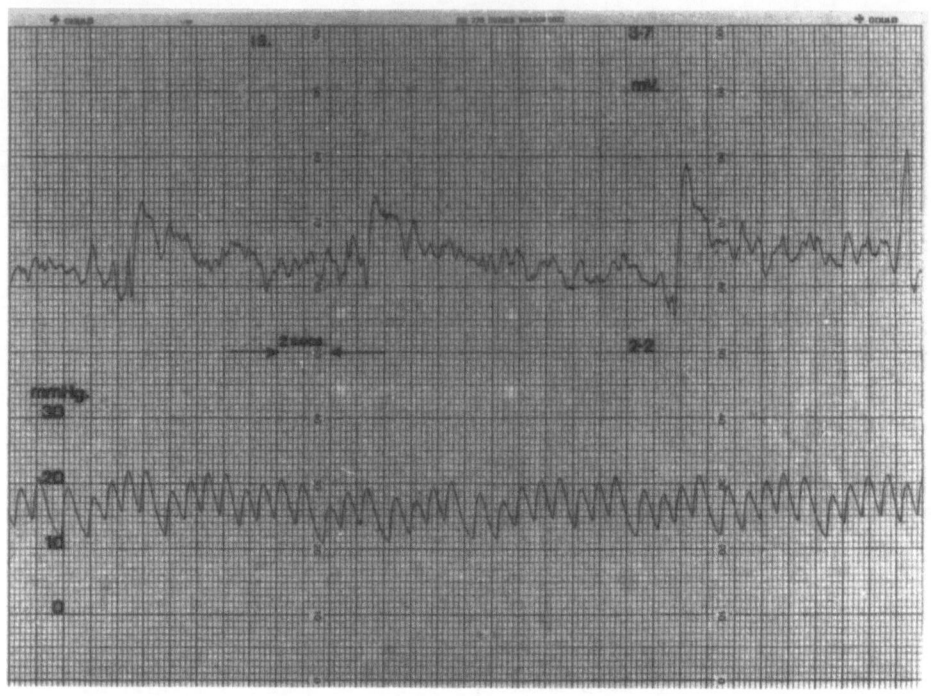

Fig. 3. Fluctuations of 0.1 mV in the P.D. signal (ventricular CSF/blood) coincident with the cardiac and respiratory component of the ICP wave from a shunted hydrocephalic child

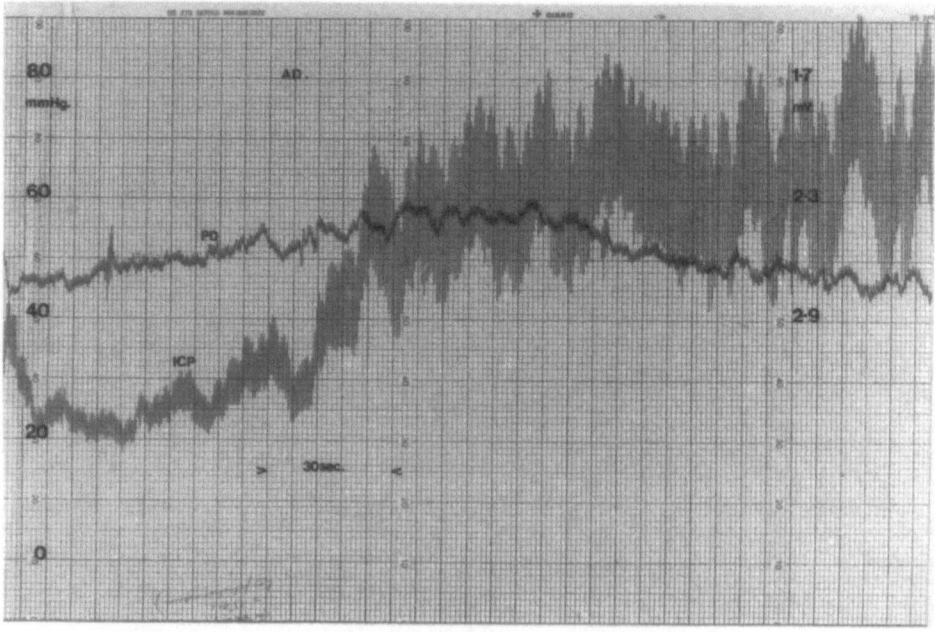

Fig. 4. Plateau (*A*) wave during sleep from boy aged 8 years 9 months with decompensated hydrocephalus (blocked VP shunt) showing a more negative change in the P.D. (0.45 mV) prior to the onset of the A wave

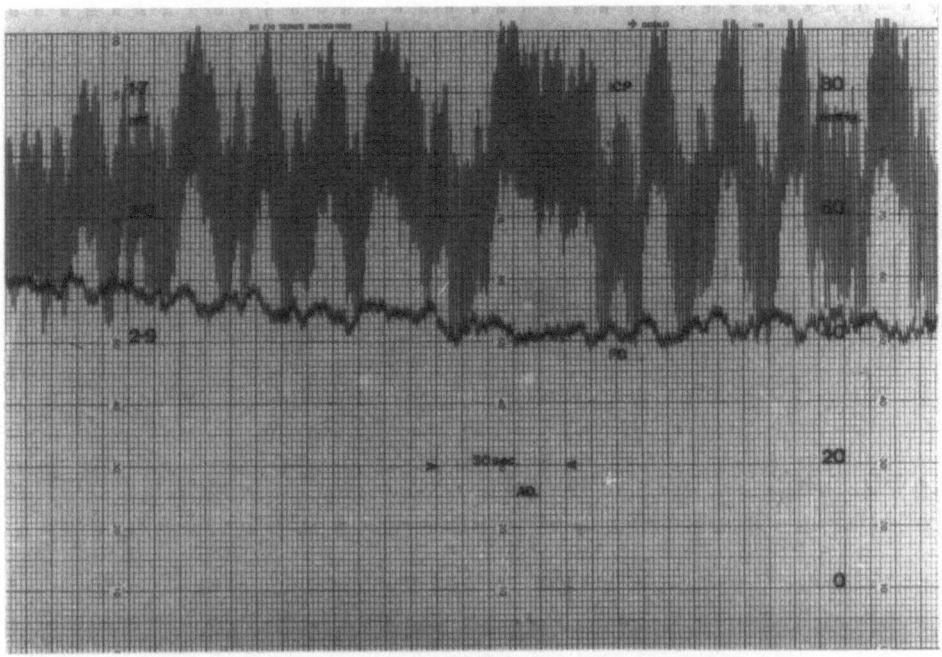

Fig. 5. C waves superimposed on a typical plateau wave with similiar electrical potential fluctuations

chart recorder (BS-272, Gould Bryans Instruments Ltd., Surrey, U.K.) and tape recorder (Racal, U.K.), as shown in Figs. 1 and 2. PD readings were taken to the nearest 0.1 mV and were corrected by 3.1 mV, to allow for the saline: blood junction potential (Sorensen et al. 1978). The study had local ethical committee agreement.

Results

During 17.5 h of recording, 2–8.5 per patient, the basal PD in the absence of abnormal pressure patterns was + 4.1 mV, range 2.5–4.9 (Table 1) with an ECG pattern, amplitude < 0.1 mV, that coincided with pulsatile fluctuations on the pressure trace and a regular fluctuation of 0.1 mV that coincided with the respiratory fluctuation on the pressure trace (Fig. 3). Asking the child to hold their breath abolished the respiratory fluctuation in both PD and pressure traces.

In two patients three episodes of plateau waves (pressure 30–70 mmHg, duration 5–30 min) occurred during sleep. In both patients these episodes were preceded, by a mean of 2 min, by a wave-like negative change in the CSF PD, amplitude of −0.3 mV, which lasted a mean total of 5 min (Fig. 4). This was followed by a positive change of +0.3 mV which lasted for the rest of the plateau wave and returned to a basal level within 1 min of the end of the pressure change. During the plateau, the pulse pressure increased up to 20 mmHg and regular fluctuations in pressure of 40 mmHg occurred at a

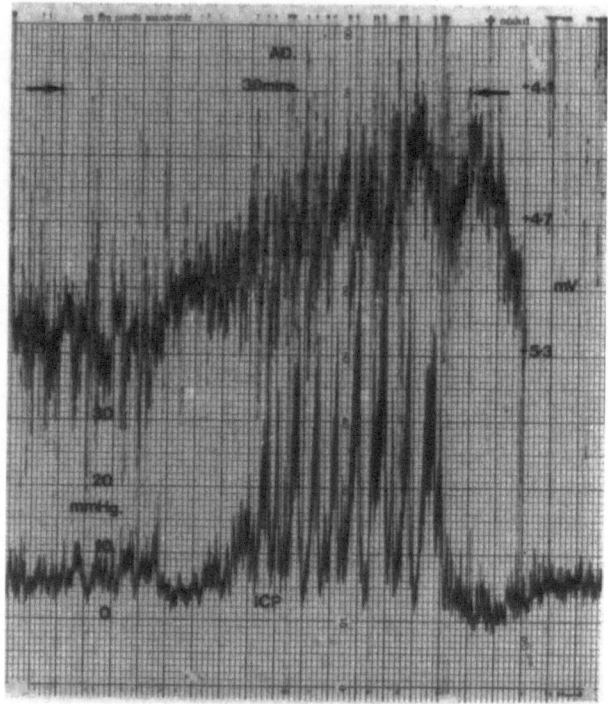

Fig. 6. Repetitive B wave activity associated with a negative trend in the P.D. signal (−1.0 mV) lasting approximately 30 min

rate of 10/min, which were accompanied by coincidental fluctuations in the PD pattern that replaced the previous respiratory fluctuation (Fig. 5).

Recurrent pressure changes typical of B waves occurred in the same two patients. Each B wave was preceded, by 0.5 min, by a negative change in the PD of −0.3 mV which ended with the pressure change. On the compressed trace a marked negative shift in PD, mean −1.0 mV, accompanied repetitive B wave activity and lasted a mean of 30 min (Fig. 6).

One patient had no plateau or B waves and had a normal basal pressure, but did have an abnormal pulse pressure of 5 mmHg. The PD trace was mainly stable, but during a ten min period there was again a negative wave-like change in PD of −0.3 mV which was associated with a widening of the pulse pressure to 15 mmHg and with headache. When the mean intracranial pressure (ICP) is consistently normal and no abnormal waveforms are seen then the P.D. signal remains stable (Fig. 7).

Discussion

Fluctuations in the PD between ventricular CSF and blood, the relations of this PD to pressure changes, and the measurement of this PD over long periods in

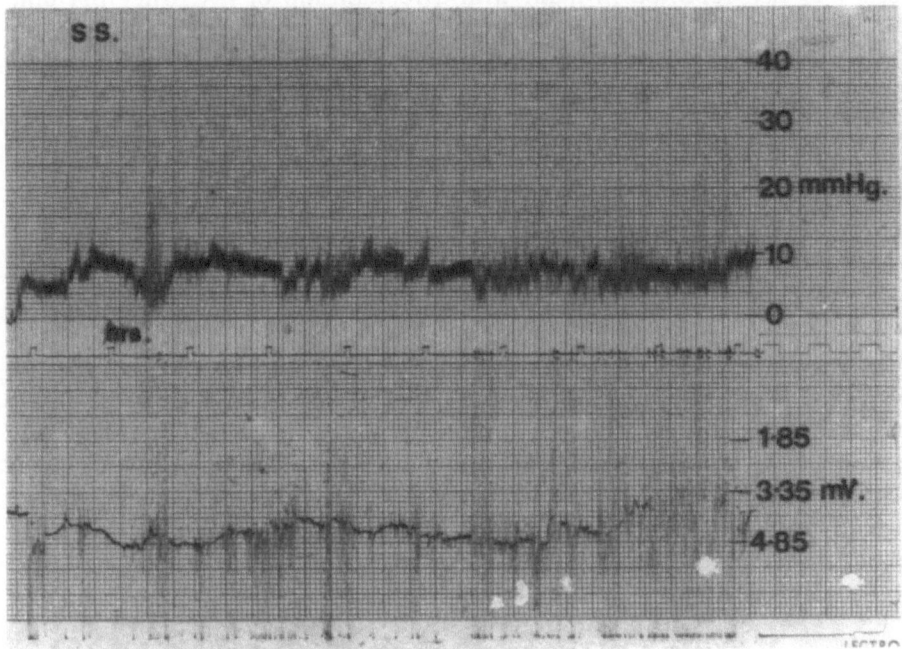

Fig. 7. A 10-h overnight recording of ICP and P.D. showing a stable basal P.D. signal and a normal mean ICP awake and asleep

the waking and sleeping states have not been reported before in man or animals. Sorensen et al. recorded the PD between lumbar CSF and blood in man, using a similar sytem, and obtained values between +1.3 and +5.1 mV over short periods (Sorensen et al. 1978). Values for the PDs in spinal and ventricular CSF in animals are comparable, with a diminishing gradient caudally (Sorensen et al. 1978; Davies et al. 1984).

The origin of the PD is undefined, but in common with other secretory epithelia must reflect ion movement, into and out of the CSF. Ionic currents occur in aqueous solution in the presence of hydrodynamic gradients (pressure, osmotic or temperature); diffusional gradients; or active transport by a tissue and/or an external electrical field (Bockris and Reddy 1970). All categories except the last could contribute to the PD across the choroid. Thus, changes in pressure gradients between the choroid capillary bed and CSF, such as the changes which occur during a plateau wave, would be expected to cause a secondary change in PD and probably account for the positive change recorded above. It has been shown that simple compression of the recording bridge has no effect on the PD (Read 1980).

However, changes in PD before any change in pressure cannot be due to this mechanism. It is recognised from perfusion experiments in animals that changes in pH concentration also cause changes in the PD of the lumbar and ventricular CSF (Davies et al. 1984). A change with respiratory alkalosis and acidosis was also reported in man, with a relationship of $-4.16\,mV/pH$ unit (Sorensen et al. 1978). Although we did not monitor arterial pH, this gradient would require arterial pH to increase by 0.1 unit and pCO_2 to decrease by about $20\,mmHg$ ($2.7\,kPa$) to account for a negative PD change of $-0.4\,mV$, which therefore seems an unlikely explanation. It is also notable that the CSF pH remains relatively constant during marked changes in arterial pH (Baxter et al. 1989), which suggests that active transport is occurring and that the PD change may not simply be due to a passive change in the bicarbonate and hydrogen ion gradients across the epithelium.

The alternative is that negative changes in the PD are due to bursts of active secretion. This is the explanation of physiological wave-like negative changes in the PD observed across the intestinal mucosa (Armstrong 1987). A negative PD change preceded pathological rises in CSF pressure in two patients, and in the third was associated with a symptomatic rise in pulse pressure, which suggests that active secretion of CSF rather than pure hemodynamic changes may precipitate these events. More research is now needed to see if this is a correct explanation, whether similar changes occur in raised intracranial pressure due to other causes and, if so, whether drugs that affect secretion could be useful in treating abnormal pressure waves.

Acknowledgments. We are grateful to the TSB Foundation, Scotland, for supporting research into Hydrocephalus at R.H.S.C. Edinburgh.

References

Armstrong WM (1987) Cellular mechanisms of ion transport in the small intestine. Chap 45 In: Johnson LR (ed). Physiology of the gastrointestinal tract Raven, New York, pp 1251–65

Baxter PS, Wilson AJ, Hardcastle J, Hardcastle PT, Taylor CJ (1989) Abnormal jejunal potential difference in cystic fibrosis. Lancet I: 464–66

Bockris JOM, Reddy AKN (1970) Modern electrochemistry: an introduction to an interdisciplinary area MacDonald, London

Carr HF (1975) Physiology of the choroid plexus. In: Netsky MG, Shuanshoti S (eds) The choroid plexus in health and disease. John Wright Bristol, pp 175–95

Davies DG, Britton SL, Gurtner GH, Dutton RE, Krasney JA (1984) Effect of carbonic anhydrase inhibition on the DC potential difference between cerebrospinal fluid and blood. Exp Neurol 86: 66–72

Read NW (1980) Kinetic study of small intestinal transport in man determined by measurements of transmucosal potential difference. MD thesis, University of Cambridge

Rosner MJ, Becker DP (1984) Origin and evolution of plateau waves. Experimental observations and a theoretical model. J Neurosurg 60: 312–324

Sorensen E, Olesen J, Rask-Madsen J, Rask-Andersen H (1978) The electrical potential difference and impedence between CSF and blood in unanaesthetised man. Scand J Clin Lab Invest 38: 203–7

23 — Cerebral Evoked Potentials in Rats with Congenital Hydrocephalus

Kozo Mutoh, Takehiko Okuno, Masatoshi Ito, and Haruki Mikawa[1]

Summary. Cerebral evoked potentials were recorded, in a congenitally hydro-cephalic rat strain, HTX, after unilateral forepaw electrical stimulation and monocular flash stimulation. In the hydrocephalic HTX rats, somatosensory evoked potentials (SEPs) were delayed in latency and reduced in amplitude, except for the first cortical positive wave, which was probably subcortical in origin. Therefore, central conduction time was prolonged. The degree of SEP abnormality was inversely correlated with the thickness of the cerebral mantle and SEPs were directly correlated to the pathological severity of hydrocephalus. By contrast, visual evoked potentials (VEPs) in the hydrocephalic group were unaltered when compared with the non-hydrocephalic group, and VEPs were considered less sensitive than SEPs. However, VEPs were abnormal in the four hydrocephalic rats that showed severe behavioral deterioration and were considered to be related to the behavioral alterations.

The HTX strain rats were considered to be appropriate for studying the clinical relevance of cerebral evoked potentials and for further elucidating the mechanism of evoked potential abnormalities in congenital hydrocephalus.

Keywords. Cerebral evoked potentials — Congenital hydrocephalus — HTX strain rat — Somatosensory evoked potentials — Visual evoked potentials

Introduction

Visual evoked potentials (VEPs) have been reported to be useful indicators in human hydrocephalus; VEP abnormalities have been related to the elevation of intracranial pressure (ICP) (Ehle and Sklar 1979; Sklar et al. 1979; York et al. 1981; McSherry et al. 1982; Alani 1985) or developmental status of the subjects (Guthkelch et al. 1982, 1984; Mutoh et al. 1988b). By contrast, somatosensory evoked potentials (SEPs) have rarely been studied in human

---

[1] Department of Pediatrics, Faculty of Medicine, Kyoto University, Kyoto, 606 Japan

hydrocephalus, although they were found to be no less useful than VEPs in our study (Mutoh et al. 1988b).

So far, experimental studies of cerebral evoked potentials using animal models of hydrocephalus has been scarce, and only a few SEP studies have been reported (Nagao et al. 1979; Sutton et al. 1986; Witzmann 1990). In the present study, we recorded VEPs and SEPs in HTX strain rats, which Kohn et al. (1981) first reported as a model of congenital hydrocephalus. In this study, we examined the significance of these cerebral evoked potentials in this animal model of congenital hydrocephalus and we correlated the results of SEPs and VEPs with the pathological severity of hydrocephalus and the behavioral alterations in each rat.

Materials and Methods

We recorded SEPs and VEPs in twenty-five (14 male, 11 female) 4-week-old HTX rats (Kohn et al. 1981), weighing between 32 and 104 g. The rats were maintained in our animal center under alternating 12-h light (6:00–18:00) and dark periods at a constant temperature (25 ± 1°C); pellets and water were supplied ad libitum. Since hydrocephalic littermates exhibited a doming of the head soon after birth (Kohn et al. 1981), hydrocephalic neonates were easily discriminated from non-hydrocephalics; 15 hydrocephalic (8 male, 7 female) and 10 non-hydrocephalic rats (6 male, 4 female) were the subjects of our study. Recording electrodes were implanted at 3 weeks old, and cerebral evoked potentials were recorded one week later, as HTX rats with the most severe hydrocephalus died at about 4 weeks of age (Kohn et al. 1981).

At 3 weeks of age, the rats were anesthesized with 20 mg/kg of sodium pentobarbital injected intraperitonealy and were secured in a stereotactic apparatus. Three epidural silver ball electrodes (0.2 mm in diameter) were implanted in each rat through holes drilled unilaterally over the cerebral hemisphere. The 3 electrodes were placed above the forelimb area of the parietal region (P, 2 mm posterior to the bregma suture and 2 mm lateral to the sagittal suture), the primary visual area of the occipital cortex (O, 6 mm posterior to the bregma suture and 3.5 mm lateral to the sagittal suture) and the nasal bone, according to Paxinos and Watson (1986). The electrode in the nasal bone served as a reference for P and O and the ground electrode, made of stainless steel (diameter 0.3 mm), was implanted in the neck muscle.

Cerebral evoked potentials were recorded as reported previously (Mutoh et al. 1988a) and recording was conducted in a shielded, sound-proof room. The room temperature was maintained between 24 and 26°C. In the present study, recordings were made without anesthetic agents, as HTX rats generally are very susceptible to anesthetics. The rats were gently restrained on a cardboard with soft adhesive tape, and recording was completed within 15 min for each rat. For both VEPs and SEPs, responses were obtained simultaneously in 2 channels from P and O, and were averaged with a Nicolet CA 1000. At least two sequential recordings were obtained to assure consistency.

To record SEPs, the forepaw contralateral to the side of electrode implantation was stimulated using two needle electrodes inserted subcutaneously on the dorsal and palmar sides of the forepaw. Isolated constant current square waves of 0.2 ms with an intensity sufficient to produce a paw twitch were delivered at the rate of 5.1 Hz. The bandpass of the amplifier was set at 5–3000 Hz (−6 dB) and 1000 responses were averaged, with an analysis time of 25 ms. VEPs were recorded after monocular stimulation with strobe flashes of 0.5 joules delivered at the rate of 1 Hz. The eye contralateral to the implanted hemisphere was dilated with Mydrin and was stimulated with a viewing distance of 30 cm. The bandpass was set at 1–100 Hz and 100 responses were averaged, with an analysis time of 250 ms.

In each rat, we observed (1) spontaneous motor activity for 15 min, (2) equilibrium responses to inclination of the floor, and (3) the way of the rat landed when tossed up above the cage, just before evoked potential recordings were made. The three behaviors were graded as 0 (not affected), 1 (moderately affected), or 2 (severely affected), and were summed to represent the behavioral severity of hydrocephalus. Therefore, the most severely affected rat had a behavioral score of 6, while a normal rat was scored as 0. After the recording, each rat was decapitated and the brain was immediately removed and frozen (−20°C) for later light microscopic investigations. Twenty-micron-thick sections of the brain, made every 200 µm, were stained with cresyl violet; the degree of hydrocephalus was then observed microscopically. That is, the slice that included the forelimb area of the parietal region was photographed in low magnification (x40), and the distance between the ventricular wall and the cortical surface (d) was measured, as illustrated in Fig. 1.

Results

Severity of Hydrocephalus

The existence of hydrocephalus in the 15 hydrocephalic rats was confirmed on gross inspection of the brain. In the non-hydrocephalic rats, the cerebral

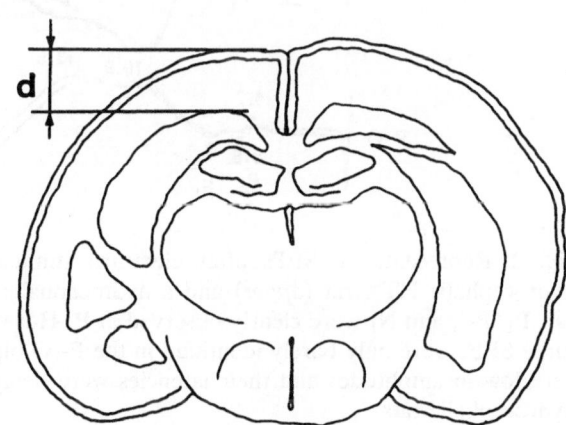

Fig. 1. Measurement of distance (*d*) between the cortical surface and the ventricular wall

thickness (d) was above 2 mm (mean 2.45; S.D. 0.25), while it ranged between 0.68 and 1.7 mm in the hydrocephalics (mean 1.15; S.D. 0.3). The mean body weight was 81.3 g in the normal rats (S.D. 17.8), but was 54.7 g, significantly lower ($P < 0.01$), in the hydrocephalics (S.D. 16.9). In the non-hydrocephalic rats, the behavioral score was 0.3 on average (S.D. 0.48), while it was significantly higher in the hydrocephalics (mean 2.9, S.D. 1.9, $P < 0.01$).

When the 15 hydrocephalic rats were divided into a group of 9 in which the cerebral thickness (d) was between 1 and 2 mm, and a group of 6 in which d

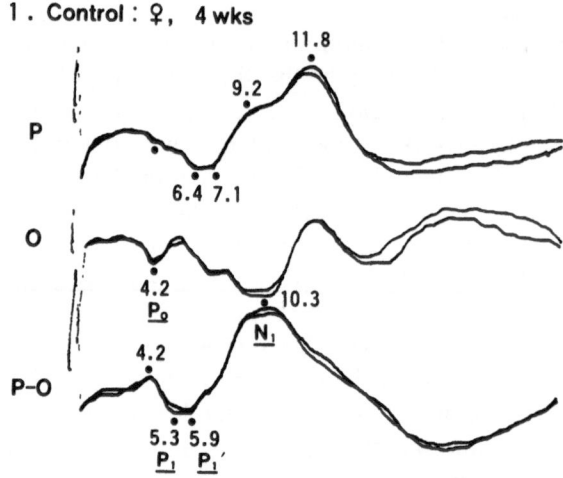

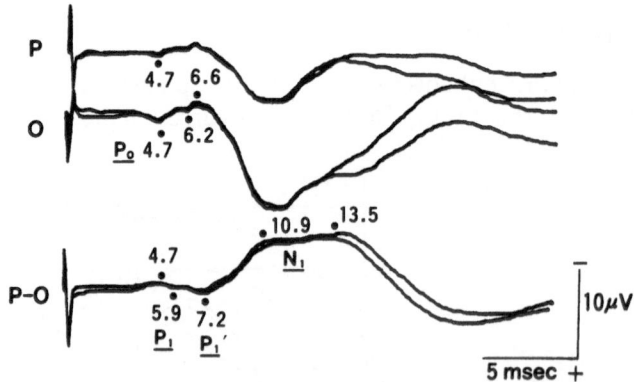

Fig. 2. Representative SEPs after electrical stimulation of one forepaw in a non-hydrocephalic HTX rat (*upper*) and a hydrocephalic HTX rat (*lower*). In the normal rat, P_1, P_1', and N_1 were clearly observed at P. However, in the hydrocephalic rat, the three SEPs were only barely identified in the P–O bipolar lead. In addition, they were very low in amplitude, and their latencies were delayed compared with those in non-hydrocephalic rats

Fig. 3. Measurements of latencies and amplitudes of respective SEP components. P_1 amplitude was measured from the negative peak preceding P_1 with $P - O$ derivation

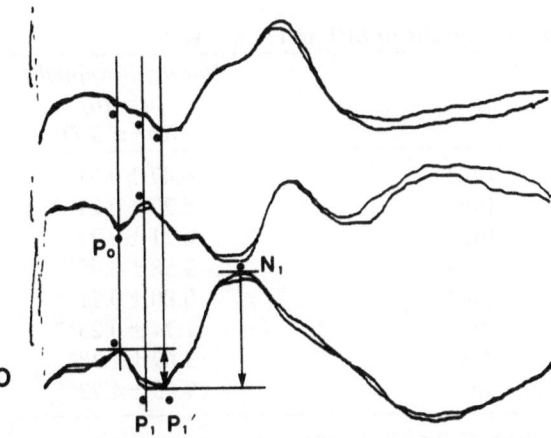

was less than 1 mm, there no difference was found between the body weights and behavioral scores of the two groups. That is, "pathologically severe" hydrocephalic rats had not necessarily deteriorated physically or behaviorally; however, their cerebral mantle was papery-thin. In the present study, the behavior and physical condition of four hydrocephalic rats, especially, had deteriorated; the rats being in the terminal stage. They were lethargic, ataxic, paraplegic, and deprived of equilibrium reactions and had the highest behavioral scores of 5 or 6. In these 4 rats, however, the thickness of the cerebral mantle, d, was not greatly reduced, being 1.16, 1.14, 0.97, and 0.9 mm, respectively.

Somatosensory Evoked Potential

In the non-hydrocephalic HTX rats, SEPs were recorded, as shown in Fig. 2. At both P and O, a positive wave with a latency of about 4 ms was recorded, which was named P_0. Following P_0, a large positive wave with two or three deflections was observed only at P, where a large negative wave followed at about 10 ms. After subtraction of P from O, a large positive wave with a latency between 5 and 7 ms remained, on which two or three deflections were similarly identified. We designated the first and second positive deflections P_1 and P_1' and the following negative wave, N_1.

In the hydrocephalic HTX rats, P_0 was similarly observed, but the following positive wave appeared to be absent at P (Fig. 2). However, after subtraction of P from O, a very low-amplitude positive wave with two deflections was observed; the two positive deflections were considered to correspond to P_1 and P_1' in the normal rats. The latencies of P_0, P_1, P_1' and N_1 and their amplitudes were measured, as shown in Fig. 3. These values were compared in the non-hydrocephalic and hydrocephalic rats (Table 1). The latencies of P_1, P_1' and N_1 were prolonged in the hydrocephalic rats, while that of P_0 was not. Accordingly, interpeak latencies (IPLs) between P_0 and P_1, and P_0 and P_1' were prolonged in the hydrocephalics. The amplitude of P_1 and the P_1-N_1 amplitude were reduced in the hydrocephalic rats.

Table 1. Results of SEP in HTX rats

		Non-hydrocephalic (n = 10) Mean ± S.D.	Hydrocephalic (n = 15) Mean ± S.D.
P_0	(ms)	4.47 ± 0.31	4.67 ± 0.42
P_1	(ms)	5.27 ± 0.21**	6.19 ± 0.60**
P_1'	(ms)	6.21 ± 0.22**	7.55 ± 0.72**
N_1	(ms)	9.58 ± 0.45*	10.72 ± 1.39*
P_0-P_1	(ms)	0.80 ± 0.21**	1.52 ± 0.56**
P_0-P_1'	(ms)	1.74 ± 0.25**	2.81 ± 0.38**
P_1	(μv)	3.69 ± 2.38*	1.43 ± 0.88*
P_1-N_1	(μv)	9.85 ± 4.72**	2.93 ± 1.95**

* $P<0.05$, ** $P<0.01$ (Student's non-paired t-test)

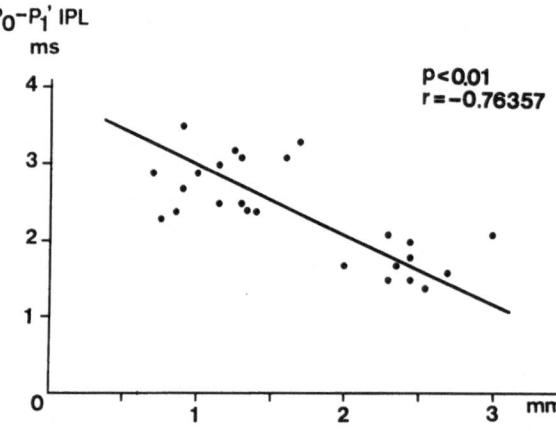

Fig. 4. Relationship between the cerebral thickness (d) and P_0-P_1' IPL. The IPL was inversely correlated with d ($n = 25$, $r = -0.76357$, $P < 0.01$)

In each hydrocephalic rat, when the latencies of P_1, P_1' and N_1 were compared with the normative values in the non-hydrocephalic rats, the P_1' latency was always over 2 S.D. of the mean for the normal rats. Similarly, the P_0-P_1' IPL, in 14 of the 15 hydrocephalic rats, exceeded 2 S.D. of the mean for the non-hydrocephalic rats. The P_0-P_1' IPL was negatively correlated with the cerebral thickness (d, Fig. 4), and the degree of SEP abnormality was positively correlated with the pathological severity of hydrocephalus.

Visual Evoked Potential

Figure 5 shows representative VEPs in non-hydrocephalic and hydrocephalic HTX rats. Within 100 ms after monocular flash stimulation, two negative and two positive VEPs were identified at contralateral O, which we named N_1, P_1, N_2, and P_2, in their order of appearance. These VEPs were identified in all but the two hydrocephalic rats whose behavior was most severely affected. We measured the latencies and amplitudes of the respective VEPs, as shown in

1. Control : ♂, 4 wks

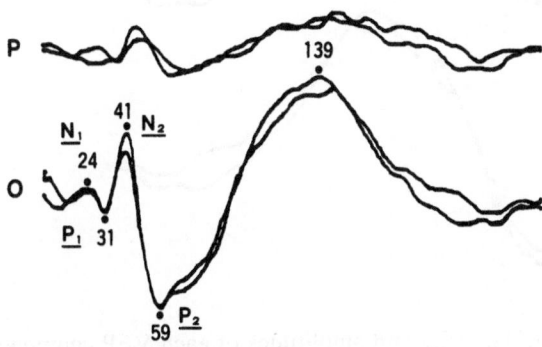

2. Hydrocephalus : ♀, 4 wks

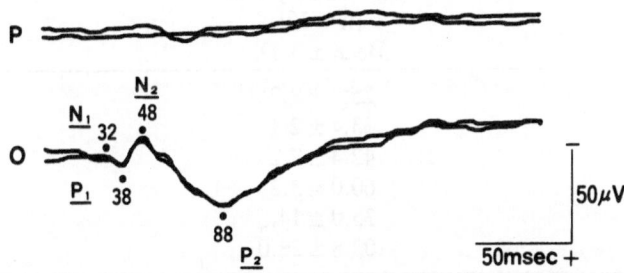

Fig. 5. VEPs after monocular flash stimulation in a non-hydrocephalic (*upper*) and hydrocephalic HTX rat (*lower*). Four VEPs, named N_1, P_1, N_2, and P_2, were identified at O within 100 ms. In some hydrocephalic rats whose behavior and physical condition had severely deteriorated, the VEPs were delayed in latency and reduced in amplitude

Fig. 6, and compared them in the non-hydrocephalic and hydrocephalic rats as groups. Unlike the results for the SEPs, the latencies and amplitudes of the VEPs were similar in the two groups (Table 2).

When the latencies of the VEPs for each hydrocephalic rat were compared with the normal values for the non-hydrocephalic rats, their values were found to have exceeded more than 2 S.D. of the mean for non-hydrocephalic rats in only two rats. These were the two remaining of the four that had the highest behavioral scores.

Discussion

The HTX strain rat was first reported by Kohn et al. (1981) as congenitally exhibiting a hydrocephalus of the communicating type, for which under-development of the veins in the periosteal-dural layers and of the pia-arachnoid

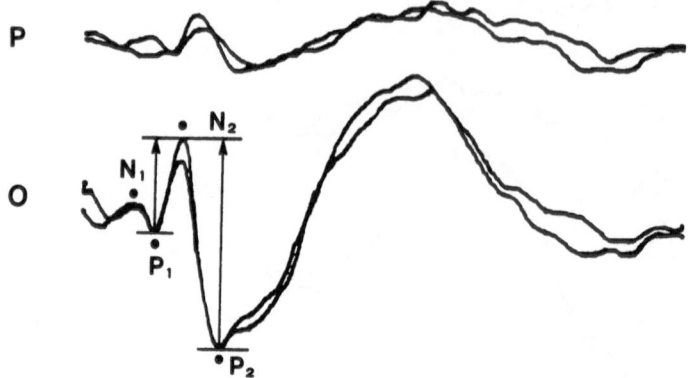

Fig. 6. Measurements of latencies and amplitudes of each VEP component

Table 2. Results of VEP in HTX rats

		Non-hydrocephalic (n = 10) Mean ± S.D.	Hydrocephalic (n = 13) Mean ± S.D.
N_1	(ms)	25.7 ± 2.7	26.5 ± 4.9
P_1	(ms)	33.4 ± 2.1	33.6 ± 2.6
N_2	(ms)	42.4 ± 2.2	43.1 ± 3.2
P_2	(ms)	60.0 ± 3.2	63.5 ± 10.3
P_1–N_2	(μv)	35.0 ± 14.3	58.5 ± 39.4
N_2–P_2	(μv)	102.8 ± 28.0	107.9 ± 65.5

cells was considered responsible. Histologically, no evidence of developmental anomalies, inflammation, or edema was noted along the aqueductal ependymal layer, although only the lateral ventricles dilated progressively, compressing cerebellar, brainstem, and periventricular substances (Kohn et al. 1981). In our observations of the hydrocephalic HTX rats, cerebral gray matter was relatively spared, with no significant neuronal loss, while cerebral white matter was extensively damaged, especially in the periventricular area of the lateral ventricles (Kohn et al. 1981).

In the present study, the hydrocephalic HTX rats were generally emaciated and deteriorated behaviorally, but the pathological severity of the hydrocephalus was not correlated with the severity of the behavioral deterioration. Such pathologico-clinical dissociation is often experienced in hydrocephalic infants and children whose cranial sutures are still unclosed and was probably secondary to the decompressing effect of the open sutures. Although not monitored in this study, intracranial pressure (ICP) might have been elevated in the four hydrocephalic rats that were in the terminal stage, while it was not elevated in the remaining hydrocephalic rats without significant behavioral deterioration.

In the 4-week-old normal HTX rats, SEPs were similar in configuration to those that were previously recorded in adult rats (Wiederholt and Iragui-Madoz 1977; Allison and Hume 1981; Mutoh et al. 1988a). As P_0 was observed at both P and O, it was considered to be subcortical in origin, while later components, P_1, P_1', and N_1, were considered to be cortical responses. P_0 probably corresponded to the P_{15} of Allison and Hume (1981) and to component III of Wiederholt and Iragui-Madoz (1977), which they also assumed to originate from the thalamus. P_1 and P_1' were considered to be analogous to P_{16} and P_{18} (or P_{20}), which Allison and Hume (1981) reported as originating rostral to the thalamus. VEPs that were recorded in the non-hydrocephalic HTX rats were also consistent with those that were previously recorded in rats by Onofrj et al. (1985) and Mutoh et al. (1988a). Onofrj et al. (1985) considered that P_1 and N_2 of the VEPs were initial cortical responses originating from the primary visual cortex.

In the present study, SEPs were abnormal in all the hydrocephalic rats, and their latencies and amplitudes were significantly altered in the hydrocephalics as a group when compared with the non-hydrocephalics as a group, except for the subcortical SEP, P_0. Therefore, sensory afferent conduction was considered to be unaffected in the peripheral nerves as well as within the central nervous system (CNS) up to the thalamus, but was probably disturbed rostral to the thalamus. The conduction disturbance rostral to the thalamus was further confirmed by the prolongation of the P_0-P_1 and P_0-P_1' IPLs that were considered to represent central conduction time between the thalamus and cerebral cortex.

These SEP findings were in line with the pathological characteristics of the hydrocephalic HTX rats, i.e., selective dilatation of the lateral ventricles, predominant white matter involvement, and strongly suspected temporal dispersion of the afferent conduction in the thalamocortical radiation. Another possibility was a lengthening of the afferent pathway between the thalamus and cortex, as the whole rostral brain should have been expanded by the enlarging lateral ventricles. In any case, the SEP abnormality was probably related to the existence of hydrocephalus itself, as it was observed in all hydrocephalic rats irrespective of the degree of behavioral deterioration. The inverse correlation between the P_0-P_1' IPL and the thickness of the cerebral mantle also supported this conclusion.

When normal and hydrocephalic HTX rats were compared as groups, VEPs were found to be unaltered and rather insensitive to the presence of hydrocephalus. However, VEPs were absent in the two rats whose behavior was most severely affected and VEP latencies were delayed in the other two hydrocephalic rats with severe behavioral deterioration. The VEP abnormalities in these four rats probably occurred in response to the elevation of ICP, as such deteriorated behaviors were likely to be secondary to the elevation of ICP, as discussed above. This consideration is in accordance with previous studies on human hydrocephalus, as many authors have reported a prolongation of VEP latencies that was related to the elevation of ICP (Ehle and Sklar 1979; Sklar et al. 1979; York et al. 1981; McSherry et al. 1982; Alani 1985).

The results of previous studies on SEPs were not in accordance with the results of the present one. Other workers all concluded that SEP changes were related to marked elevation of ICP (Nagao et al. 1979; Sutton et al. 1986; Witzmann 1990). The reason for the discrepancy is not known precisely, but may be due to differences in the animal models employed. Nagao et al. (1979) studied cats with acute intracranial hypertension, while Witzmann (1990) studied rats with acute intracranial hypertension; neither of these studies dealt with hydrocephalus proper. Only Sutton et al. (1986) studied cats with kaolin hydrocephalus, but they used only adult cats. Therefore, SEPs might have been different in the HTX strain rats, in which hydrocephalus was congenital and its onset was fetal in nature (Kohn et al. 1981). Considering that hydrocephalus is a disease that occurs mainly during the neonatal or infantile period (O'Brien 1982), the HTX strain rat was considered to be an optimal model of hydrocephalus and is considered to be appropriate for use in the further study of the VEP and SEP values in predicting the neurological and intellectual outcome of hydrocephalus.

References

Alani AM (1985) Pattern-reversal visual evoked potentials in patients with hydrocephalus. J Neurosurg 62: 234–237

Allison T, Hume AL (1981) A comparative analysis of short-latency somatosensory evoked potentials in man, monkey, cat, and rat. Exp Neurol 72: 592–611

Ehle A, Sklar F (1979) Visual evoked potentials in infants with hydrocephalus. Neurology (NY) 29: 1541–1544

Guthkelch AN, Sclabassi RJ, Vries JK (1982) Changes in the visual evoked potentials in hydrocephalic children. Neurosurgery 11: 599–602

Guthkelch AN, Sclabassi RJ, Hirsch RP, Vries JK (1984) Visual evoked potentials in hydrocephalus: Relationship to head size, shunting, and mental development. Neurosurgery 14: 283–286

Kohn DF, Chinookoswong N, Chou SM (1981) A new model of congenital hydrocephalus in the rat. Acta Neuropathol (Berl) 54: 211–218

McSherry JW, Walters CL, Horbar JD (1982) Acute visual evoked potential changes in hydrocephalus. Electroencephalogr Clin Neurophysiol 53: 331–333

Mutoh K, Okuno T, Ito M, Mikawa H (1988a) Effects of pentobarbital on visual and somatosensory evoked potentials in adult rats. Ann Paediatr Jpn 34: 73–79

Mutoh K, Okuno T, Nakano S, Mikawa H, Moritake K, Kikuchi H (1988b) Visual and somatosensory evoked potentials in hydrocephalus. Ann Paediatr Jpn 34: 1–3

Nagao S, Roccaforte P, Moody RA (1979) Acute intracranial hypertension and auditory brain-stem responses. Part 1: Changes in the auditory brain-stem and somatosensory evoked responses in intracranial hypertension in cats. J Neurosurg 51: 669–676

O'Brien MS (1982) Hydrocephalus in children. In: Youmans JR (ed) Neurological surgery, 2nd edn. Saunders, Philadelphia, pp 1381–1422

Onofrj M, Harnois C, Bodis-Wollner I (1985) The hemispheric distribution of the transient rat VEP: A comparison of flash and pattern stimulation. Exp Brain Res 59: 427–433

Paxinos G, Watson C (1986) The rat brain in the stereotaxic coordinates, 2nd edn. Academic, Sydney

Sklar F, Ehle A, Clark WK (1979) Visual evoked potentials: A noninvasive technique to monitor patients with shunted hydrocephalus. Neurosurgery 4: 529–534

Sutton LN, Cho B, Jaggi J, Joseph PM, Bruce DA (1986) Effects of hydrocephalus and intracranial pressure on auditory and somatosensory evoked responses. Neurosurgery 18: 756–761

Wiederholt WC, Iragui-Madoz VJ (1977) Far field somatosensory potentials in the rat. Electroencephalogr Clin Neurophysiol 42: 456–465

Witzmann A (1990) Changes of somatosensory evoked potentials with increase of intracranial pressure in the rat's brain. Electroencephalogr Clin Neurophysiol 77: 59–67

York DH, Pulliam MW, Rosenfeld JG, Watts C (1981) Relationship between visual evoked potentials and intracranial pressure. J Neurosurg 55: 909–916

24 — Clinical Significance of ICP Measurement in Infants Part I: Normal Intracranial Pressure

Shigetaka Anegawa, Takashi Hayashi, and Ryuichiro Torigoe[1]

Summary. Intracranial pressure (ICP) was monitored in 32 infants with an aplanation transducer while they were either awake or asleep. When they were conscious, the baseline pressure was $85.0 \pm 10.3 \, \text{mmH}_2\text{O}$ and various types of activity affecting ICP were noted. During non REM sleep, the baseline pressure was $89.3 \pm 12.9 \, \text{mmH}_2\text{O}$ and no large waves were seen except for fine oscillations recorded at $30 \, \text{mmH}_2\text{O}$ above the ICP level. In the REM period, infants older than 2.5 months showed ICP wave forms similar to the A and B waves described by Lundberg. The amplitude of ICP waves from normal infants correlated to their age until they were about 5 months old.

In this paper we present the characteristics of ICP in normal infants. We also discuss the possible mechanisms for the occurrence of pressure waves during the REM period.

Keywords. Intracranial pressure — Aplanation principle — Normal infant — Baseline pressure — Pressure wave

Introduction

Continuous monitoring of the intracranial pressure (ICP) would be useful in the diagnosis, treatment, and observation of infants with intracranial disorders. Since the use of invasive measuring devices carries the risk of serious complications, such devices are not used as widely in infants as in adults. To reduce the risks of monitoring, a simple noninvasive method of measuring the ICP, using the aplanation principle, was developed by Wealthal and Smallwood (1974). They obtained excellent correlations between the results of their tonometric method and direct ICP measurements. Although several studies using the aplanation principle for ICP measurement have been published since then (Donn and Philip 1978; Edwards 1974; Myerberg et al. 1980; Robinson et al.

---

[1] Department of Neurosurgery, Institute of Neurosciences, St. Mary's Hospital, Kurume, Fukuoka, 830 Japan

1977; Salmon 1981; Vidyasagar and Raju 1977), no report on the continuous observation of ICP in normal subjects has appeared.

In this paper we report on changes in the ICP which occur during REM and non-REM sleep, as well as those which occur due to age in normal infants. The results of our study may provide a good index for the evaluation of ICP in infants.

Subjects and Methods

Thirty-two normal infants aged from day 1 to 11 months were studied. All the infants underwent detailed neurological examination and CT scanning if necessary. Those infants who showed abnormalities on neurological examination and/or CT scan or had respiratory problems were excluded from the study. The ICP was recorded using an aplanation transducer, the details of which have been published elsewhere (Hayashi et al. 1987). In order to record ICP, all infants were placed in a supine position with the head supported by pillows on both sides, and the body was kept horizontal. Measurements were performed for 4–12 h during waking and sleeping. No sedation was used. Because so many factors can disturb natural sleep, REM sleep was identified only by the appearance of REM. Pressure was calibrated in mmH_2O and continuous ICP tracings were registered on a polygraph operating at a chart speed of 0.5 cm/s. The effects of stimulation and activity on the ICP were accurately recorded on a chart. Baseline pressure was defined as the pressure represented by the distance from the horizontal line at $0 mmH_2O$ to the minimum value of the cerebral pulse wave.

Results

Intracranial Pressure During Waking (Fig. 1)

As shown in Fig. 1, it was almost impossible to make continuous recordings during the waking period due to the movements of the infants, since body movements such as crying produced ICP spikes. The baseline pressure at rest was 85.0 ± 10.3 mmH_2O, which was almost the same as that during sleep. No pressure waves were observed during waking. In the initial stage of feeding, the ICP increased from $30 mmH_2O$ to $50 mmH_2O$, but it soon returned to its original level.

Intracranial Pressure During Sleep

In all cases, the ICP was higher during sleep than during waking. The baseline pressure was 89.3 ± 12.9 mmH_2O. Smaller fluctuations of less than $30 mmH_2O$, synchronized mainly with respiration, were often observed, especially in the

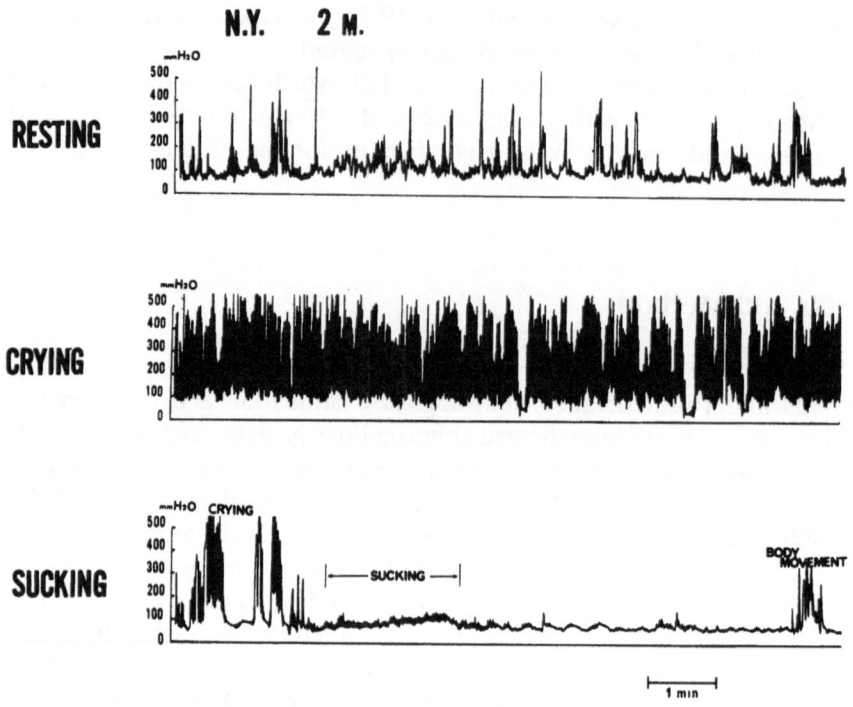

Fig. 1. Intracranial pressure during waking. Resting, crying, and sucking states are presented

older infants. Changes in the baseline pressure took place gradually, however, and did not exceed 40 mmH$_2$O (Fig. 2).

Although the baseline pressure was slightly lower in infants under one month of age, little change attributable to age was observed in the baseline pressure.

The amplitude was below 10 mmH$_2$O for all infants under one month of age, and it increased in proportion to age until 5 months (Fig. 3).

During non REM sleep, the amplitude changed little, whereas it increased markedly during REM sleep (Fig. 4).

A relation between age and presure waves was also noted. In subjects under 2.5 months of age, fine and irregular oscillations occurred only in the REM phase of sleep without any increase in ICP. Moreover, subjects older than 2.5 months had marked increases of ICP, due to pressure waves, throughout REM sleep. The ICP rose rapidly and remained high for several minutes in some cases. Other cases showed irregular pressure changes with superimposed fluctuations of large amplitude occurring in a short time period of 1–2 min. These waves appeared to be similar to the A and B waves described by Lundberg (1960). After these changes, the ICP returned rapidly to its original level and in some cases provoked or spontaneous arousal took place after this. The maximum pressure during this period exceeded 250 mmH$_2$0 and the peak of the superimposed fluctuations surpassed 300 mmH$_2$0. Both the onset and the

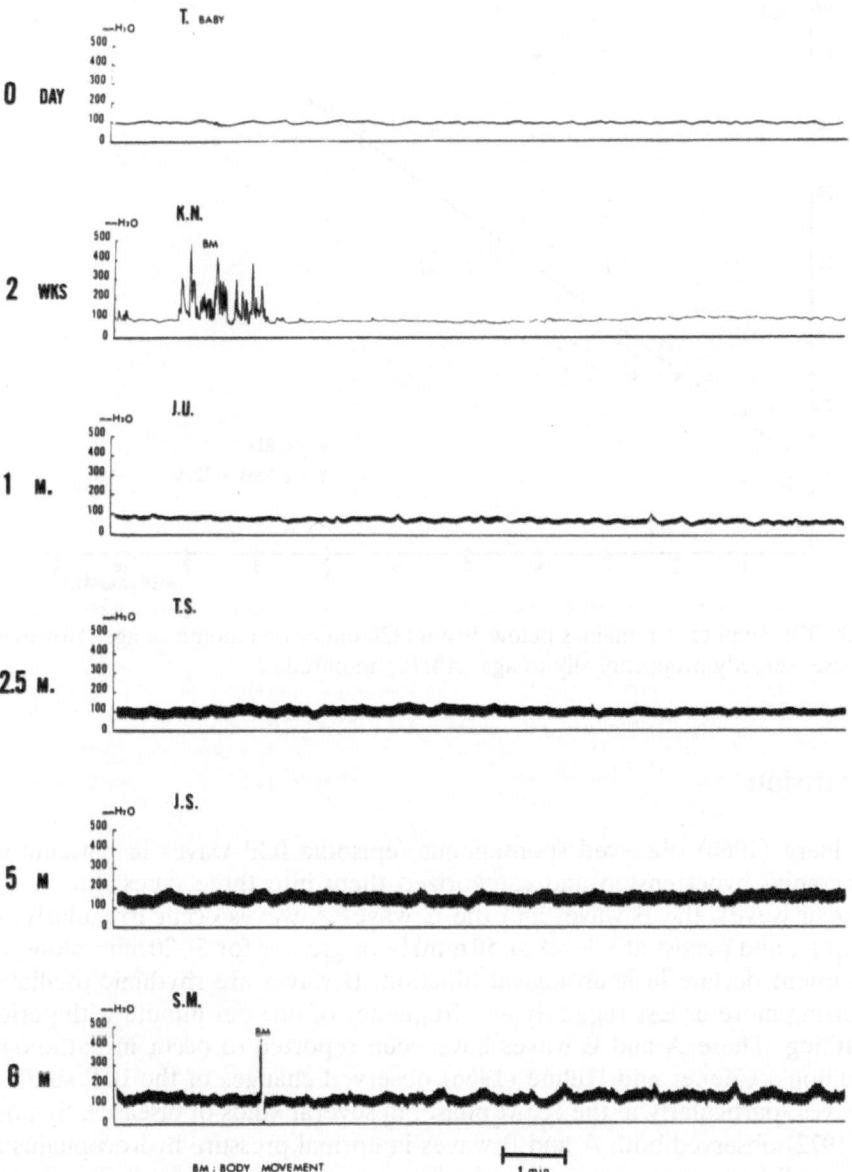

Fig. 2. Intracranial pressure during non REM phase of sleep. No apparent pressure waves are noted, except for fine oscillations. Note the increase of the amplitude directly proportional to age

end of the pressure waves coincided with the onset and the end of REM sleep. Although there was some tendency for older infants to have stronger pressure waves, the height, duration, and form of the wave varied in each individual and from one point in time to another.

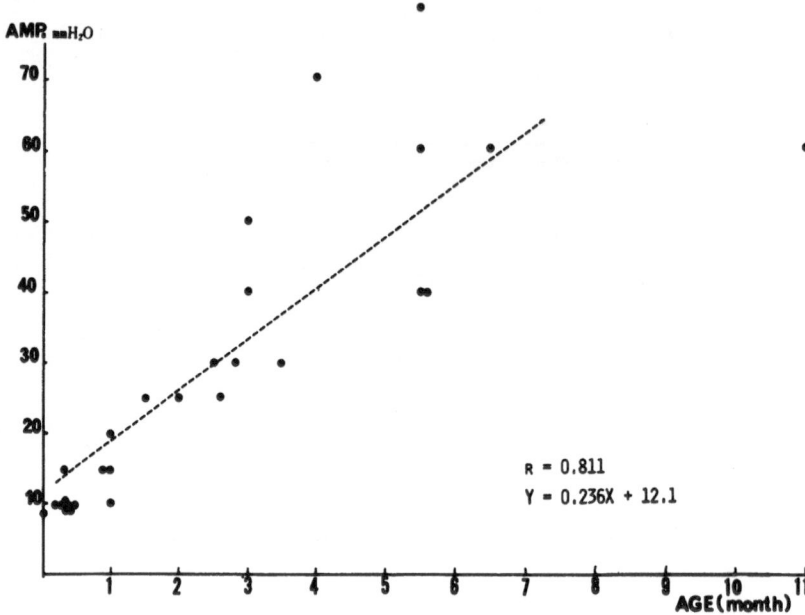

Fig. 3. The amplitude remaines below 10 mmH20 under one month of age. However, it increases directly proportionally to age. *AMP.*, amplitude

Discussion

Lundberg (1960) observed spontaneous, episodic ICP waves in patients with intracranial hypertension and categorized them into three types: the A wave (plateau wave), the B wave, and the C wave. A waves occur irregularly, end abruptly, and persist at a level of 50 mmHg or greater for 5–20 min, along with a transient decline in neurological function. B waves are rhythmic oscillations occurring more or less regularly at a frequency of one per minute with periodic breathing. These A and B waves have been reported to occur in pathological conditions. Cooper and Hulme (1966) observed changes of the ICP similar to A waves, particularly in the REM phase, in several kinds of diseases. Symon et al. (1972) observed both A and B waves in normal pressure hydrocephalus and suggested the term "episodically raised pressure hydrocephalus." Chawla et al. (1974) also demonstrated the presence of these waves in normal pressure hydrocephalus and indicated that the presence of such waves provides the most reliable criterion for the effect of shunt operations. Di Rocco et al. (1975) reported the existence of episodic pressure increases during REM sleep in hydrocephalic children whose ICP at rest was within the normal range. They suggested that these episodic changes in ICP could be a pathogenic factor in ventricular dilatation. Pierre-Kahn et al. (1976) also observed pressure waves during REM sleep in borderline hydrocephalus and suggested that the iden- tification of these waves could more precisely indicate the prognosis and the

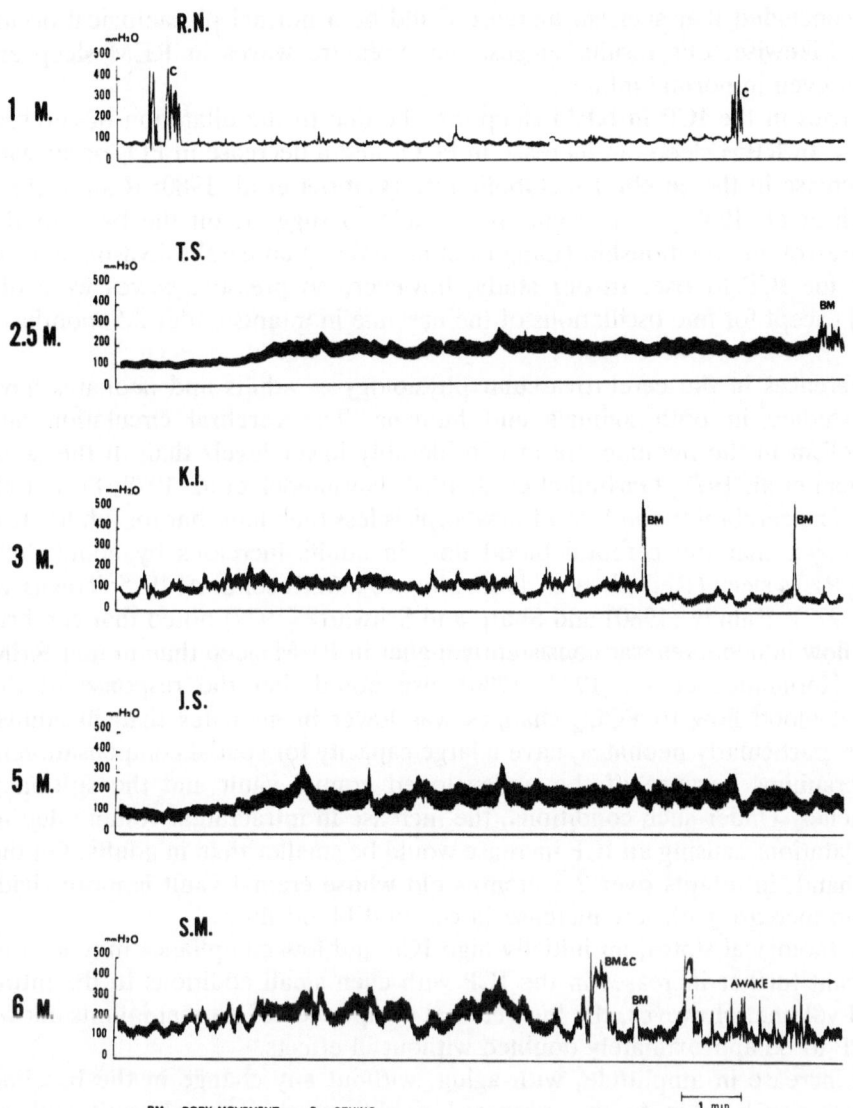

Fig. 4. Intracranial pressure during REM phase of sleep. Note the marked increase of the baseline pressure that corresponded to an increase in amplitude

appropriate therapy. In all these reports, pressure waves observed in REM sleep have been regarded as a pathological phenomenon.

However, Martin (1978) reported a patient who had a hysterical episode, in whom the ICP was measured because of the suspected existence of an intracranial lesion. B waves were observed in the early morning but not necessarily while the patient was sleeping. Gücer and Viernstein (1979) studied ICP changes in normal monkeys who were asleep and awake, and found the pressure rise during REM sleep to about double the normal baseline pressure.

They concluded that such an increase could be a normal physiological occurrence. Likewise, our results suggest that pressure waves in REM sleep are present even in normal infants.

Changes in the ICP in REM sleep may be due to the dilatation of cerebral arteries. In REM sleep, an increase in PCO_2 and a decrease in PO_2 occur with the increase in the cerebral metabolic rate (Gabriel et al. 1980; Rahilly 1980; Reivich et al. 1968), so it seems reasonable to suggest, on the basis of the pressure-volume relationship (Langfitt et al. 1965), that cerebral vasodilatation causes the ICP to rise. In our study, however, no pressure waves were observed except for fine oscillations of the baseline in infants under 2.5 months of age.

Differences in the cerebrovascular physiology of adults and neonates have been studied in both animals and humans. The cerebral circulation and metabolism in the neonate are at considerably lower levels than in the adult (Brennan et al. 1971; Garfunkel et al. 1954; Hernandez et al. 1978; Lou et al. 1979). The cerebral blood flow of newborns is less than half that for adults. It is also known that the cerebral blood flow in adults increases by about 36% during REM sleep (Reivich et al. 1968; Shapiro and Rosendorff 1975; Townsent et al. 1973). Rahilly (1980) and Sharp and Schwartz (1977) noted that cerebral blood flow in neonates was consistently higher in REM sleep than in non-REM sleep. Hernandez et al. (1978, 1980) also noted that the response of the cerebral blood flow to PCO_2 changes was lower in neonates than in adults. Infants, particularly neonates, have a large capacity for spatial compensation in their craniums because of the undeveloped cranial vault and the still-open fontanelles. Under such conditions, the increase in intracranial volume due to vasodilatations causing an ICP increase would be smaller than in adults. On the other hand, in infants over 2.5 months old whose cranial vault is more rigid, ICP can increase with any increase in cerebral blood flow.

In pathological states, an initially high ICP and low compliance may lead to significant further increases in the ICP with even small additions to the intracranial volume. However, the high cranial compliance of normal infants allows the ICP to be approximately doubled without ill effects.

The increase in amplitude, with aging, without any change in the baseline pressure may be due to the increased rigidity of the cranial vault and an increase of the cerebral blood flow.

Neonates have small cerebral pulse waves because of their immature cranial vaults and cerebral vasculature; as the cranium and cerebrovascular system develop the amplitude of the pressure waves becomes larger.

Some values for normal ICP have been reported (Welch 1980). It is known that normal ICP varies according to age and the phase of sleep. The ICP in some infants with progressive hydrocephalus has also been found to be within the normal range. Thus, evaluating the ICP on the basis of the baseline pressure alone is not adequate; continuous monitoring of the ICP during waking and sleeping is indispensable for properly assessing a patient's state. The results of our study may provide a good index for such monitoring.

Conclusions

1. Intracranial pressure was monitored during waking and sleeping in 32 normal infants, using an aplanation transducer.
2. The baseline pressure during waking was $85.0 \pm 10.3\,mmH_2O$. Changes of the ICP due to physiological processes were observed.
3. The baseline pressure during non-REM sleep was $89.3 \pm 12.9\,mmH_2O$ and no changes were observed, except for small changes of below $30\,mmH_2O$ in the baseline pressure. A correlation between amplitude and age was seen until the infants were 5 months old.
4. During REM sleep, episodic increases of ICP as high as $300\,mmH_2O$, with or without a superimposed pressure rise, were noted.
5. The relationship between normal ICP, pressure waves, and cerebral blood flow was discussed.

References

Brennan RW, Patterson RH, Kessler J (1971) Cerebral blood flow and metabolism during cardiopulmonary bypass: Evidence of microembolic encephalopathy. Neurology 21: 665–672

Chawla JC, Hulme A, Cooper R (1974) Intracranial pressure in patients with dementia and communicating hydrocephalus. J Neurosurg 40: 376–380

Cooper R, Hulme A (1966) Intracranial pressure and related phenomena during sleep. J Neurol Neurosurg Psychiatry 29: 564–570

Di Rocco C, McLone DG, Shimoji T, Raimondi AJ (1975) Continuous intraventricular cerebrospinal fluid pressure recording in hydrocephalic children during wakefulness and sleep. J Neurosurg 42: 683–689

Donn SM, Philip AGS (1978) Early increase in intracranial pressure in preterm infants. Pediatrics 61: 904–907

Edwards J (1974) An intracranial pressure tonometer for use on neonates. Preliminary report. Dev Med Child Neurol (Suppl) 16: 38–39

Gabriel M, Helmin V, Albani M (1980) Sleep-induced PO2 changes in preterm infants. Eur J Pediatr 134: 153–154

Garfunkel JM, Baird HW, Ziegler J (1954) The relationship of oxygen consumption to cerebral functional activity. J Pediatr 44: 64–72

Gucer G, Viernstein LJ (1979) Intracranial pressure in the normal monkey while awake and asleep. J Neurosurg 51: 206–219

Hayashi T, Kuramoto S, Honda E, Anegawa S (1987) A new instrument for noninvasive measurement of intracranial pressure through the anterior fontanel. I. Preliminary report. Nerv Syst Child 3: 151–155

Hernandez MJ, Brennan RW, Vannucci RC, Bowman GS (1978) Cerebral blood flow and oxygen consumption in the newborn dog. Am J Physiol 234: 209–215

Hernandez MJ, Brennan RW, Bowman GS (1980) Autoregulation of cerebral blood flow in the newborn dog. Brain Res 184: 199–202

Langfitt TW, Kassell NF, Weinstein JD (1965) Cerebral blood flow with intracranial hypertension. Neurology (NY) 15: 761–773

Lou HC, Lassen NA, Friis-Hansen B (1979) Impaired autoregulation of cerebral blood flow in the distressed newborn infant. J Pediatr 94: 118–121

Lundberg N (1960) Continuous recording and control of ventricular fluid pressure in neurosurgical practice. Acta Psychiatr Scand 33 (Suppl 149): 1–193

Martin G (1978) Lundberg's B waves as a feature of normal intracranial pressure. Surg Neurol 9: 347–348

Myerberg DZ, York C, Chaplin ER, Gregory GA (1980) Comparison of noninvasive and direct measurement of intracranial pressure. Pediatrics 65: 473–476

Pierre-Kahn A, Gabersek V, Hirsch J (1976) Intracranial pressure and rapid eye movement sleep in hydrocephalus. Childs Brain 2: 156–166

Rahilly PM (1980) Effect of sleep state and feeding on cranial blood flow of the human neonate. Arch Dis Child 55: 265–270

Reivich M, Isaacs G, Evarts E, Kety S (1968) The effect of slow wave sleep and REM sleep on regional cerebral blood flow in cat. J Neurochem 15: 301–306

Robinson RO, Rolfe P, Sutton P (1977) Non-invasive method for measuring intracranial pressure in newborn infants. Dev Med Child Neurol 19: 305–308

Salmon JH (1981) Intracranial pressure. Am J Dis Child 135: 502

Shapiro CM, Rosendorff C (1975) Local hypothalamic blood flow during sleep. Electroencephalogr Clin Neurophysiol 39: 365–369

Sharp FR, Schwartz WJ (1977) Proposed effect of brain noradrenaline on neuronal activity and cerebral blood flow during REM sleep. Experientia 33: 1618–1620

Symon L, Dorsch NWC, Stephens RJ (1972) Pressure waves in so-called low-pressure hydrocephalus. Lancet II: 1291–1292

Townsent RE, Printz PN, Obrist WD (1973) Human cerebral blood flow during sleep and waking. J Appl Physiol 35: 620–625

Vidyasagar D, Raju TNK (1977) A simple noninvasive technique of measuring intracranial pressure in the newborn. Pediatrics 59: 957–961

Wealthall SR, Smallwood R (1974) Method of intracranial pressure via the fontanelle without puncture. J Neurol Neurosurg Psychiatry 37: 88–96

Welch K (1980) The intracranial pressure in infants. J Neurosurg 52: 693–699

25 — Clinical Significance of ICP Measurement in Infants
Part II: Intracranial Pressure in Infants with Hydrocephalus

Shigetaka Anegawa, Takashi Hayashi, and Ryuichiro Torigoe[1]

Introduction

Despite the advantage of intracranial pressure (ICP) measurement in infants, many surgeons are still reluctant to use it because of possible operative complications. Abnormal ICPs in hydrocephalic infants have often been reported, where pressure waves, observed particularly in REM sleep, seem to be a pathological phenomenon due to the decrease in ability for spatial compensation (Chawla et al. 1974). Furthermore, one of the problems in evaluating ICP data in infants is uncertainty in the definition of true normal ICP, which changes simultaneously with the natural development of infants (Welch 1980). In part I of this study, the authors tried to delineate the characteristics of normal ICP in infants. In reviewing ICP measurements in 32 normal infants, pressure waves similar to the A and B waves first described by Lundberg (1960) were found, particularly in REM sleep. It was also noted that increase in amplitude was directly proportional to increase in age. In this study, our concern is to evaluate one of the current adjunctive procedures in pediatric neurosurgery, continuous intracranial pressure monitoring of patients with hydrocephalus, and to evaluate its efficacy as a factor to be taken into account when making decisions on treatments. Although several papers on hydrocephalus and ICP have been published (Symon et al. 1972; Symon and Dorsch 1975; Di Rocco et al. 1975; Di Rocco et al. 1976; Pierre-Kahn et al. 1976; Venes 1979), the problem of the way ICP changes in these patients and the kinds of spontaneous fluctuation that can be expected still remains.

It is the purpose of our study to elucidate the pathological occurrence of ICP in infants with hydrocephalus.

Keywords. Hydrocephalus — Intracranial pressure — Baseline pressure — Pressure wave — Amplitude

---

[1] Department of Neurosurgery. Institute of Neurosciences, St. Mary's Hospital, Kurume, Fukuoka, 830 Japan

Subjects and Methods

Forty-nine hydrocephalic infants ranging from 2 days to 13 months in age were studied. Measurements were made for 2–24 hours, using an aplanation transducer placed on the anterior fontanelle by means of adhesive. Multiple measurements were carried out in 31 patients at regular intervals and for a maximum of nine times. All infants were kept horizontal in the supine position. Measurements were made under spontaneous respiration except in the cases of three patients under operation.

To identify the phase of sleep and the effect of respiration, electroencephalograms, electro-myograms of the chin, electro-oculograms, respiration, and electro-cardiograms were also monitored polygraphically in 32 patients. In these patients, REM sleep was identified by the following four signs — low voltage EEG activity, rapid eye movement, absence of tonic EEG activity, and REM appearance (Fig. 1). In the remaining 17 patients, REM sleep was identified by REM appearance alone.

Pressure was calibrated in mmH_2O and continuous ICP tracings were registered on a polygraphic instrument operating at a chart speed of 0.5 cm/second. Baseline pressure was defined as the pressure represented by the distance from the horizontal line at $0 mmH_2O$ to the minimal value of the cerebral pulse wave.

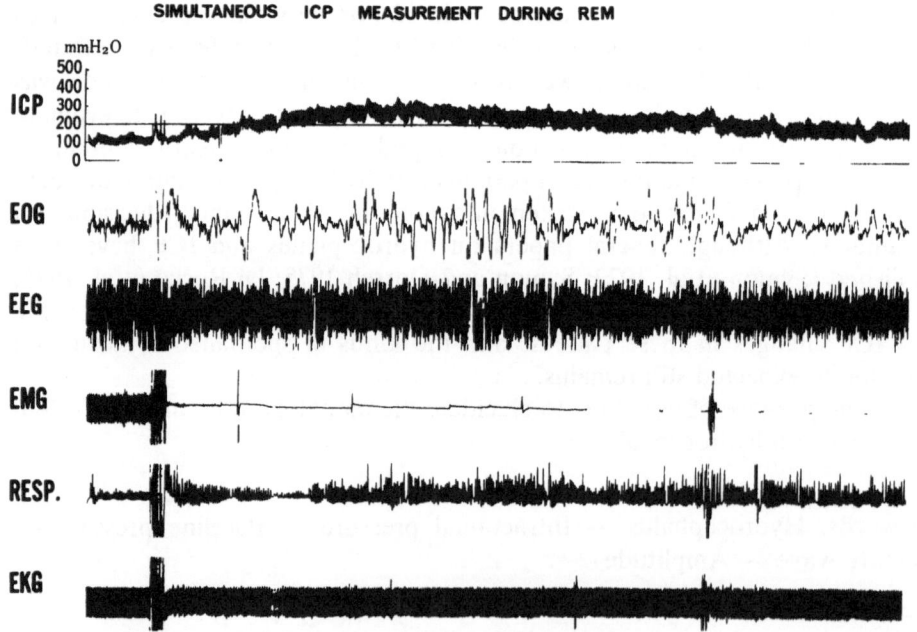

Fig. 1. Polygraphic recording of ICP. Electroencephalogram (*EEG*), electromyogram of the chin (*EMG*), electro-oculogram (*EOG*), respiration (*RESP.*), and electrocardiogram (*EKG*) were monitored to identify the sleep phase

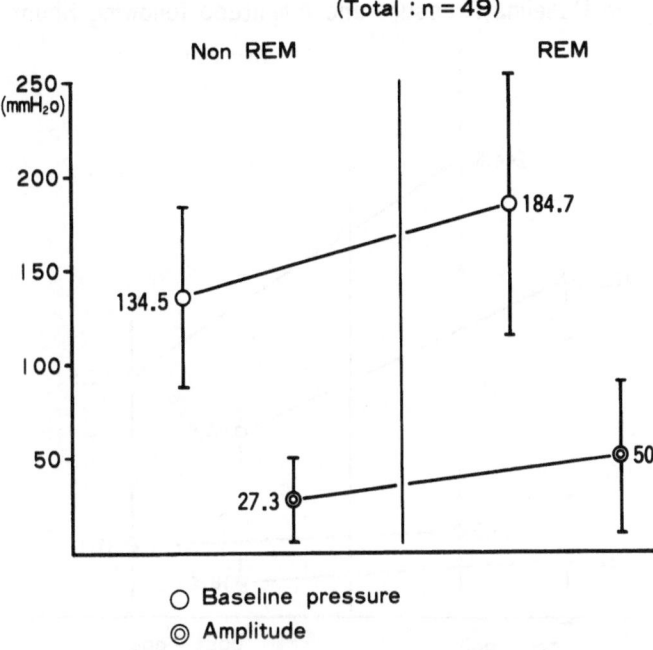

Fig. 2. ICP in non-REM and REM sleep

Results

The baseline pressure in Non-REM sleep was 134.5 ± 48.6 mmH$_2$O and that in REM sleep showed an elevation of up to 184.7 ± 69.1 mmH$_2$O. The amplitude in non-REM sleep was 27.3 ± 22.1 mmH$_2$O and that in REM sleep was 50.0 ± 40.5 mmH$_2$O. The baseline pressure fluctuated within a wide range and sometimes showed normal values (Fig. 2). Furthermore, in all the patients the amplitude increased along with the pressure increase in REM sleep. No significant differences in etiologies of the hydrocephalus were noted. Amplitude exhibited parallel changes. Eighty-six percent of the cases with hydrocephalus showed normal baseline pressures during certain recording periods. No correlation was found between amplitude, age, and baseline pressure. In 12 patients for whom ICP monitorings before and after ventriculo-peritoneal shunt (VP shunt) were available, changes in the baseline pressure were significant: Preoperative baseline pressures were 182.2 ± 33.2 mmH$_2$O in non-REM and 244.8 ± 60.6 mmH$_2$O in REM sleep, whereas postoperative baseline pressures were 90.8 ± 22.9 mmH$_2$O in non-REM and 129.5 ± 36.3 mmH$_2$O in REM sleep. The amplitude also decreased postoperatively (Fig. 3). Intra-operative monitoring of ICP was done in three patients. Just after the placement of a ventricular catheter, a sudden decrease in baseline pressure and amplitude was observed, and the pressure waves seen in the preoperative period were almost completely eliminated post-operatively (Fig. 4).

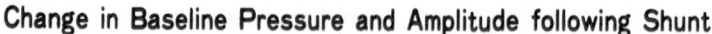

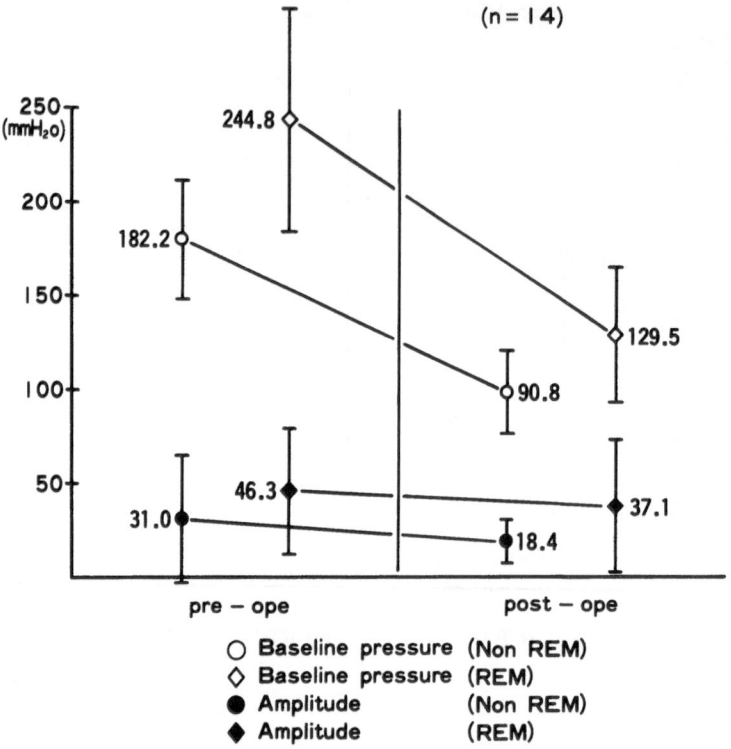

Fig. 3. Changes in pre- and postoperative ICP

Different types of pressure waves were observed; these were classified into four major types (Fig. 5). A Type I wave was similar to the A wave described by Lundberg and appeared only in REM sleep. The duration of the Type I wave was about 5–10 min and this was accompanied by a sudden decrease in ICP to the original baseline pressure at the end of REM sleep. The younger the patient, the smaller the increase of ICP. Although the peak value for ICP was 500 mmH$_2$O during REM sleep, no clinical deteriorations were noted. Type I waves were observed in every patient during every REM sleep and the shape of the waves varied from one REM sleep to another, even in the same patient (Fig. 6). Moreover, Type II waves were frequently observed together with a Type I wave. In one patient with slit ventricle, a significant increase in ICP during REM sleep suggested low intracranial compliance. The peak value was 500 mmH$_2$O and the amplitude was over 200 mmH$_2$O (Fig. 7).

Type II waves occurred most frequently, even in non REM sleep, and were observed in all patients. These waves always appeared with changes in respiration. Furthermore, it was noted that Type II waves appeared more frequently before and after REM sleep in all patients. In one patient with isolated fourth ventricle, huge Type II waves were observed in non-REM sleep when

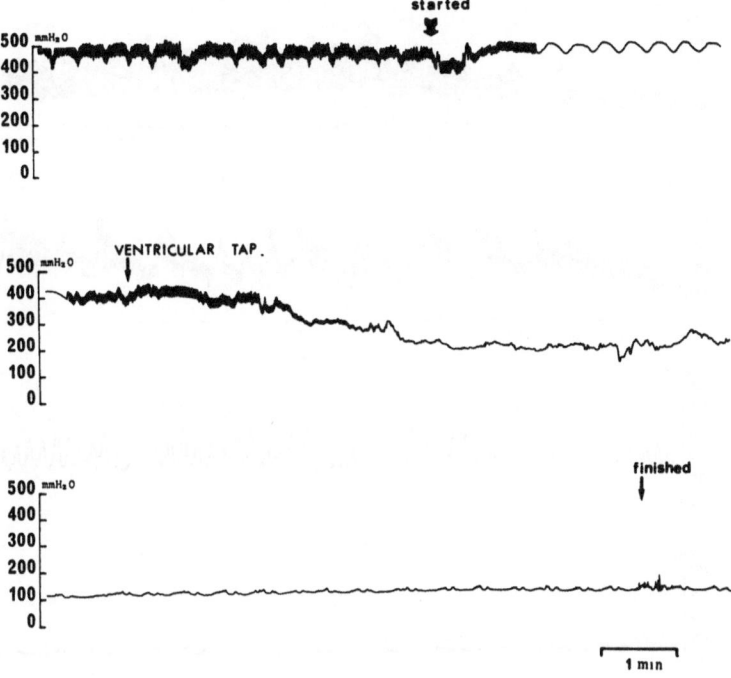

Fig. 4. ICP tracing during operation

shunt malfunction occurred (Fig. 8). In one patient with postmeningitic hydro-cephalus where the initial baseline pressure was 180 mmH$_2$O, Type II waves disappeared gradually, concomitant with decrease of the baseline pressure and normalization of the ventricle (Fig. 9).

Type III waves were observed only in two hydrocephalic patients: the patients with Crouzon's disease and subdural empyema. The respiratory pattern of these patients was similar to that of Cheyne-Stokes respiration. The appear-ance of Type III pressure waves was found to be synchronized with respiratory patterns. The periodic respiration of these patients was interrupted by periods of hyperventilation when the baseline pressure decreased (Fig. 10). The base-line pressure with Type III waves was over 300 mmH$_2$O and the patients' condition was critically ill. In the subdural empyema case, follow-up ICP monitoring showed that Type II waves replaced Type III waves.

Type IV waves were observed in patients with marked ventriculomegaly. Figure 11 indicates a case whose initial amplitude of over 20 mmH$_2$O dropped to below 10 mmH$_2$O about a month later. Moreover, irregular shapes of press-ure waves not related to respiration or to body movements were observed. Even though this patient's amplitude returned to the previous level again after the installation of a VP shunt, the shape of the ventricle did not change (Fig.

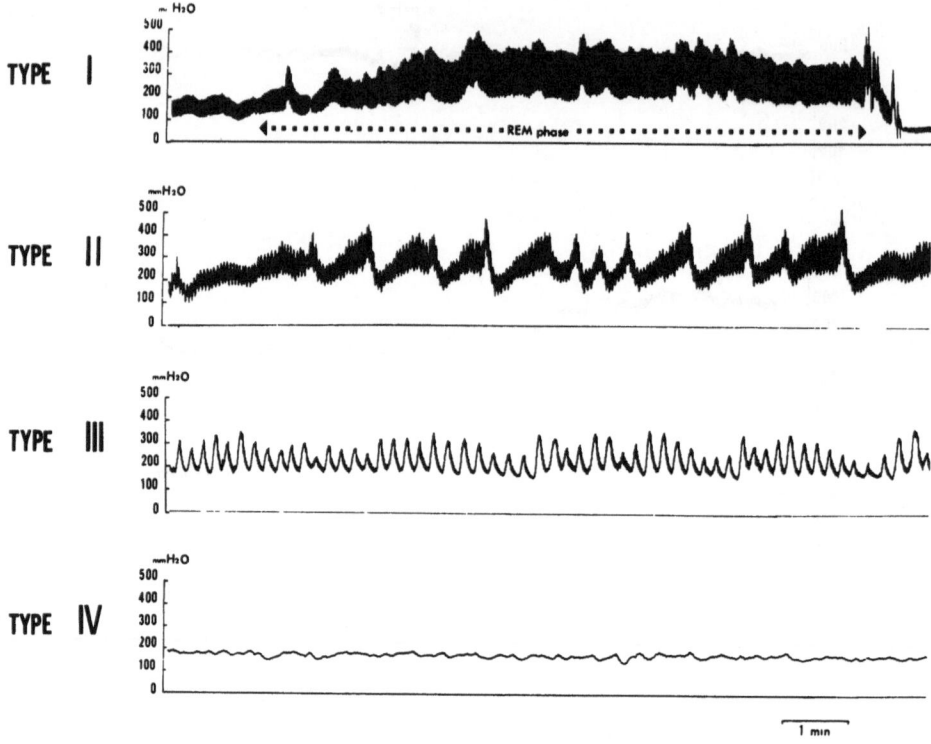

Fig. 5. Four types of pressure waves observed in infants with hydrocephalus

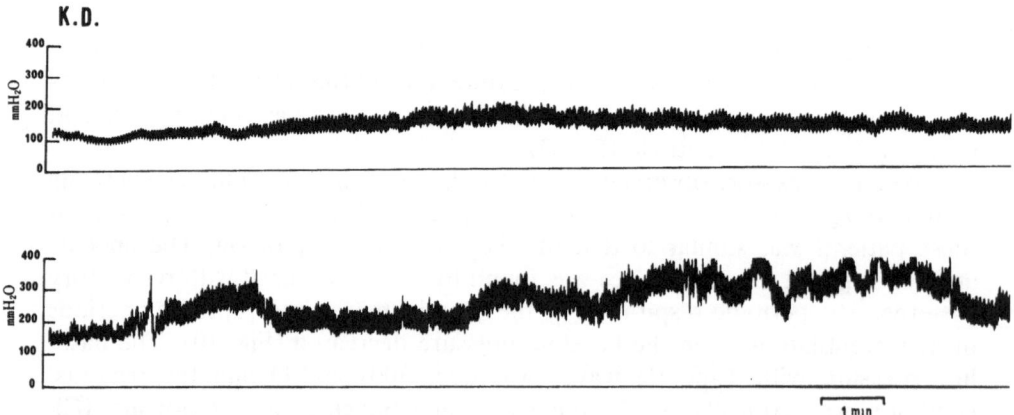

Fig. 6. Degrees of the increase in ICP vary from one REM sleep to another, even in the same patient

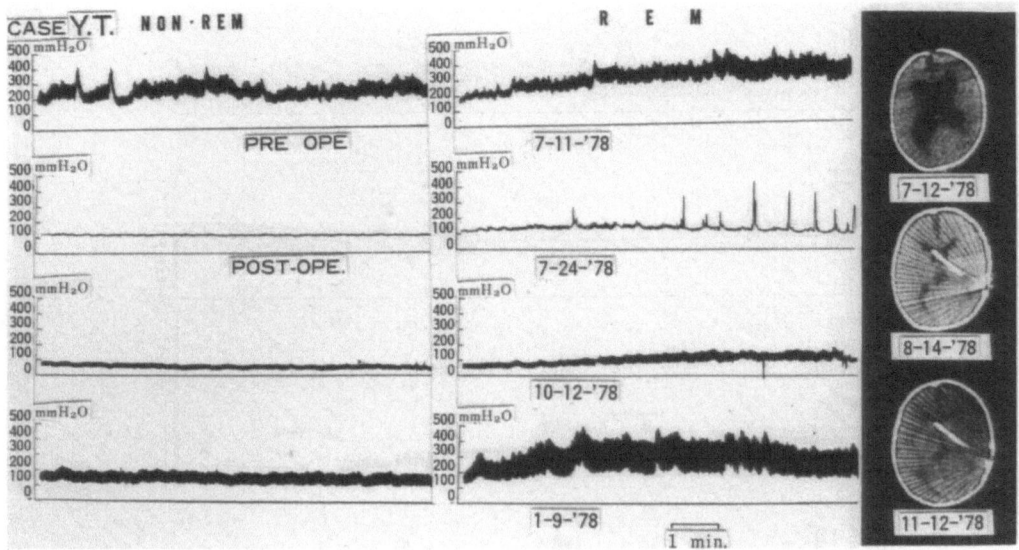

Fig. 7. ICP in a patient with "slit" ventricle syndrome. Note the marked elevation in the baseline pressure and augmented cerebral pulse amplitude in REM sleep

11). In the case of marked ventriculomegaly, the amplitude was quite small even when a high baseline pressure was observed.

Discussion

Baseline Pressure and Amplitude

The baseline pressure in hydrocephalus was found to be 134.5 mmH$_2$O in non-REM sleep and 184.7 mmH$_2$O in REM sleep. Even in the shunted patients, preoperative pressure was 182.2 mmH$_2$O. These values were not so high as expected. Furthermore, our data show that the baseline pressure in patients with hydrocephalus can vary within a wide range and can sometimes even show normal values. In fact, in over 80% of our patients ICP was found to be normal during some recording periods.

The origin of the amplitude is still controversial. It has been agreed that the major pulsation determining amplitude depends upon the pulsatile component in the cerebral blood flow (Bering 1955; Sibayan et al. 1970). Cerebral pulse waves have also been thought to depend upon intracranial compliance. Furthermore, it has been pointed out that changes in amplitude correspond to changes in the spatial buffering capacity of the brain. Venes (1979) suggested that the alteration of cerebral pulse wave amplitude form might be a sufficient indicator to predict and therefore impede neurological deterioration. We also

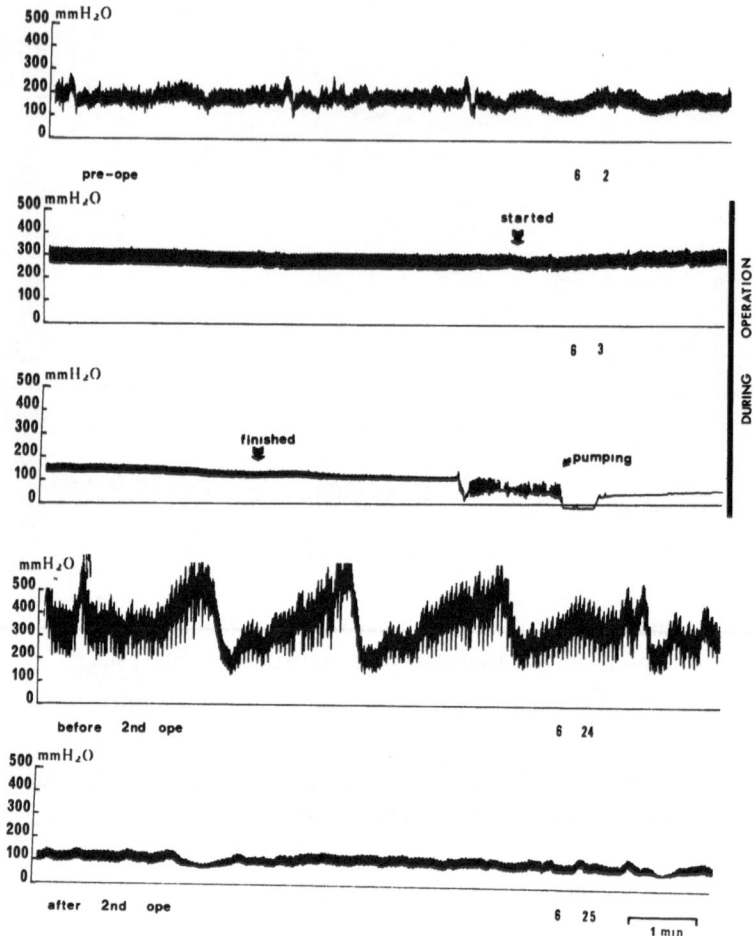

Fig. 8. ICP in a patient with isolated fourth ventricle when the shunt was obstructed. Note huge Type II waves

found that the amplitude increased concomitantly with the increase of ICP during REM sleep. In a case of "slit" ventricle, Nichols and Sklar (1989) suggested that decreased CSF volume, resulting in an augmented cerebral pulse amplitude, might be responsible for this syndrome. In summary, amplitude must reflect intracranial compliance and cerebrovascular resistance as well as developmental changes. Hence, it remains to be demonstrated how amplitude can be evaluated in infants with hydrocephalus.

Pressure Waves (Fig. 12)

Three kinds of pressure waves were first described by Lundberg in 1960: an A (plateau) wave, a B wave, and a C wave. Lundberg observed that A waves occurred in various diseases other than hydrocephalus; diseases that were

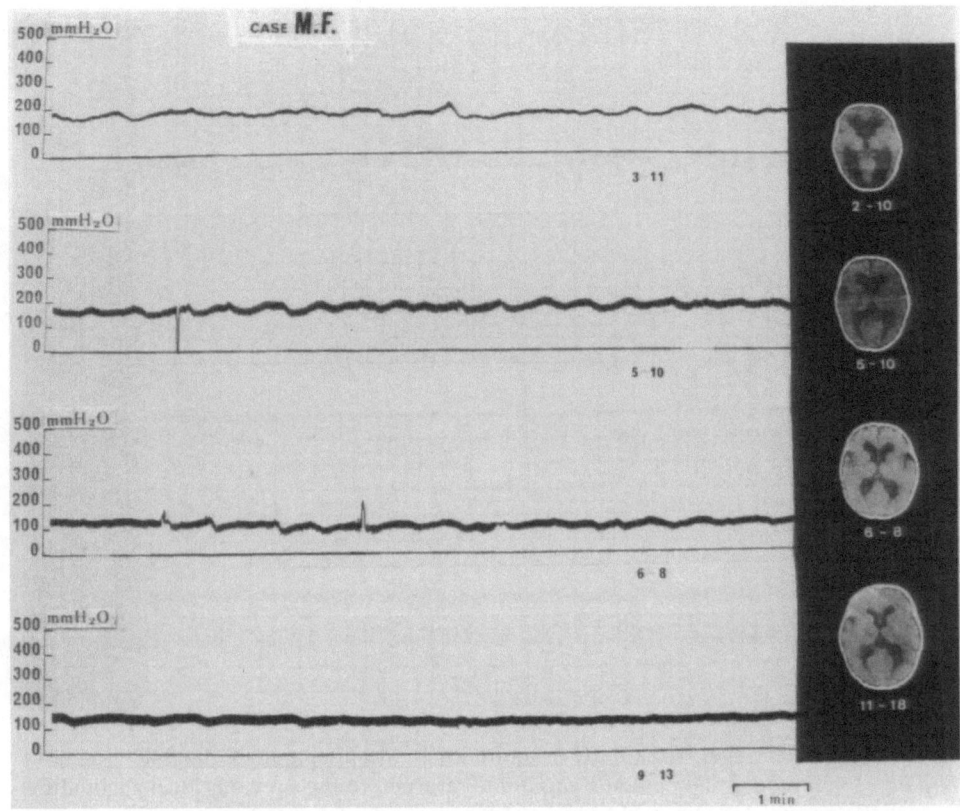

Fig. 9. ICP monitorings in a patient with postmeningitic hydrocephalus. The patient was followed without installation of VP shunt. Note disappearance of Type II wave as the baseline pressure decreased and the size of the ventricle became normal

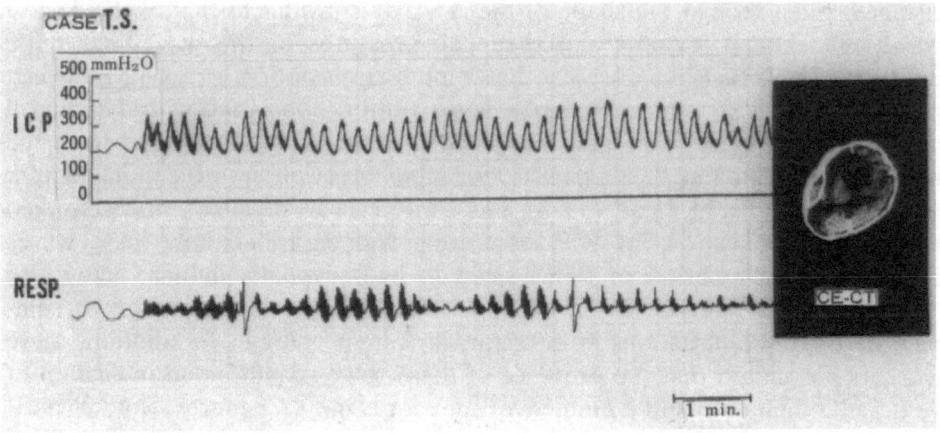

Fig. 10. Type III wave seen in an infant with subdural empyema. The pattern of the pressure waves is synchronized with the respiratory (*RESP.*) pattern

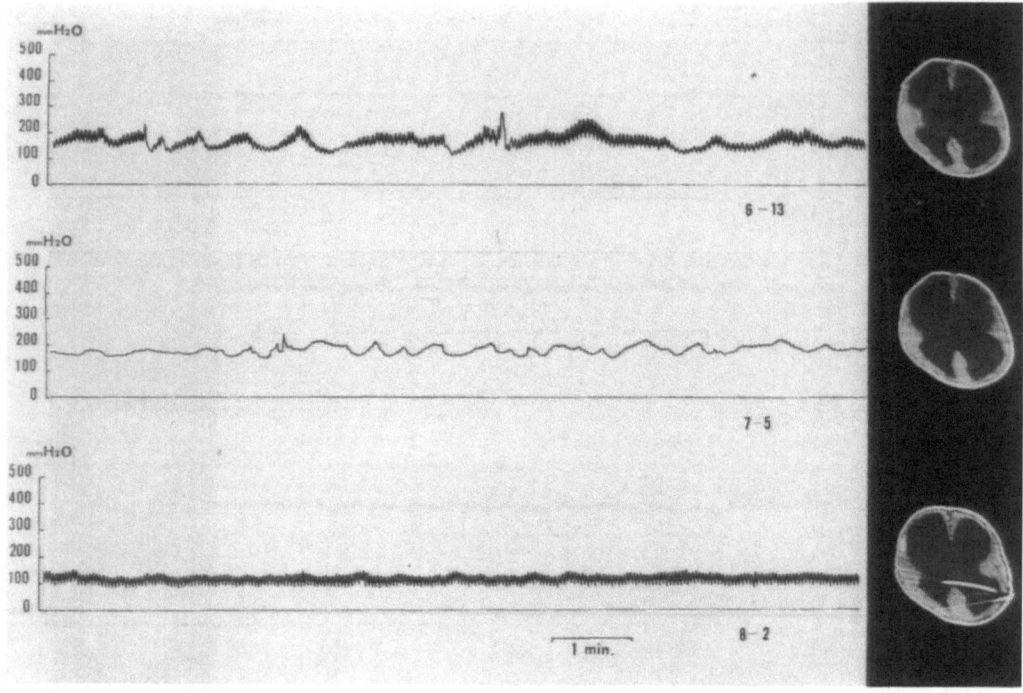

Fig. 11. Type IV wave. Amplitude is quite small despite a high baseline pressure (*middle*). Even though the patient's amplitude returned to the previous level again after the installation of a VP shunt, the shape of the ventricle did not change

accompanied by intracranial hypertension and frequently associated with transient neurological deterioration. He thought that A waves must reflect changes in cerebral blood volume secondary to alterations in the cerebrovascular resistance. Even though the shape of the A wave is similar to that of the Type I wave, the clinical features and the peak pressures of the waves are quite different. These facts may suggest that Type I waves and A waves have distinct pathophysiological origins. However, some authors concerned with the clinical applications of these facts have suggested that these waves resulted from the inability of the patient to compensate for rapid variation in intracranial content volume. Pierre-Kahn et al. (1976) and Di Rocco et al. (1975, 1976) studied the clinical applications of ICP monitoring and described how these waves occurred in each period of REM sleep in hydrocephalic infants. They also suggested that these waves resulted from the inability of the patient to compensate for rapid variations in intracranial content volume. In addition, these workers postulated that the presence of these waves could be an indication of ventricular dilatation and a predictive index for shunt procedures. Both Type II and III waves should be included into the B wave described by Lundberg (1960). The B wave was defined by Lundberg (1960) as rhythmic oscillations,

Fig. 12. Mechanism of the appearance of pressure waves in hydrocephalus

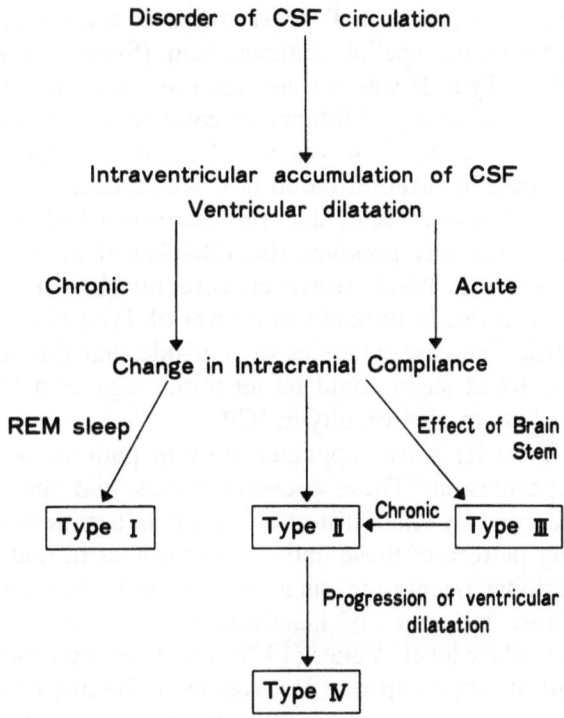

related to respiratory changes, occurring regularly at a frequency of about one per min. He proposed that they reflected cardiorespiratory dynamics. Venes (1979) presented evidence that B waves reflected changes in the cerebral blood flow, possibly secondary to alterations in cerebrovascular resistance. Pickard et al. (1980) and Chawla et al. (1974) concluded that the presence or absence of B waves provided the best predictive assessment for shunt procedure.

In Part I of our study we were able to provide evidence that Type I and Type II waves were normal features of ICP, even in infants, as reported by some authors (Martin 1978; Gücer and Viernstein 1979; Mautner et al. 1989). Hence, the singular presence of these pressure waves does not provide any definitive indication of abnormal ICP. In addition, even though others have reported consistent values for baseline pressures in normal children (Welch 1980), our data indicate that the baseline pressures of patients with intracranial hypertension can vary within a wide range and can sometimes show normal values. In fact, in over 80% of our patients with hydrocephalus, ICP was found to be normal during some recording period. The question then remains, what is the difference between normal and abnormal ICP. The form and duration of Type I waves changed considerably in REM sleep. So Type I waves cannot be used as predictive indicators, since they lack the consistency necessary to effectively discriminate between normal and abnorma ICP. It has also been proposed that the appearance of Type II waves is the result of a decrease in the brain's capacity for spatial compensation (Symon et al. 1972; Symon and Dorsch 1975). Type II waves were observed in both non-REM and REM sleep in the abnormal group of infants, in contrast to normal infants, in whom the appearance of Type II waves was limited to REM sleep. In normal infants, an increase in cerebral blood flow which occurs during REM sleep may result in an increase of ICP, and the increase which occurs in non-REM sleep may not cause any pressure rise (Reivich et al. 1968; Rahilly 1980; Shapiro and Rosendorff 1981). However, cerebral blood flow in non-REM sleep may also allow a rise in pressure as a form of Type II wave. Hence, our observation of borderline cases leads us to conclude that the appearance of Type II waves in non-REM sleep could be an initial sign of a low compliance state and does present an abnormality in ICP.

Type III waves appeared only in patients wih acute or severe intracranial hypertension. These pressure waves had the same characteristics as those recorded by Kjällquist et al. (1964) in a patient with brain tumor. The respiratory pattern of these patients was similar to that of Cheyne-Stokes respiration. Periodic respiration such as Cheyne-Stokes respiration has been related to different degrees of inactivation of the regulatory mechanism at the supramedullary level. Venes (1979) suggested that the periodic nature of respiration and the appearence of B waves might be due to an intrinsic brain stem rhythm. Hence, the presence of Type III waves must be an indicator that ICP is high enough to damage the brain stem.

In a hydrocephalic infant with marked ventriculomegaly, amplitude became smaller without any change in baseline pressure over a short term. We have insufficient data to explain what is responsible for this interesting phenomenon. However, the fact that there were no morphological changes before or after the placement of a VP shunt suggests that irreversible changes in the compliance of the brain due to long-standing compression of the ventricular wall and marked dilatation of the ventricle may remain, even after the baseline pressure becomes normal.

Conclusions

The baseline pressure in infants with hydrocephalus was found to be within the normal range. Moreover, those who showed ICP hypertension were often found to have normal baseline pressures. In addition, various forms of pressure waves which have been observed in adult cases were also noted in the infants. Since these pressure waves and amplitudes are assumed to reflect intracranial compliance and cerebrovascular dynamics, more detailed investigation of pathophysiological changes in the intracranial environment may be possible by further analysis of pressure waves and amplitudes.

References

Bering EA Jr (1955) Choroid plexus and arterial pulsation of cerebrospinal fluid. Demonstration of the choroid plexuses as a cerebrospinal fluid pump. Arch Neurol Psychiat 73: 165–172

Chawla JC, Hulme A, Cooper R (1974) Intracranial pressure in patients with dementia and communicating hydrocephalus. J Neurosurg 40: 376–380

Di Rocco C, McLone DG, Shimoji T, Raimondi AJ (1975) Continuous intraventricular cerebrospinal fluid pressure recording in hydrocephalic children during wakefulness and sleep. J Neurosurg 42: 683–689

Di Rocco C, Maira G, Rossi GF, Vignati A (1976) Cerebrospinal fluid pressure studies in normal pressure hydrocephalus and cerebral atrophy. Eur Neurol 14: 119–128

Gücer G, Viernstein LJ (1979) Intracranial pressure in the normal monkey while awake and asleep. J Neurosurg 51: 206–210

Kjällquist Å, Lundberg N, Pontén U (1964) Respiratory and cardiovascular changes during rapid spontaneous variations of ventricular fluid pressure in patients with intracranial hypertension. Acta Neurol Scand 40: 291–317

Lundberg N (1960) Continuous recording and control of ventricular fluid pressure in neurosurgical practice. Acta Psychiatr Scand (Suppl 149)36: 1–193

Martin G (1978) Lundberg's B waves as a feature of normal intracranial pressure. Surg Neurol 9: 347–348

Mautner D, Dirnagl U, Haberl R, Schmiedek P, Garner C, Villringer A, Einhaupl KM (1989) B-waves in healthy persons. In: Hoff JT, Betz AL (eds) Intracranial pressure VII. Springer, Berlin Heidelberg New York, pp 209–212

Nichols JS, Sklar FH (1989) Cerebral pulse amplitude in a canine model of "slit" ventricle syndrome. In: Hoff JT, Betz AL (eds) Intracranial pressure VII. Springer, Berlin Heidelberg New York, pp 201–202

Pickard JD, Teasdale GM, Matheson M, Lindsay K, Galbraith S, Wyper D, Macpherson P (1980) Intraventricular pressure waves — the best predictive test for shunting in normal pressure hydrocephalus. In: Shulman K, Marmarou A, Miller JD, Becker DB, Hochwald GM, Brock M (eds) Intracranial pressure IV. Springer, Berlin Heidelberg New York Tokyo, pp 488–491

Pierre-Kahn A, Gabersek V, Hirsch JF (1976) Intracranial pressure and rapid eye movement sleep in hydrocephalus. Childs Brain 2: 156–166

Rahilly PM (1980) Effect of sleep state and feeding on cranial blood flow of the human neonate. Arch Dis Child 55: 265–270

Reivich M, Isaacs G, Evarts E, Kety S (1968) The effect of slow wave sleep and REM sleep on regional cerebral blood flow in cat. J Neurochem 15: 301–306

Shapiro CM, Rosendorff C (1981) Local hypothalamic blood flow during sleep. Electroencephalogr Clin Neurophysiol 39: 365–369

Sibayan RQ, Begeman PC, King AI, Gurdjian ES, Thomas LM (1970) Experimental hydrocephalus. Arch Neurol 23: 165–172

Symon L, Dorsch NWC (1975) Use of long-term intracranial pressure measurement to assess hydrocephalic patients prior to shunt surgery. J Neurosurg 43: 332–344

Symon L, Dorsch NWC, Stephens RJ (1972) Pressure waves in so-called low-pressure hydrocephalus. Lancet II: 1291–1292

Venes JL (1979) B-Waves — A reflection of cardiorespiratory or cerebral nervous systems rhythm? Childs Brain 5: 352–360

Welch K (1980) The intracranial pressure in infants. J Neurosurg 52: 693–699

26 — A Volume–Blood Flow Velocity Response (VFR) Relationship Derived from CSF Compartment Challenge as an Index of Progression of Infantile Hydrocephalus

Robert A. Minns[1], Day-eel Goh[1], Steven D. Pye[2], and A. James W. Steers[1]

Summary. Optimal management in childhood hydrocephalus requires prevention of secondary ischemic damage and reliable indication for surgical treatment to prevent long-term shunt related complications. Transcranial Doppler ultrasound provides a noninvasive means of monitoring cerebrohemodynamic response. Cerebral blood flow velocity (CBFV) and intracranial pressure (ICP) was measured during 38 CSF taps in 11 patients (6 neonates, 5 children). The Resistance Index (RI = S − D/S) (where S — peak systolic velocity and D — end diastolic velocity) decreased significantly ($P < .001$) after all taps, mainly due to a larger percentage increase in diastolic velocity and mean flow velocity (MFV) which increased in 89% of taps, suggesting a significant reduction in cerebrovascular resistance and increased flow after cerebrospinal fluid (CSF) depletion. There was a significant positive correlation of RI to ICP ($r = 0.63$, $P < .001$) in older children. Exponential decay of RI with volume depletion allows estimation of "critical" volume buffering capacity. Serial volume flow velocity response (VFR) in individual infants may indicate progression or arrest of the hydrocephalic process and may help to select more precisely those who will benefit from surgical intervention.

Keywords. Cerebral blood flow — Intracranial pressure — Transcranial doppler — Hydrocephalus

Introduction

It is important to differentiate progressive hydrocephalus in children from those cases which will arrest spontaneously or those that may require only temporary cerebrospinal fluid (CSF) removal. The aim of management is to prevent further ischemic damage due to increasing ventricular dilatation and

---

[1] Department of Paediatric Neurology, Royal Hospital for Sick Children, Edinburgh, EH9 1LF, Scotland, UK
[2] Department of Medical Physics, Western General Hospital, Edinburgh, EH4 2XU, Scotland, UK

raised intracranial pressure (ICP) while avoiding unnecessary surgical procedures and the long term complications of shunting such as craniocerebral disproportion from overdrainage. Single measurements of ICP, even when repeated on separate occasions, do not provide information on intracranial dynamics and compliance to separate those who have reached a critical point on the exponential intracranial volume — pressure curve with limited available volume buffering capacity. Shulman and Marmarou (1971) and Miller et al. (1973) have characterised ICP dynamics with the Pressure-Volume Index (PVI) and the Volume-Pressure Response (VPR), respectively, using volume challenge techniques. However, infants with hydrocephalus were reported to have elevated PVI compared to predicted normal values (Shapiro et al. 1985) due to altered brain biomechanics as a result of the hydrocephalic process.

The Doppler principle can be applied to measurement of cerebral blood flow velocity (CBFV). Hill and Volpe (1982) first reported a decrease in pulsatile flow of anterior cerebral arteries in infantile hydrocephalus using Doppler ultrasound. Resistance Index (RI = (S −D)/S where S — peak systolic velocity and D — end diastolic velocity) as an index of cerebrovascular resistance adapted by Bada et al. (1979) from Pourcelot's Index of Resistance (Pourcelot 1976) was significantly raised. Transcranial Doppler ultrasound techniques (Aaslid et al. 1982) now provide a noninvasive means of repeated assesment of cerebrohamodynamic change for all ages.

The aim of our study was to examine a direct blood flow velocity response to volume manipulation in children with hydrocephalus, as ICP rise causes ischemic damage due to its secondary effect on cerebral perfusion. A volume — flow velocity response (VFR) could theoretically estimate residual volume buffering capacity before an "ischemic" point is reached and serial VFRs should therefore indicate progression or arrest of the hydrocephalic process. There have been no previous reports on sequential CBFV change with volume manipulation in hydrocephalic children.

Patients and Methods

Eleven patients (7 males, 4 females) with hydrocephalus of varying etiology, age range 35 weeks gestation–118 months, were assesed. Table 1 describes their clinical details and indications for CSF taps. They are divided into two groups. Group I were all neonates ($n = 6$) while group 11 patients were between 12–118 months old, because the "normal" range of cerebral Doppler indices are age dependent with less change after the first year of life (Bode 1989; Chadduck and Seibert 1989). Four patients in group 11 had existing ventricular peritoneal shunts in situ. Indications for CSF taps were signs or symptoms of raised ICP, evidence of increasing ventricular dilatation, e.g., from imaging evidence (ultrasound or computed tomography (CT) scan) or increasing head circumference measurements in young infants.

A total of 38 CSF taps (33 in group 1; 5 in group 11) were performed. ICP was measured directly through a ventriculostomy reservoir where available

Table 1. Clinical details and indications for CSF taps

Patient	Age	Etiology	Clinical
Group 1: Neonates			
(1) LF	C.A — 2 weeks	Perinatal Infection	Progressive vent dilation
(2) MG	Term	X-linked Congenital	Gross hydrocephalus
(3) NB	Term	Occlp encephalocele	Vent dilat postrepair
(4) FR	35/40	Posthemmorhagic	Vent dilat and p.cysts
(5) RA	Term	Prenatal PHH	Progressive vent dilatation
(6) JM	Term	Myelomeningocele	Vent dilat postrepair
Group 2: Children			
(7) CM	17 months	PHH	Vent dilatation, mild dev delay, not shunted
(8) CJ	4 years	PHH	Broken VP shunt
(9) PB	12 months	Myelomeningocele	Increased vent dilat
(10) LH	10 years	Post-meningitis	Slit vent, ataxia
(11) IF	14 months	PHH	Vomiting, ICP raised

C.A, corrected age; vent dilat, ventricle dilatation; occip, occipital; PHH, posthemorraghic hydrocephalus; p.cysts, porencephalic cysts; VP, ventriculo-peritoneal, ICP, intracranial pressure

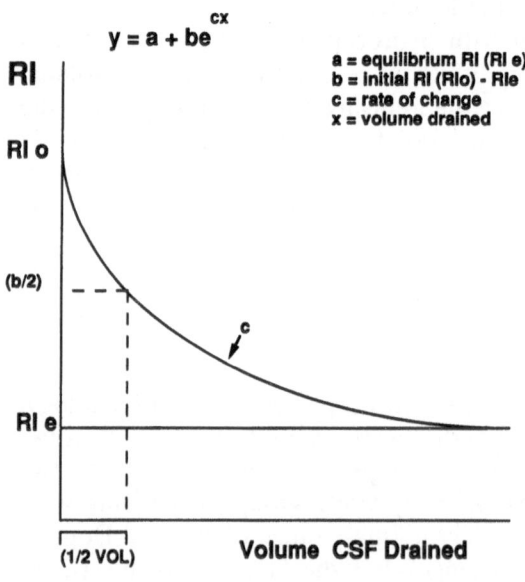

$$y = a + be^{cx}$$

a = equilibrium RI (RI e)
b = initial RI (RIo) - RIe
c = rate of change
x = volume drained

Fig. 1. A predicted exponential curve fit $y = a + be^{cx}$ for serial observed Resistance Index (RI) decay with volume depletion during CSF taps. *Half-volume* = −0.7/c, i.e., the volume drained when 1/2 change in RI has occurred

[1/2 VOL = volume when RI = RI e + (RI o - RI e)/2]

(Leggate et al. 1988) or through ventricular (n = 4) or lumbar (n = 1) puncture, using a non-displacement method with a strain gauge pressure transducer (Gaeltec) connected to a butterfly or spinal needle. CSF was drained in 1-ml increments with repeated ICP measurements until a normal value for age range was achieved (Minns et al. 1989).

Continous CBFV in the middle cerebral artery (MCA) insonated through the thin temporal squamous bone (methodolgy as described by Aaslid 1982) was recorded throughout the tap using pulsed-wave Doppler (Decoder — Doptek Ltd., Chichester, UK) with a 2 or 4 MHz probe. This allowed unhindered access for ICP measurement and CSF removal; the MCA was chosen also for accesibility, easy identification, and reliability using the transcranial approach. CBFV signals were recorded onto audiotape and reviewed separately; only good quality consecutive waveforms were analyzed. Incorporated computer calculation of RI, MFV (time averaged mean of maximum velocity envelope) were used to characterise the Doppler waveforms and a mean value of at least 10 waveforms was obtained. RI was mainly used to minimize error in CBFV measurement due to variability in angle of insonation.

Pre- and post-tap ICP, RI, MFV, PSFV (peak systolic flow velocity) and EDFV (end diastolic flow velocity) were compared using Student's paired t-test. Plots of RI (y) against volume CSF drained (x) were fitted to an exponential curve $y = a + be^{cx}$ (a = equilibrium RI, i.e., RIe, atb = initial RI i.e. RIo, b = change in RI i.e., RIo-RIe, and c = rate of exponential decay), (see Fig. 1). A "half-volume" when half the change in RI had occurred was obtained by calculation, i.e., "half-volume" = $-0.7/c$.

Results

Tables 2 and 3 summarise the pre-and post-tap ICP and Doppler indices from group 1 and 11 patients. In all taps there was, as expected, a statistically significant change in ICP and also a highly significant decrease in RI ($P < .001$) after volume withdrawal. After 34 taps (89%), there was an increase in MFV — this was statistically significant only in group 1. The percentage increase in EDFV was greater and more significant than PSFV change in both groups, thus the decrease in RI was due primarily to improved diastolic flow. There was a significant positive correlation of RI to increased ICP ($r = +0.63, P < .001$) in group 11 patients — see Fig. 2. In the neonatal group, overall correlation between RI and ICP was poor but in two neonates who had sufficient repeated measurements, there was a significant correlation ($r = +0.61$ and $0.40, P < .001$) in their individual measurements.

Data were available for 36 serial RI and volume plots. Figure 3 shows the sequential parallel decrease in RI and ICP with CSF volume depletion from a patient who was not shunted. Only two taps did not fit an exponential curve. RI was significantly lower in the children compared to the neonates. The rate of exponential decay was slowest in the child (aged 17 months) who was not shunted, i.e., largest "half-volume," suggesting increased volume buffering in

Table 2. Doppler and ICP change pre- and post-CSF taps in Group I (neonates) patients

Doppler indices and ICP	No. of paired obs	Pre-tap	Post-tap	% Change	P value
Mean RI (SD)	33	0.78 (.06)	0.69 (.06)	11.5%	<.001
Mean MFV (SD) cm/s	33	45.2 (9.4)	52.6 (9.2)	16.3%	<.001
Mean PSFV (SD) cm/s	23	82.8 (8.9)	87.4 (10.8)	5.6%	<.02
Mean EDFV (SD) cm/s	23	15.8 (5.4)	25.1 (5.7)	59%	<.001
Mean ICP (SD) mmHg	31	9.8 (2.6)	4.6 (1.6)	53%	<.001

Table 3. Doppler and ICP changes pre- and post CSF taps in Group II (children) patients

Doppler indices and ICP	No. of paired obs	Pre-tap	Post-tap	% Change	P value
Mean RI (SD)	5	0.61 (.08)	0.5 (.06)	18%	<.001
Mean MFV (SD) cm/s	5	54.9 (17)	66.5 (16)	21%	NS
Mean PSFV (SD) cm/s	5	86.0 (26)	93.7 (24)	9%	NS
Mean EDFV (SD) cm/s	5	33.2 (11)	45.7 (15)	37.7%	<.05
Mean ICP (SD) mmHg	5	15.4 (3.8)	5.8 (1.8)	62.2%	<.02

Fig. 2. Plot of RI versus ICP during CSF taps in Group 11 patients (>12 months old) shows significant positive correlation ($r = 0.63$, $P < .001$)

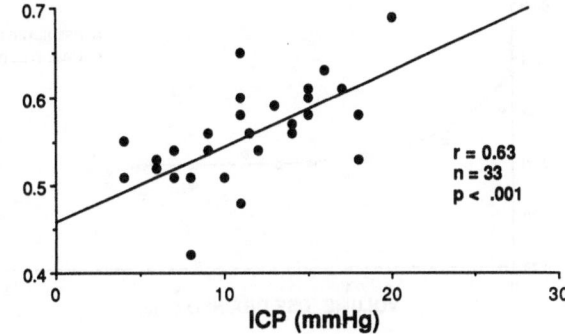

Fig. 3. Plot of parallel RI and ICP change against volume CSF drained in patient CM with unshunted hydrocephalus

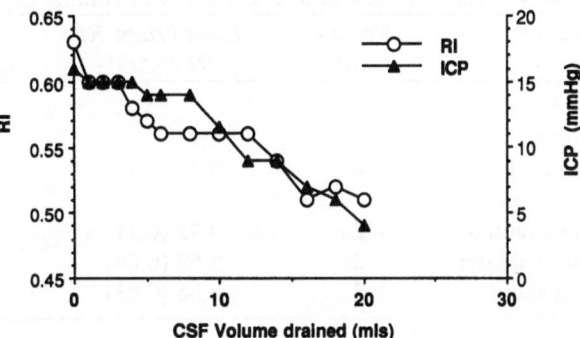

Fig. 4. Plot of predicted RI (*open triangle*) and observed RI (*closed circles*) against CSF volume drained in child (CM) with unshunted hydrocephalus shows slow exponential decay in RI

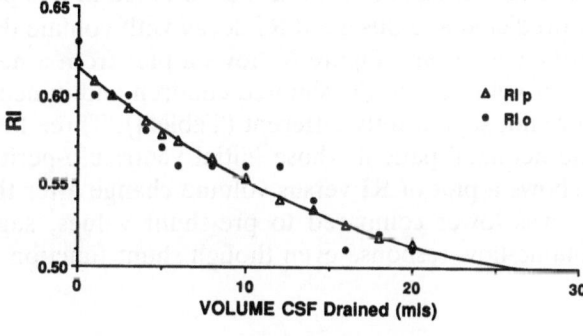

Fig. 5. Plot of predicted and observed RI against volume drained in a child who presented with a broken shunt shows rapid exponential decay in RI

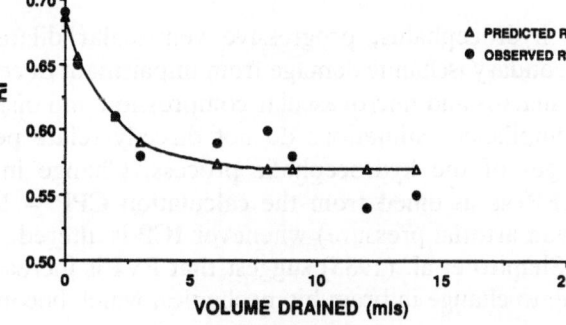

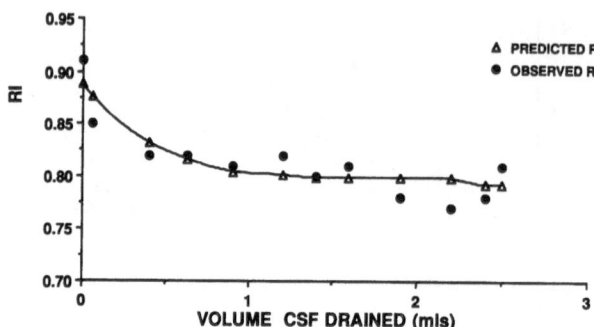

Fig. 6. Plot of predicted and observed RI with volume drained in a neonate (NB) who was not shunted

Table 4. '*Half-volumes*' and RI change with volume depletion during CSF taps

Patients	No. obs (n)	Equilibrium RI RI e (SD)	Change in RI (RI o – RI e) SD	Half-vol (mls)
Children				
Non-shunted	1	0.47	0.15	11.9
Shunted	4	0.48 (0.1)	0.13 (.03)	2.1 (1)
Neonates				
Not shunted	2	0.72 (0.1)	0.13 (.05)	1.97
Shunted later	24	0.69 (0.04)	0.08 (.03)	1.75 (2)
Post shunt	3	0.66 (0.03)	0.08 (.04)	0.81 (0.3)

the absence of a ventricular shunt. Figure 4 shows a plot of observed and predicted RI against volume CSF drained in this patient. Figure 5 shows a plot of predicted and observed RI decay with volume depletion in a child who had a broken shunt and Figure 6 shows a plot from a neonate who was not shunted. "Half-volumes" in the shunted children and in neonates with or without shunts were not significantly different (Table 4). Three further taps were performed in one neonatal patient whose initial ventriculo-peritoneal shunt blocked. Figure 7 shows a plot of RI versus volume change after this initial shunt. Equilibrium RI was lower compared to pre-shunt values, suggesting that shunting alters volume-flow response even though shunt function was not adequate.

Discussion

In hydrocephalus, progressive ventricular dilatation and raised ICP causes secondary ischamic damage from impairment of cerebral perfusion with changes of macro- and microvascular compression and distortion (Wozniak et al. 1975). Compliance estimations do not directly relate perfusion responses at various stages of the hydrocephalic process. Change in cerebral perfusion pressure (CPP) is assumed from the calculation CPP = MAP − ICP (where MAP is mean arterial pressure) whenever ICP is altered.

Shapiro et al. (1985) suggest that PVI is increased in hydrocephalic children due to change in brain biomechanics, which becomes a perpetuating factor that

Fig. 7. Plot of predicted and observed RI with volume drained from a CSF tap performed after initial unsuccessful ventriculo-peritoneal shunting in a neonatal patient (RA). Equilibrium RI was lower than pre-shunt values

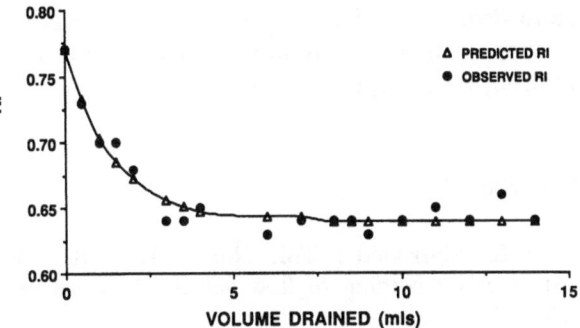

allows ventricular enlargement to occur by encouraging storage of volume. This, however, does not distinguish those patients whose hydrocephalic process arrests spontaneously before significant ischemic insult occurs and whose indications and optimal timing for intervention remain controversial. CSF shunting proceedures disrupt normal CSF absorption and most patients with CSF shunts become shunt-dependent and thus remain at risk from long-term complications such as ventriculitis and slit ventricle syndrome.

Archer et al. (1986), using hypercapnia-induced increase in CBF, showed a significant correlation with decrease in RI as an index of distal cerebrovascular resistance. Our results suggest that CSF depletion reduces ICP and distal resistance to CBF, as there was a highly significant reduction in RI which was due to a more significantly increased EDFV after CSF taps. Previous studies reporting decrease in RI after CSF taps have not utilized direct ICP measurements (Van Bel et al. 1988) or have not related RI to ICP and volume manipulation (Seibert et al. 1989).

We have shown that decrease in RI with volume depletion generally followed an exponential curve similar to the ICP/volume-relationship (VPR or PVI), suggesting that there is similarly a "critical" volume buffered before blood flow response is significantly altered. In neonates and young infants with wide open sutures, single ICP measurements do not predict those who require shunting. There was a poor overall correlation of ICP to RI in the neonatal group and those with elevated RI did not necessarily have increased ICP (Hill and Volpe 1982). Thus some infants may have considerably raised cerebrovascular resistance with reduced perfusion without significantly raised ICP. Repeated RI measurements can provide an estimate of cerebrovascular resistance and its rate of change with volume manipulation (VFR) for individual patients. If RI remains elevated compared to the normal range for age and serial VFR shows deterioration or no change with time, surgical intervention would be indicated, as there is no development of natural arrest. Repeated RI measurements showing an improvement toward normal values for age would encourage non-interventional management. Noninvasive transcranial Doppler monitoring of cerebrohemodynamic change in hydrocephalus, in particular serial change with volume manipulation (VFR), may help to select more precisely those who require intervention.

Acknowledgment. We are grateful to the Earl of Elgin and the TSB Foundation for supporting research into hydrocephalus at the Royal Hospital for Sick Children, Edinburgh, Scotland, UK

References

Aaslid R, Markwalder TM, Nornes H (1982) Noninvasive transcranial Doppler ultrasound recording of flow velocity in basal cerebral arteries. J Neurosurg 57: 769–774

Archer LNJ, Evans DH, Paton JY, Levene MI (1986) Controlled hypercapnia and neonatal cerebral artery Doppler ultrasound waveforms. Pediatrics 20: 218–221

Bada HS, Hajjar W, Chua C, et al. (1979) Noninvasive diagnosis of neonatal asphyxia and intraventricular hamorrhage by Doppler ultrasound. J Pediatr 95: 775

Bode H (1989) Transcranial Doppler sonography in children. J Child Neurol 4: S68–S76

Chadduck WM, Seibert JJ (1989) Intracranial duplex Doppler: Practical uses in pediatric neurology and neurosurgery. J Child Neurol 4: S77–S86

Hill A, Volpe JJ (1982) Decrease in pulsatile flow in the anterior cerebral arteries in infantile hydrocephalus. Pediatrics 69: 4–7.

Leggate JRS, Baxter P, Minns RA, et al. (1988) Role of a separate subcutaneous cerebrospinal fluid reservoir in the management of hydrocephalus. Br J Neurosurg 2: 327–338

Miller JD, Garibi J, Pickard JD (1973) Induced changes of cerebrospinal fluid volume: Effects during continous monitoring of ventricular fluid pressure. Arch Neurol 28: 265

Minns RA, Engleman HM, Stirling H (1989) Cerebrospinal fluid pressure in pyogenic meningitis. Arch Dis Child 64: 814–820

Pourcelot L (1976) Diagnostic ultrasound for cerebral vascular diseases. In: Donald I, Levi S (eds) Present and future of diagnostic ultrasound. Kookyer, Rotterdam, pp 141–147

Seibert JJ, McCowan TC, Chadduck WM (1989) Duplex pulsed Doppler US versus intracranial pressure in the neonate: clinical and experimental studies. Radiology 171: 155–159

Shapiro K, Fried A, Marmarou A (1985) Biomechanical and hydrodynamic character ization of the hydrocephalic infant. J Neurosurg 63: 69–75

Shulman K, Marmarou A (1971) Pressure volume considerations in infantile hydrocephalus. Dev Med Child Neurol 13: 90

Van Bel F, Van de Bor M, Baan J, et al. (1988) Blood flow velocity patterns of the anterior cerebral arteries before and after drainage of posthamorraghic hydrocephalus in the newborn. J Ultrasound Med 7: 553–559

Wozniak M, Mclone DG, Raimondi AJ (1975) Micro- and macrovascular changes as the direct cause of parenchymal destruction in congenital murine hydrocephalus. J Neurosurg 43: 535–545

27 — The Role of Altered Brain Properties in Ventricular Dilatation

Futoshi Takei, Kaoru Ito, and Osamu Sato[1]

Summary. Factors which contribute to the development of the venticulomegaly seen in hydrocephalus are being studied but have not yet been clarified. In this situation, the alteration of brain parenchymal properties has been thrust into the limelight; this alteration seems to be one of the establishing causes of the development of hydrocephalus. Under these circumstances, our study focused on brain parenchyma itself; we aimed to document whether any alteration of brain parenchymal properties influenced ventricular dilatation.

We used 59 adult mongrel cats in this study. Unilateral saline infusion was performed on the feline brain parenchyma to change brain properties, in 19 animals of groups three and four ($n = 19$: groups 3 ($n = 5$) and 4 ($n = 14$) in contrast to 40 animals which were not infused ($n = 40$: groups 1 ($n = 30$) and 2 ($n = 10$). Pressure volume index (PVI), local tissue compliance (LTC), and intracranial compliance (IC), used as indicators of neural axial conditions, were obtained before and after infusion in the cisterna magna and lateral ventricle. After initiating the process to alter brain properties, a kaolin injection was made into the cisterna magna in 14 animals ($n = 14$: groups 2 and 4) in contrast to animals which were not injected with kaolin ($n = 5$: groups 1 and 3). Visual assessment of ventricular dilatation was made 10–14 days after the initial preparations. In the ventriculomegaly which developed, we found different degrees of ventricular dilatation in the kaolin injected cats. In group 4 in particular, both symmetrical and asymmetrical ventricular dilatation and unilateral ventricular dilatation in the lateral ventricle on the side of the infusion were observed, while in group 2 only symmetrical ventriculomegaly was seen; no ventriculomegaly was observed in group 3. Saline infusion caused spatial independence between the cisterna magna and lateral ventricle and measured PVI values were enhanced after infusion. Local tissue compliance (LTC) increased during infusion and IC was reduced. According to these results, the alteration of brain parenchymal properties, providing "softening" tissue,

---

[1] Department of Neurosurgery, Tokai University, School of Medicine, Isehara, Kanagawa, 259–11, Japan

may play an important role as a factor contributing to the development of hydrocephalus.

Keywords. Experimental — Hydrocephalus — ventriculomegaly — Brain property — Pathogenesis

Introduction

In the past, many efforts have been made to solve the problem of the mechanism of ventricular dilatation and its influence on hydrocephalus (Granholm 1966; Edvinsson and West 1971; James et al. 1973; Rowlatt 1978; D'Avell et al. 1980; Kaufman et al. 1980; Matsumoto et al. 1983–90; Shapiro et al. 1984, 1987; Takei et al. 1987) However, these data in both clinical and experimental settings, appear no to be sufficient to clarify this important issue. Under such circumstances, the alteration of brain parenchymal properties has been thrust into the limelight. Obviously, the various materials contained within the cranial cavity exhibit different physiological characteristics. In our previous reports (Shapiro et al. 1985a,b; Shapiro et al. 1986), we have documented the biomechanical role of the container properties of the brain, such as the calvarium and dura mater, in kaolin-induced hydrocephalus. We found that the degree of ventricular dilatation was far advanced when animals were made hydrocephalic by kaolin injection into the cisterna magna after the calvarium and dura mater were removed. These results illustrate the fact that impairment of CSF dynamics is not the sole cause of hydrocephalic ventricular dilatation. Therefore, in this study we focused on the brain parenchyma itself and investigated whether any alteration of brain parenchymal properties influenced hydrocephalic ventricular dilatation.

Material and methods

Classification of the Animals

Fifty-nine adult mongrel cats, each weighing 2.5–4.5 kg, were used in this study. The cats were divided into two groups: those with and those without unilateral infusion of physiological saline into the brain parenchyma. These two groups were subdivided into two groups; those with and those without kaolin injection into the cisterna magna (i.e., group 1 ($n = 30$): without infusion and without kaolin injection as control; group 2 ($n = 10$): without infusion and with kaolin injection as comparison for group 4; group 3 ($n = 5$): with infusion and without kaolin injection as a comparison for group 4; group 4 ($n = 14$): with infusion and with kaolin injection).

Preparation of the Animals

The cats were anesthetized with intraperitoneal pentobarbital (30 mg/kg) by endotracheal intubation. They were then placed in a stereotactic frame in the sphinx position. A Starling respirator was applied to maintain anesthesia during surgical and monitoring manipulation, as reported previously. (Takei et al. 1987)

Using a sterile technique, two 1mm burrholes were made over the calvarium, one for the ventricular needle at 3.5mm behind the bregma, 3.5mm lateral from the midline, and 10–11mm depth into the brain surface and one for the infusion of physiological saline into the brain parenchyma at 6mm behind the bregma, 8.5mm lateral and 13mm depth into the brain surface. In all animals, 23G needles were inserted into the lateral ventricle for pressure monotoring as well as into the brain parenchyma for infusion and 21G needles were inserted into the cisterna magna for pressure monotoring. A Harvard infusion pump was used to deliver the physiological saline into the brain parenchyma in order to establish altered biomechanical properties in the brain parenchyma. The rates of infusion were 0.0014ml/min for the 1st hour, 0.0029ml/min. for the 2nd hour and 0.0074ml/min. for the 3rd hour. After the manipulations outlined below, kaolin suspension (250mg/ml) was injected into the cisterna magna. The cats were then allowed to recover and were supported as required during the development of hydrocephalus. Ten to fourteen days after initiation of hydrocephalus, animals underwent in vivo perfusion for assessment of lateral ventricle size.

Measurement of the Pressure Volume Index (PVI), Local Tissue Compliance (LTC), and Intracranial Compliance (IC) and Assessment of Lateral Ventricle Size

The pressure in the cisterna magna and the lateral ventricle and tissue pressure at the same infusion site were monitored. PVI, as an indicator of altered brain property, was measured simultaneously in the cisterna magna and lateral ventricle, using the bolus injection technique before and after intraparenchymal fluid infusion. The number of animals measured for PVI were: group 1: $n = 18$; group 2: $n = 18$; group 3: $n = 5$; group 4: $n = 14$. The PVI in the pre- and post-infused conditions in both measured sites were then compared. Local tissue compliance was calculated by dividing the change in inflow volume (Δv) by the inflow pressure and correcting for gauge compliance ($n = 6$). Intracranial compliance was calculated using the formula C = 0.4343 PVI/Po ($n = 14$). Assessments of the size of the ventriculomegaly, based on the coronal section through the foramen of Monro, were made by visual inspection and by A/B ratio, as previously reported (Takei et al. 1987). The number animals assessed for A/B ratio were: group 1: $n = 30$; group 2: $n = 10$; group 3: $n = 5$; and group 4: $n = 8$. To obtain this ratio, the measured minimum width of the floor of the lateral ventricle (A) was divided by the maximum span of the ventricle(B). Our established A/B ratio for normal lateral ventricle size was less than 0.30; hydrocephalic was more than 0.40.

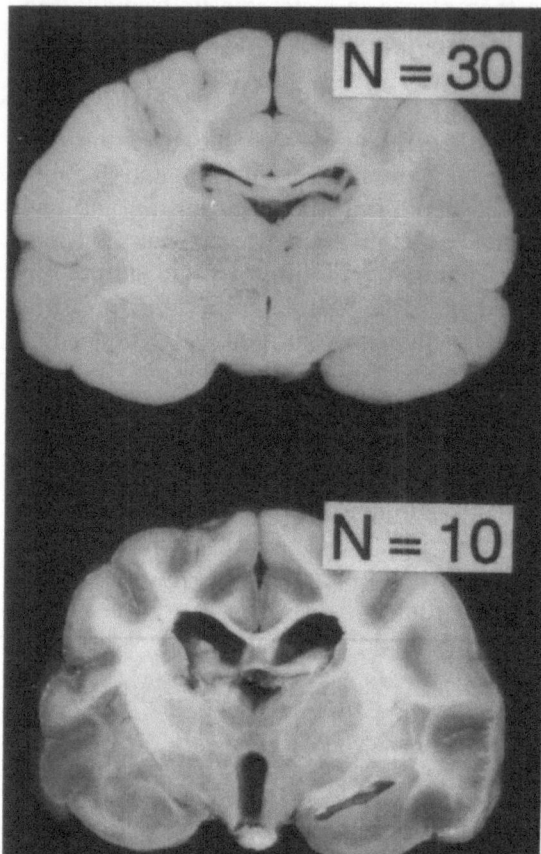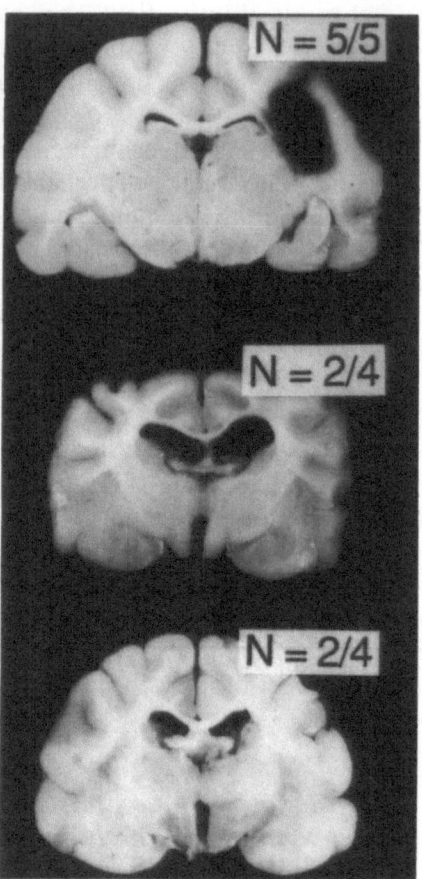

Fig. 1. These photographs show the different degrees of ventricular dilatation in the group with no intraparenchymal saline infusion. *Upper*, group 1 (control) without kaolin injection; no ventricular dilatation is seen and average A/B ratio is less than 0.30 *Lower*; group 2 with kaolin injection; symmetrical ventricular dilatation is seen and average A/B ratio is more than 0.40. *Numbers* above specimens indicate the number of animals observed

Fig. 2. These photographs show the different degrees of ventricular dilatation in the group with intraparanchymal saline infusion. *Upper*, group 3 without kaolin injection; there is no ventricular dilatation and average A/B ratio is less than 0.30. The spot in the brain parenchyma is the place where the saline was infused. *Middle* and *lower*, group 4 with kaolin injection; two different degrees of ventricular dilatation are seen. *Middle*, asymmetrical ventriculomegaly is seen; *lower*, symmetrical ventriculomegaly is seen. The average A/B ratio in this group is more than 0.40 *Numbers* above the specimens indicate the number of animals which developed either asymmetrical or symmetrical ventricular dilatation over animals categorized as hydrocephalus

Results

Degree of Ventricular Dilatation

Different degrees of ventricular dilatation were observed among these groups. (Figs. 1,2) No ventricular dilatation was observed in group 1 and the control values for the average A/B ratio were less than 0.30, as we had established previously. In group 2, symmetrical ventricular dilatations were observed and its average A/B ratio was more than 0.40. The animals in group 3 showed no ventricular dilatation, even when the saline infusion into the brain parenchyma was performed. No structural abnormalities were seen where the saline was infused. The average A/B ratio was less than 0.30. In group 4, ventricular dilatation was developed and revealed two different patterns in its configuration: two symmetrical and two asymmetrical ventricular dilatations were obtained in eight cats. The average A/B ratio in this group was more than 0.40 and the sizes of the ventricular dilatations seen in the asymmetrical pattern were greater on the side of infusion. No mechanical obstruction of the foramen of Monro or structural alteration at the site of infusion were observed in group 4.

Influence of Saline Infusion Into Brain Parenchyma on Measured PVI, LTC, and IC

In group 3 and 4, 79% of the animals (15/19) showed an increment of intracisternal PVI measurement, as shown in Fig. 3 (60% (3/5) of group 3 and 86% (12/14) of group 4 were measured in the cisterna magna). Sixty eight precent of these animals (13/19) had intraventricular PVI measurements as shown in Fig. 4 (60% (3/5) of group 3 and 71% (10/14) of group 4 were measured in the lateral ventricle. These profiles of measured PVI alteration are depicted in Fig. 3. The local tissue compliance was increased as a function of infusion in all animals infused (Fig. 5) and intractranial compliance, (IC) measured both in the cisterna magna (reduction rate 27%) and the lateral ventricle (reduction rate 14%), was reduced after infusion (Fig. 6). Before saline infusion, as in the normal condition, some correlation was found between the alteration of PVI measured simultaneously in the cisterna magna and lateral ventricle, as shown in Fig. 7 (upper); $0.1 > P > 0.05$. In contrast, no correlation was revealed after infusion; $0.4 > P$ (Fig. 7 lower). In group 4, all cats developed ventricular dilatation with A/B ratios of more than o.40 and showed alteration of PVI. No correlations were observed between the degree of ventriculomegaly and the rate of alteration in measured PVI, local tissue compliance, and intracranial complicance.

Discussion

Various studies, in both clinical and experimental settings have been made to solve the mechanism of ventricular dilatation in hydrocephalus (Granholm

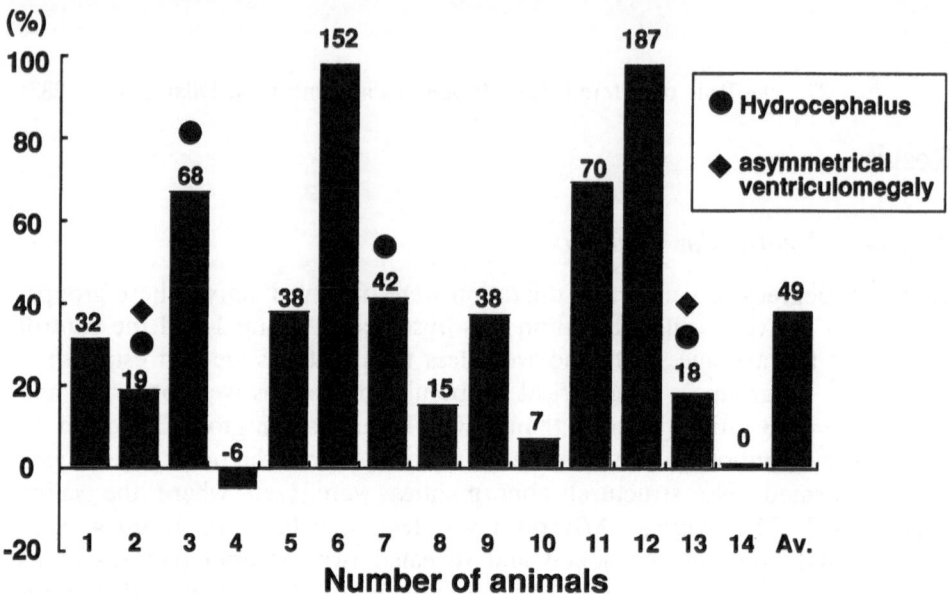

Fig. 3. Alteration of the PVI measured in the cisterna magna in group 4. In this group, 79% of the animals showed an increment of measured PVI values and all animals which developed either symmetrical or asymmetrical ventricular dilatation also showed increments of measured PVI. ●, hydrocephalus including both symmetrical and asymmetrical ventriculomegaly; ◆, hydrocephalus with asymmetrical ventriculomegaly

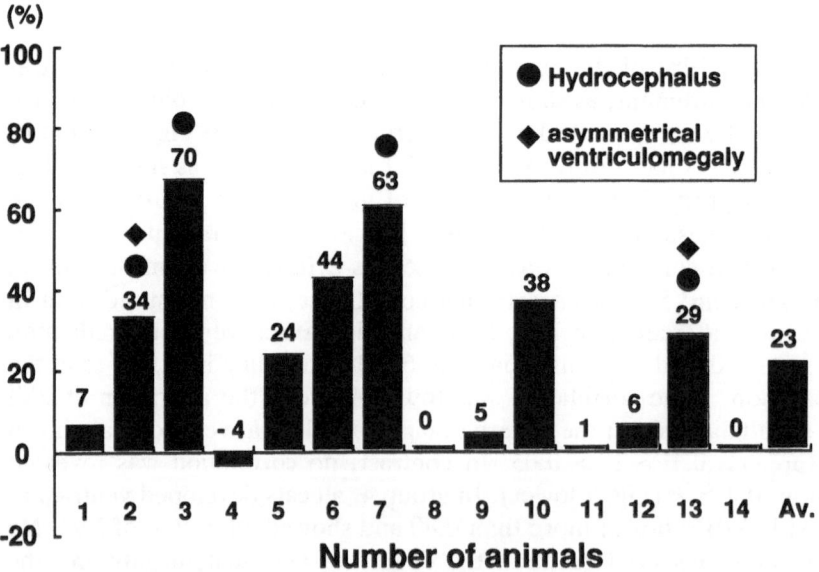

Fig. 4. Alteration of the PVI measured in the lateral ventricle in group 4. In this group, 68% of the animals showed increments of measured PVI values and all animals which developed either symmetrical or asymmetrical ventricular dilatation showed increments of the measured PVI. ●, hydrocephalus including both symmetrical and asymmetrical ventriculomegaly, ◆, hydrocephalus with asymmetrical ventriculomegaly

Fig. 5. Increment of the values of local tissue compliance (LTC) during saline infusion

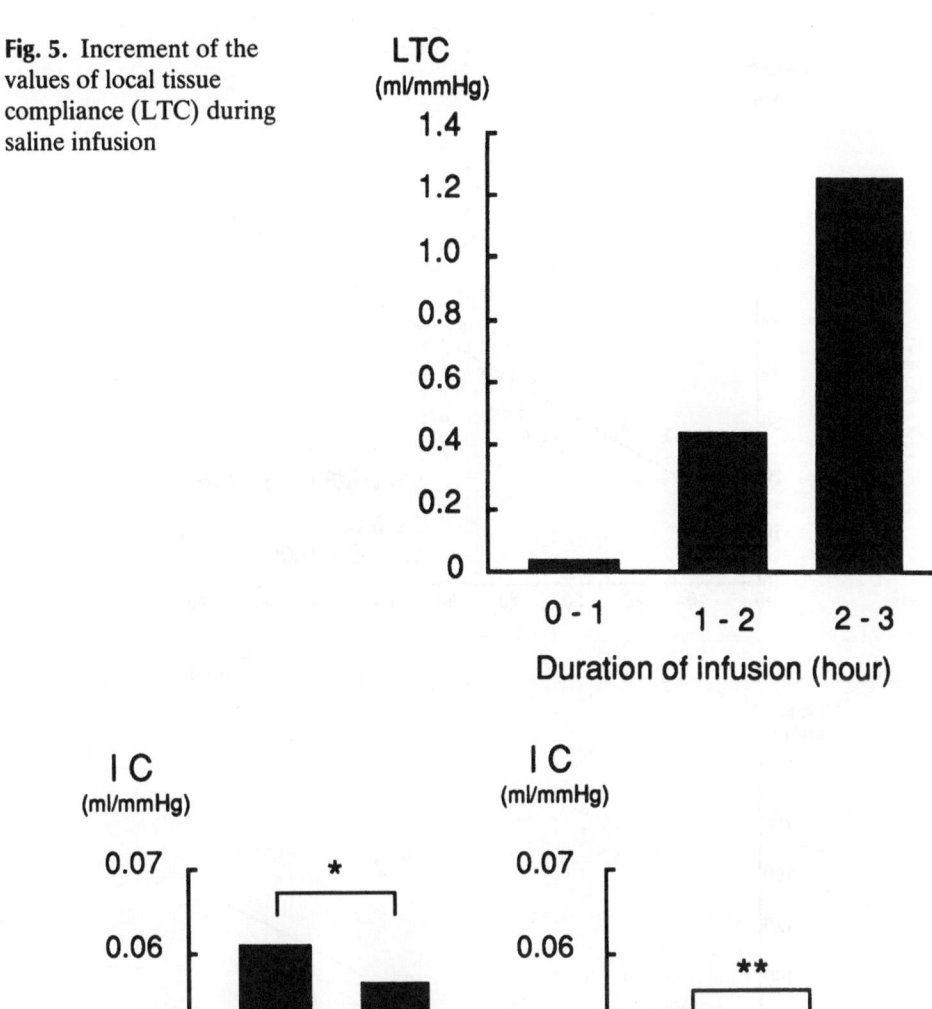

Fig. 6. Alteration of intracranial compliance measured in both cisterna magna (*left*) and lateral ventricle (*right*). More significant reduction of IC was observed in the cisterna magna than in the lateral ventricles. *P = 0.058, **P = 0.26

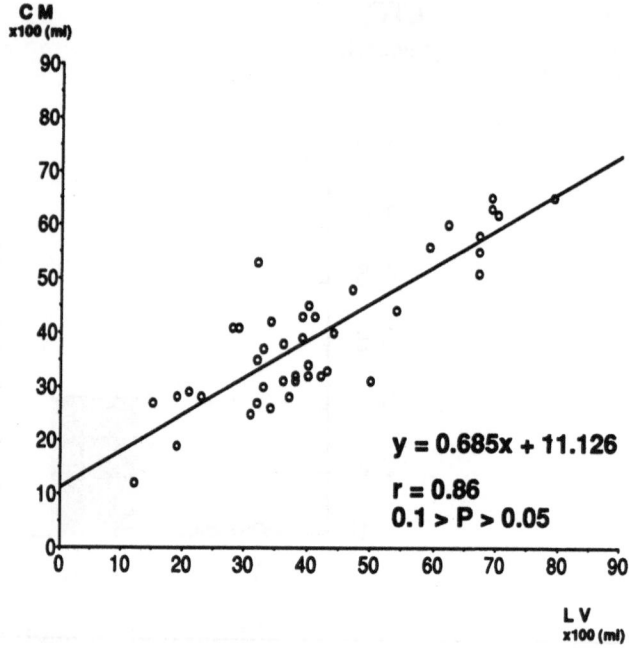

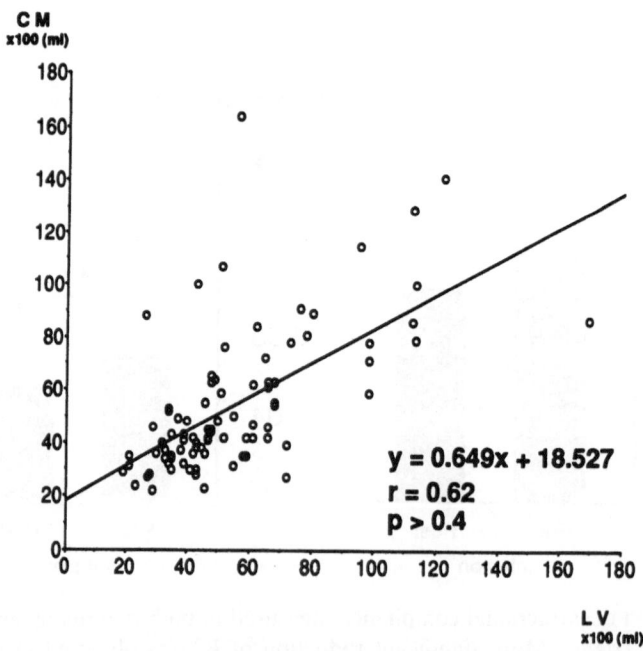

Fig. 7. Scattergrams depicting the correlation between PVI measured in the cisterna magna and lateral ventricle. *Upper*, pre-infusional condition, *lower*, post-infusional condition. A more significant correlation is observed in the pre-infusional condition $(0.1 > P > 0.05)$ than in the post-infusional condition $(0.4 > P)$

1966; Edvinsson and West 1971; James et al. 1973; Rowlatt 1978; D'Avell et al. 1980; Kaufman et al. 1980; Matsumoto et al. 1983–90; Shapiro et al. 1984, 1987; Takei et al. 1987; Hochwald et al. 1972). Among numerous such efforts, our previous study emphasized the biomechanical role of the container property in hydrocephalic ventricular dilatation. This was done by observation of the PVI, which is widely utilized as an indicator of intracranial hydrodynamics. In that report, PVI increased to 170% in animals which had undergone removal of the calvarium and to 480% in animals which had undergone removal of the calvarium and dura mater. (Shapiro et al. 1985a and b; Takei et al. 1987) (Table 1) Furthermore, the degree of ventricular dilatation, assessed by measurement of the A/B ratio, showed a different pattern when the covering tissues were removed (Fig. 8). From these results, we concluded that as the alteration of PVI seen in these models was different from the alteration of PVI seen in ventriculomegaly in kaolin-induced hydrocephalus then impairment of CSF dynamics was not the sole cause of hydrocephalic ventricular dilatation.

As far as pressure dynamics is concerned, 86% of the animals in group 4 in this study ($n = 12/14$) showed decreased intracranial compliance, calculated either in the cisterna magna or lateral ventricle. All animals with developed ventricular dilatation in group 4 showed the same reduction of intracranial compliance, while some enhancement of measured PVI was observed in the same group. Furthermore, values for local tissue compliance in all animals, no matter whether ventriculomegaly had developed or not, tended to increase during infusion. This characteristic softening of tissue and reduction of intracranial compliance which take place as the result of infusion may affect each other; buffering processes following the Monroe-Kellie doctrine should take place in these observed alterations (Marmarou et al. 1980; Rapoport 1984; Walstra et al. 1980). On the basis of such circumstances, symmetrical ventricular dilatation was seen in both groups 2 and 4 and asymmetrical hydrocephalus, in which dilatation was seen on the infusion side was observed in group 4. Asymmetrical ventricular dilatation, so called unilateral hydrocephalus, is commonly reported in a clinical setting as the result of obstruction of the foramen of Monro, (Bhagwati 1964; Salomon 1970; Anderson et al. 1974; Matsumori and Beppu 1976; Wilberger et al. 1983; Eller and Pasternak 1985; Oi and Matsumoto 1985; Nakamura and Tsubokawa 1986; Nakamura et al. 1989; Venkataramana et al. 1989) However, in this study no such morphological changes were found in group 4 and both lateral ventricles were basically dilated. This differs from the unilateral hydrocephalus obtained by obstruction of the foramen of Monro, in which the ventricle on the opposite side of the dilated ventricle is usually normal in size.

The most curious result in this study was that greater enlargement of ventriculomegaly was found on the same side of the infusion and the pathogenesis for the presence of both symmetrical and asymmetrical ventricular dilatation found in the same group. In morphological observations of the infusion model made by Hirano et al. (1984), expansion of the extracellular space was observed without any breakdown of the blood-brain barrier. Those tissue alterations resembled vasogenic edema and it was revealed by Marmarou et al. (1980)

Table 1. PVI and degree of ventriculomegaly in the model of altered container property

		PVI (ml) m ± S.E.	% changes of PVI (%)	Lateral Ventricle A/B ratio		
				2wk	3wk	4wk
Control		0.76 ± 0.04	—	< 0.30		
Altered container property model	Craniectomy performed	1.30 ± 0.07	170	0.44	0.48	0.60
	Craniectomy & dural removal performed	3.60 ± 0.17	480	0.53	0.59	0.57

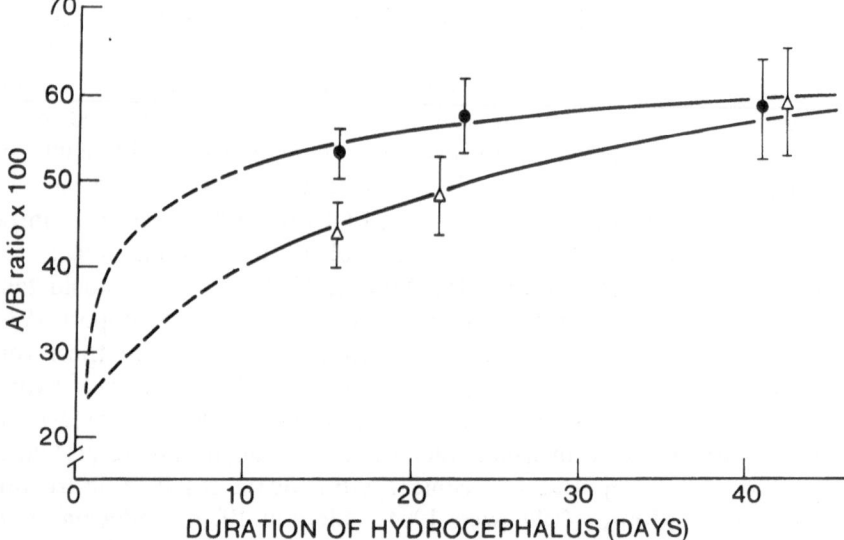

Fig. 8. Graph depicting ventricular size, estimated by the A/B ratio as a function of time after initiation of hydrocephalus with kaolin injection. These curves show that different degrees of ventricular dilatation were observed in the first 2–3 weeks in animals with calvarial and dural openings (●, PVI alteration 480%) and in animals with calvarial openings only (△, PVI alteration 170%)

and Walstra (1980) that tissue compliance created by intraparenchymal fluid infusion altered as a function of infusion. In such a background, our measured local tissue compliance on the same side as the infusion increased in all animals infused. Consequently, both normal and "looser" tissues continued compressing the neural axis by steady state intracranial pressure during and after infusion. Comparing the elasticity of normal and "looser" tissue, it is obvious that "looser" tissue becomes compressed more easily than normal tissue. However, only softening of tissue is not sufficient to act as a contributing factor in the development of ventriculomegaly, as shown by results for the animals in group 3, in which no ventricular dilatations were observed even the "looser" tissue was obtained. It should be required another factor like as intra-cisternal injections of the kaolin for promoting the ventricular dilatations. Under those conditions, asymmetrical ventricular dilatation might be developed. The significance of the presence of both symmetircal and asymmetrical ventricular dilatation in the same group of kaolin-injected and saline-infused animals is uncertain. According to our initial speculation, asymmetrical ventricular dilatation should have developed in all animals in which the same manipulations were performed as in group 4; however, in actuality only half of the animals developed asymmetrical ventricular dilatation. We must reconsider the nature of this infused model in terms of the disappearance of the infused fluid and the nature of kaolin-induced hydrocephalus and its initiating period of ventriculomegaly. Considering these factors, the alteration of brain parenchymal properties, namely the newly established altered biomechanical brain properties created by infusion, could be a significant factor in ventricular dilatation.

The spatial independence of PVI measured after infusion is also curious. In normal conditions, PVI measurements in the cisterna magna and lateral ventricle correlated with each other, in contrast to post-infusion measurements which revealed no such relationship. If these fluids infused into the brain parenchyma may lead to the alteration of biomechanical character, whether directly or indirectly, at sites of PVI measurement such as the cisterna magna and lateral ventricle, special caution must be exercised when dealing with these values, especially in pathologic conditions. We speculate that this alteration of biomechanical character was caused by the difference in "buffering" structure surrounding the site of PVI measurement in pathologic conditions. Takizawa et al. (1986) also emphasized the "buffering" effect in the CSF space on PVI measurement. Several points still need attention but will be discussed in the future. Our conclusions from this study were:

1. The alteration of brain parenchymal properties created by saline infusion into the parenchyma resulted in the enhancement of PVI measurments in the neural axis. In contrast to this, calculated tissue compliance increased while intracranial compliance was reduced.

2. Measurements of PVI differed from one site to another when there were any changes of brain intraparenchymal properties.

3. The degree of ventricular dilatation cannot be predicted by measured PVI values, local tissue compliance, and intracranial compliance.

4. Dynamic alterations of CSF and disparity of CSF production and absorption, cannot be the sole explanation for hydrocephalic ventricular dilatation. Changes in the tissues covering the brain such as the calvarium and dura mater, as well as changes in the characteristics of brain parenchyma itself may be contributing factors in the development of ventricular dilatation.

Acknowledgments. We express our appreciation to Mrs. Shinozaki, Miss Takahari, and Miss Kobayashi for technical assistance.

References

Anderson H, Carlsson CA, Gomes SP (1974) Unilateral hydrocephalus. Neurochirurgia (Stuttg) 17: 63–67

Bhagwati S (1964) A case of unilateral hydrocephalus secondary to occlusion of one foramen of Monro. J Neurosurg 21: 226–229

D'Avell D, Greenberg RP, Mingrino S, Scanarini M, Pardatscher K (1980) Alterations in ventricular size and intractranial pressure caused by sagittal sinus pathology in man. J Neurosurg 53: 656–661

Eller TW, Pasternak JF (1985) Isolated ventricles following intraventricular hemorrhage. J Neurosurg 62: 357–362

Edvinsson L, West KA (1971) Relation between intracranial pressure and ventricular size at various stages of experimental hydrocephalus. Acta Neurol Scand 47: 451–457

Granholm L (1966) Induced reversibility of ventricular dilatation in experimental hydrocephalus. Acta Neurol Scand 42: 581–588

Hirano A, Marmarou A, Nakamura T, Inoue A (1984) The fine structural study of brain response to intracerebral infusion of serum in the cat. In: Inaba Y, Klatzo, I, Spatz M (eds) Brain Edema. Springer, Berlin Heidelberg NY Tokyo, pp 32–39

Hochwald GM, Lux WE, Sahar A, Ransonoff J (1972) Experimental hydrocephalus: Changes in CSF dynamics as a function of time. Arch Neurol 26: 120–129

James AE, Strecker EP, Novok G, Burns B (1973) Correlation of serial cisternogram and cerebrospinal fluid pressure measurement in experimental communicating hydrocephalus. Neurology (NY) 23: 1226–1233

Kaufman HH, Dujovny M, Huchton JD, Kossovsky N, Miller M, Carmel PC (1980) "Natural" canine model of infantile hydrocephalus. Neurosurgery 6: 142–148

Marmarou A, Takagi H, Shulman K (1980) Biomechanics of brain edema and effects on local cerebral blood flow. In: Eds J. Cervós-Navarro R. Fecszt. Advances in neurology. Raven, New York, pp 345–358 (Brain edema, vol 28)

Matsumori K, Beppu T (1976) Non-active, non-obstructive, congenital unilateral hydrocephalus. Brain Nerve 28: 597–604

Matsumoto S, Sato K, Tamaki N (1983–1990) Annual review of hydrocephalus, vol 1–vol. 8. Neuron, Tokyo

Nakamura S, Tsubokawa T (1986) Destructive hydrocephalus: proposed new category. Nerv Syst Child 2: 101–104

Nakamura S, Makiyama H, Miyagi A, Tsubokawa T, Ushinohama H (1989) Congenital unilateral hydrocephalus. Nerv Syst Child 5: 367–370

Oi S, Matsumoto S (1985) Pathophysiology of obstruction of foramen of Monro in unilateral hydrocephalus. Neurosurgery 17: 891–896

Rapoport SI (1984) A model for brain edema. In: Inaba Y, Klatzo I, Spatz M (eds) Brain Edema. Springer, Benlin Heidelberg NY Tokyo, pp 59–71

Rowlatt U (1978) The microscopic effects of ventricular dilatation without increases in head size. J Neurosurg 48: 957–961

Salomon JH (1970) Isolated unilateral hydrocephalus following ventriculo-arterial shunt. J Neurosurg 32: 219–22

Shapiro K, Marmarou A, Portnoy H (1984) Hydrocephalus. Raven, New York

Shapiro K, Fried A, Takei F, Kohn I (1985a) Effect of skull and dura on neural axis pressure-volume relationships and CSF hydrodynamics. J Neurosurg 63: 76–81

Shapiro K, Takei F, Fried A, Kohn I (1985b) Experimental feline hydrocephalus. The role of biomechanical changes in ventricular enlargement in cats. J Neurosurg 63: 82–87

Shapiro K, Takei F, Fried A, Kohn I (1986) Independence of compliance and CSF hydrodynamics as an explanation for volume preservation in the neural axis. In: Miller JD, Teasdale GM, Rowan JO, Galbraith SL, Menddelow AD (eds) Intracranial pressure VI. Springer, Berlin Heidelberg NY Tokyo, pp 74–78

Shapiro K, Kohn I, Takei F, Zee C (1987) Progressive ventricular enlargement in cats in the absence of transmantle pressure gradients. J Neurosurg 67: 88–92

Takei F, Shapiro K, Kohn I (1987) Influence of the ventricular enlargement on the white matter water content in progressive feline hydrocephalus. J Neurosurg 66: 577–583

Takizawa H, Sanders TG, Miller JD (1986) Variations in pressure-volume index and CSF outflow resistance at different locations in the feline craniospinal axis. J Neurosurg 64: 298–303

Venkataramana NK, Kolluri S, Swamy KSN, Arya BYT, Das BS, Reddy GNN (1989) Neurosurgery 24: 282–284

Walstra G, Takagi H, Marmarou A, Shapiro K, Shulman K (1980) The time course of brain tissue compliance and resistance in a controlled model of brain edema. In: Shulman K Marmarou A, Miller JD; Becker DP, Hochwald GM, Brock M (eds) Intracranial pressure IV. Springer, Berlin Heidelberg NY Tokyo, pp 253–255

Wilberger JE, Vertosick FT, Vries JK (1983) Unilateral hydrocephalus secondary to congenital atresia of the foramen of Monro. J Neurosurg 59: 899–901

28 — Biomechanical Analysis of Hydrocephalus by Different Physical Models

Tatsuya Nagashima, Seiji Hamano, Norihiko Tamaki,
Satoshi Matsumoto[1], and Yukio Tada[2]

Summary. The finite element method (FEM), an advanced numerical method supported by computer technology, was introduced to the biomechanical research on hydrocephalus. In the present study, comparative analysis of intra-cerebral biomechanics in hydrocephalus was conducted using different physical models.

First, two dimensional finite element analysis with elastic models was performed to clarify the intracerebral stress distribution in hydrocephalus. It showed a characteristic tensile stress concentration at the anterolateral angle of the lateral ventricle. The distribution of stress concentration coincided with the distribution of periventricular lucency on computed tomography (CT) scan. The periventricular tensile stress concentration was decreased by the enlargement of the ventricle. Second, simulation using a hyper-elastic model showed the same pattern of intracerebral stress distribution as the elastic model. However, the former showed wider distribution than the latter. Third, a poroeleastic model was introduced. The poroelastic model is a first approximation of Hakim's concept of the "open cell sponge", and it describes cerebro-spinal fluid (CSF)/tissue interaction in the hydrocephalic process. The progress of ventricular dilatation and the extension of periventricular cerebrospinal fluid edema were well represented by the poroelastic model.

Keywords. Hydrocephalus — Computer simulation — Cerebrospinal fluid — Biomechanics

Introduction

The interaction between cerebrospinal fluid (CSF) and brain tissue plays a central role in the pathophysiology of hydrocephalus. However, little attention

---

[1] Department of Neurosurgery, Kobe University School of Medicine, Kobe University, Kobe, 650 Japan
[2] Department of System Engineering, Faculty of Engineering, Kobe University, Kobe, 657 Japan

has been paid to the properties of the brain tissue and the interaction of tissue properties with CSF parameters in the study of the hydrocephalic process.

Hakim stated that it is important to examine intracranial pathophysiology in the light of certain physics concepts. He reviewed concepts dealing with factors which govern resting intracranial pressure and he conceptualized the brain as a submicroscopic sponge of viscoelastic material (Hakim and Hakim 1984). Marmarou (1984) pointed out the importance of mathematical models of hydrocephalus that incorporate both tissue and CSF analysis.

We have since attempted to formulate mathematical models to describe the hydrocephalic process (Nagashima et al. 1984, 1987). Starting from elastic models, we extended our models to hyperelastic, viscoelastic, and poroelastic models. Meanwhile advanced neuroimaging techniques such as magnetic resonance imaging (MRI) enabled us to see the in vivo movement of cerebrospinal fluid into the periventricular parenchyma, the change of ventricular size, and the change of gray and white matter volume in hydrocephalic process. The accumulation of imaging data begged to be studied in the light of biomechanics. In the present study, computer simulations of hydrocephalus were conducted using different physical models and the finite element method.

Material and Methods

1. Intracerebral Stress Analysis by Elastic Models

The elastic model was based on the principle of the linear stress-strain relationship and the principle of infinitesimal deformation. Horizontal CT scans of (1) normal adult, (2) adult hydrocephalus, and (3) pediatric hydrocephalus were used to construct two dimensional finite element models. Because of the symmetry of the brain, the left half of a horizontal slice of human brain was used for modeling in the following study. The values for Young's modulus and Poisson's ratio for brain tissue were assumed to be $3.0 \times 10^{-1} \mathrm{N/m^2}$ and 0.49 respectively, according to reported values (Aoyagi et al. 1980; Ommaya 1968; Walsh and Alfonso 1976). That means the brain tissue is assumed to be almost incompressible. Intraventricular CSF pressure was transformed to the nodal forces that work perpendicularly to the ventricular wall. Nodes on the midline were restricted to perpendicular displacement.

First, intracerebral stress distributions were simulated in three different models under the same intraventricular CSF pressure. Second, the effect of bone defect on intracerebral stress distribution was simulated by changing the Young's modulus of the frontal bone to that of dura. Third, the effect of the disproportionally enlarged ventricle on intracerebral stress distribution was then simulated.

2. Comparative Analysis of Intracerebral Stress Distribution by the Hyperelastic and Elastic Models

A two dimensional hyperelastic finite element model (Mooney's hyperelasticity) was constructed from a horizontal slice of normal brain. The hyperelastic model is an approximation of the brain as "gum-like material". Intracerebral stress distribution was simulated under the same intraventricular CSF pressure and boundary conditions as in the elastic model.

3. Biomechanical Analysis Using the Poroelastic Model

The poroelastic model was based on Biot's theory of linear consolidation (Nagashima et al. 1987). Consolidation is the phenomenon of deformation of a porous medium, accompanied by the flow of fluid in pores through the medium. The theory is based on five principles: (a) conservation of fluid mass; (b) Darcys law for the flow of fluid; (c) mechanical equilibrium of the porous medium as a whole; (d) Hooke's law for the deformation of the solid skeleton; and (e) Terzhagi's principle of effective stress. In this study, brain was assumed to be a porous medium containing fluid in the extracellular space.

A two dimensional finite element model was constructed from a horizontal slice of human brain. Each element of the finite element model was assigned six material properties according to the literature (Davson 1967; Fenstermacher and Patlack 1976; Rall et al. 1962; Rapoport 1978; Reulen et al. 1977; Rosenberg et al. 1980): Young's modulus for the brain, $3.0 \times 10 \text{N/m}^2$ for gray matter, $3.0 \times 10^{-1} \text{N/m}^2$ for white matter; Poisson's ratio for the brain, 0.4999 for gray and white matter; extracellular space of the brain, 0.2 for white and gray matter; and viscosity and compressibility of the extracellular fluid, the same as those of pure water. Changes of ventricular configuration, intracerebral stress, and interstitial pressure were simulated by an ACOS 1000 computer system (Information Processing Center, Kobe University, Japan). The result of computer simulation was compared with CT scans of a patient with hydrocephalus due to subarachnoid hemorrhage.

Results

1. Intracranial Stress Distribution by Elastic Models

The elastic model analysis showed marked tensile stress concentration at the anterolateral angle of the lateral ventricle under increased intraventricular CSF pressure (Fig. 1). The intracerebral stress was maximum at the subependymal white matter and diminished toward the brain surface. The distribution of tensile stress coincided with the distribution of the periventricular hypodensity on CT scan. When the ventricle was enlarged by increased CSF pressure, the periventricular tensile stress concentration was dispersed. The tensile stress around the ventricle disappeared, with marked ventricular dilatation, in pediatric hydrocephalus. On the other hand, shear stress remained in the white matter after marked dilatation of the ventricle (Fig. 1).

When a bone defect was made at the frontal area, the distribution of the tensile stress projected toward it (Fig. 2). The magnitude of intracerebral tensile and shear stresses was increased by the bone defect.

Fig. 1a–c. Simulated intracerebral stress distribution using elastic models of normal (**a**), moderately enlarged (**b**), and markedly enlarged ventricle (**c**). The distribution of shear, compressive, and tensile stresses is shown in each model. The mesh represents the finite element model that is constructed with triangular elements

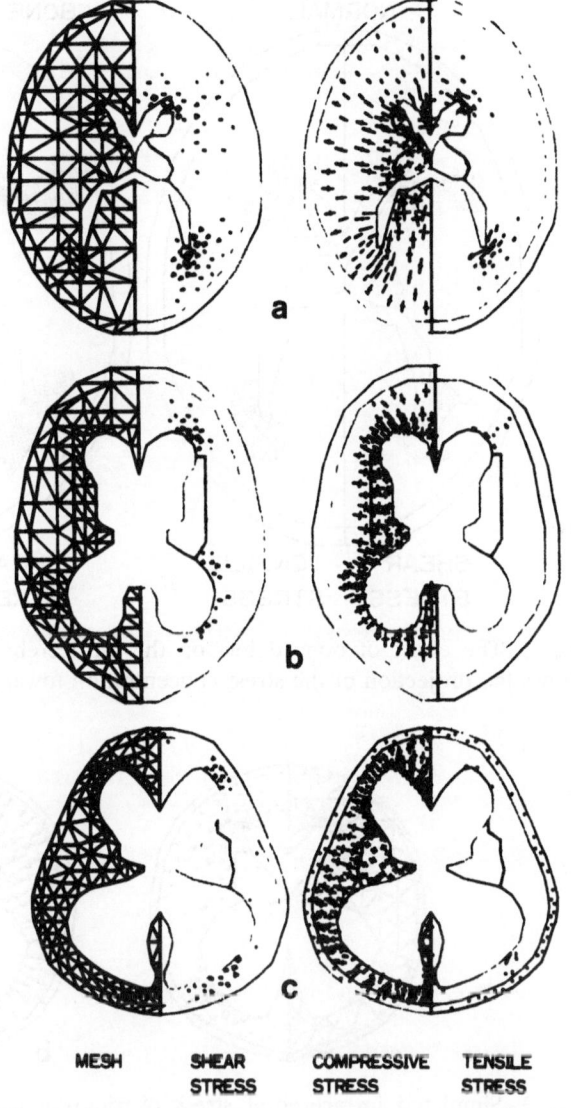

MESH   SHEAR   COMPRESSIVE   TENSILE
            STRESS   STRESS   STRESS

In the case of the hydrocephalic brain with a disproportionally enlarged ventricle, tensile stress concentrated more around the anterolateral angle than the posterior horn of the lateral ventricle (Fig. 3b).

2. Comparative Analysis of Intracerebral Stress Distribution by the Hyperelastic and Elastic models

The hyperelastic model showed the same pattern of intracerebral stress distribution as the elastic models. However, the former showed wider distribution of stress concentration than the latter. The hyperelastic model showed larger

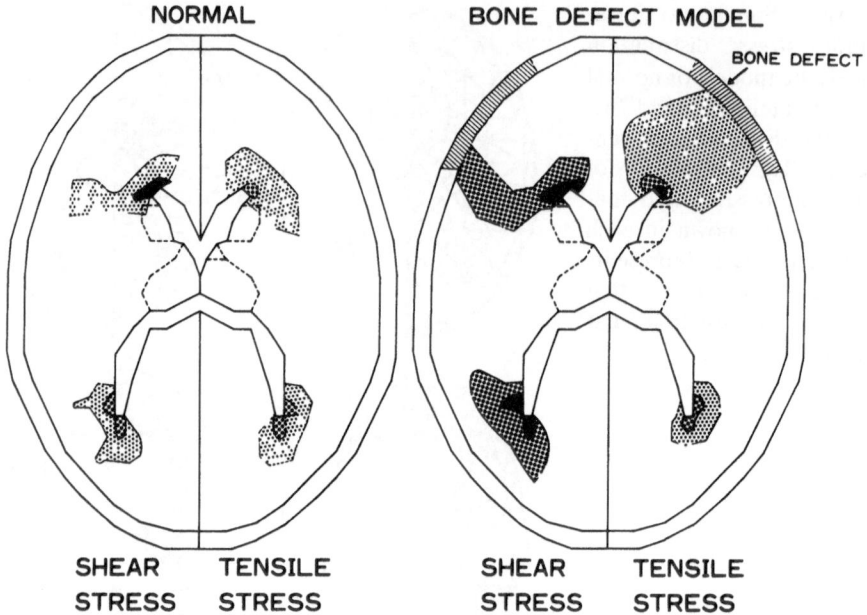

Fig. 2. The effect of bone defect on the intracerebral stress distribution. The figure shows the projection of the stress concentration toward the bone defect

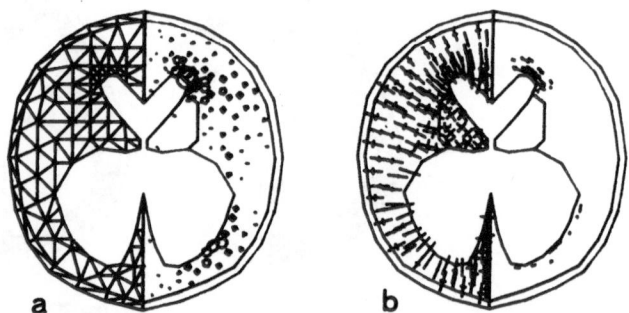

Fig. 3. Simulated intracerebral stress distribution using the elastic model of a disproportionally enlarged ventricle

deformation than the elastic model (Fig. 4). On the other hand, shear stress remained around the posterior horn of the lateral ventricle.

3. Biomechanical Analysis Using the Poroelastic Model

The poroelastic model showed time-dependent change of the periventricular tissue pressure, represented as circles in Fig. 5. The periventricular tissue pressure started to increase after the elevation of intraventricular CSF pressure to 20 mmHg, and a hydrostatic pressure gradient was generated from the

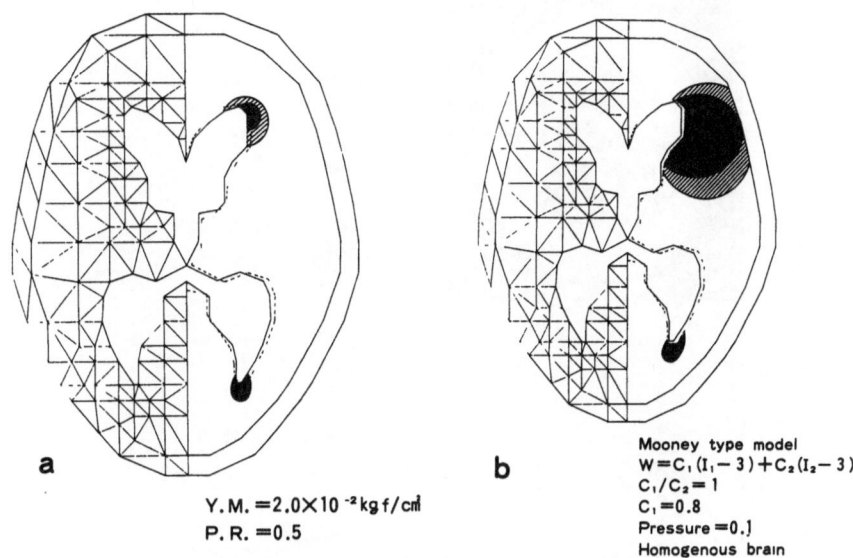

a

Y.M. =2.0×10^{-2}kgf/cm²
P.R. =0.5

b

Mooney type model
$W = C_1(I_1-3) + C_2(I_2-3)$
$C_1/C_2 = 1$
$C_1 = 0.8$
Pressure $= 0.1$
Homogenous brain

Fig. 4. Comparative study of intracerebral stress distribution using the elastic and the hyperelastic models, **a** Elastic model **b** hyperelastic model

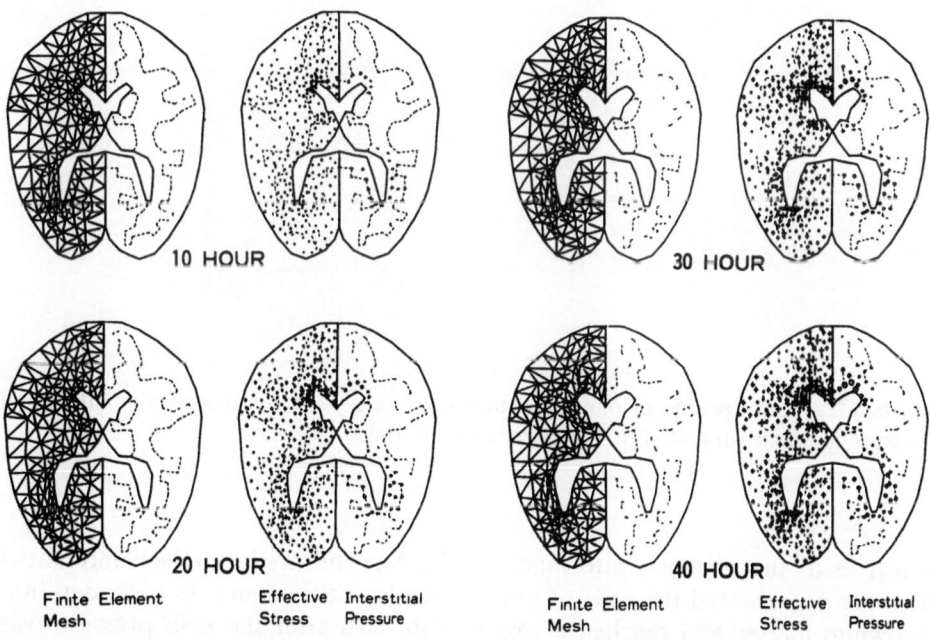

10 HOUR

30 HOUR

20 HOUR

40 HOUR

| Finite Element | Effective | Interstitial | | Finite Element | Effective | Interstitial |
| Mesh | Stress | Pressure | | Mesh | Stress | Pressure |

Fig. 5. Simulation of the hydrocephalic process using the poroelastic model. Changes of the finite element mesh, intracerebral stress, and interstitial pressure are represented

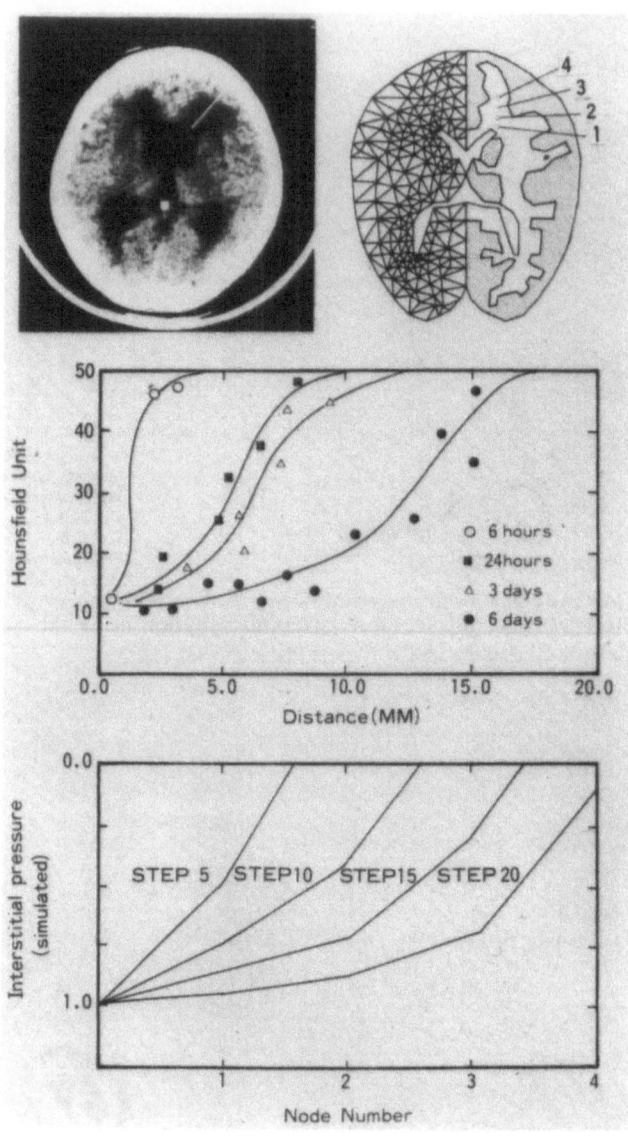

Fig. 6. CT density profile of periventricular low density and periventricular interstitial pressure gradient simulated by the poroelastic model

ventricle to the distant white matter (Fig. 5). The area of raised interstitial pressure represented the area of periventricular CSF edema. In extended into the white matter and reached a steady state 40h after the CSF pressure was raised. The extension of the periventricular CSF edema clearly resided in the white matter.

In Fig. 5, the effective stress is represented by crosses. The size of the crosses represents the magnitude of the stress. The effective stress was concentrated in the periventricular white matter, most prominently at the anterior and posterior angle of the lateral ventricle. The effective stress progressively increased, accompanied by ventricular enlargement. The area of effective stress concentration coincided with the distribution of the simulated periventricular CSF edema, which is represented by circles (Fig. 5).

In the left column of Fig. 5, the change of ventricular configuration after increases of CSF pressure was well represented by the poroelastic model. After 40 h, the simulation represented a moderately enlarged ventricle. However, the limited deformation of a single triangular element restricted the further deformation of the ventricle: indicating that the collapse of small triangular elements by further enlargement of the ventricle breaks the simulation.

Serial CT scans made after the occurrence of subarachnoid hemorrhage showed the change of ventricular size and the extension of periventricular CSF edema. Intraventricular CSF pressure, recorded simultaneously, showed a peak 24 h after the hemorrhage and a gradual fall after 48 h. The PVL appeared 24 h after the hemorrhage began and subsequently extended through the periventricular white matter. It finally reached the cortical gray matter 5 days after the hemorrhage. The CT density profile of the low density periventricular area obtained from a hydrocephalic brain was compared with the simulated gradient of periventricular interstitial pressure. The CT density profile of the hydrocephalic brain was well represented by the simulated interstitial pressure gradient (Fig. 6).

Discussion

Biomechanical analysis of hydrocephalus must be based on the correct understanding of the mechanical properties of the brain. However, it is usually difficult to determine the material properties of brain tissue because of its material heterogeneity and its complex boundary conditions. Our approach to this problem has been to use computer simulation with the finite element method (Nagashima et al. 1984, 1987). We first applied the FEM to the study of vasogenic brain edema in 1984. Its basic concept is that a continuum (total structure) can be analytically modeled by subdividing it into regions (finite elements), each of whose behavior can be described by a separate set of assumed functions (Zienkiewicz 1970). If the total structure is heterogeneous like the brain, being represented by distinct differential equations, the FEM is applicable. Its special advantage is that it represents highly irregular and complex structures and loading and boundary conditions.

Hakim indicated the stress concentration in the periventricular tissue of hydrocephalic brain by a two dimensional photoelastic analysis using a hollow sphere model (Hakim and Hakim 1984). The photoelastic study showed circumferential stress distribution, with the level of stress farther away from the ventricular wall being much lower than that at the ventricular wall. His simple model, however, did not represent the complex geometry of the brain.

Finite element analysis of intracerebral stress distribution using elastic models showed stress concentration around the anterior and posterior horns of the lateral ventricle, which supported the result of Hakim's photoelastic analysis. The distribution of the periventricular stress concentration coincided with the distribution of PVL on the CT scan and with the distribution of a histologically proven spongy change of the periventricular white matter in hydrocephalus (Fitz et al. 1978; Hiratsuka et al. 1979; Milhorat et al. 1970; Mosely 1979; Pasquini et al. 1977; Sahar et al. 1970; Weller and Michel 1980). The similarity of the distribution of the periventricular stress concentration and the spongy change in the brain suggests that the stress concentration plays an important role in destroying the periventricular white matter and in generating CSF edema. The dispersion and dimininution of the stress concentration by ventricular enlargement support the observation that the PVL does not appear in cases with markedly enlarged ventricle. Although the elastic models were based on a simple linear stress-strain relationship, they described the basic pattern of stress distribution in the hydrocephalic brain well.

In animal experimental hydrocephalus, ventricular enlargement occurred more severely at the side of the bone defect than at the side of the intact calvarium. The simulation provided a mechanical interpretation of the asymmetrical ventricular dilatation caused by a unilateral bone defect in hydrocephalus. That is, the increased intracerebral stress generated by the bone defect causes asymmetrical ventricual dilatation.

The elastic model is based on the principle of infinitesimal deformation, therefore it does not describe visible enlargement of the ventricle. On the other hand, the hyperelastic model permits large deformation of the ventricle. The hyperelastic model supported the intracerebral stress distribution simulated by the elastic model.

The poroelastic model is a first approximation of Hakim's (1984) concept of the "submicroscopic open cell sponge" (Penn and Bucus 1984). This model described the intracerebral stress distribution, the tissue pressure change, and the change of ventricular configuration in the hydrocephalic process. The simulated intracerebral stress distribution in the poroelastic model supported the result of the simulation by the elastic model. Consequently, the elastic model, the hyperelastic model, and the poroelastic model showed the typical pattern of stress concentration around the anterolateral angle of the lateral ventricle.

The simulated gradient of the interstitial pressure coincided with the CT density profile of periventricular low density on the CT scan (Fig. 6). The result shows that CSF migration into periventricular tissue depends on the interstitial pressure gradient. These results support the hypothesis that the stress concentration and the hydrostatic pressure gradient generate periventricular CSF edema.

The results of the computer simulation represented the change of ventricular configuration fairly well as compared with the serial CT scans of hydrocephalus. MRI study of hydrocephalus has shown that the deformation of the brain is due mainly to the compression of white matter (Nagashima et al.

1987). According to Hakim (1984), maximal deformation of the brain occurred close to the ventricle in their experimental study. These clinical and experimental findings support the results of our computer simulation.

Finally, development from the elastic model to the poroelastic model gave us a more realistic simulation of the hydrocephalic process. Further progress of FEM analysis with model refinement will provide further understanding of the pathophysiology of hydrocephalus.

References

Aoyagi N, Masuzawa H, Sano K, Kobayashi S (1980) Compliance of the brain. No To Shinkei 32: 47–56

Davson H (1967) Physiology of the cerebrospinal fluid. Churchill, London

Fenstermacher JD, Patlak CS (1976) The movement of water and solute in the brain of mammals. In: Pappius HM, Feindel W (eds) The dynamics of brain edema. Springer, New York. pp 87–94

Fitz CR, Harwood-Nash DC, Chung S, Siesjo IM (1978) Metrizamide ventriculography and computed tomography in infants and children. Neuroradiology 16: 6–9

Hakim S, Hakim C (1984) A biomechanical model of hydrocephalus and its relationship to treatment. In: Shapiro K, Marmarou T, Portnoy H (eds) Hydrocephalus. Raven, New York, pp 143–160

Hiratsuka H, Keigo F, Kodai O, Tskasato Y, Matsushita T, Yutani I (1979) Modification of periventricular reflux in metrizamide CT cisternography. J Comput Assist Tomogr 3: 204–208

Marmarou T (1984) Biomechanics and theoretical models of hydrocephalus: Summary. In: Shapiro K, Marmarou T, Portnoy H (eds) Hydrocephalus. Raven, New York, pp 193–195

Marmarou A, Shapiro K, Poll W, Shulman K (1978) Study of kinetics of fluid movement within brain tissue. In: Bek JWF, Bosch DA, Brock M (eds) Intracranial Pressure III. Springer, New York, pp 1–4

Milhorat TH, Clark RG, Hammock MK, McGrath PP (1970) Structural, ultrastructural, and permeability changes in ependyma and surrounding brain favoring equilibration in progressive hydrocephalus. Arch Neurol 22: 397–407

Mosely IF (1979) Factors influencing the development of periventricular lucencies in patients with raised intracranial pressure. Neuroradiology 17: 65–69

Nagashima T, Tamaki N, Matsumoto S, Seguchi Y, Tamura T (1984) Biohmechanics of vasogenic brain edema: An application of the finite element method. In: Klazo I, Spaz M (eds) Brain edema. Springer, Berlin, pp 92–98

Nagashima T, Tamaki N, Matsumoto S, Horwits B, Seguchi Y (1987) Biomechanics of hydrocephalus: A new theoretical model. Neurosurgery 21: 898–904

Ommaya AK (1968) Mechanical properties of tissue of the nervous system. J Biomech 1: 127–138

Pasquini U, Bronzini M, Gozzol E, Mancini F, Salvolini U (1977) Periventricular hypodensity in hydrocephalus: A clinicopathological and mathematical analysis using computed tomography. J Comput Assist Tomogr 1: 443–448

Penn RD, Bucus JW (1984) The brain as a sponge: a computed tomographic look at Hakim's hypothesis. Neurosurgery 14: 670–675

Rall DP, Oppelt WW, Patlak CS (1962) Extracellular space of brain as determined by diffusion of inulin from the ventricular system. Life Sci 1: 43–48

Rapoport SI (1978) A mathematical model for vasogenic brain edema. J Theor Biol 74: 439–467

Reulen HJ, Graham R, Spatz M, Klazo I (1977) Role of pressure gradients and bulk flow in dynamics of vasogenic brain edema. J Neurosurg 46: 24–35

Rosenberg GA, Kyner WT, Estrada E (1980) Bulk flow of brain interstitial fluid under normal and hyperosmolar conditions. Am J Physiol 238: f42–49

Sahar A, Hochwald GM, Ransohoff J (1970) Experimental hydrocephalus: Cerebrospinal fluid formation and ventricular size as a function of intraventricular pressure. J Neurosci 11: 81–91

Walsh EK, Alfonso S. (1976) Elastic behavior of brain tissue in vivo. Am J Physiol 260: 1058–1062

Weller RO, Michell J (1980) Cerebrospinal fluid edema and its sequellae in hydrocephalus. In: Cervos-Navaro J, Ferszt R (eds) Brain edema. Raven, New York, pp 111–123

Zienkiewicz OC (1970) The finite element method. McGraw Hill, London

Treatment
of Hydrocephalus

I. Hydrocephalus of Various Etiologies

29 — Management of Hydrocephalus Secondary to Posterior Fossa Tumor in Childhood

Tadanori Tomita and Szymon S. Rosenblatt[1]

Summary. A series of 112 children with cerebellum — fourth ventricle tumors treated surgically from 1980 through 1989 is presented. Pathology of these tumors consists of 52 medulloblastomas, 46 astrocytomas, and 14 ependymomas. All patients had a radical tumor resection, and patients with insufficient tumor resection or with other tumor histology are not included in this study. Neuroimaging studies showed hydrocephalus in all but 10 patients. For the management of associated hydrocephalus, a precraniotomy shunt was placed in 38 patients; 5 of them were complicated by upward herniation or intratumoral hemorrhage. After radical resection of the tumor, the precraniotomy shunt was successfully removed in 14 patients (36.8%). The remaining patients had posterior fossa craniotomy without shunt: 46 had intraoperative ventriculostomy and postoperative external ventricular drainage (EVD) and intracranial pressure (ICP) monitoring, while 20 had no postoperative EVD. Of 66 patients without precraniotomy shunts, 13 (20%) needed a permanent shunt after tumor resection. Hydrocephalus associated with a resectable posterior fossa tumor is best managed by intraoperative ventriculostomy and postoperative EVD and ICP monitoring, which provide a smooth postoperative course and avoid multiple surgical procedures and shunt-dependency.

Keywords. Hydrocephalus — CSF shunt — Cerebellar neoplasms — Intracranial pressure monitor — Upward herniation

Introduction

Hydrocephalus is frequently associated with posterior fossa tumors. The mechanism of the hydrocephalus is typically obstructive in nature, disturbing the communications between the fourth ventricle and the subarachnoid space or between the third and fourth ventricles. Removing a mass lesion restores the

[1] Division of Pediatric Neurosurgery, Children's Memorial Hospital and Northwestern University Medical School, Chicago, IL 60614, USA

cerebrospinal fluid (CSF) circulation and results in the resolution of associated hydrocephalus. Hydrocephalus associated with surgically resectable mass lesions, particularly tumors in the cerebellum or fourth ventricle, has been managed differently in the past. Some workers recommend decompressing the hydrocephalus by CSF diversion shunt prior to definitive surgery and others perform the surgery without a shunt. During the period from 1980 through 1989, we have practiced three different methods in managing patients with hydrocephalus secondary to cerebellum — fourth ventricle tumors: 1. precraniotomy shunt, 2. no perioperative CSF diversion, 3. intraoperative ventriculostomy and postoperative external ventricular drainage and ICP monitoring. These three methods are compared, and the incidence of shunt requirement after radical tumor resection is also studied.

Clinical Material and Methods

This series consist of 112 infants and children with cerebellum — fourth ventricle tumors which were radically (totally or subtotally) resected at posterior fossa craniotomy. Those with insufficient resection (partial resection or biopsy) were not included. This study was limited to cases with medulloblastomas (52 cases), astrocytomas (46 cases), and ependymomas (14 cases).

Earlier in this series, before 1984, most patients recieved a precraniotomy shunt and had posterior fossa craniotomy 1–2 weeks after shunting. Precraniotomy shunts were placed in 38 patients (36 ventriculo-peritoneal (V-P) shunts and 2 EVD). Pathology of the tumors consisted of medulloblastomas in 18, astrocytomas in 12, and ependymomas in 8.

From 1984 through 1985, 20 patients were given dexamethasone therapy at initial diagnosis, and a posterior fossa craniotomy was undertaken, without precraniotomy shunting or postoperative EVD, at the earliest convenient time. Three patients had intraoperative ventriculostomy which was converted to an Ommaya device at the end of the surgery. Pathology of these patients' tumors included medulloblastoma in 8, astrocytoma in 10, and ependymoma in 2.

From 1986, patients with hydrocephalus secondary to surgically resectable brain tumors were almost exclusively treated with dexamethasone therapy at diagnosis, followed by craniotomy at the earliest convenient day, with intraoperative ventriculostomy, postoperative EVD, and ICP monitoring. This group had 46 patients, with medulloblastoma in 22, astrocytoma in 20, and ependymoma in 4.

Results

Of 38 patients with precraniotomy shunts, 5 had serious complications directly related to shunt placement. Three patients had upward herniation, which, in the case of 2 of them, resulted in death, despite an emergency posterior fossa craniotomy. Pathology of these tumors was medulloblastoma in one and ependymoma in 2. These patients developed acute lethargy and respiratory arrest several hours after the shunting procedure. Computed tomography (CT) scans demonstrated a massive upward herniation with collapsed ventricular system. The other two patients had a hemorrhage into the posterior fossa tumor, causing acute coma and respiratory arrest. They had medulloblastoma and ependymoma, respectively. Both patients survived after emergency craniotomy, though they needed a prolonged recovery time. Another patient, who had fourth ventricular astrocytoma, died 10 days after tumor resection due to E. coli sepsis related to precraniotomy shunt infection.

The precraniotomy shunt was removed between 2 weeks and 2 months postoperatively after the preceding shunt ligation for testing as to whether or not patients needed a shunt. Fourteen (36.8%) of 38 precraniotomy shunts were removed in this fashion. They were from eight patients with medulloblastoma, five with astrocytoma, and one with ependymoma.

Other patients without precraniotomy shunts had dexamethasone therapy and underwent an elective posterior fossa craniotomy at the earliest convenient time. The craniotomy was performed within 24–72 hours, during which time close clinical observation and further tests, such as magnetic resonance imaging (MRI) were done. Only 2 patients needed urgent craniotomy due to clinical deterioration such as increasing lethargy or development of bradycardia prior to the scheduled surgery. All posterior fossa craniotomies were done with patients in a prone position.

Of 20 patients who did not have postoperative EVD, 3 needed a shunt insertion after craniotomy: one with ependymoma needed this urgently on the same night, and other two with medulloblastomas needed shunt insertion 2 days later due to sudden neurological deterioration.

Ten patients with intraoperative ventriculostomy and postoperative EVD and ICP monitoring had an internal shunting converted from EVD. These were 6 patients with medulloblastoma and 4 patients with astrocytoma. A shunt was inserted when neurological deterioration, changes in vital signs and/or sustained elevation of the ICP occurred after closing the EVD. When clinical deterioration occurred after closing the EVD, these patients had the EVD opened, allowing the ventricular fluid to drain; shunt insertion was done electively. Another 36 patients had the EVD removed at their bedsides between 3 and 10 days after operation. There were no infections related to EVD.

Discussion

When the size of posterior fossa tumors was maximally reduced, 13(20%) of 66 patients without precraniotomy shunts required a permanent shunt. This rate is less than that appearing in the data provided by Hudgins and Edwards (1987) which showed that approximately 35% of their patients required a shunt. Restoring the CSF pathway is one of the goals of posterior fossa craniotomy. Various factors explain the necessity for postoperative shunting in these patients. As all patients without precraniotomy shunts had posterior fossa craniotomy in the prone position, intraoperative manipulations of the posterior fossa contents permitted blood to enter the third and lateral ventricles or the subarachnoid space, which causes hydrocephalus. Another factor was the possibility of cerebellar edema vesulting from surgical manipulation. About half of the patients who needed postoperative shunting showed cerebellar mutism, thus cerebellar swelling may have been the cause of failure to restore the CSF pathways. However, the pathomechanism of cerebellar mutism is not well understood, and cerebellar mutisms are not necessarily related to post-operative hydrocephalus (Ferrante et al. 1990). The third factor was the possibility that the subarachnoid space was obliterated by chronic hydrocephalus or by CSF dissemination of the malignant tumor cells.

Although symptoms related to the increased intracranial pressure are re-solved in a great majority of patients after a precraniotomy shunt (Raimond: and Tomita 1981), one should not ignore the potential risks of the serious complications, such as upward herniation or hemorrhage into the tumor. The benefits of precraniotomy shunting are as follows: it improves the patient's general condition; definitive surgery can be scheduled at a more flexible time; and posterior fossa craniotomy can be done with patients in a sitting position as the ventricle size is already reduced in size: the posterior is slack at opening the posterior fossa dura.

However, for large posterior fossa tumors, these benefits will be out-weighed by the above-mentioned potential risks of precraniotomy shunts. Even though patients with precraniotomy shunts do not develop full-blown upward hernia-tion, tumors in the fourth ventricle tend to shift rostrally and ventrally so that the rostral portion of the fourth ventricle and the caudal portion of the aqueduct of Sylvius are obliterated by the tumor mass (Tomita et al. 1988). Surgical resection thus becomes more difficult than when there is a CSF space in the rostral and ventral aspect of the tumor in the fourth ventricle. We prefer operating on patients who are in the prone position; this provides a more comfortable position for the operating surgeon and there is less risk of air embolism. Hence, the sudden loss of CSF caused by opening the aqueduct can be controlled. Although clinical worsening of the patient due to hydrocephalus is indeed a serious concern while awaiting definitive surgery, dexamethasone therapy provides a temporary improvement and stabilization of neurological signs and symptoms. However, these patients should be monitored carefully and definitive craniotomy should be done at the earliest possible time.

We found that postoperative EVD was beneficial for patients because sudden deterioration due to postoperative hydrocephalus could be easily pre-vented. In particular, in cerebellar mutisms which occur 48–72 h after surgery, patients present with irritability and lethargy in the initial stage, so that one may not be able to distinguish this condition from acute hydrocephalus. Blood-tinged ventricular CSF and intracranial air are drained through the EVD postoperatively; this reduces the risk of chemical meningitis and, perhaps, the development of hydrocephalus. EVD, by monitoring the ICP, also guides the clinician to the decision as to whether or not a postoperative shunt is needed.

This last point is important because, from our experience, patients tend to become shunt-dependent and the ventricles tend to become slit-like once a shunt is installed.

Although CT scanning is recommended to evaluate changes of ventricular size at intervals after craniotomy, the size of the ventricle may not show significant change despite a restoration of the CSF pathway. Persistent postoperative ventriculomegaly is not an indication for shunting. Without shunting, ventriculomegaly usually needs several weeks to months to become smaller. Clinical correlation with patient symptoms and ICP changes dictates whether postoperative shunting is indicated. Persistently elevated ICP, associated with patient symptoms such as headaches, lethargy, and bradycardia, is a definite indicator for shunting, while intermittent rises of ICP are not indicators for shunting when the patient is otherwise stable. Occasionally, swelling of the posterior fossa would due to the development of pseudomeningocele or CSF leakage from the wound may necessitate shunting.

Another benefit of EVD is the reduction in the number of surgical procedures and therefore the reduction in the use of anesthesia, as the EVD can be removed at the bedside and the patient will, most likely, need only one surgical intervention.

References

Ferrante L, Mastronardi L, Acqui M, Fortuna A (1990) Mutism after posterior fossa surgery in children. Report of three cases. J Neurosurg 72: 959–963

Hudgins RJ, Edwards MSB (1987) Management of infratentorial brain tumors. Pediatr Neurosci 13: 214–222

Raimondi AJ, Tomita T (1981) Hydrocephalus and infratentorial tumors. Incidence, clinical picture, and treatment. J Neurosurg 55: 174–182

Tomita T, McLone DG, Das L, Brand WN (1988) Benign ependymomas of the posterior fossa in childhood. 14: 277–285

30 — Traumatic Brain Edema in the Pathogenesis of Post-traumatic Hydrocephalus

J. Tjuvajev, J. Eelmäe, T. Tomberg, and A. Tikk[1]

Summary. The subjects of this prospective study were 64 consecutively admitted severely head injured patients with Glasgow coma scale (GCS), scores of <8. In 25 surviving patients the rate of ventricular dilatation was estimated by Evans index (EI) one month after injury and compared with the volume of brain edema, measured by the volumetric edema index (VEI), on computerized tomography (CT) (16–22 HU) in the acute period. A repetitive 2 ml bolus injection method was used for calculating the viscoelastic parameters of the craniospinal system (CSS). This study showed that the rate of post-traumatic hydrocephalus, defined as an EI >0.3, correlated more with the volume of brain edema measured during post-trauma days 3–5 and did not significantly correlate with the VEI of the first 36 h post injury. Throughout the period of study the CSF resorption resistance (R) remained within the normal range (<10 mmHg/ml per min). At 1 month after injury intracranial pressure (ICP), pressure volume index (PVI), and elastance (E) showed the increase of the volume buffering capacity of the CSS. These data support the view that post-traumatic hydrocephalus development is mainly caused by the atrophy of injured and edematous brain tissue. Thus, in such cases shunting procedures are not appropriate.

Keywords. Head injury — Post-traumatic hydrocephalus — Brain edema — CSF dynamics

Introduction

Post-traumatic hydrocephalus (PTH) is considered to be one of the late sequelae of severe craniocerebral injury. However, as most of the descriptions of series of PTH patients in the literature deal with the results of various shunting procedures, the incidence of posttraumatic communicative hydro-cephalus is documented very differently, from 0.25% to 90% (Lewin 1968;

[1] Department of Neurosurgery, Tartu University Hospital, Tartu, Estonia

Pedersen 1979; Foroglou 1976; Koo and LaRoge 1977; French and Dublin 1977; Gudeman et al. 1981; Busch 1989; Croswasser et al. 1988). In contrast, in hydrocephalic patients the incidence of head injury in anamnesis varies from 2% to 50% of cases (Salmon 1972; Wieser and Probst 1975; Laws and Mokri 1977; Symon and Hinzpeter 1977; Jensen and Jensen 1979). Such large variations might occur because of the different criteria used for determination of PTH.

It has also been shown that the rate of ventriculomegaly in PTH correlates with residual disturbances in neurological (Kaas and Lonnum 1978; Gradeur et al. 1979), verbal and social-adaptative (Kishore et al. 1978; Van Dogen and Braakman 1980), and cognitive functions (Levin et al. 1981; Meyers et al. 1983; Cullum and Bigler 1986), and in verbal and graphic memory (Buschke and Fuld 1974; Hannay et al. 1979; Dikmen et al. 1987). Thus PTH is a vital subject for the practitioner caring for patients with traumatic encephalopathy, as a large number of brain trauma patients develop ventricular enlargement. The managing physician should understand which ventriculomegalic patients are suffering from hydrocephalus, which have cerebral atrophy, and which stand a reasonable chance of improvement on surgical placement of a ventricular shunt. From this point of view the investigation of the pathogenesis of PTH is still very important.

During the last decade studies on the pathogenesis of PTH have given rise to two main concepts. One postulates that the main pathogenetic factor is the impairment of CSF-dynamics, especially of CSF resorption after traumatic subarachnoid hemorrhage (SAH) and secondary leptomeningitis (Tans 1979; Borgesen et al. 1979; Tans and Poortvliet 1984; Kosteljanez and Ingstrup 1985; Kosteljanez 1986; Borgesen and Gjerris 1987).

The other concept of PTH pathogenesis emphasizes the role of diffuse axonal injury and degenerative and atrophic processes in the brain after severe head injury (Strich 1956; Adams et al. 1977; Pilz 1983; Jane et al. 1985; Levin et al. 1985; Wilson et al. 1988; Blumbergs et al. 1989).

This study describes the role of brain edema and changes of CSF-dynamics in the pathogenesis of PTH in severely head injured patients and also tries to answer the question, "To shunt or not to shunt?".

Clinical Materials and Methods

Patient Population

This prospective study population consisted of 64 severely head injured patients (41 males and 23 females) who were admitted to the intensive care unit during the first 24 h after injury with Glasgow Coma Scale (GCS) scores (Teasdale and Jennett 1974) ≤8 measured up to 6 h after injury (Table 1). The average GCS was 5.88 ± 1.8 and the age range of the population was 5–89 years (39.5 ± 19.6). All patients underwent CT, continuous monitoring of intracranial pressure (ICP), and CSF-dynamics studies as a part of a standard

Table 1. Statistical summary of general parameters in 64 severely head injured patients on admission to the intensive care unit

Variable	Average	Median	STD	STE
Age	39.52	35.0	19.61	2.55
GCS	5.88	6.0	1.8	0.23
Hematoma volume	81.77	68.54	67.42	9.94
Edema volume	48.01	45.73	18.92	2.48
ICP	10.41	9.0	6.16	0.8

GCS, Glasgow coma scale; ICP, intracranial pressure

clinical protocol. This protocol was carried out three times: during the first 24 h, on days 3–5 post trauma, and 1 month after trauma in survivors. Such timing of dynamical studies was based on data which showed that the brain edema volume increased significantly during the 3–5-day post trauma period and that the major posttraumatic changes in brain morphology were found one month after trauma (Levin et al. 1981; Wilson et al. 1988).

Computed Tomography

CT scans were performed parallel to the orbito-meatal line; 7–12 scans of 10 mm thickness were obtained and several linear and volumetric measurements were made.

From the linear measurements the Evans index (EI) was calculated (Evans 1942) — the ratio of maximum distance between the frontal horns of the lateral ventricles divided by the maximum skull circumference, measured on a scan at the level of the foramen of Monro. Hydrocephalus was defined as an Evans index greater than 0.30.

Volumetric measurements included intracranial hematoma volume and volumetric edema index (VEI), this latter was calculated as the total volume of measured brain edema divided by the number of scans performed in a concrete case to exclude differences in scan numbers between patients. The volume of edema was evaluated by the summation of the volumes measured as irregular regions of interest on tomodensitometrically hilighted areas having a range of 16–22 Hounsfield Units (HU) (Fig. 1).

ICP Monitoring and CSF-Dynamics Testing

ICP was measured by means of an epidural transducer (Statham P 50 Gould) attached to a monitoring system (SMC-108 Hellige). Then a constant rate repeated intrathecal 2 ml bolus injection method was used for calculating the visco-elastic properties of the cranio-spinal system (CSS) and the CSF-dynamics parameters. These parameters were obtained from lumbarly registered CSF pressure changes (Tikk and Eelmae 1985) measured by Statham P 23 Gould transducer connected by tubing system to the needle and referenced

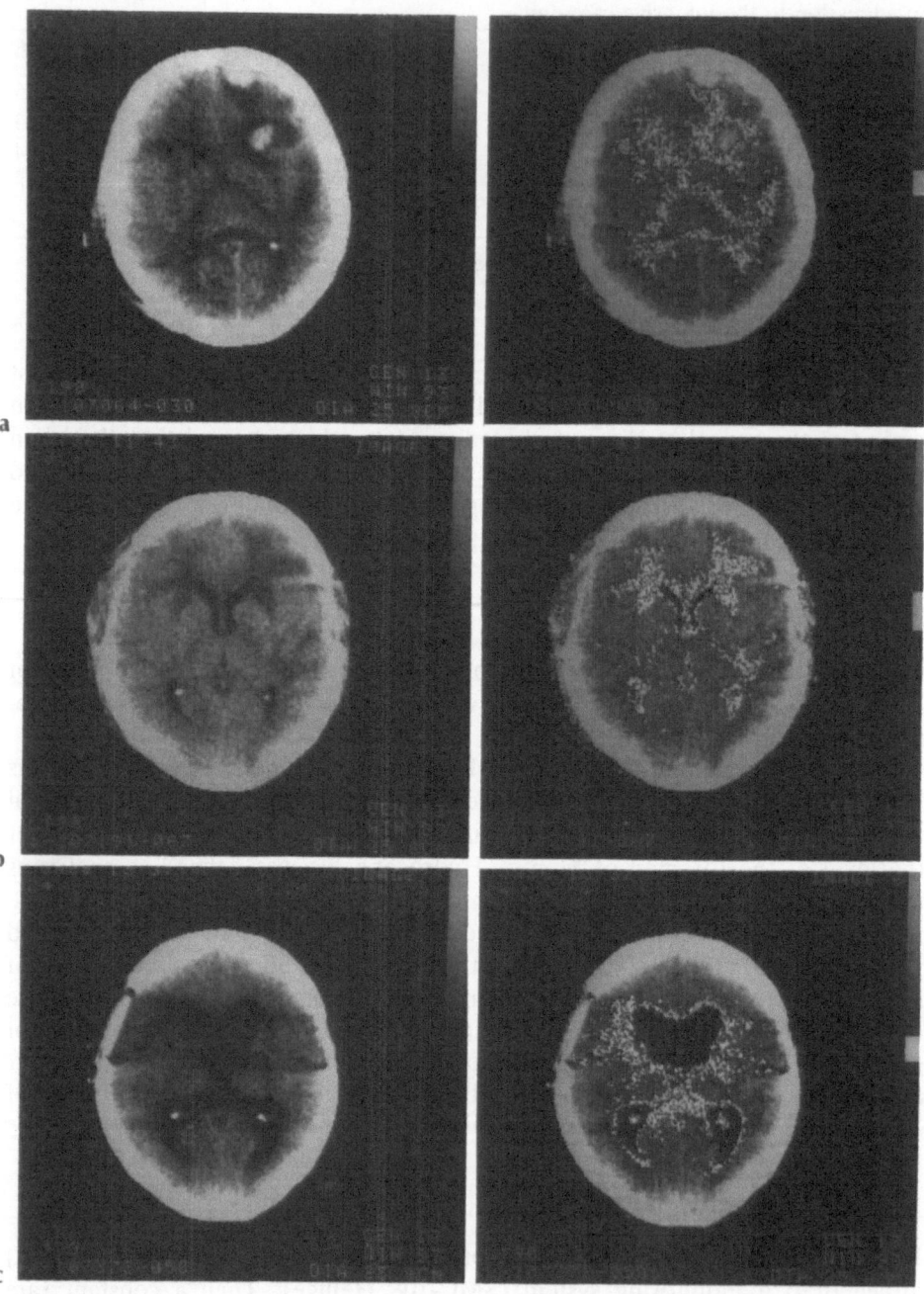

Fig. 1 a–c. Dynamic changes of ventricular dimensions and brain edema volume in a patient with severe head injury. **a** first 24 h after injury EI = 0.07; VEI = 46.28; R = 0.75 **b** 3–5-day posttrauma period EI = 0.26; VEI = 58.42; R = 1, 8 **c** 1 month after head injury EI = 0.45; VEI = 39.64; R = 0.46; EI, Evans index; VEI, volumetric edema index; R, CSF, resorption resistance

to the level of the midline. The total volume of saline to be injected according to this method is 20 ml, but for loading the CSS in the acute period of head injury the pressure-volume index (PVI), elastance (E), and CSF resorption resistance (R) were calculated after the injection of 10 ml (5th bolus) to prevent a severe increase of ICP. Formulas used for the calculations were according to Marmarou et al. (1978).

Management of Patients

All patients with traumatic intracranial hematomas were operated and the ICP was controlled so as not to exceed 20–25 mmHg. Artificial ventilation was to a $PaCO_2$ of 24–34 mmHg. Other features of management have been described elsewhere (Alberico et al. 1987); high doses of barbiturates were avoided.

Results

Of the 64 patients included in the study, 43 patients survived until the 3–5-day post trauma period (mortality 32.8%) and 25 patients survived 1 month after the trauma (mortality 60.9%). Preventive dehydratation therapy was performed before operation and the average ICP remained at 10.4 ± 6.2 mmHg. It was found that in the acute period of head injury the visco-elastic parameters of the CSS showed decreased PVI (16.21 ± 14.31 ml), increased E (2.1 ± 1.87 mmHg/ml), and normal R (1.7 ± 1.6 mmHg/ml per min). On the CT the average volume of hematomas (VSum) was 75.2 ± 16.37 ml and the average VEI was 48.1 ± 18.9 ml/scan.

Relationship Between VEI, PVI, and E

Using a multiplicative model of regression analysis of PVI on VEI from the data of the first 24 h and the 3–5-day post-trauma period it was found that PVI decreased with the increase of VEI (Fig. 2), indicating a decrease of CSS volume buffering capacity and a corresponding increase of E (Fig. 3), reflecting the increase of brain tissue stiffness in brain edema. It must be noted that some patients, in spite of a high VEI, had an increased PVI and decreased E. This phenomenon was observed in older patients especially and can be explained by a premorbid age-dependent increase of CSF spaces and CSS volume buffering capacity or a more profound impairment of vascular autoregulative mechanisms and a higher compliance to brain tissue compression.

Temporal Course of VEI Related to ICP, PVI, and E

Analysis of the influence of edema volume on ICP, PVI, and E was carried out in surviving patients. Patients were divided into two groups: in the first group VEI during the 3–5-day posttrauma period increased from 42.92 ± 20.21 ml/scan to 51.46 ± 18.23 ml/scan and in the second group VEI decreased

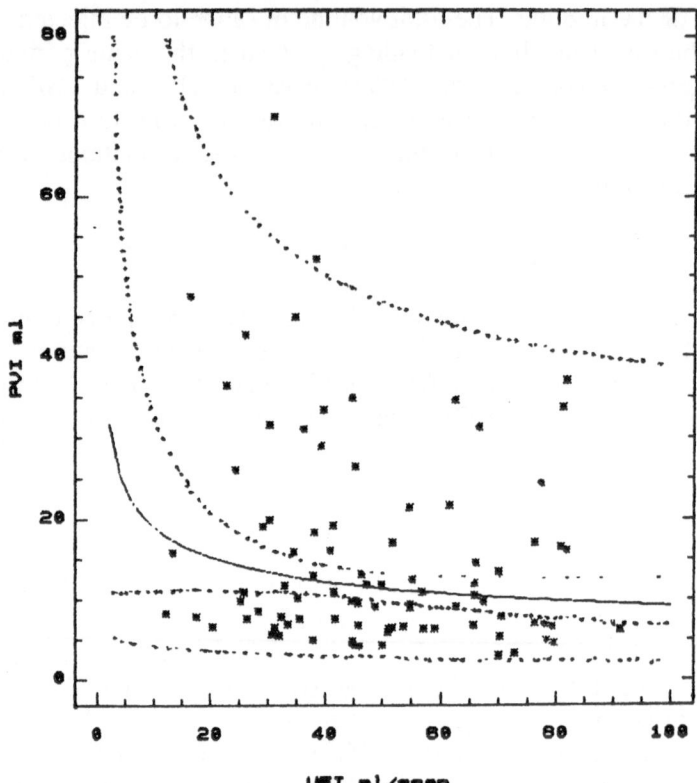

Fig. 2. Multiplicative model of regression PVI vs VEI (equation PVI = a*VEI^b). Intercept = 3.67 (Intercept is equal to Log a); Slope = −0.32; Probability level = 0.07. It can be seen that increases of the brain edema volumetric index (*VEI*) cause decreases of the pressure-volume index (*PVI*) of the cranio-spinal system, due to the decrease of volume-buffering capacity

from 49.24 ± 19.84 ml/scan to 38.16 ± 19.14 ml/scan. Figure 4 shows that, in spite of successful ICP control, in the group with VEI increase PVI tended to decrease, from 15.04 ± 6.94 ml to 10.55 ± 4.04 ml and E increased from 1.43 ± 1.0 mmHg/ml to 1.49 ± 1.27 mmHg/ml, due to the decrease of volume-buffering capacity and an increase of CSS rigidity related to the growth of brain edema. In the other group with a relative decrease of VEI and resolving brain edema, PVI was also found to decrease, from 18.09 ± 17.8 ml to 14.02 ± 13.28 ml, and the decrease of E was relatively small — from 1.41 ± 1.06 mmHg/ml to 1.2 ± 0.45 mmHg/ml. One month after head injury VEI was greater in the first group than in the second group, corresponding to 43.6 ± 16.3 ml/scan and 35.15 ± 9.6 ml/scan, respectively, but the groups did not differ statistically in low ICP (6.88 ± 0.38 mmHg and 6.42 ± 0.44 mmHg), lowered E (1.04 ± 0.51 mmHg/ml and 0.89 ± 0.16 mmHg/ml), relatively normalizing PVI in comparison with the 3–5-day post trauma period (14.26 ±

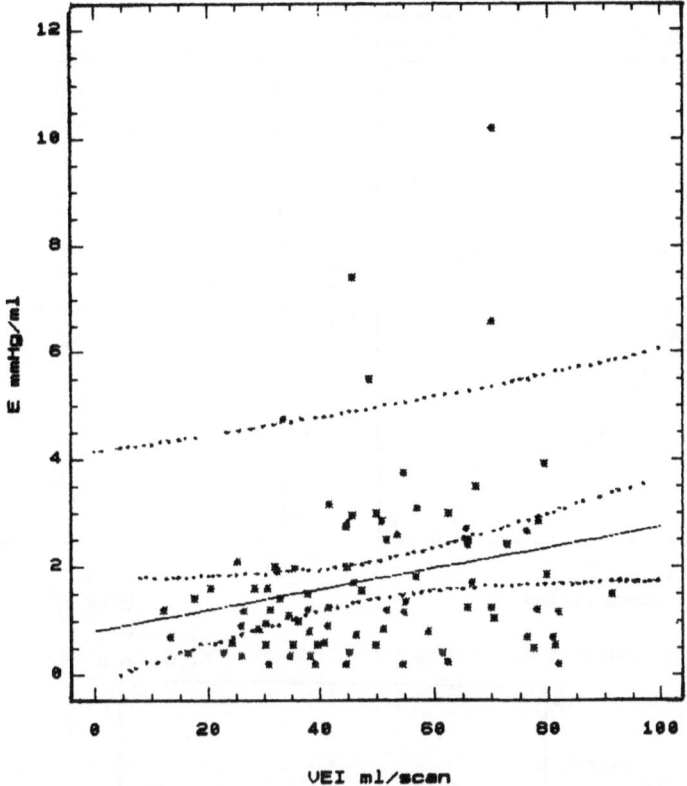

Fig. 3. Linear regression model of E vs VEI (equation E = a + b*VEI). Intercept = 0.81; Slope = 0.019; Probability level = 0.037 It can be seen that increases of the brain edema volumetric index (*VEI*) cause increases of elastance (*E*), due to increase of brain tissue stiffness

2.23 ml and 16.21 ± 1.56 ml), and low R values (1.17 ± 0.73 mmHg/ml per min and 0.73 ± 0.57 mmHg/ml per min).

Temporal Course of EI Related to VEI and R

Patients were divided into two groups according to dynamic changes in the EI. In the first group, EI during the 3–5-day day post-trauma period increased from 0.23 ± 0.06 to 0.27 ± 0.05; in the second group EI decreased from 0.24 ± 0.04 to 0.21 ± 0.06 (Fig. 5). Correspondingly, in the first group, the average VEI and R were relatively decreased — VEI from 46.36 ± 20.8 ml/scan to 44.43 ± 16.47 ml/scan and R from 1.21 ± 0.27 mmHg/ml per min to 1.03 ± 0.08 mmHg/ml per min. In the second group, VEI and R were relatively increased — VEI from 47.19 ± 21.55 ml/scan to 55.57 ± 22.31 ml/scan and R from 1.69 ± 0.23 mmHg/ml per min to 2.02 ± 0.39 mmHg/ml per min. One month after injury ventricles in the first group were smaller (EI 0.29 ± 0.03); in the second group they were larger (EI 0.33 ± 0.06).

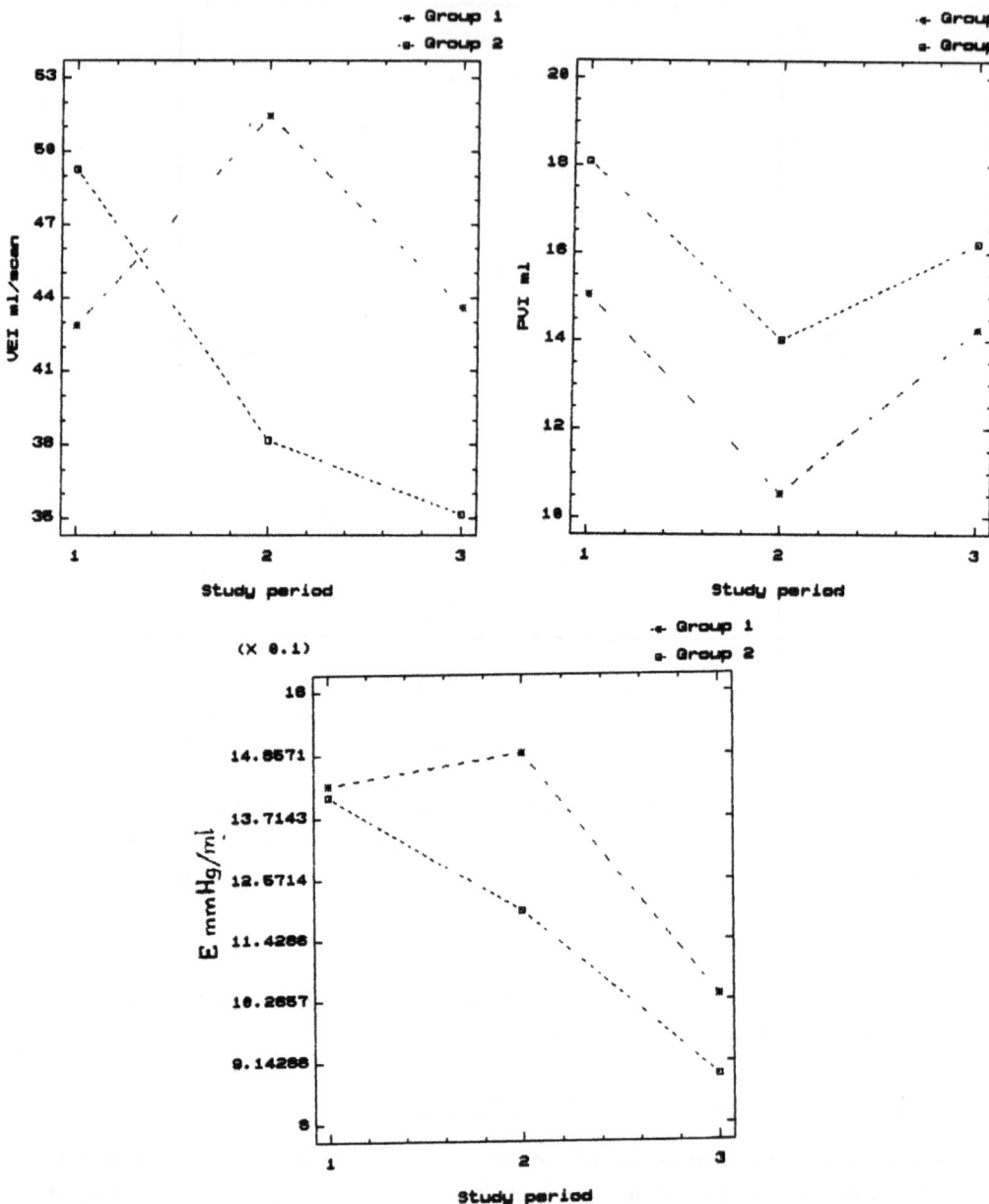

Fig. 4. Temporal course of VEI related to PVI and E. Trends of average values of VEI, PVI, and E determined in two dynamic groups according to the periods of study: (1) first 24 h after injury; (2) 3–5-day posttrauma period; (3) 1 month after injury. VEI, volumetric edema index; PVI, pressure volume index; E, elastance

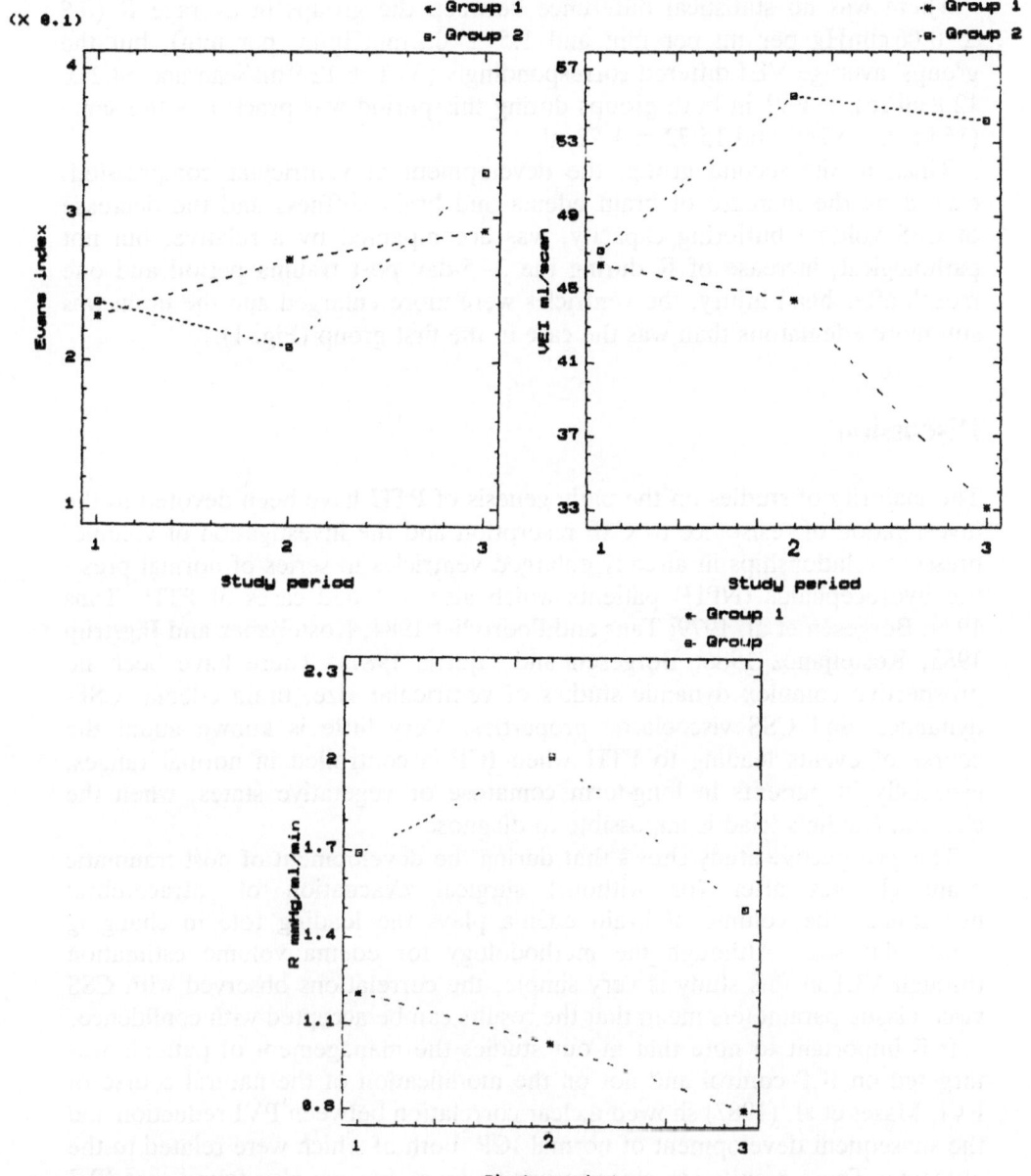

Fig. 5. Temporal course of EI related to VEI and R. Trends of average values of EI, VEI, and R determined in two dynamic groups according to the periods of study: (1) first 24 h after injury; (2) 3–5-day posttrauma period; (3) 1 month after injury. EI, Evans index; VEI, volumetric edema index; R, CSF resorption index

There was no statistical difference between the groups in average R (0.8 ± 0.06 mmHg per ml per min and 1.5 ± 0.2 mmHg/ml per min), but the groups' average VEI differed correspondingly (33.1 ± 12.9 ml/scan and 54.2 ± 12.8 ml/scan). PVI in both groups during this period was practically the same (16.08 ± 1.85 ml and 15.72 ± 1.72 ml).

Thus, in the second group, the development of ventricular compression, caused by the increase of brain edema and brain stiffness and the decrease of CSS volume buffering capacity, was accompanied by a relative, but not pathological, increase of R during the 3–5-day post trauma period and one month after head injury, the ventricles were more enlarged and the brain was still more edematous than was the case in the first group (Fig. 1).

Discussion

The majority of studies on the pathogenesis of PTH have been devoted to the investigation of resistance to CSF resorption and the investigation of volume/pressure relationships in already enlarged ventricles in series of normal pressure hydrocephalus (NPH) patients which also included cases of PTH (Tans 1979; Borgesen et al. 1979; Tans and Poortvliet 1984; Kosteljanez and Ingstrup 1985; Kosteljanez 1986; Borgesen and Gjerris 1987). There have been no prospective complex dynamic studies of ventricular size, brain edema, CSF-dynamics, and CSS viscoelastic properties. Very little is known about the course of events leading to PTH when ICP is controlled in normal ranges, especially in patients in long-term comatose or vegetative states, when the classical Hakim's triad is impossible to diagnose.

This prospective study shows that during the development of post-traumatic brain changes after (or without) surgical evacuation of intracerebral hematomas the volume of brain edema plays the leading role in changing ventricular size. Although the methodology for edema volume estimation through VEI in this study is very simple, the correlations observed with CSS visco-elastic parameters mean that the results can be accepted with confidence.

It is important to note that in our studies the management of patients was targeted on ICP control and not on the modification of the natural course of PVI. Maset et al. (1987) showed a clear correlation between PVI reduction and the subsequent development of normal ICP, both of which were related to the outcome. These results are close to our findings, but we also found that PVI reduction and increase of E developed even when ICP was held within the normal ranges (lower than 20 mmHg), and that PVI reduced nonlinearly and E increased linearly during the growth of brain edema volume. These factors also emphasize the importance of monitoring the temporal course of the PVI.

The growth of brain edema volume and the depletion of CSS volume buffering capacity observed during the 3–5-day post trauma period, confirm data gathered on brain edema dynamics by several other authors using other methods (Kobrine and Kempe 1973; Hase et al. 1978; Auer 1979; Reulen et al. 1980; Cao et al. 1984).

Our data on the temporal courses of ventricular size and brain edema volume showed a predominant ventricular enlargement in the group of patients who had an increase of brain edema volume during the 3–5-day post trauma period. It must be emphasized that CSF resorption resistance remained low and within the normal ranges during the whole period of study, but there was a relative nonpathologic increase of R during the 3–5-day post trauma period, as described by Marmarou et al. (1987). As the result of this study we conclude that the leading role in the mechanism of hydrocephalic ventricular enlargement in patients with PTH is not impairment of CSF resorption, as is postulated in the literature, but is the degeneration and atrophy (hydrocephalus *ex vacuo*) of injured and edematose brain tissue, as shown by several microscopic studies (Strich 1956; Adams et al. 1977; Pilz 1983; Jane et al. 1985; Blumbergs et al. 1989) and recently confirmed by magnetic resonance imaging (MRI) (Levin et al. 1985; Wilson et al. 1988).

Management of severely head injured patients must be focused not only on the control of ICP and PVI, but also on the prevention of the growth of brain edema due to secondary ischemic processes. According to this concept of PTH pathogenesis, shunting operations are not appropriate. Nevertheless, in every case with suspected developing ventricular enlargement or other PTH symptoms, CSF resorption resistance must be measured and in cases with a pathological increase of R, shunting operations are recommended.

References

Adams J, Mitchell D, Graham D (1977) Diffuse brain damage of immediate type. Brain 100: 489–502

Alberico A, Ward J, Choi S, Marmarou A, Young H (1987) Outcome after severe head injury. J Neurosurg 67: 648–656

Auer L (1979) Long term monitoring of ventricular fluid pressure in patients with head injury problems and indications. Neurosurg Rev 2: 73–77

Blumbergs P, Jones N, North J (1989) Diffuse axonal injury in head trauma. J Neurol Neurosurg Psychiatry 52: 838–841

Borgesen S, Gjerris F, Sorensen S (1979) Intracranial pressure and conductance to outflow of CSF in normal pressure hydrocephalus. J Neurosurg 50: 489–493

Borgesen S, Gjerris F (1987) Relationships between intracranial pressure, ventricular size, and resistance to CSF outflow. J Neurosurg 67: 535–539

Busch G (1989) Post-traumatic defects in computed tomography. Neurosurg Rev 10: 269–73

Buschke H, Fuld P (1974) Evaluating storage, retention, and retrieval in disordered memory and learning. Neurology (NY) 24: 1019–1025

Cao M, Lisheng H, Shouzheng S (1984) Resolution of brain edema in severe brain injury at controlled high and low intracranial pressures. J Neurosurg 61: 707–712

Cullum C, Bigler E (1986) Late effects of hematoma on brain morphology and memory in closed head injury. Int J Neurosci 28: 279–283

Dikmen S, Temkin N, McLean A, Wyler A, Machamer J (1987) Memory and head injury severity. J Neurol Neurosurg Psychiatry 50: 1613–1618

Evans W (1942) An encephalometric ratio for estimating ventricular enlargement and cerebral atrophy. Arch Neurol Psych 47: 931–937

Foroglou G (1976) L'Hydrocephalie post-traumatique. Neurochirurgie 22: 108–111

French B, Dublin A (1977) The value of computerized tomography in the management of 1000 consecutive head injuries. Surg Neurol 7: 171–183

Gradeur D, Allal R, Pidelievre C (1979) Etude tomodensitometrique des lesions cerebrales post-traumatiques. J Radiol 60: 79–86

Groswasser Z, Cohen M, Reider-Groswasser I, Stern M (1988) Incidence, CT findings and rehabilitation out-come of patients with communicative hydrocephalus following severe head injury. Brain Inj 2: 267–72

Gudeman S, Kishore P, Becker D, Lipper M, Girevendulis A, Jeffries B (1981) Computed tomography in the evaluation of post-traumatic hydrocephalus. Radiology 141: 397–402

Hannay H, Levin H, Grossman R (1979) Impaired recognition memory after head injury. Cortex 15: 269–283

Hase U, Reulen H, Fenske A (1978) Intracranial pressure-volume in patients with subarachnoid hemorrhage (SAH). Acta Neurochir (Wien) 44: 69–80

Jane J, Stewart O, Genarelli T (1985) Axonal degeneration induced by experimental noninvasive minor head injury. J Neurosurg 62: 96–100

Jensen F, Jensen FM (1979) Acquired hydrocephalus. Acta Neurochir (Wien) 46: 243–257

Kaas B, Lonnum A (1978) Long-term prognosis of patients with central cerebral ventricular enlargement: A fifth follow-up study of 100 patients with third ventricle measuring 12 mm or more in width. Acta Neurol Scand 57: 19–30

Kishore P, Lipper M, Miller J (1978) Posttraumatic hydrocephalus in patients with severe head injury. Neuroradiology 16: 261–265

Koo A, LaRoge R (1977) Evaluation of head trauma by computed tomography. Radiology 123: 345–346

Kobrine A, Kempe L (1973) Studies in head injury — Part 1.: An experimental model of closed head injury. Surg Neurol 1: 34–37

Kosteljanez M (1986) CSF dynamics and pressure-volume relationships in communicating hydrocephalus. J Neurosurg 64: 45–52

Kosteljanez M, Ingstrup H (1985) Normal pressure hydrocephalus: Correlation between CT and measurements of cerebrospinal fluid dynamics. Acta Neurochir (Wien) 77: 8–13

Laws E, Mokri B (1977) Occult hydrocephalus: Results of shunting correlated with diagnostic tests. Clin Neurosurg 24: 316–333

Levin H, Meyers C, Grossman R, Sarwar M (1981) Ventricular enlargement after closed head injury. Arch Neurol 38: 623–629

Levin H, Handel S, Goldman A, Eisenberg H, Guinto F (1985) Magnetic resonance imaging after 'diffuse' nonmissile head injury. Arch Neurol 42: 963–968

Lewin W (1968) Preliminary observations on external hydrocephalus after severe head injury. Br J Surg 55: 747–751

Marmarou A, Shulman K, Rosende R (1978) A nonlinear analysis of the cerebrospinal fluid system and intracranial pressure dynamics. J Neurosurg 48: 332–344

Marmarou A, Maset A, Ward J, Choi S, Brooks D, Lutz H, Moulton R, Muizellaar P, DeSales A, Young H (1987) Contribution of CSF and vascular factors to elevation of ICP in severely head-injured patients. J Neurosurg 66: 883–890

Maset A, Marmarou A, Ward J, Choi S, Lutz H, Brooks D, Moulton R, DeSales A, Muizellaar P, Turner H, Young H (1987) Pressure-volume index in head injury. J Neurosurg 67: 832–840

Meyers C, Levin H, Eisenberg H (1983) Early versus late ventricular enlargement following closed head injury. J Neurol Neurosurg Psychiatry 46: 1092–1097

Pedersen H, Gyldensted M, Gyldensted C (1979) Measuring normal ventricular system and supratentorial subarachnoidal spaces in children with computer tomography. Neuroradiology 17: 231–237

Pilz P (1983) Axonal injury in head injury. Acta Neurochir [Suppl] (Wien) 32: 119–123

Reulen H, Tsuyumu M, Prioleau G (1980) Further results concerning the resolution of vasogenic brain edema. In: Vlieger M, Lange S, Becks J (eds) Brain edema: Pathology, diagnosis and therapy. Adv Neurol 28: 375–381

Salmon J (1972) Adult hydrocephalus. Evaluation of shunt therapy in 80 patients. J Neurosurg 37: 423–428

Strich S (1956) Diffuse degeneration of nerve fibres as a cause of brain damage due to head injury. A pathological study of twenty cases. J Neurol Neurosurg Psychiatry 19: 163–185

Symon L, Hinzpeter T (1977) The engima of normal pressure hydrocephalus: tests to select patients for surgery and predict shunt function. Clin Neurosurg 24: 285–315

Tans J (1979) Differentiation of normal pressure hydrocephalus and cerebral atrophy by CT and spinal infusion test. J Neurol 222: 109–118

Tans J, Poortvliet D (1984) Comparison of ventricular steady-state infusion with bolus infusion and pressure recording for differentiation between arrested and nonarrested hydrocephalus. Acta Neurochir (Wien) 72: 15–29

Teasdale G, Jennett B (1974) Assessment of coma and impaired consiousness: A practical scale. Lancet II: 81–84

Tikk A, Eelmae J (1985) CSF hydrodynamics studied by means of a simple constant volume injection technique. In: Abstracts of the 6th International Symposium on Intracranial Pressure and Mechanisms of Brain Damage. June 9–13, Glasgow, Scotland, pp 10–11

Van Dogen K, Braakman R (1980) Late computed tomography in survivors of severe head injury. Neurosurgery 7: 14–22

Wieser H, Probst C (1975) Clinical observations on hydrocephalus with special regard to the post-traumatic malresorptive form. J Neurol 212: 1–21

Wilson J, Wiedmann K, Hadley D, Condon B, Teasdale G, Brooks D (1988) Early and late magnetic resonance imaging and neuropsychological outcome after head injury. J Neurol Neurosurg Psychiatry 51: 391–396

31 — Treatment of Postmeningitic Hydrocephalus

Yasuo Yamanouchi, Takasumi Yasuda, Yutaka Nonoyama,
Yasuo Kawamura, and Hiroshi Matsumura[1]

Summary. Even with the advent of antibiotics, treatment of postmeningitic hydrocephalus has been a difficult problem. Early surgical intervention based on new diagnostic modalities has improved mortality and morbidity. We reviewed 43 cases of postmeningitic hydrocephalus treated at our Institute over the past 20 years so that we could determine an effective therapeutic regimen. The subjects were 43 patients who had hydrocephalus following purulent meningitis. The results of our review were: 1. Thirty cases occurred during the first 10 years, while 13 occurred during the last 10 years, indicating a decline in the number of cases. 2. Meningitis was due to delayed treatment for myelomeningocele in 5 cases or encephalocele (1 case) 3. Complications such as brain abscess (4 cases) and subdural abscess (2 cases) or effusion (3 cases) were factors for poor prognoses. 4. Twenty five percent of the patients had multiloculated ventricular systems, resulting in a grave outcome. 5. Shunt operations should be postponed until ventricular fluid improves in accordance with these parameters: protein, less than 300 mg/dl, preferably less than 100 mg/dl; glucose, more than 30 mg/dl; cell counts, less than 200/3 cells per mm^3. 6) Prognoses for the first 30 patients were poor, while those for the last 13 were improved. The present review indicates that early diagnosis and early treatment of meningitis are the keys to promising prognosis. Close communication with pediatricians is most important.

Keywords. Hydrocephalus — Meningitis — Complications — Treatment regimen

Introduction

With the development of chemotherapy, the survival rate of children with meningitis has been improved; however, the mortality and morbidity is occasionally influenced by various complications. Although complications

---

[1] Department of Neurosurgery, Kansai Medical University, Moriguchi, 570 Japan

which require surgical intervention are now detected at an early stage with diagnostic tools such as computerized tomography, magnetic resonance imaging, and ultrasound, resulting in more improved treatments, various issues still remain. Among these complications requiring surgical intervention hydrocephalus occurs most frequently. We retrospectively reviewed cases of postmeningitic hydrocephalus in children in order to establish an effective regimen for the treatmen of this condition.

Subjects and Methods

We reviewed 43 cases of hydrocephalus following purulent meningitis which were treated at our Institute during the past 20 years. The patients were under the age of 15 and included 20 boys and 23 girls. We treated 30 patients during the first 10 years and 13 patients during the last 10 years, which fact indicates an apparent decrease in the number of patients during the last 10 years. We have treated only three patients during the last 5 years. Treatments included a ventricular tap, external ventricular drainage (EVD), ventriculo-peritoneal (V-P) shunt following EVD, or V-P shunt alone.

Results

As shown in Fig. 1, the age when diagnosis of meningitis was confirmed was mainly during the neonatal and infantile periods. We could not evaluate the interval between the onset of meningitis and the manifestation of the clinical state of hydrocephalus. Causative organisms are listed in Table 1. A gram-negative bacillus was the bacteria most responsible for infection in neonates and infants, being involved in 50% of all cases in which a causative organism was verified. Six patients were born with central nervous system malformation; namely, 5 patients had myelomeningocele and 1 patient had encephalocele. Four patients out of 5 with myelomeningocele were operated on at 1 month, 2 months, 20 days, and 6 days after birth, respectively. As the parents' consent was hard to obtain, surgery was delayed, resulting in the development of meningitis during this period.

0−30 D	24 cases (55%)	89 %	95 %
31 D−1 Y	15 cases		
<2 Y	2 cases		
>2 Y	2 cases		

Fig. 1. Age at diagnosis of meningitis

Table 1. Causative organisms of meningitis in our series

Micrococcus	3
Proteus mirabilis	2
Staphylococcus epidermidis	2
Staphylococcus aureus	2
Pseudomonas aeruginosa	2
Haemophilus influenzae	2
Mycobacterium tuberculosis	2
Staphylococcus faecalis	1
Bacillus	1
Escherichia coli	1
Candida	1
α-Streptococcus	1
β-Streptococcus	1
Klebsiella	1
negative	8
unknown	11

Complications other than hydrocephalus, derived from infections, occurred in 9 lesions in 8 patients (19%); there were 4 cases of brain abscess, 2 cases of subdural abscess, and 3 cases of subdural effusion; 63% of these patients had been affected by meningitis during the neonatal period. These complications were difficult to treat because of the coexistence of two different clinical states, and, therefore, the prognosis for these patients was extremely poor; 6 patients remained in a vegetative state, 1 patient died, and the fate of 1 patient was unknown.

A so-called multiloculated ventricular system was found in 11 patients (25%) (Fig. 2). Ten of these 11 patients had been affected by meningitis during the neonatal period. The interval between the onset of meningitis and initiation of treatment following the definite diagnosis of meningitis was 27 days for patients with multiloculated ventricular system, while that for patients without multi-loculation was 8 days on the average, showing an apparent delay of treatment for the former. Among patients with multiloculated ventricular systems the incidence of complications due to brain abscess and subdural abscess was very high, 6 cases in 5 patients (45%); 3 cases of brain abscess and 3 cases of subdural effusion. We treated 2 patients by resecting the septa through a craniotomy and 4 patients were treated by ventriculostomy using a ventriculoscope. Two patients underwent a bilateral shunting procedure. The prognoses for these 11 patients were miserable: 1 remained in a vegetative state; 8 died; and the fate of 2 is unknown. Histological examination of six biopsy or autopsy septa samples confirmed the presence of glial tissues and myelin sheath in 2 cases (Fig. 3).

In 1977 we made a retrospective study of 128 shunts for postmeningitic hydrocephalus in order to evaluate the laboratory examination of CSF at the

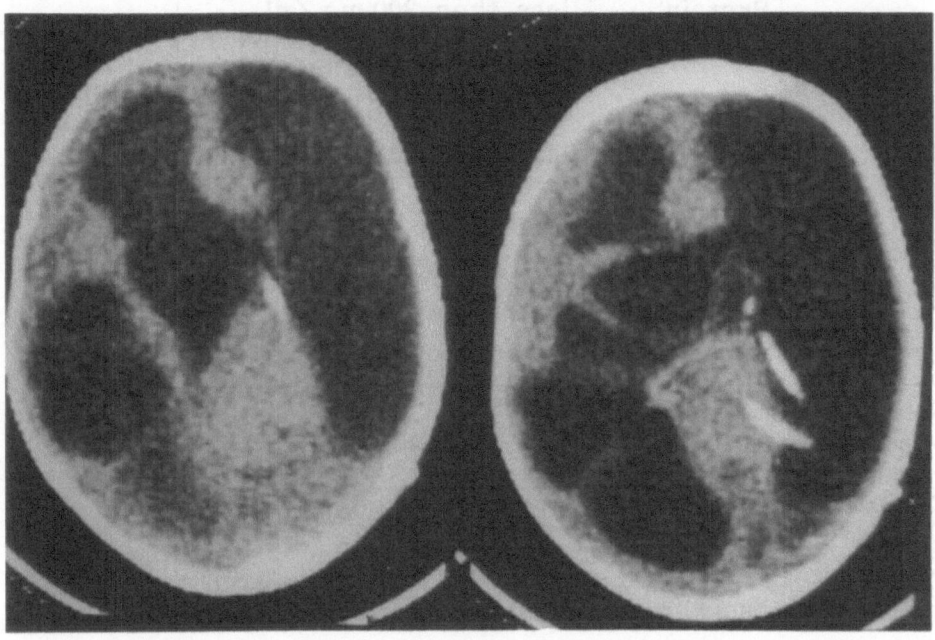

Fig. 2. CT scan of a patient with so-called multiloculated ventricular system

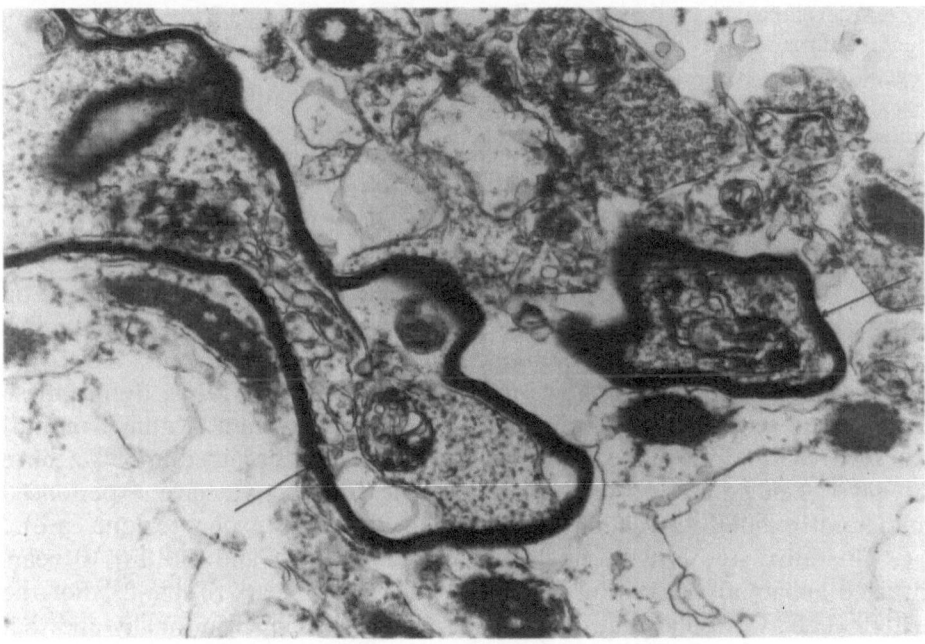

Fig. 3. Electron micrograph of the septa at surgery in one case. Despite poor tissue preservation, myelin sheath is noted. (× 22,000)

Protein	less than 300 mg/dl
	(hopefully 100 mg/dl)
Sugar	more than 30 mg/dl
Cell count	less than 200/3 cells/mm³

Fig. 4. Criteria of CSF for shunting

Table 2. Patient outcome

	First 10 years	Last 10 years	Total
Normal development	2	5	7
Mental retardation	3	6	9
Vegetative state	1	1	2
Dead	14	1	15
Unknown	10	0	10
Total	30	13	43

Table 3. Patient outcome according to age of onset of meningitis

Age of onset	~30 days	~1 year	1 year~
Normal development	4	3	
Mental retardation	4	5	
Vegetative state	0	1	1
Dead	8	4	3
Unknown	8	2	
Total	24	15	4

time of the shunting procedure. We proposed a treatment regimen based on our results indicating that shunting procedure should be postponed until a negative culture of CSF was obtained for 1 month and until the ventricular fluid data were improved as shown in Fig. 4 (Someda et al. 1977). Before these criteria were settled on early obstruction of the initial shunt (within 1 month) was observed in 57% of cases and recurrent infection occurred in 35%. Since we have been strictly observing our present criteria, we have experienced neither early shunt obstruction, nor recurrent infection (expect for one case).

Comparative study of the final outcome for the first and the last 10 years revealed apparently successful results for the last 10 years (Table 2). For the first 10 years, we found that only 2 patients had developed normally and that 14 patients out of 30 had died. Thus, the result was miserable. For the last 10 years, in contrast, we found that 5 patients out of 13 had developed normally and the mortality rate was only 8%.

Outcome by age is shown in Table 3. Patients who were affected during the neonatal period were likely to show poor prognosis.

Discussion

Meningitis occasionally induces various complications and may influence mortality and morbidity. Complications such as hydrocephalus, brain abscess, subdural abscess, and subdural effusion require surgical treatment; among these, the incidence of hydrocephalus is high (Karan 1986; Lorber and Pickering 1966), about 30%. Other reports have described incidences of 56% in autopsies (Berman and Banker 1966) and 67% in neonatal meningitis (Diebler and Dulac 1987). Most patients in our series were affected with meningitis during the neonatal period. Potential hydrocephalus should be kept in mind during the management of meningitis, especially in the neonatal period. As shown in Fig. 2, the causative organisms in our series varied, and this reflects the well-known fact that causative organisms for meningitis in children differ according to the age of onset (Snyder 1989; Weil 1990).

Infantile hydrocephalus is characterized by the frequent accompaniment of ventriculitis, especially in neonatal patients; the incidence has been reported as 67% (Salmon 1972) and 92% (Berman and Banker 1966) in autopsy series. Affected infants admitted to neurosurgical services occasionally need management of the cerebrospinal fluid (CSF) because of 1. incomplete healing of meningitis and/or ventriculitis, and 2. increased CSF protein content in spite of the inflammation having healed. In order to excrete infected CSF, floating debris, and high protein CSF, and in order to deliver antibiotics into the ventricle, ventricular puncture, ventricular drainage, and placement of an Ommaya reservoir have been carried out. However, since punctured porencephaly is often associated with ventricular puncture, and since recurrent infection was induced by placement of the Ommaya reservoir, ventricular drainage exclusively has been carried out during the last 10 years in this Institute. We analyzed 128 shunts in postmeningitic hydrocephalus and proposed criteria (Fig. 4) (Someda et al. 1977) for application to shunt operations taking into consideration the patency of the shunt system and the recurrence of infection. Good surgical results were obtained after observing our criteria, indicating their usefulness.

Multiloculated ventricular systems were observed in at least 25% of patients, but this rate is not conclusive and could be increased if the older cases had been examined more accurately. Ten out of 11 these patients were affected by meningitis during the neonatal period, and this complication may contribute to the poor prognosis of neonates with postmeningitic hydrocephalus. In neonates some immune mechanisms are deficient and incidences of sepsis (Snyder 1989; Weil 1990) and ventriculitis (Berman and Banker 1966; Salmon 1972) are high, and infection is readily spread because of the wide extracellular space. Additionally, neonatal meningitis is most frequently induced by gram-negative bacilli, especially *Escherichia coli*. *Escherichia coli* and K1 capsular antigen are

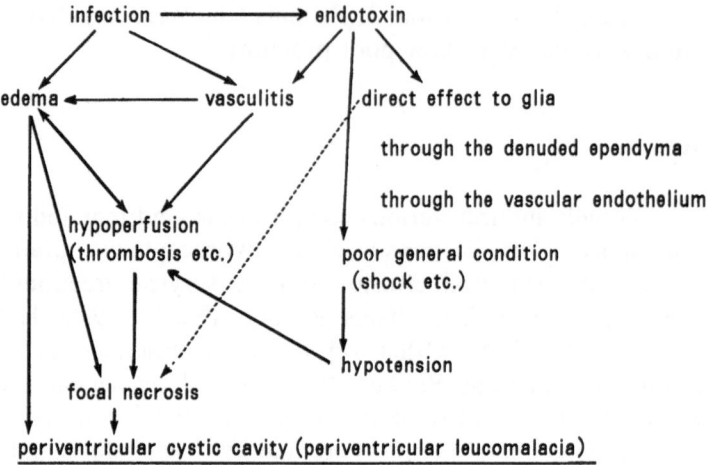

Fig. 5. Pathogenesis of the multiloculated ventricular system

known to be associated with this organism's invasiveness (Robbins et al. 1974). These multiple factors may be related to the formation of multilocular ventricular systems and may contribute to the high incidence of this phenomenon in neonatal postmeningitic hydrocephalus. Our present study revealed that delayed treatment for meningitis was closely connected with the formation of these ventricular systems. The difficulty of diagnosing meningitis in neonatal patients may also result in multiloculation.

The mechanism of the formation of multilocular ventricle systems was first reported by Berman and Banker (1966). Many studies have reported that intraventricular protrusions of the glial tissue, referred to as glial tufts or glial bridges, might contribute to their formation (Sakata et al. 1978; Schultz and Leeds 1973; Wolf and Kerstan 1974; Yamada et al. 1982). Sakata et al. (1978) in an autopsy examination of one case, proposed that multilocular formation in a broad sense might be due to a porencephalic cyst adjacent to the ventricle.

We have reported elsewhere (McLone et al. 1982; Yamanouchi et al. 1984) on our speculations regarding one mechanism for the development of a multi-loculated ventricular system. These speculations arose from the experimental study of mice; we suggested that edema, after an inflammatory extension into the brain parenchyma, coalesces in the paraventricular white matter, fuses, and forms a paraventricular cavitation, and the resultant cavitation grows large enough to form a pseudoventricle, — a "loculated ventricle". Histological examination of human specimens supported our speculation. In consideration of vascular factors the formation mechanism of the paraventricular cystic cavity should be discussed. According to Friede (1973), the main factor involved, other than infarction, which is frequently seen in neonatal meningitis, is thrombophlebitis of the subependymal vein. The association of endotoxin has also been reported. Gilles et al. (1976) reported that injection of sterile *E. coli* endotoxin into the peritoneal cavity of neonatal kittens produced severe leucoencephalopathy and cavitation. We carried out similar experiments in mice and confirmed edema in the paraventricular white matter. Figure 5 shows our schema for the pathogenesis.

The so-called multiloculated ventricular system includes intraventricular septation and paraventricular cysts; in the case of paraventricular cysts, membranectomy must be avoided (Naidich et al. 1983; Yamanouchi et al. 1984). Multiloculation is clinically confirmed by the following facts: in spite of obvious shunt malfunction the anterior fontanelle is not so tense, the head circumference does not increase rapidly, and the general condition of the patient is not so bad. Generally, a multiloculated ventricular system is considered to be the terminal stage of infection of the brain parenchyma and the ventricle resulting from delay in initiating appropriate treatment.

We have described our treatment of postmenigitic hydrocephalus and have reconfirmed that early detection of and early initiation of treatment for meningitis is most crucial to obtain successful prognoses, because delayed treatment for myelomeningocele or cephalocele may cause meningitis and delayed conservative management of meningitis was prominent in patients with multiloculated ventricular systems. Keeping in close contact with pediatricians, neurosurgeons should resect the infected lesion and remove contagious CSF promptly and thoroughly without wasting time.

References

Berman PH, Banker BO (1966) Neonatal meningitis. A clinical and pathological study of 29 cases. Pediatrics 38: 6–24

Diebler C, Dulac O (1987) Pediatric neurology and neuroradiology. Springer, Tokyo, pp 139–144

Friede RL (1973) Cerebral infarcts complicating neonatal leptomeningitis. Acute and residual lesions. Acta Neuropathol (Berl) 23: 245–253

Gilles FH, Leviton A, Kerr CS (1976) Endotoxin leucoencephalopathy in the telencephalon of the newborn kitten. J Neurol Sci 27: 183–191

Karan S (1986) Purulent meningitis in the newborn. Nerv Syst Child 2: 26–31

Lorber J, Pickering D (1966) Incidence and treatment of post-meningitic hydrocephalus in the newborn. Arch Dis Child 41: 44–50

McLone DG, Killion M, Yogev R, Sommers MW (1982) Ventriculitis of mice and men. In: Concepts in pediatric neurosurgery II. Karger, Basel, pp 112–126

Naidich TP, McLone DG, Yamanouchi Y (1983) Periventricular white-matter cysts in a murine model of gram-negative ventriculitis. AJNR 4: 461–465

Robbins JB, McCracken GH Jr, Gotschlich EC, Ørskov F, Ørskov I, Hanson LA (1974) Escherichia coli K1 capsular polysaccharide associated with neonatal meningitis. N Engl J Med 290: 1216–1220

Sakata K, Yamada H, Funakoshi T, Abe T (1978) On pathogenesis of intraventricular septations. Nerv Syst Child 3: 295–302

Salmon JH (1972) Ventriculitis complicating meningitis. Am J Dis Child 124: 35–40

Schultz P, Leeds NE (1973) Intraventricular septations complicating neonatal meningitis. J Neurosurg 38: 620–626

Snyder RD (1989) Bacterial infections of the nervous system. In: Swaiman KF (ed) Pediatric neurology. Principles and practice. Mosby, St Louis, pp 447–473

Someda K, Yamanouchi Y, Miki K, Kawamura Y, Matsumura H, Ogata M, Yamamoto T, Inuzuka N, Chokyu M, Ban S, Sato S, Nagasawa S (1977) Postmeningitic hydrocephalus — Analysis of factors predisposing early shunt obstruction. Neurol Surg 5: 445–452

Weil ML (1990) Infections of the nervous system. In: Menkes JH (ed) Textbook of child neurology. Lea and Febiger, Philadelphia, pp 327–423

Wolf H, Kerstan J (1974) Neugeborenenmeningitis, kompliziert durch 'Ventrikulitis'. Monatsschr Kinderheilkd 122: 402–404

Yamada H, Abe T, Tanabe Y, Sakai N (1982) Experimental and clinical studies on pathogenesis of intraventricular septations following meningoventriculitis in childhood. Monogr Neural Sci 8: 81–85

Yamanouchi Y, Kawamura Y, Matsumura H, McLone DG (1984) New concept of the pathogenesis of multiloculated ventricular system. Nerv Syst Child 9: 9–16

32 — "Benign"* Intracranial Hypertension and Polyradiculitis — Two Varieties of One Disease?

Yanko Yankov[1]

Summary. In our experience with 20 children who had polyradiculitis type Guillain-Barré syndrome (GBS) and 2 children who had "benign" intracranial hypertension (BIH) we found neurological sequelae in 3 out of 13 followed patients with GBS and full recovery of the 2 children with BIH. Those patients who had slow involution of the disease were monitored by threshold vibrometry and we used mannitol and Collagenan successively. In our discussion we suggest some striking similarities between the two conditions: (1) GBS and BIH are generally expressed 1–3 weeks after viral infection and both regress after treatment in the majority of patients; (2) Both conditions have similar pathogenic mechanisms; (3) Some patients with GBS also demonstrate papillaedema which may be interpreted as a sign of analogy between the two conditions. The advantage of regarding the conditions as analogous is that therapy would be better monitored. The experience of the neurosurgons who generally first confront BIH can be enriched by experience of the neurologists and pediatricians who treat patients with GBS.

Keywords. "Benign" intracranial hypertension — Polyradiculitis — Impaired CSF absorption — Monitoring of treatment

Introduction

Polyradiculitis type Guillain-Barré syndrome (GBS) is a well known neurological entity. In the majority of patients there is a definite history of preceding illness of a viral type having occurred 1–3 weeks before the neurological signs. Cranial nerve involvement occurs in 10%–40% of patients. Papillaedema has been reported in a few patients.

---

* "Benign" intracranial hypertension is used in the sense of idiopathic intracranial hypertension, excluding intracranial hypertension of other known etiologies.
[1] Clinic of Child Neurology, Institute of Neurology, Psychiatry and Neurosurgery, Medical Academy, Sofia, Bulgaria

"Benign" intracranial hypertension (BIH) describes a heterogenous group of disorders that are characterized by increased intracranial pressure, excluding intracranial mass lesions, obstructive hydrocephalus, intracranial infection, and hyper-tensive encephalopathy (Brodie 1974; Jefferson and Clark 1976; Baker et al. 1989). According to Johnston and Paterson (1974) BIH results from the following major causes in children: middle ear infection (24.3%), non-specific infections (13.9%) minor head injuries (4.4%), withdrawal of steroid therapy (1.2%), and others. After presenting the results of our monitored treatment of GBS and BIH we suggest some analogies between the two conditions.

Subjects and Methods

Between 1987 and 1989, 20 children aged 4–16 years were admitted to the Child Neurology Clinic of Sofia with diagnosed GBS. All of them underwent a full complex of clinical, electromyographic, CSF, otoneurologic, ophthal-mologic, neuroradiologic, and threshold vibrometry investigations. We intro-duced an original method of threshold vibrometry, using a routine audiometer for determining even small problems in the sense of balance. This method is atraumatic, easy, and informative. Thirteen of the children (six boys and seven girls) were treated, with periodic monitoring of neurological signs and vibration threshold, for a period of 1–3 years.

The condition of two of our patients, a 5-year-old and a 6-year-old, with BIH corresponded to conditions of idiopatic BIH. Their signs of hypertension, blurred vision, and papillaedema appeared 10 and 15 days after non-specific infections in the 5-year-old and 6-year-old, respectively. The 5-year-old patient had been treated with Erythran for this infection. He and the second patient, the 6-year-old, recovered from the BIH after treatment.

Results

The evolution, involution, and treatment of GBS in 13 children are rep-resented schematically in Fig. 1. At first we treated these children with steroids (1–1.5 mg/kg), vitamins, and early rehabilitation complex. In patients 2, 3, 4, 8, 9, and 12 all clinical and subclinical signs estimated by motor conduction velocity and threshold vibrometry were fully restored. If clinical or subclinical signs of neuropathy persisted we treated with mannitol 10%, 1 g/kg i.v. for 30 minutes. After 10 days this treatment was repeated (Patients 1, 5, 7, and 10). Patients 6 and 13 were on assisted ventilation and their treatment was carried out by other colleagues. If, in the next control examination, the patients still demonstrated clinical or subclinical signs of neuropathy we used Collagenan, following the dosage recommended by the manufacturer (Laboratoires Sobio, Paris). In its list of indications five autoimmune diseases are cited, but not Guillain-Barré. This double antimalaric was used for 3 months in patients 1, 5, and 7 whose clinical manifestations persisted even after osmotic treatment

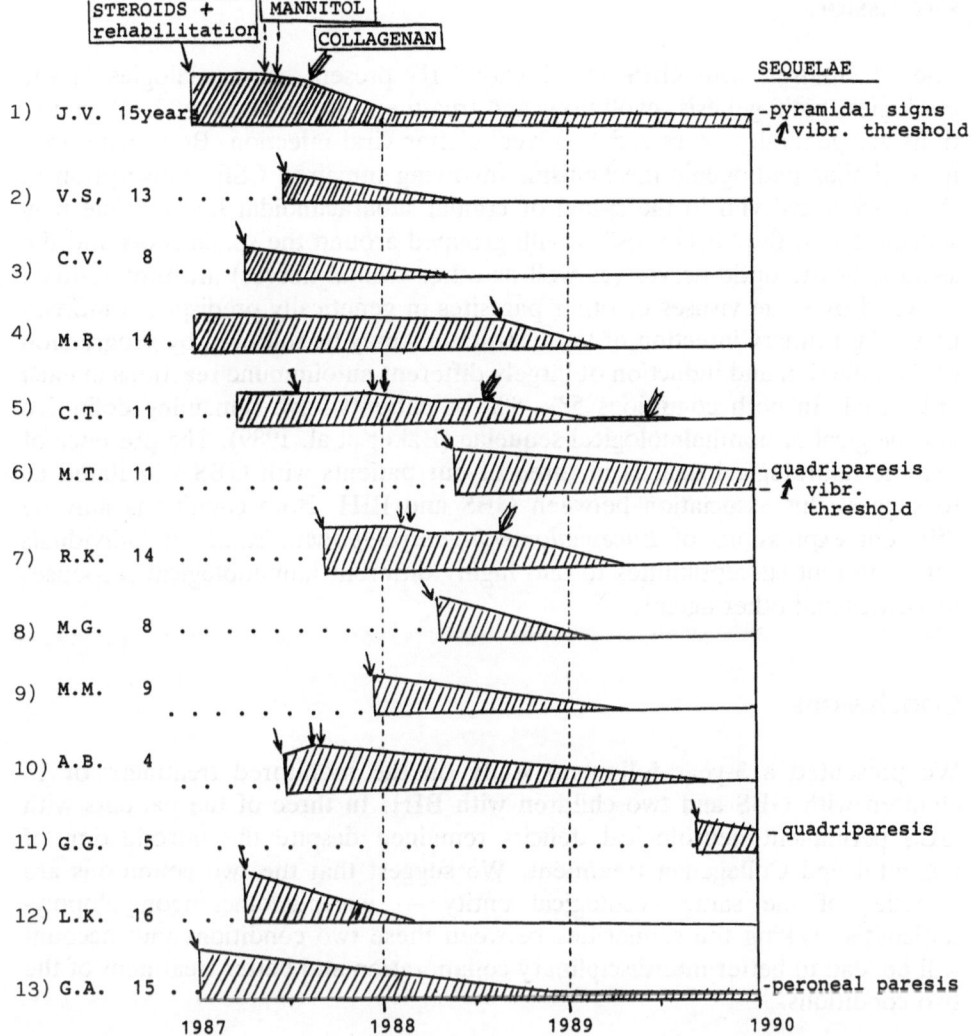

Fig. 1. Clinical course in 13 children with GBS follow-up study and monitoring of treatment

with mannitol. The results, documented by periodic clinical examinations, electromyogram (EMG), and threshold vibrometry, showed marked improvement 2–4 weeks after the beginning of Collagenan treatment and complete restoration 6 months later.

The two children with BIH were treated by daily lumbar puncture and with mannitol. The complaints of severe headache and blurred vision diminished after the 3rd day of treatment and disappeared after 10 days. On the day of admission to the clinic, papillaedema was expressed in both children; 3.0 and 2.5 d, respectively. With treatment, the papillaedema showed involution and disappeared completely 4 months later in both children.

Discussion

The 13 children with GBS and 2 with BIH present some analogies in the etiologies, pathogenesis, evolution, and treatment of the diseases. Both conditions are generally expressed 1–3 weeks after viral infection. Both conditions have similar pathogenic mechanisms involving impaired CSF reabsorption at the arachnoidal villi in the spinal or cranial subarachnoidal spaces. One may speculate that the "packages" of villi grouped around the spinal roots and the sheaths of the optic nerves (as well as other cranial nerves) are preferentialy attacked by some viruses or other parasites in genetically predisposed individuals. The primary infection of these structures may be followed by progression of the infection and induction of largely different autoimmune reactions in each individual. In both conditions 5%–8% of patients have remaining definitive neurological or ophthalmological sequelae (Baker et al. 1989). The presence of definite neurological deficits in three of our patients with GBS stimulated us to suggest this association between GBS and BIH. Both conditions may be different expressions of *Encephalomeningomyelopolyradiculitis* in individuals with different susceptibilities to and highly different immunological responses to viruses and other agents.

Conclusions

We presented a 3-year follow-up study on the monitored treatment of 13 children with GBS and two children with BIH. In three of the patients with GBS permanent neurological deficits remained despite the introduction of mannitol and Collagenan treatment. We suggest that the two conditions are varieties of the same nosological entity — encephalomeningomyelopolyradiculitis. Taking the similarities between these two conditions into account will be lead to better interdisciplinary collaboration and better treatment of the two conditions.

References

Baker RS, Baumann RJ, Buncic JR (1989) Idiopathic intracranial hypertension (pseudotumor cerebri) in pediatric patients. Pediatr Neurol 5: 5–15
Brodie HG (1974) Benign intracranial hypertension: A survey of the clinical and radiological features and long term prognosis. Brain 97: 313–326
Jefferson A, Clark J (1976) Treatment of benign intracranial hypertension by dehydration agents with particular reference to the measurement of the blind spot area as a means of recording improvment. J Neurol Neurosurg Psychiatry 39: 627–639
Johnson I, Paterson A (1974) Benign intracranial hypertension. Diagnosis and prognosis. Brain 97: 289–298

33 — Surgical Management of Hydrocephalus Accompanying Cystic Lesions in Infancy

Tetsuhiko Asakura, Masaki Niiro, Fumiaki Yuhi, and Kanetaka Kimotsuki[1]

Summary. We report four cases of acute hydrocephalus caused by cystic lesions in infancy and discuss the therapeutical problems involved in the management of this type of hydrocephalus. The mass lesions were an astrocytoma, a choroid plexus papilloma, an angioma, and an arachnoid cyst. Cystic tumors in infancy are always large by the time they are diagnosed, so that intracranial pressure (ICP) is always high and general condition is sometimes poor. It is preferable that ICP is reduced gradually when preparing for operation. Therefore, a stepwise procedure is recommended, that is, a draining procedure prior to the radical operation. In a baby with a fairly enlarged head, rapid reduction of ICP is danger, along with massive bleeding. Conditions are more favorable for us if we have enough time to carry out further examinations, such as cerebral angiography, MRI, and more detailed evaluations of the patient's general condition. Cyst drainage is effective for managing hydrocephalus in cystic tumors. If the production of fluid in the cyst is not great, a repeated tap through the reservoir is always sufficient for managing the increased ICP. Also, echography, in addition to conventional computed tomography (CT) scanning and magnetic resonance imaging (MRI), is useful in observing the size of the cyst or the ventricle.

Keywords. Hydrocephalus — Cystic tumors — In infancy — Cyst drainage — Cranial cchography

Introduction

Infantile hydrocephalus caused by cystic tumors or cysts is considered to be rare and in some therapeutical problems are involved in its management. An enlarged head or increased intracranial pressure (ICP) is always seen by the time the condition is diagnosed. Emergency operation is sometimes necessary

---

[1] Department of Neurosurgery, Faculty of Medicine, University of Kagoshima, Kagoshima, 890 Japan

but the general condition of the infant is sometimes poor and, in some tumors, massive bleeding occurs during operation. Therefore, we usually carry out a stepwise procedure, that is, a draining procedure prior to the radical operation. In this paper we report the results of our surgical therapy and discuss the surgical management problems.

Patients and Methods

Four infants (under 1-year-old) with acute hydrocephalus caused by cystic mass lesions were the subjects (Table 1). All patients had CT scans and cranial echograpy and three had MRI and cerebral angiography. Two brain tumors and an angioma were treated by drainage procedure prior to the radical operation, and an arachnoid cyst was treated by cyst-peritoneal shunt. The echograms were obtained with a static or real-time scanner in the coronal and sagittal planes. A 3.5 or 5.0 MHz transducer was used.

Results

The lesion masses were a plexus papilloma, an angioma, an arachnoid cyst and an astrocytoma. Varying degrees of hydrocephalus accompanied each lesion. In three of the four cases, an enlarged head or signs of increased ICP were seen when diagnosed. CT scans and MRI showed mass lesions clearly and accurately. Echograms also showed the tumor masses and adjacent structures, demonstrating the distinction between cysts and ventricle particularly clearly. After operation, subdural effusion appeared and a mild residual ventricular dilatation resulted in some cases, but the clinical results after 6 months–3½ years were satisfactory.

Case 1: 10-Month-Old Female

About three months before admission, her large head was noted when she

Table 1. Summary of findings in hydrocephalus with cystic lesions in infancy

Case age and sex	Location	Character of neuroimaging	Angiogram	Surgical procedure	Diagnosis
1. 10M. F.	Lt. lateral ventricle	Homogenously enhanced mass with cystic ventricular dilatation	Tumor blush	Repeated tap removal	Plexus papilloma
2. 7M. M.	Lt. the thalamus ~ basal ganglia	Nodular enhancement in the medial wall of the cyst Mild ventricular dilatation	Vascular	Repeated tap removal	Capillary hemangioma
3. 4M. F.	Paracollicular	Huge cyst with marked hydrocephalus	None	C-P shunt	Arachnoid cyst
4. 9M. F.	Rt. Frontal	Nodular enhancement with multiple cyst Contralateral hydrocephalus	Avascular	Continuous drainage removal	Malignant astrocytoma

visited the nearest hospital. Several days before admission, her mother found that she could not grasp her bottle or toys with her right hand.

Physical and Neurological Examination

The circumference of her head was 48.5 cm, the size of the anterior fontanelle was 4.2 × 3.7 cm and its tension was high. Neurological examination showed right hemiparesis and mental and physical retardation of two or three months.

Neuroradiological Findings

1. CT scan revealed a left hemispheric large cystic lesion which was separated into two spaces by a membranous structure. A round isodensity mass mixed with a low density spot was observed in the medial side of the cyst. The mass lesion was homogenously enhanced by the contrast medium. The midline structure was shifted to the right side (Fig. 1).
2. On MRI, T1 weighted images showed a mass of isointensity mixed with low intensity and T2 weighted images showed a slightly high intensity mass bordered by a low intensity band from the surrounding structure. On the cranial margin of the large cyst, MRI showed thin cerebral cortex. On the T2 weighted images, the signal intensity of the cystic parts was slightly higher than that of the contralateral ventricle. The solid mass situated in the trigone of the left lateral ventricle was homogenously enhanced by the contrast medium (Fig. 2).
3. On the left cerebral angiogram, performed after drainage, the tumor stain was seen from the arterial phase to the venous phase. The tumor was fed by the anterior and lateral posterior choroidal arteries and the posterior temporal artery.

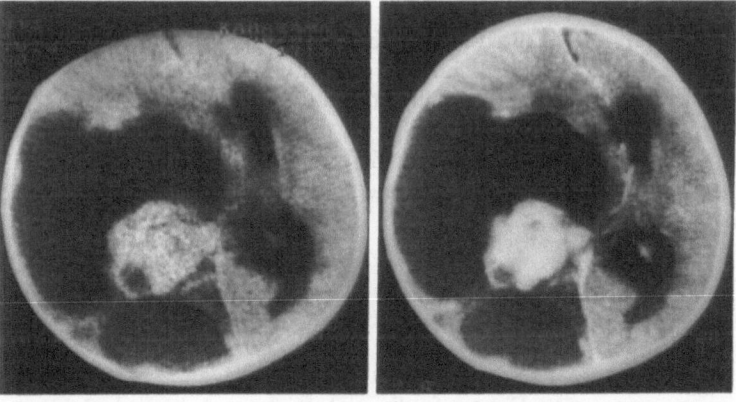

Fig. 1. Case 1: CT scan revealing a left hemispheric large cystic lesion separated into two spaces by a membranous structure. A round isodensity mass mixed with a low density spot was observed in the medial side of the cyst. The mass lesion is enhanced homogenously by the contrast medium

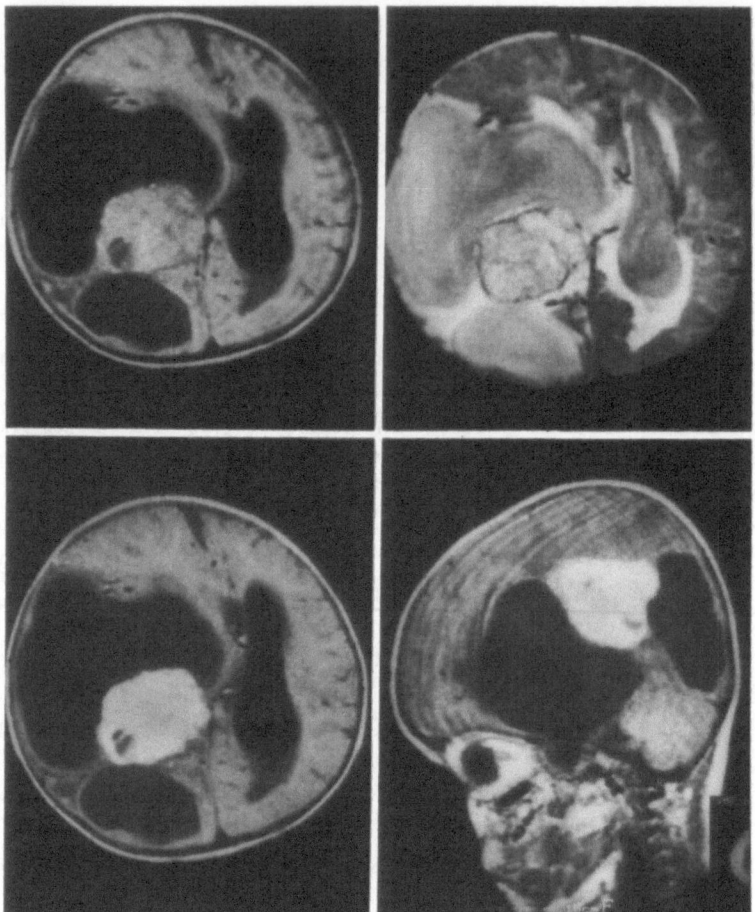

Fig. 2. Case 1: MRI, T1 weighted images showing a mass of isointensity mixed with low intensity and T2 weighted images showing a slightly high intensity mass bordered by a low intensity band from the surrounding structure. On the cranial margin of the large cyst, the thin cerebral cortex is shown. On the T2 weighted images, the signal intensity of the cystic parts is slightly higher than that of the contralateral ventricle. The solid mass situated in the trigone of the left lateral ventricle is homogenously enhanced by the contrast medium

Clinical Course After Admission

After admission, clinical signs due to increased ICP, such as vomiting and poor temper, were apparent. First of all, a left frontal burr hole was opened. Xanthochromic fluid was aspirated and an Ommaya reservoir was set up. After continuous draining, the clinical signs due to increased ICP improved. But as the cysts were reduced, a subdural effusion appeared (Fig. 3), so that cyst fluid had to be aspirated every two or three days through the reservoir; this was observed by cranial echography. Some residual examinations such as

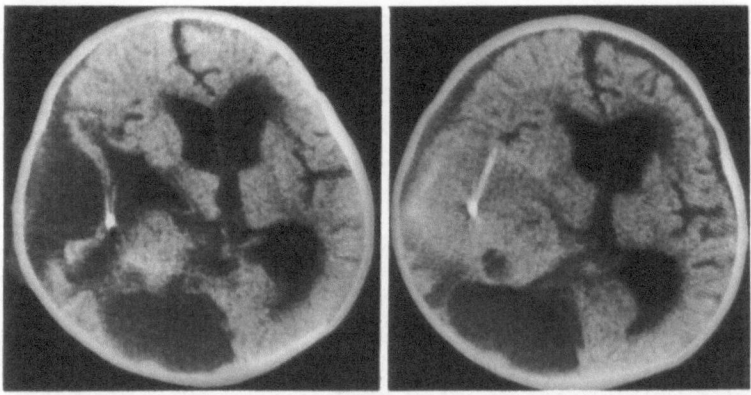

Fig. 3. Case 1: post-drainage CT scan showing the subdural effusion in the left temporal region (*left*). Cystography showing the isolated cystic cavity (*right*)

angiography, for example, were then completed. After that, the radical operation was done. The cyst wall was the ependyma of the ventricle and the cyst was divided into two spaces by a membranous structure. During the operation the distinction between the solid mass and the cystic part was well visualized by echogram. Ultimately, the cystic part of the tumor seen on the images was found to be in the partially dilated inferior horn of the lateral ventricle obstructing the trigone. The histological diagnosis was choroid plexus papilloma. After removal of the tumor, head enlargement ceased, but ventricular dilatation and slight subdural effusion continued.

Case 2: 7-Month-Old Male

One month after birth, a disturbance of ocular movement, that is, conjugate deviation to the left side, was found. Four months after birth, disturbed movement was found in his right hand. Three weeks before admission, when visiting the neurosurgical hospital, the abnormal CT scan finding was noted.

Physical and Neurological Findings

The circumference of his head was 43.5 cm; the anterior fontanelle was not enlarged, but tension its was slightly high. Neurological examination showed right hemiparesis.

Neuroradiological Findings

1. CT scan revealed a cystic mass lesion in the left basal ganglia. By contrast medium, a nodularly enhanced lesion was seen in the left thalamus; this was the medial side of the cyst. The lateral ventricle was moderately enlarged and the left side was compressed and deformed (Fig. 4).
2. On MRI, the nodular lesion showed isointensity with mixed low and high intensity spots on the T1 weighted images. On the T2 weighted images the

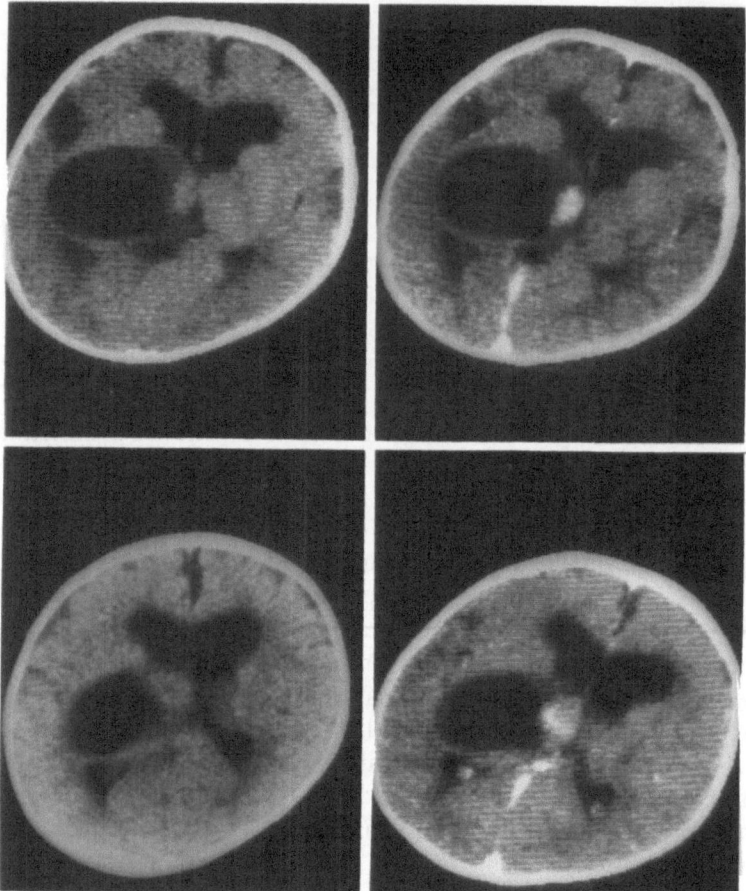

Fig. 4. Case: CT scan revealing a cystic mass lesion in the left basal ganglia. By contrast medium, a nodularly enhanced lesion is seen in the left thalamus; this is the medial side of the cyst. The lateral ventricle is moderately enlarged and the left side is compressed and deformed

lesion also showed isointensity with mixed contrasting high and low intensity spots. The lesion was homogenously enhanced by the contrast medium. The signal intensity of the cyst was slightly higher than that of the ventricle. The third ventricle was compressed by the tumor and the lateral ventricle was mildly dilated (Fig. 5).

3. On the left cerebral angiogram, performed after drainage, a small stain fed by the anterior choroidal artery was seen (Fig. 6).

Clinical Course After Admission

First of all, a left frontal burr hole was opened. Xanthochromic fluid was aspirated and an Ommaya reservoir was set up. When aspiration was dis-

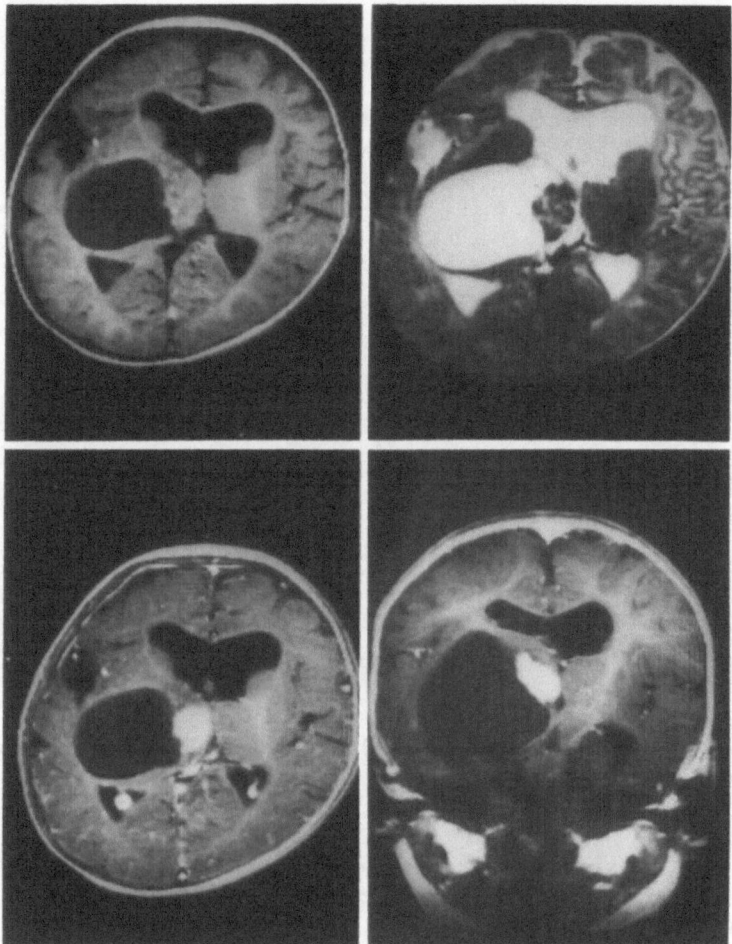

Fig. 5. Case 2: MRI showing the nodular lesion which shows isointensity with mixed low and high intensity spots on the T1 weighted images. On the T2 weighted images the lesion also shows isointensity with mixed contrasting high and low intensity spots. The lesion is homogenously enhanced by the contrast medium. The signal intensity of the cyst is slightly higher than that of the ventricle. The third ventricle is compressed by the tumor and the lateral ventricle is mildly dilated

continued, signs of increased ICP such as vomiting and poor temper appeared. Echography was useful for revealing the enlarged cyst and the compression of the ventricle (Fig. 7). After that, cyst fluid was aspirated every day under echography. After the necessary examinations were completed, the radical operation was done. Histological examination revealed the angiomatous malformation like capillary hemangioma. After the removal of the angioma, the subdural effusion was appeared and continued.

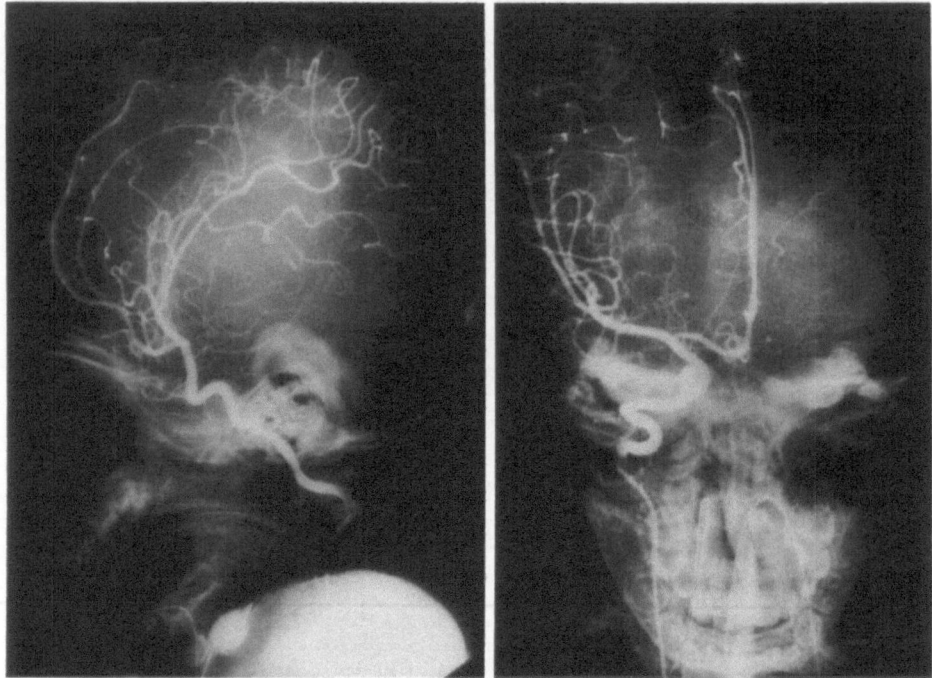

Fig. 6. Case 2: left cerebral angiogram (*CAG*) showing a small stain fed by the anterior choroidal artery

Case 3: 4-Month-Old Female

Four days before delivery, echography indicated suspected hydrocephalus. After a normal delivery, CT scan revealed a paracollicular cystic mass without hydrocephalus. Because the circumference of her head was normal, no treatment was given. Four months after birth, her head gradually became enlarged.

Physical and Neurological Findings

The circumference of her head was 48.5 cm, the size of the anterior fontanelle was 2.5 × 4.5 cm and its tension was high.

Neuroradiological Findings

1. MRI obtained after birth showed a paracollicular cystic mass without hydrocephalus (Fig. 8).
2. CT scan before admission showed a large cystic mass lesion, which occupied the midline structure and spread diffusely from the infratentorial to the supratentorial region.
3. On MRI after admission, the cyst extended from the superior cerebellum to the interhemispheric space and the corpus callosum was displaced archedly.

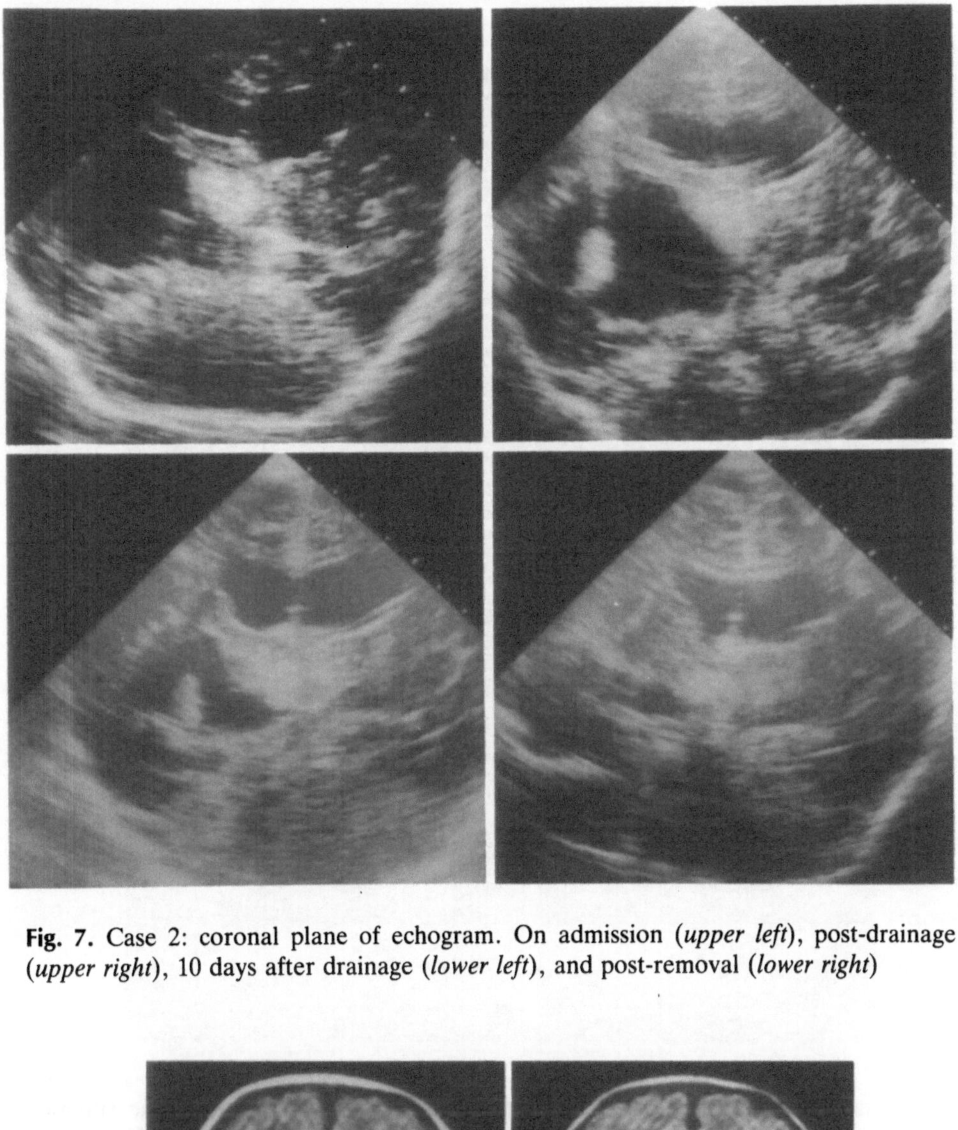

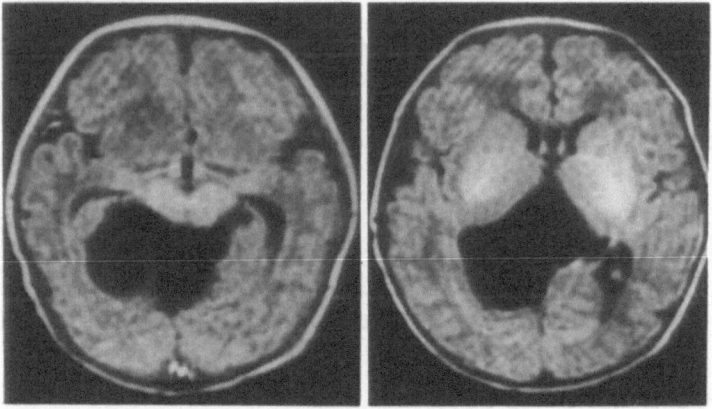

Fig. 7. Case 2: coronal plane of echogram. On admission (*upper left*), post-drainage (*upper right*), 10 days after drainage (*lower left*), and post-removal (*lower right*)

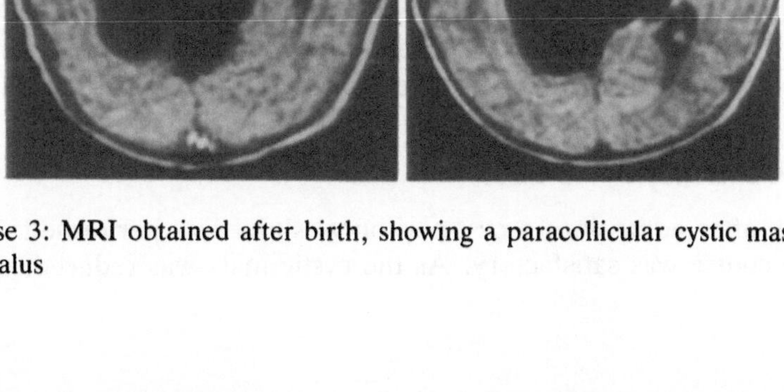

Fig. 8. Case 3: MRI obtained after birth, showing a paracollicular cystic mass without hydrocephalus

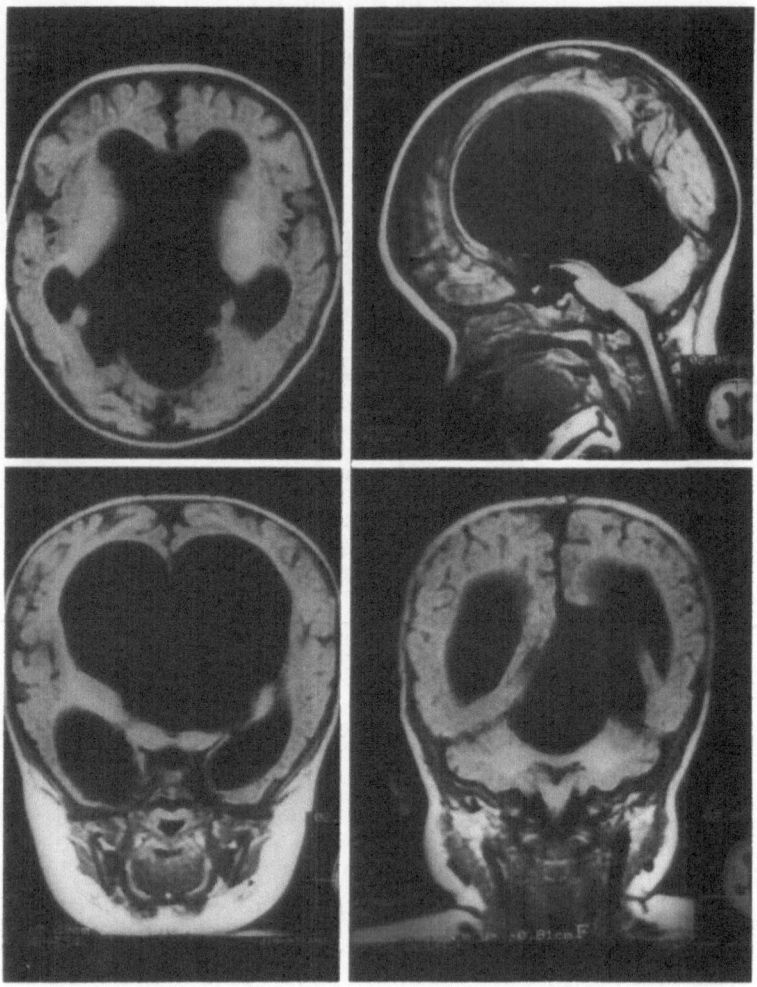

Fig. 9. Case 3: MRI after admission, showing the cyst extending from the superior cerebellum to the interhemispheric space. The corpus callosum is displaced archedly. The third ventricle and the inferior horn are remarkably dilated, but the anterior horn and the body of the lateral ventricle are compressed

The third ventricle and the inferior horn were remarkably dilated, but the anterior horn and the body of the lateral ventricle were compressed (Fig. 9).
4. Echogram obtained through the anterior fontanelle showed an enlarged lateral ventricle and a cystic mass situated between the ventricles.

Clinical Course After Admission

One week after admission, a cyst-peritoneal shunt was performed. The post-operative course was satisfactory. As the cystic mass was reduced, the hydro-

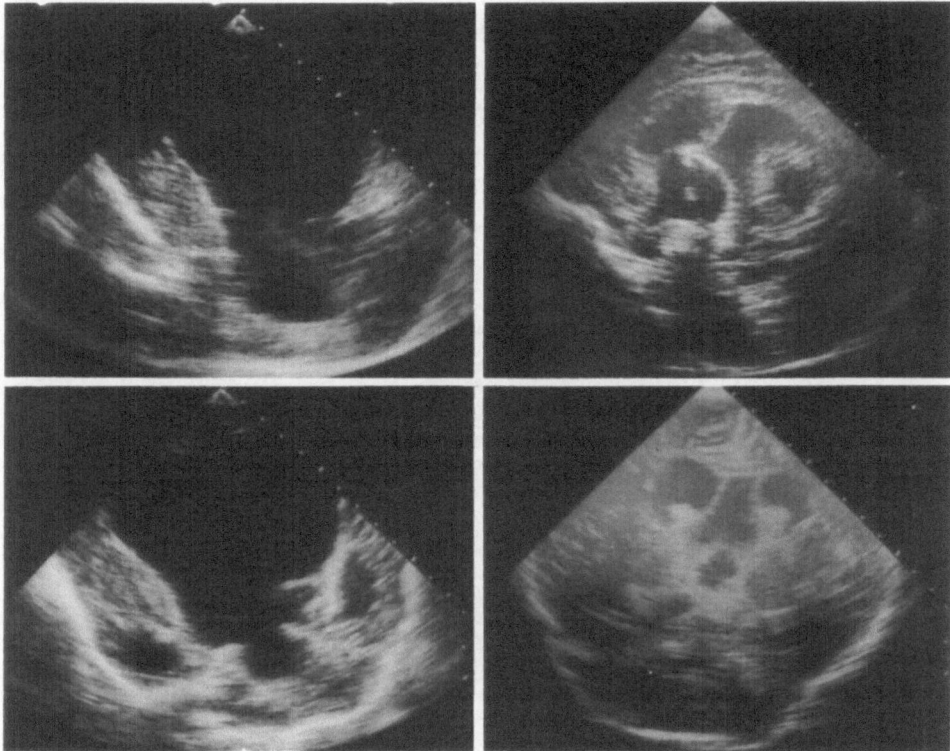

Fig. 10. Case 3: preoperative (*left*) and postoperative (*right*) echograms. The *upper* ones show the sagittal and the *lower* show the coronal plane. The echogram shows the course of cyst and ventricle reduction well. The distinction of cyst from ventricle was visualized better by postoperative echogram

cephalus improved. The course of the cyst and ventricle reduction was well followed by echography and, furthermore, distinction of cyst from ventricle was visualized better than by other means (Fig. 10). Post-operative cystography revealed that the cystic cavity did not communicate with the CSF pathway. The final diagnosis of this case was paracollicular arachnoid cyst.

Case 4: 9-Month-Old Female

Five months after birth, her mother found that movement of her left extremities was poor when she crawled on all fours. One week before admission, she was seen to be somewhat ill. Three days before admission, she vomited suddenly and from that time her consciousness gradually became impaired. She vomited frequently and on the night prior to admission she had frequent tonic convulsions.

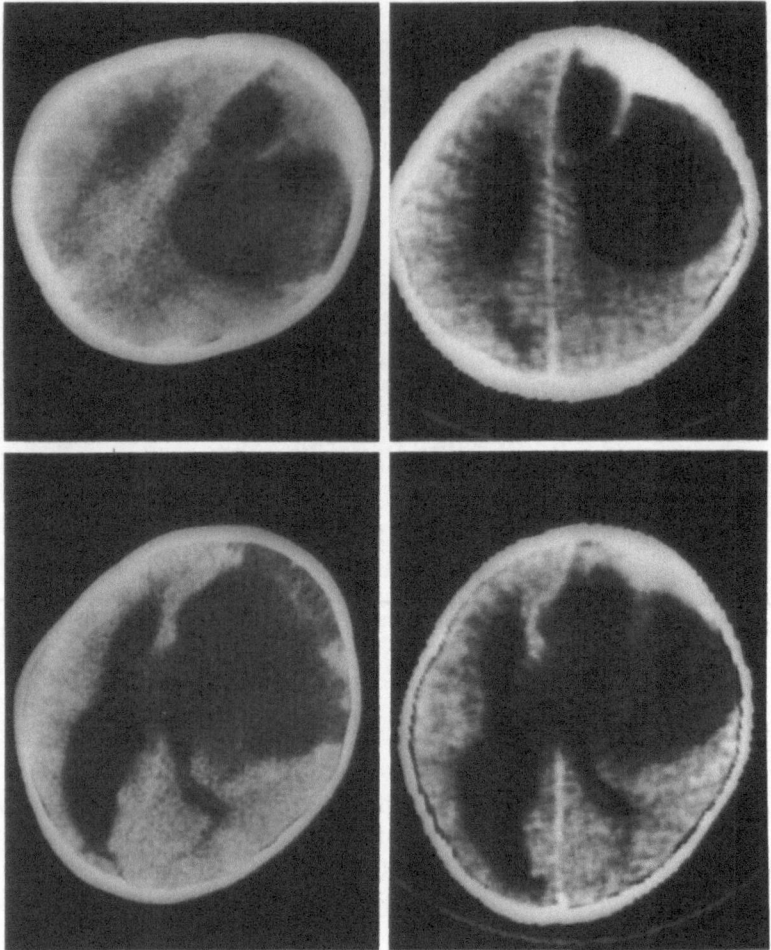

Fig. 11. Case 4: CT scan showing right frontal multicystic mass lesion and antero-lateral part of cyst wall enhanced nodularly. Midline structure shifted to the left and contralateral ventricular dilatation is also seen

Physical and Neurological Findings

The circumference of her head was 48 cm, the size of the anterior fontanelle was 1.5 × 2.0 cm and its tension was high. Neurological examination showed disturbance of consciousness (J.C.S.: 1-1-restless) and left hemiparesis.

1. CT scan showed a right frontal multicystic mass lesion and nodular enhancement of the antero-lateral part of the cyst wall. The midline structure was shifted to the left and contralateral ventricular dilatation was also seen (Fig. 11).

Fig. 12. Case 4: Echogram through the anterior fontanelle, showing the multicystic mass lesion more clearly than on the CT scan

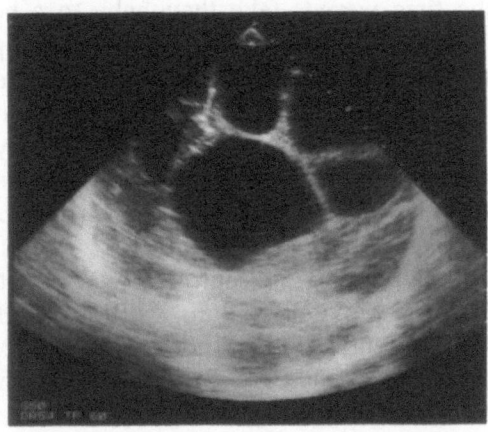

2. Echogram through the anterior fontanelle showed the multicystic mass lesion more clearly than on CT scan (Fig. 12).

3. Right cerebral angiogram, performed after drainage, showed a large right frontal avascular mass accompanied by severe mass effects.

Clinical Course After Admission

An emergency operation was performed on the day of admission. A right frontal burr hole was opened. Xanthochromic and viscous fluid was aspirated and continuous cyst drainage was set up. After drainage, signs of increased ICP such as vomiting, convulsions, and disturbance of consciousness disappeared. After these procedures further examination was completed. Nine days after drainage, the radical operation was performed. The tumor was removed and the cystic cavity was opened. Histological diagnosis was malignant astrocytoma. Post-operative radiation therapy was carried out. At present, 3½ years after operation, she shows no neurological deficits.

Discussion

Brain tumors in infants are considered to be rare. According to the Brain Tumor Registry in Japan (1982), the incidence of brain tumors in childhood is almost 15% of total brain tumors and the proportion of infants is 2% of childhood brain tumors. Reported brain tumors in infancy are astrocytomas, teratomas, plexus papillomas, ependymomas or ependymoblastomas, glioblastomas, and oligodendrogliomas (Iwasaki et al. 1980; Hayashi et al. 1983; Kikuchi et al. 1985; Kawano et al. 1986; Uematsu et al. 1986). Astrocytomas, teratomas, and plexus papillomas are more common. The clinical diagnosis of brain tumors in infancy is often difficult because focal neurological deficits are lacking as an initial sign (Han et al. 1984). An enlarged head or signs of increased ICP or convulsion are the most common chief complaints. But by the time parents take their baby to a hospital, the tumor has often become extremely large and is sometimes accompanied by obstructive hydrocephalus. In our reported cases, except for a case of angioma, enlarged heads and signs of increased ICP were the chief clinical manifestations on admission.

The locations of brain tumors in infancy differ from those in childhood. They are more common in the supratentorial region in infants than in older children (Iwasaki et al. 1980). In three of our four cases tumors were located in the supratentorial region and one, a paracollicular arachnoid cyst, extended both supratentorially and infratentorially. Obstructive hydrocephalus originating from the supratentorial mass seems to differ slightly from that originating from the infratentorial mass. In our case of plexus parilloma, the tumor occupied the trigone of the lateral ventricle and the inferior horn was dilated cystically. In our case of angioma, a large cyst compressed the third ventricle and the CSF flow from the foramen of Monro to the aqueduct was thought to be disturbed. In our case of astrocytoma, tentorial herniation was thought to be the origin of the contralateral obstructive hydrocephalus. In our case of paracollicular arachnoid cyst, the aqueduct was obstructed by the huge arachnoid cyst. In infratentorially located brain tumors in older children, hydrocephalus due to obstruction of the aqueduct or fourth ventricle is common. However, in infants, partial or unilateral dilatation of the lateral ventricle and third ventricular compression seems to occur relatively rarely.

We will now discuss the therapy used and the therapeutical problems encountered in each of our cases. In arachnoid cysts, when there are signs of increased ICP and accompanied obstructive hydrocephalus, or when there are focal signs due to arachnoid cysts, surgical therapy is considered necessary. (Hayashi et al. 1987). Craniotomy with membranectomy and ventriculoperitoneal or cyst-peritoneal shunt has always been carried out (Hayashi et al. 1987; Karube et al. 1985), but there is no definite consensus about which method is the best. A paracollicular arachnoid cyst which sometimes begins in infancy does not present an enlarged head at birth. Several months after birth, the infant's head becomes rapidly enlarged, as was the case with our patient (Karube et al. 1985). Because the clinical course is always rapid, a shunting procedure should be performed first of all. In a non-communicating paracolicullar cyst, the cyst-peritoneal shunt is preferable. But if only the shunt operation is performed, as some authors have pointed out (Hayashi et al. 1987), there is some danger of overshunting and resulting, subdural effusion or hematoma; small head size may also result from overshunting. The obstruction of the shunt is also a danger. In our case, after the operation, a thin subdural effusion without any neurological signs was seen on the CT scan. Careful observation was necessary. The echogram through the anterior fontanelle was useful for evaluating the size of the cyst and the ventricle, and the membranous wall between the cyst and the ventricle was well visualized.

In the case of plexus papilloma, overproduction of CSF is thought to be the cause of hydrocephalus. In younger children there were some cases which showed partial cystic dilatation of the lateral ventricle caused by the obstruction of the tumor (Kawano et al. 1986; Uematsu et al. 1986). In these cases, it was preferable to do cyst drainage first. In operating on plexus papillomas, massive bleeding is always seen. Therefore it is necessary to ensure that ICP is reduced gradually before operation and that the patient's general condition is well maintained. In our case, a subdural effusion occurred after drainage and continued after the radical operation. After operation, there may be a problem in that the dilated ventricle is not reduced. A V-P shunt is sometimes necessary (Kawano et al. 1986). In our case, the thin subdural effusion continued, along with the ventricular dilatation. No clinical signs are seen now, but careful observation is necessary.

In the case of cystic angioma, which is very rare, ventricular dilatation was moderate. When cyst drainage was discontinued, the cyst and lateral ventricle became enlarged and signs of ICP became apparent. In this situation, changes of the cyst and ventricle were clearly observed by echograpy. A subdural effusion occurred after operation in this case also.

In the case of astrocytoma, ICP was considered to be so high that transtentorial herniation was impending. Emergency operation was necessary to reduce the ICP. The echogram was useful for evaluating the multiple nature of the cyst and it enabled us to visualize the septums between the cysts more clearly than the CT scan. We were able to drain the largest cyst guided by the echogram.

As mentioned above, there are some characteristic findings in cystic tumors in infancy. They are always large by the time they are diagnosed, so that ICP is always high and general condition is sometimes poor. Tumors often have rich vascularity; during operation, bleeding is massive and we should be careful of hypotensive shock (Kawano et al. 1986). It is preferable that ICP is reduced gradually when preparing for operation. In a baby with a fairly enlarged head, there is a danger of hypotensive shock along with massive bleeding if ICP is reduced rapidly. Conditions are more favorable for us if we have enough time to carry out further examinations, such as cerebral angiograms, MRI, and more detailed evaluations of the patient's general condition. There are two methods for reducing increased ICP temporarily. One is continuous drainage, and the other is repeated tapping through a set reservoir. As compared with solid tumors, cyst drainage is effective for managing the hydrocephalus in cystic tumors. Because the production of fluid in the cyst is not great, repeated tapping through the reservoir is always sufficient for managing the increased ICP. For preventing infections, it is important to avoid drainage which lasts too long. After the radical operation, subdural effusion often appeared and ventricular dilatation was residual. Careful observation was necessary for these post-operative problems.

There are some merits in echography (Han et al. 1984; Slovis and Kuhns 1981). It is a non-invasive method and it is possible to use it repeatedly at the bedside. Echography makes it possible to show lesions with passing time. It can accurately demonstrate the location and extent of the tumors, show the mass effect to adjacent structures, visualize the septum of the cysts and make a distinction between cyst and ventricle. Echography is said to be useful as a screening procedure in infants who have a large head or abnormal neurological findings and it is a useful guiding tool in operations (Han et al. 1984; Slovis and Kuhns 1981).

In managing hydrocephalus with cystic lesions in infancy, a stepwise procedure, that is, a draining procedure prior to the radical operation is recommended. Echography, in addition to conventional CT scanning and MRI, is useful in the management of this condition.

References

Han BK, Babcock DS, Oestreich AE (1984) Sonography of brain tumors in infants. AJNR 5: 253–258

Hayashi R, Hashimoto T, Fukusumi A (1983) A case of teratoma in newborn. Nerv Syst Child 8: 17–24

Hayashi T, Honda E, Anegawa S, Kuramoto S (1987) Clinical evaluation of children with intracranial arachnoid cysts treated surgically. Nerv Syst Child 12: 185–192

Iwasaki Y, Wakai S, Matsutani M, Takakura K, Sano K (1980) Brain tumors in infants. Nerv Syst Child 5: 391–398

Karube T, Yano S, Miyao M, Kamoshita S, Iwasa H, Shimabukuro H, Yamada N, Murase I (1985) Three cases of arachnoid cyst of the quadrigeminal cistern. Nerv Syst Child 10: 347–352

Kawano H, Hayashi M, Kubota T, Ishikura A, Kobayashi H, Tsuji T (1986) Infantile choroid plexus papilloma. Nerv Syst Child 11: 193–198

Kikuchi K, Kamisato N, Kowada M, Mineura K (1985) Large cystic oligodendroglioma in childhood. Nerv Syst Child 10: 329–334

Slovis TL, Kuhns LR (1981) Real-time sonography of the brain through the anterior fontanelle. AJR 136: 277–286

The committee of the Brain Tumor Registry in Japan (1982) Brain tumors in children. pp 26–30

Uematsu Y, Kuwata T, Iwamoto M, Kuriyama T, Shizuki K (1986) Choroid plexus papilloma of the lateral ventricle with relapsing intraventricular hemorrhage in an infant. Nerv Syst Child 11: 415–420

34 — Pathophysiological Considerations of Subdural Fluid Collection in Childhood

Hiroshi Itoh and Tetsuro Miwa[1]

Summary. In childhood, subdural fluid collection often affects the developing brain, but the clinical significance of various states of hydrocephalus is imperfectly understood. This study consists of 61 patients under three years of age who had subdural fluid collection. The subjects were classified as follows: Group A (posttraumatic) 41 cases, Group B (unknown origin) 12 cases, Group C (complicated with cerebral dysgenesis) 8 cases. Subdural fluid pressure was high (more than 180 mmH$_2$O) in Group A. Continued low or normal pressure was observed in 10 out of 19 cases from Groups B and C. Ventricular reflux and delayed clearance of metrizamide on computed tomography (CT)-cisternography was seen in 11 out of 15 cases in Groups B and C. In 8 of the 61 cases two-space communication, including late filling of the subdural space with contrast medium, was observed. Magnetic resonance imaging (MRI) and CT scans showed enlarged ventricles and subdural spaces with a sulcal pattern in most cases in Group B. The prognosis varied significantly, and severe brain dysfunction was common in Group B. This may have been due to the prolonged suppression of the brain by the large amounts of subdural fluid retained for more than three months, and to brain anomalies such as holoprosencephaly. We concluded that determination of subdural fluid pressure was significant for estimating the degree of brain damage with craniocerebral disproportion and for providing information for therapeutic purposes. The pathophysiological condition of hydrocephalus and brain atrophy accompanied by subdural fluid collection is discussed in detail.

Keywords. Subdural fluid collection — Intracranial CSF pressure — CT scan — Cisternography — Craniocerebral disproportion

Introduction

In childhood, subdural fluid collection affects the developing brain and can disturb physical and mental development. Some cases show poor clinical

[1] Department of Neurosurgery, Tokyo Medical College, Shinjuku-Ku, Tokyo, 160 Japan

353

courses and results despite treatment that by conventional standards would be considered sufficient. From the literature, it is apparent that there is considerable confusion regarding the pathogenesis of subdural fluid collection in childhood. This is well illustrated by the terms "external hydrocephalus" or "benign subdural effusion".

However, all these terms seem to describe similar cases or conditions. The pathological causes can be classified as posttraumatic, postmeningitic, various complicated congenital cerebral anomalies, and those of unknown origin. On a pathophysiological basis there is no clear correlation between subdural fluid collection and the stage of hydrocephalus. The aim of this paper is to present an analysis of the pathophysiological conditions of subdural fluid collection in childhood.

Subjects and Methods

This study examined 61 patients under three years of age who had subdural fluid collection. The subjects were classified as follows: Group A consisted of 41 cases with known causes (posttraumatic, postmeningitic); Group B consisted of 12 cases of unknown origin; Group C consisted of 8 cases accompanied by cerebral dysgenesis (holoprosencephaly, cerebral dysgenesis).

All subjects were treated in the Tokyo Medical College hospital, Tokyo, from 1980 to 1990. Figures in parentheses in Table 1 are the number of children who had craniocerebral disproportion. A total of 61 patients were investigated by neurological examination before and after surgery, neuroradiological studies of CT scan and MR images, intracranial pressure (ICP) monitoring, and metrizamide CT-cisternography. Regional cerebral blood flow (CBF) study revealed the following distribution of IMP-SPECT.

Results

Perinatal abnormalities were observed in 10 patients in Groups B and C. The head size increased steadily in 10 patients in Group A. However, there were 4 cases of decreased head size in Group B. Patients in Group B had the highest mean age at admission. Clinical symptoms and signs are shown in Table 2.

Table 1. Cases of subdural fluid collection in patients under 3 years of age (Sept. 1990)

	No. of cases (n)	Survival	Death
A Original disease (trauma, meningitis)	41	40	1
B Unknown origin	12	9 (4)	3 (1)
C Associated with cerebral anomaly	8	4 (2)	4 (1)
Total	61	53 (6)	8 (2)

Figures in parentheses indicate numbers of children who had craniocerebral disproportion

Table 2. Perinatal history and clinical findings

	A (n = 41)	B (n = 12)	C (n = 8)
Perinatal history			
Abnormal delivery	1	2	3
asphyxia	1	2	1
SFD	1	1	1
Age at admission	3.0 months	5.0 months	2.7 months
Head circumference			
>2SD	10	1	4
<2SD	4	4	0
Clinical sings and Symptoms			
Convulsion	15(37%)	7(58%)	3
Irritability	9	5(42%)	4(50%)
Vomiting	23(56%)	3	6(75%)
Tense fontanelle	21(51%)	1	4(50%)
Impaired conscious.	4	0	1

SFD, small for date; SD, standard deviation

In Group A, 21 out of 41 patients had increased tension of the fontanel and vomiting. In Group B, 7 out of 12 patients had general convulsions at admission and the other 5 patients were in an irritable state. Patients in Group B had the least tendency to show increased ICP.

The patients with poor prognoses in Groups B and C in particular had indications of possible intrauterine problems or irreversible brain damage suffered during the perinatal period.

Despite treatment, there were 8 cases of craniocerebral disproportion in Groups B and C. In all patients except one, no shrinkage was observed in the subdural space after repeated operation. Six of these patients were suspected of having slight psychomotor retardation and 2 patients died.

Generally, in Group A, large amounts of fluid volume over the surface of the brain healed without any trouble.

In most cases, CT scans revealed accumulations of varying amounts of fluid within the subdural and subarachnoid spaces. In 11 out of 20 cases in Groups B

Table 3. CT Scan

	A (n = 41)	B (n = 12)	C (n = 8)
Width of subdural space (more than 10 mm)	7	6	5
Dilatation of cerebral sulci (sulcal pattern)	6	7	4
Enlargement of interhemisph. fissure	5	6	5
BC index >25	8	7	5
Cranial deformity and others	7	4	3

BC, bicaudate index

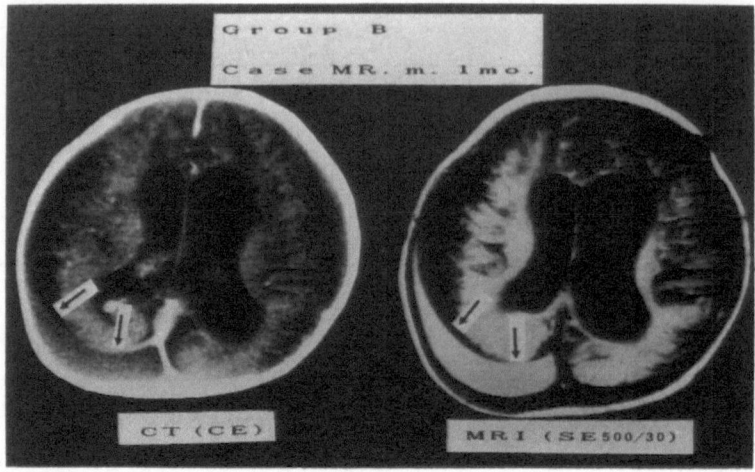

Fig. 1. Case 1:1-month-old male. MRI shows high signal in subdural space and low signal in subarachnoid space (*right*) The sulcal pattern of CT images indicates the possibility of secondary brain atrophy (*left*)

and C, a sulcal pattern and enlargement of subarachnoid spaces were observed. On CT images the width of the bifrontal caudate index was clearly seen to have increased more than 25% (Table 3).

After CT scans, MRI in 35 cases clearly revealed widened subarachnoid spaces bilaterally, frontally, and parietally, with a high signal for slightly bloody fluid in the subdural space. Figure 1 shows a case with large ventricles and subdural space with enlarged subarachnoid space. This case showed a high signal for bloody fluid in the parietoposterior region and a low signal for subarachnoid spaces, bilaterally throughout the brain surface. We were not able to obtain a significant correlation between the volumes of subdural or subarachnoid fluid in the two compartments or to determine prognosis.

ICP monitoring was performed by pressure transducer. Table 4 shows 22 Group A patients that demonstrated either continuous or intermittent high pressure. However, in 10 out of 19 patients in Groups B and C, the baseline pressure was continuously normal or low. It is interesting that there was a significant difference between the high pressure and low pressure cases.

From the results of the pressure study, good operative results can be expected in high pressure cases, while in cases showing low pressure with monophasic waves results are poor.

Table 4. ICP monitoring in subdural fluid collection

	A (n = 22)	B (n = 11)	C (n = 8)
1. High (base-line) pressure ($\geqq 180\,mmH_2O$)	8	0	0
2. Intermittent high pressure	14	3	6
3. Low (base-line) pressure ($\leqq 90\,mmH_2O$)	0	8	2

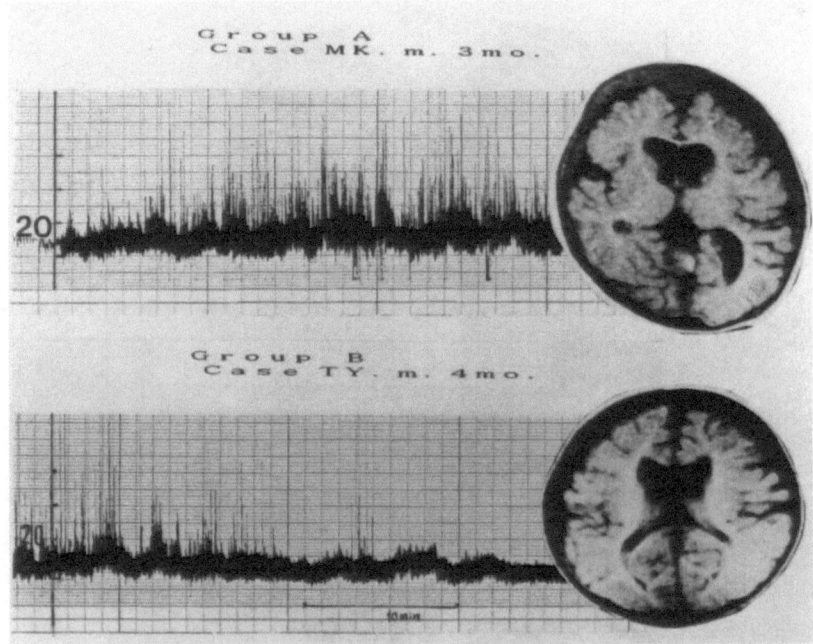

Fig. 2. ICP monitoring *Upper*, case 2:3-month-old male (group A), *Lower*, case 3:4-month-old male (group B). Base line pressure shows constant high pressure with B-like waves. MRI shows subdural fluid collection with slightly enlarged ventricles in both cases

Table 5. Metrizamide CT-cisternography

	A (n = 15)	B (n = 9)	C (n = 6)
Ventricular reflux ~ delayed clearance	6	6	5
Contrast block on convexity or basal cisterns	7	2	2
Two space communication (SDS → SAS), late filling of SDS	3	3	2
Ventricular enlargement	5	7	6

SDS, subdural space; SAS, subarachnoid space

Figure 2 shows two cases of high pressure with B-like waves and MR images. Metrizamide-CT cisternography was performed in 30 patients (Table 5). In 11 out of 15 patients in Groups A and C, ventricular reflux and delayed clearance was seen. However, 7 out of 15 patients in Group A showed blockage of the subarachnoid space and delayed absorption. Eight out of the 30 patients showed two-space communication, including late filling of the subdural space by contrast medium.

After the first surgery, the ventricular reflux disappeared. However, clearance of the contrast medium did not improve immediately. Using IMP-SPECT,

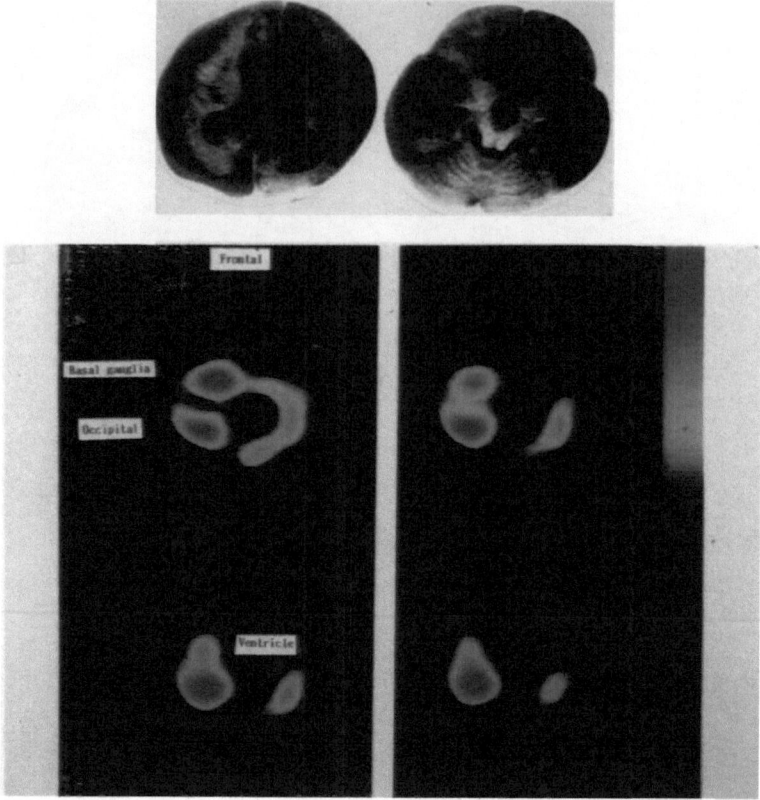

Fig. 3. Iodoamphetamine single photon emission computed tomography (IMP-SPECT). Case 4:7-month-old male (group B). Marked decrease of CBF is shown in a case of craniocerebral disproportion

we also attempted to determine changes in regional cerebral blood flow after surgery. In Group A and in recovery cases in Group B, the slight decrease of CBF was recovered in both frontal areas at 3 weeks after surgery. However, as seen in Fig. 3, a marked decrease of CBF was seen in a Group B case of severe craniocerebral disproportion in both hemispheres.

Discussion

Generally, pathological subdural fluid collection is located in the expanded subdural space, due to various pathological causes and processes. In our study, some cases revealed cerebrospinal fluid in the pathologically dilated subarachnoid space and enlargements of the ventricular system. In the literature, many authors have described a similar pathological condition by the use of terms such as benign communicating hydrocephalus (Forey 1955; Ito et al. 1987; Kendall et al. 1981), external hydrocephalus, and pseudohydrocephalusmegalocephaly. Anderson et al. (1984) interpreted results for the 7 patients that they studied as "abnormal fluid accumulation in the subarachnoid space under increased pressure, with slight widening of ventricles". Robertson et al. (1979) pointed out that the widening of the subarachnoid channel appears to occur during the first stage in the development of congenital hydrocephalus. From the literature (Barlow 1984; Chapman 1983; Robertson et al. 1979), it is apparent that there is considerable confusion regarding the pathogenesis of external hydrocephalus or subdural fluid collection.

A history of trauma, meningitis, perinatal causes and other factors have been reported (Ito et al. 1987; Matumoto and Tamaki 1986; Ment et al. 1981) in subdural fluid collection or so-called external hydrocephalus. The prognosis of this condition, when caused by subdural fluid collection of unknown origin was poor (Ito et al. 1987). Abnormal head growth or small head for the age of the child reflect evidence of pathologically increased intracranial pressure or secondary brain atrophy. Among infants with pathologically increasing head size, Anderson et al. (1984) and Mori et al. (1980) found a group with external hydrocephalus and a benign clinical course. In our series, all but 4 of our patients with subdural fluid collection of known origin developed normally.

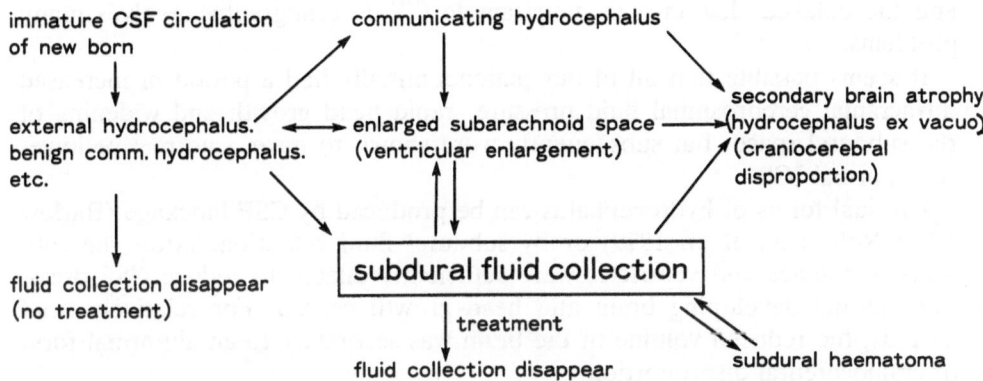

Fig. 4. Various pathogeneses of subdural fluid collection (or external hydrocephalus) and correlation of various states. A case showing subdural space enlargement (more than 10 mm in width) with wide subarachnoid space (sulcal pattern) and ventricle (BFI more than 30%) seemed to indicate brain atrophy (craniocerebral disproportion) in CT findings. BFI, bifrontal index

However, 5 out of 12 of our patients with subdural fluid collection of unknown origin developed abnormally.

The latter group of patients showed a small head and markedly widened subarachnoid space with dilated ventricles. All of our cases of craniocerebral disproportion showed similar changes. Robertson et al. (1979) reported that the dilatation of the subarachnoid space is due to mechanical blockage produced by abnormal retention of subdural fluid, while on the other hand, CSF communication between the ventricles and the dilated subarachnoid space is due to secondary brain atrophy. In our series, the disproportionate brain showed that re-expansion of the brain was not obtained postoperatively. Accordingly, differential diagnosis between an advanced condition of subdural fluid collection and brain atrophy is difficult. The clinical and radiological findings for chronic stage subdural fluid collection indicated decreased intracranial pressure. We have found that a pressure study can reveal the indications for operation and allow evaluation of cerebral function.

Metrizamide CT cisternography study of CSF dynamics in children with subdural fluid collection showed delayed clearance and delayed absorption of CSF (Maytal et al. 1987; Mori et al. 1980). Barlow (1984) reported that the isotope pattern seen in RI cisternography, which included delayed absorption and CSF reflux into the ventricles, was similar to that seen in communicating hydrocephalus, which led Maytal (1987) to call this condition "External obstructive hydrocephalus".

Metrizamide CT cisternography showed two-space communication of the subdural and subarachnoid spaces, with early inflow or late outflow of contrast medium. The pattern of radiologic findings in these patients, as regards the presence of the two-space communication, appears to suggest a tear in the arachnoid membrane. The absence of flow over the cerebral convexity and the delayed clearance in metrizamide CT cisternography involves many problems.

It seems possible that all of our patients initially had a period of increased intracranial cerebrospinal fluid pressure, rapid head growth and widening of the subdural space, but subsequently were shown to have a normal or lower than normal ICP.

Unusual forms of hydrocephalus can be produced by CSF blockage (Barlow 1984; Robertson et al. 1979) or by subdural fluid retention. After the subarachnoid space and ventricles were sufficiently dilated to reduce CSF pressure, normal developing brain and head growth ceased. For relatively brief periods, the reduced volume of the brain was secondary to an abnormal form of craniocerebral disproportion.

In our study, in those patients whose recovery was good CBF had returned to normal by three weeks after operation. However, there was marked decreas of CBF in patients who had severe craniocerebral disproportion of both hemispheres. Similar findings were seen in cases of severe cerebral atrophy after anoxic changes in the brain. Perinatal damage and the suppressive retention of large amounts of fluid in the subdural space due to unknown causes or combined cerebral dysgenesis are poor prognostic factors. Moreover, in patients in whom the condition has existed for more than 3 months prior to treatment, it is difficult to complete treatment and good results cannot be expected. The brain cannot be expected to recover in cases showing subdural space enlargement of more than 10 mm in width with wide subarachnoid space and ventricles suggesting brain atrophy. In the final stage, it becomes clear on CT scans that marked craniocerebral disproportion will continue.

Not only morphological studies of CT scans, but also further functional studies are necessary for evaluation of the effects of subdural fluid collection.

References

Andersson H, Elfverson J, Svensdsen P (1984) External hydrocephalus. Childs Brain 11: 389–402

Barlow CF (1984) CSF dynamics in hydrocephalus with special attention to external hydrocephalus. Brain Dev 6: 119–127

Chapman HP (1983) External hydrocephalus. In: Concepts in Pediatric Neurosurgery, vol. Karger, Basel, pp 102–118

Forey J (1955) Benign forms of intracranial hypertension. Brain 78: 1–41

Ito H, Takeda Y, Suzuki N, Inaba I, Asamoto M, Miwa T (1987) Clinical consideration of extreme craniocerebral disproportion due to severe subdural fluid collection in childhood. Nervous system in children (Tokyo) English abst. 12:151–159

Kendall B, Holland I (1981) Benign communicating hydrocephalus in children. Neuroradiology 21: 93–96

Matumoto S, Tamaki N (1986) Extracerebral collection. In: Vigouroux VP (ed), Advances in neurotraumatology. Springer, Wien, pp 135–146

Maytal J, Alvarez LA, Elkin CM, Shinnar S, (1987) External hydrocephalus; Radiologic spectrum and differentiation from cerebral atrophy. AJNR 8: 271–278

Ment LR, Ducan CC, Geehr R (1981) Benign enlargement of the subarachnoid space in the infant. J Neurosurg 54: 504–508

Mori K, Handa H, Itoh M, Okuno T (1980) Benign subdural effusion in infants. J Comput Assist Tomogr 4: 466–471

Robertson W, Chun R, Orrison W, Sackett J (1979) Benign subdural collection of infancy. J Pediatr 94: 382–385

35 — Hydrocephalus
Revision of its Classification

Koreaki Mori[1]

Summary. Progress in neuroimaging techniques has led to accumulation of an extensive body of information on hydrocephalus. Whereas most of the current classifications of this disorder are oversimplified, others are either not sufficiently specific or do not adequately reflect the variability of its characteristics, and as such, are of little help for pragmatic purposes and for patient prognostication. In this communication, a contemporary classification of hydrocephalus is presented, bearing in mind its role in the clinical management of cases, and its place in further research of the disorder.

Keywords. Hydrocephalus — Classification — Cerebrospinal fluid pathways — Pathophysiology — Revision

Introduction

Recent breakthroughs in neuroradiology have given a remarkable boost to our general understanding of the pathophysiology of hydrocephalus; this disorder is no longer regarded as a single disease entity, but rather as a sign resulting from disturbances in cerebrospinal fluid (CSF) dynamics — which disturbances themselves are induced by other disease processes. With the establishment of shunting operations for the treatment of hydrocephalus and the use of computed tomography (CT) scans for the follow-up of cases, conventional concepts of hydrocephalus have undergone considerable modification over the years (Matsumoto 1976; Raimondi 1986; Sato 1986). Conventional classifications of hydrocephalus describe the condition in such terms as "communicating" and "non-communicating", which refer to various forms of obstruction in the major CSF pathways. In many cases, however, (especially in congenital hydrocephalus, which constitutes the majority), studies of the CSF dynamics have often failed to demonstrate the presence of any verifiable obstruction. Furthermore, the CT scan, by virtue of its non-invasiveness, has made it possible

[1] Department of Neurosurgery, Kochi Medical School, Nankoku, Kochi, 783 Japan

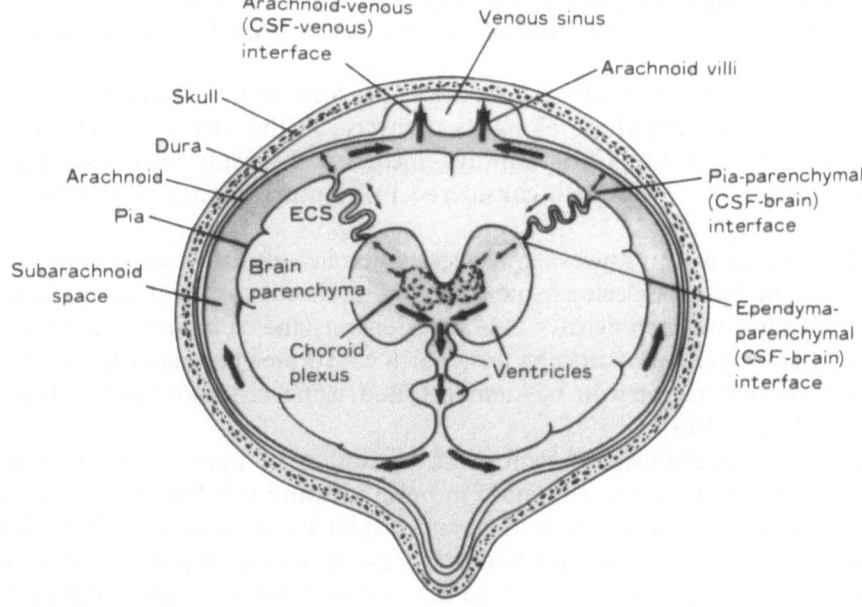

Fig. 1. Schematic drawing of CSF circulation ◀, bulk flow in "major pathway"; ←, "lesser pathway"; ECS, extracellular space in the white matter (glia-capillary complex)

for us to observe the morphological changes of hydrocephalus from its very beginning to the final stages. In the light of these factors, it has become necessary to revise the conventional classification of hydrocephalus.

Pathophysiology

The mechanisms of CSF production and absorption are still not clearly under-stood. Some studies have shown that choroidal and extrachoroidal production of CSF occurs simultaneously (Sato et al. 1972). The conventional concept is that CSF is absorbed through arachnoid villi in the pachionian granulations. Other possible routes that have been proposed include transependymal (Wislock and Putnum 1921; Bering and Sato 1976; Hopkins et al. 1977; Mori et al. 1977), transpial (Brightman 1968; Morse and Low 1972), and into the choroid plexus. By virtue of their connection with the ventricle through cell junctions, intracellular and extracellular spaces also serve as possible CSF pathways (Brightman 1965; Mori and Raimondi 1975; Raimondi 1986) (Fig. 1).

Diffuse white matter damage with consequent glial and capillary damage (Hassler 1964; Wozniak et al. 1975; Oka et al. 1985) accompanied by intracel-lular and extracellular fluid accumulation may be a possible mechanism for the occurrence of intraparenchymal hydrocephalus. Changes at this stage may correspond to brain edema; and increase in intraparenchymal fluid collection may lead to extraparenchymal collection (Reulen et al. 1978; Cao et al. 1984; Raimondi 1987). Ventricular dilatation may result from both of these processes.

Disturbances in CSF dynamics either take the form of impaired CSF absorption or obstruction anywhere along its pathways in the face of an unaltered rate of formation. Major CSF pathways, including the ventricular system and subarachnoid space, have been considered to be possible sites of obstruction (Milhorat 1972).

Such obstruction can, however, be ascertained in only a few conditions such as obstruction by mass lesions, membranous occlusion of ventricular outlets by ependymitis or meningitis, and adhesions in the subarachnoid spaces. However, in congenital hydrocephalus, which constitutes the majority of cases, no apparent obstruction can be demonstrated using cisternography (Drayer and Rosenbaum 1978).

The precise mechanism of ventricular dilatation in hydrocephalus is not known. In the early stages, alteration in pulse pressure (Di Rocco et al. 1978) and viscoelasticity of the brain (Hakim and Hakim 1984), against the back-flow due to CSF retention in subarachnoid spaces, may play important roles. In intraparenchymal hydrocephalus there may be increase in brain compliance, with the result that pulse waves originating from the choroid plexus may cause ventricular dilatation, even under normal intraventricular pressure. Prolonged parenchymal damage under pressure from collected fluid may lead to thinning of the cerebral mantle; and finally the ventricle and subarachnoid spaces may dilate because of brain atrophy — a condition known as "hydrocephalus *ex vacuo*."

Whereas ventriculomegaly might be absent in the early stages of hydrocephalus, there might be marked dilatation of the subarachnoid spaces (Raimondi 1987), with the latter leading to subdural fluid collection which might, however, be transient.

In congenital hydrocephalus, there is a disturbance of CSF absorption associated with increased CSF volume. Raimondi (1987) postulated the stages of progression of hydrocephalus, from intraparenchymal through extraparenchymal. These may correspond to changes in the main site of fluid collection. They include:

1. Intracellular fluid collection
2. Extracellular fluid collection
3. Subarachnoid fluid collection
4. Intraventricular fluid collection
5. Intraventricular and subarachnoid fluid collection.

Stages 1 and 2, which correspond to early changes of parenchymal destruction, may not be observed on neuroimaging. Dilatation of the subarachnoid spaces may be seen on CT and magnetic resonance imaging. Stage 4 corresponds to the typical picture of hydrocephalus. In stage 5, brain atrophy results in whole extraparenchymal fluid collection, which corresponds to late changes of parenchymal destruction.

Brain parenchymal damage may be diffuse or focal. Both types may, however, be combined, as occurs in such conditions as infarction, intracerebral hematoma, and brain contusion. Ventricular dilatation with inappropriate focal dilatation may occur as a result of these.

Classifications

Even though intracranial retention of CSF occurs in all forms of hydrocephalus, it is not always accompanied by ventricular dilatation or increased intracranial pressure (Raimondi 1986; Raimondi 1987). Hydrocephalus has been classified from various standpoints because of the broad variety of its etiology and characteristics. Some of the more common classifications include:

1. Non-communicating vs communicating. This classification is based on the suspected site of obstruction along the CSF pathways. Non-communicating hydrocephalus is due to intraventricular obstruction and is characterized by absence of communication between the ventricular and subarachnoid spaces. In the communicating type, the obstruction is believed to be in the subarachnoid space. It may, however, also be due to agenesis of arachnoid villi (Ellington and Margolis 1969; Gilles and Davidson 1971; Gutierrez et al. 1975) or, rarely, to venous sinus occlusion (Kinal 1962; Saint-Rose et al. 1984).
2. Intrauterine vs extrauterine.
3. Congenital vs acquired. Hydrocephalus present at birth is congenital hydrocephalus. Since it may, however, present later in life, it is not always possible to distinguish between the congenital and acquired types.
4. Infantile vs adult. Primarily, this refers to the time of onset of hydrocephalus. Infantile hydrocephalus is mostly congenital, whereas adult hydrocephalus mostly tends to be acquired. The latter may, however, be congenital hydrocephalus with onset occurring during the adult period.
5. Mild vs severe. The key feature to be taken into consideration in making this distinction is the ventricular size. Here, it is assumed that the severity of hydrocephalus is in direct proportion to the size of the ventricles.
6. Acute vs chronic. This classification depends on the time interval between onset of hydrocephalus and its diagnosis.
7. Rapid vs slowly progressing.
8. Progressive vs arrested. Arrested or compensated hydrocephalus occurs as the result of a balance between the production and absorption of CSF (Laurence and Coats 1962; Hemmer and Böhm 1976; Whittle et al. 1985). This may occur following a shunt operation or, rarely, it may be shunt independent (Holtzer and deLange 1973; Johnston et al. 1984).
9. Simple vs complicated. This classification is based on the presence or absence of congenital intracranial parenchymal malformations with hydrocephalus, and is useful in prognostication. The "complicated" variety includes dysgenetic hydrocephalus, hydroencephalodysplasia and destructive hydrocephalus.

10. Intraventricular vs extraventricular. The relationship of the obstruction site to the ventricular system forms the core of this classification, which indicates the site of obstruction more clearly than "non-communicating vs communicating."

11. Internal vs external. The former refers to hydrocephalus in which there is ventricular enlargement with retention of CSF in the ventricular system. In external hydrocephalus, CSF retention is more prominent in the subarachnoid space than in the ventricular system.

12. Hypertensive vs hypotensive.

13. Tumoral vs non-tumoral.

14. Treatable vs non-treatable. Whereas simple hydrocephalus is amenable to treatment and generally carries better prognosis, hydrocephalus associated with severe malformations such as severe porencephaly, alobar holoprosencephaly, and hydranencephaly is a severe form of complicated hydrocephalus and is said to be non-treatable.

Proposed Pathogenetic Classification (Table 1)

By virtue of their connection with the ventricular system through ependymal cell junctions, intracellular and extracellular spaces serve as possible CSF pathways, and their obstruction (as occurs in parenchymal damage) may cause hydrocephalus even when the major pathway is patent (Osaka et al. 1979; Mori 1990). The stages of progression of hydrocephalus, from intraparenchymal through extraparenchymal, may correspond to changes in the main sites of fluid collection.

Most forms of hydrocephalus are characterized by the presence of an "obstruction" in the intraparenchymal compartment. Included in this group are simple hydrocephalus, dysgenetic hydrocephalus, and destructive hydrocephalus resulting from disturbance in the cerebral blood flow. Non-communicating hydrocephalus and some types of communicating hydrocephalus may be classified as extraparenchymal hydrocephalus. Some cases of intraparenchymal hydrocephalus may also be associated with a blockage in the extraparenchymal compartment and may therefore fall into the intra- and extraparenchymal combined hydrocephalus group. Intraparenchymal hydrocephalus probably represents an early stage of hydrocephalus, and encompasses a stage similar to

---

Table 1. Pathogenetic classification of hydrocephalus. (Modified from Raimondi, 1987)

1. Intraparenchymal hydrocephalus
    (a) Intracellular hydrocephalus
    (b) Extracellular hydrocephalus
2. Extraparenchymal hydrocephalus
    (a) Subarachnoidal hydrocephalus
    (b) Intraventricular hydrocephalus
3. Intra- and extraparenchymal combined hydrocephalus

brain edema (Raimondi 1987) or benign intracranial hypertension in which ventriculomegaly is usually absent (Sklar et al. 1979; Raimondi 1987).

Conclusion

Hydrocephalus is regarded as the retention of CSF anywhere along its pathways. It results from an imbalance between CSF production and absorption, and may or may not be accompanied by ventricular dilatation and/or increased intracranial pressure. Of the several classifications that have been proposed, one of the best is that proposed by Raimondi (1987). From a purely pathophysiological standpoint, this classification embraces all the possible routes of CSF absorption and highlights the precise location of fluid collection, in recognition of the fact that the cause of fluid retention varies with its location.

References

Bering EA Jr, Sato O (1976) Hydrocephalus: changes in formation and absorption of cerebrospinal fluid within the cerebral ventricles. J Neurosurg 20: 1050–1063

Brightman MW (1965) The distribution within the brain of ferritin injected into cerebrospinal fluid compartments. 1. Ependymal distribution. J Cell Biol 26: 99–123

Brightman MW (1968) The intracerebral movement of proteins injected into blood and cerebrospinal fluid of mice. Prog Brain Res 29: 19–37

Cao M, Lisheng H, Shouzheng S (1984) Resolution of brain edema in severe brain injury at controlled high and low intracranial pressures. J Neurosurg 61: 707–712

Di Rocco C, Pettorossi VE, Caldarelli R, Mancinelli R, Velardi F (1978) Communicating hydrocephalus induced by mechanically increased amplitude of the intraventricular cerebrospinal fluid pressure: Experimental study. Exp Neurol 59: 40–52

Drayer BP, Rosenbaum AE (1978) Studies of the third circulation: Ampipaque CT cisternography and ventriculography. J Neurosurg 48: 946–956

Ellington E, Margolis G (1969) Block of arachnoid villi by subarachnoid hemorrhage. J Neurosurg 30: 651–657

Gilles FH, Davidson RI (1971) Communicating hydrocephalus with deficient dysplastic parasagittal arachnoidal granulations. J Neurosurg 35: 421–426

Gutierrez Y, Friede RL, Kakiney WJ (1975) Agenesis of arachnoid granulations and its relationship to communicating hydrocephalus. J Neurosurg 43: 553–558

Hakim S, Hakim C (1984) A biomechanical model of hydrocephalus and its relationship to treatment. In: Shapiro K, Marmarou A, Portnoy H (eds) Hydrocephalus. Raven, New York, pp 143–160

Hassler O (1964) Angioarchitecture in hydrocephalus. An autopsy and experimental study with the aid of microangiography. Acta Neuropathol (Berlin) 4: 65–74

Hemmer R, Böhm B (1976) Once a shunt, always a shunt? Dev Med Child Neurol 18 (Suppl 37): 69–73

Holtzer GJ, deLange SA (1973) Shunt-independent arrest of hydrocephalus. J Neurosurg 39: 698–701

Hopkins LN, Bakay L, Kinkel WR, Grand W (1977) Demonstration of transventricular CSF absorption by computerized tomography. Acta Neurochir (Wien) 39: 151–157

Johnston IH, Howman-Giles R, Whittle JR (1984) The arrest of treated hydrocephalus in children. A radionucleotide study. J Neurosurg 61: 752–756

Kinal ME (1962) Hydrocephalus and the dural venous sinuses. J Neurosurg 19: 195–201

Laurence KM, Coats S (1962) The natural history of hydrocephalus: Detailed analysis of 182 unoperated cases. Arch Dis Child 37: 345–362

Matsumoto S (1976) Pathogenesis of hydrocephalus. Neurol Med Chir (Tokyo) 16: 287–295

Milhorat TH (1972) Hydrocephalus and the cerebrospinal fluid. Williams and Wilkins, Baltimore

Mori K (1990) Hydrocephalus — revision of its definition and classification with special reference to "intractable infantile hydrocephalus". Nerv Syst Child 6: 198–204

Mori K, Raimondi AJ (1975) Submicroscopic changes in the periventricular white matter of hydrocephalic ch mouse. Arch Jpn Chir 44: 159–168

Mori K, Murata T, Nakano Y, Handa H (1977) Periventricular lucency in hydrocephalus on computerized tomography. Surg Neurol 8: 337–340

Morse DE, Low FN (1972) The fine structure of the pia mater of the rat. Am J Anat 133: 349–368

Oka N, Nakada J, Endo S, Takaku A, Shinohara H, Morisawa S (1985) Angioarchitecture in experimental hydrocephalus. Neurol Med Chir (Tokyo) 25: 701–706

Osaka K, Mori K, Handa H (1979) New classification of hydrocephalus based on recent concepts of cerebrospinal fluid circulation. Brain Nerv 7: 475–485

Raimondi AJ (1986) Hydrocephalus: Definition and classification. Presented at the 14th Annual Meeting of the Japanese Society for Pediatric Neurosurgery, Kochi, Japan

Raimondi AJ (1987) Pediatric neurosurgery. Theoretical principles, art of surgical techniques. Springer, New York Berlin Heidelberg

Reulen HJ, Tsuyamu M, Tack A, Fenske AR, Prioleau GR (1978) Clearance of edema fluid into cerebrospinal fluid. A mechanism for resolution of vasogenic brain edema. J Neurosurg 48: 754–764

Saint-Rose C, La Combe J, Pierre-Kahn T, Renier D, Hirsch J (1984) Intracranial venous sinus hypertension: Cause or consequence of hydrocephalus in infants? J Neurosurg 60: 727–736

Sato O (1986) Changes in concept: Mechanisms of genesis in hydrocephalus. Nerv Syst Child 11: 195–202

Sato O, Asai T, Amano Y, Hara M, Tugane R, Yagi M (1972) Extraventricular origin of the cerebrospinal fluid: Formation rate quantitatively measured in the spinal subarachnoid space of dogs. J Neurosurg 36: 276–282

Sklar FH, Beyer CW, Ramananthan M, Cooper PR, Clark WK (1979) Cerebrospinal fluid dynamics in patients with pseudotumor cerebri. Neurosurgery 5: 208–216

Whittle IR, Johnston IH, Besser M (1985) Intracranial pressure changes in arrested hydrocephalus. J Neurosurg 62: 77–82

Wislock GB, Putnum TJ (1921) Absorption from the ventricles in experimentally produced internal hydrocephalus. Am J Anat 29: 313–320

Wozniak M, McLone DG, Raimondi AJ (1975) Micro- and macrovascular changes as the direct cause of parenchymal destruction in congenital murine hydrocephalus. J Neurosurg 43: 535–545

II. Shunt Systems

36 — The Effectiveness of a Siphon Control Device in Preventing the Complications of Overshunting

Donald D. Horton, Greg Williams, and Michael Pollay[1]

Summary. Most available cerebrospinal fluid diversion systems utilize differential-pressure valves that often allow overshunting, resulting in complications due to the siphoning of fluid from the ventricular system. A new siphon-control device has been designed to address the problem of cerebrospinal fluid overdrainage. This study evaluates the effectiveness of this device in reducing complications of the "siphon" phenomenon. The siphon control device was found to reduce the incidence of post shunt subdural fluid collections and slit ventricle syndrome while not increasing the occurrence of shunt obstruction or infection.

Keywords. Shunt complications — Siphon control device — Hydrocephalus — Anti-Siphon device

Introduction

The phenomenon of cerebrospinal fluid overdrainage in patients treated with ventricular shunts has been shown to result in significant clinical complications including subdural fluid collections, craniostenosis, slit ventricle syndrome, orthostatic hypotension, and shunt obstruction (Foltz and Blanks 1988; Fox et al. 1973; Kaufman et al. 1973; Kiekens et al. 1982; Sainte-Rose et al. 1989). Effective elimination of cerebrospinal fluid (CSF) overdrainage in patients with ventricular shunt systems has been somewhat difficult. The first commercially available anti-siphon valve, designed as an anti-siphon device (ASD) for ventricular shunting, was reported by Portnoy et al. in 1973. Previous reports have shown a less than ideal success rate with the use of an anti-siphon valve (McCullough and Wells 1982). In the present paper, we discuss a new device designed to address the problem of cerebral spinal fluid overdrainage (see Fig. 1). The purpose of this study is to evaluate the effectiveness of this new

[1] Division of Neurological Surgery, University of Oklahoma Health Sciences Center, Oklahoma City, OK 73126, USA

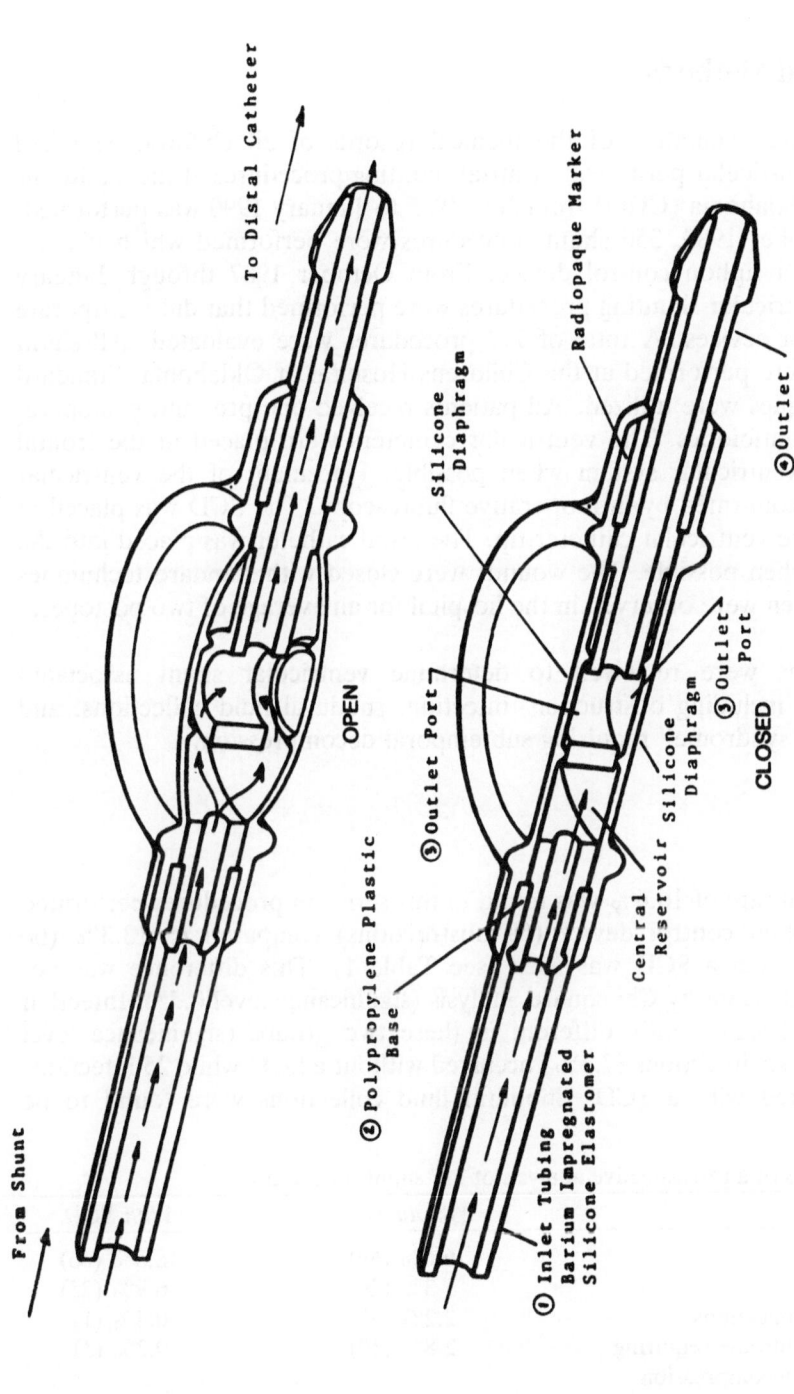

Fig. 1. Cross-sectional diagram of the PS Medical CSF siphon-control device. *Arrows* represent the direction and route of fluid flow. (From Horton and Pollay 1990)

siphon control device (SCD) in reducing complications of cerebrospinal fluid overdrainage.

Subjects and Methods

A retrospective evaluation of the medical records of all children who had undergone ventricular peritoneal or atrial shunting procedures at the Childrens Hospital of Oklahoma (CHO) from July 1985 to January 1990 was performed. Prior to October 1987, 356 shunt procedures were performed which did not incorporated a siphon control device. From October 1987 through January 1990, 361 ventricular shunting procedures were performed that did incorporate siphon control devices. A total of 717 procedures were evaluated. All shunt procedures were performed at the Childrens Hospital of Oklahoma. Standard sterile techniques were utilized. All patients received one pre- and postoperative dose of antibiotics. The ventricular catheters were placed in the frontal horn of the ventricular system when possible. Placement of the ventricular catheter was confirmed by intraoperative fluoroscopy. The SCD was placed at the level of the ventricular catheter tip. The distal catheter was placed into the peritoneum when possible. The wounds were closed with standard techniques and the children were observed in the hospital for an average of two postoperative days.

The records were reviewed to determine ventricular shunt associated complications including obstruction, infection, subdural fluid collections, and "slit-ventricle syndrome" requiring subtemporal decompression.

Results

An obstruction rate of 16.6% was found in this series in procedures performed without a siphon control device (59 obstructions) compared to 18.3% (66 obstructions) when a SCD was used (see Table 1). This difference was not statistically significant by Chi-square analysis (significance level 0.55). Infection rates were not significantly different in these two groups (significance level 0.84). Twenty-six infections (7.3%) occurred without a SCD while 25 infections (6.9%) occurred with a SCD. Subdural fluid collections were found to be

Table 1. Results of a retrospective analysis of 717 shunt procedures

	Without SCD	*With SCD*
Obstruction	16.6% (59)	18.3% (66)
Infection	7.3% (26)	6.9% (25)
Subdural fluid collections	2.2% (8)	0.3% (1)
Slit ventricle syndrome requiring subtemporal decompression	2.8% (10)	0.3% (1)

SCD, Siphon-control device

statistically different in these two groups (Chi-square significance level 0.18). Eight patients (2.2%) were found to have developed subdural fluid collections requiring surgical treatment when a SCD was not incorporated into the system compared to one patient (0.3%) when the SCD was used as a component in the shunt system. Slit-ventricle syndrome resulting in subtemporal decompression was reduced significantly (significance level .005). Ten patients (2.8%) underwent subtemporal decompression in the group without a SCD, while one patient (0.3%) required a decompression when a SCD was incorporated into the shunt system.

Discussion

The resting pressure within the ventricular cavity varies considerably with age, body activity, respiratory phase, and body position. It has been shown that in the sitting or standing position, the intraventricular pressure becomes sub-atmospheric. These observations become clinically relevant when a differential-pressure valve is required to provide adequate removal of CSF from obstructed ventricular cavities. Significant subatmospheric pressures may be produced in shunted patients as a result of the "siphon" phenomenon. The addition of an anti-siphon valve to the outlet of a differential-pressure valve eliminates the siphoning phenomenon in the upright position and allows the valve to operate in response to a positive inlet pressure (see Fig. 2) (Horton and Pollay 1990). Anti-siphon regulation of inlet pressure has been shown to substantially but not completely eliminate the complications that are associated with overdrainage of cerebrospinal fluid (Portnoy 1973).

The in vitro pressure-flow characteristics of the SCD have been previously reported by the authors. In that study the anti-siphon device (Heyer-Schulte anti-siphon device, American V. Mueller, Chicago. Ill.) and the siphon control device (PS Medical siphon-control device, PS Medical, Santa Barbara, Calif.) were substantially equivalent in performance characteristics and surgical implantation techniques and essentially eliminated the "siphon" phenomenon.

The results of this retrospective analysis suggest that incorporation of the SCD significantly reduced the rate of post shunt subdural fluid collections and the necessity for subtemporal decompression. The incidence of post shunt infection and obstruction was not significantly altered in this study.

Conclusions

The use of a siphon control device had no adverse effect on post shunt obstruction or infection rates.

The use of a siphon control device significantly reduces some of the deleterious effects of cerebrospinal fluid overdrainage.

We recommend that the siphon control device be used with low resistance valves to reduce the sequelae of cerebrospinal fluid overdrainage.

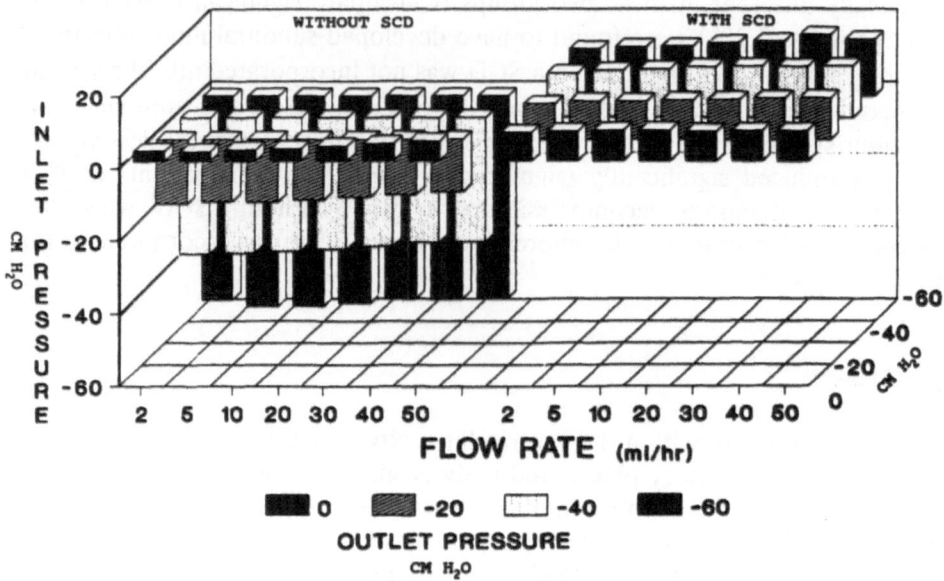

Fig. 2. The effect of outlet pressure on inlet pressure of the perfused PS Medical low-pressure valve with and without an attached siphon-control device (*SCD*). (From Horton and Pollay 1990)

References

Foltz EL, Blanks JP (1988) Symptomatic low intracranial pressure in shunted hydro-cephalus. J Neurosurg 68: 401–408

Fox JL, McCullough DC, Green RC (1973) Effect of cerebrospinal fluid shunts on intracranial pressure and on cerebrospinal fluid dynamics. 2. A new technique of pressure measurement: Results and concepts. 3. A concept of hydrocephalus. J Neurol Neurosurg Psychiatry 36: 302–312

Horton D, Pollay M (1990) Fluid flow performance of a new siphon-control device for ventricular shunts. J Neurosurg 72: 926–932

Kaufman B, Weiss MH, Young HF, Nulsen FE (1973) J Neurosurg 38: 288–297

Kiekens R, Mortier W, Pothmann R, Bock WJ, Seibert H (1982) The slit-ventricle syndrome after shunting in hydrocephalic children. Neuropediatrics 13: 190–194

McCullough DC, Wells M (1982) Complications with antisiphon devices in hydro-cephalics with ventriculoperitoneal shunts. In: Epstein F, Raimondi AJ (eds) Con-cepts in pediatric neurosurgery, vol. 2. Karger, Basel, pp 63–75

Portnoy HD, Schulte RR, Fox JL, Croissant PD, Tripp L (1973) Anti-siphon and reversible occlusion valves for shunting in hydrocephalus and preventing subdural hematomas. J Neurosurg 38: 729–738

Sainte-Rose C, Hoffman HJ, Hirsch JF (1989) Shunt failure. In: Marlin AE (ed) Concepts in pediatric neurosurgery, vol. 9. Karger, Basel, pp 7–20

37 — Importance of Anti-Siphon Devices in Shunt Therapy of Pediatric and Adolescent Hydrocephalus

Yasuhiro Chiba, Kazuhiko Tokoro, and Hiroyuki Abe[1]

Summary. A Slit-like ventricle (SLV) is occasionally observed on computerized tomography (CT) scans in pediatric hydrocephalus. The incidence of SLV was investigated in 64 pediatric and adolescent patients with cerebrospinal fluid (CSF) shunts in relation to their activity of daily living (ADL) and to the presence or absence of an anti-siphon device (ASD). Patients were divided into three groups. Group A had full ADL and shunt systems with ASDs. Group B had full ADL and shunt systems without ASDs. Group C consisted of bedridden patients without ASDs in their shunt systems. All patients had hypertensive hydrocephalus. All but two had ventriculoperitoneal shunts. Medium pressure valves were inserted in all. The average follow-up period was 8.8 years. The incidence of SLV was 7.4% in group A, 53.1% in group B, 20% in group C, and 31.3% for all groups. Group A had a signicantly lower incidence of SLV than group B (X^2 test, $P < 0.001$). One patient in group B developed slit ventricle syndrome. The CSF flow patterns through the shunt were examined using our thermosensitive technique. A rapid flow pattern was observed in most of group B. By contrast, this pattern was observed in only a few cases in group A. SLV appeared in only one out of four cases in group C despite the rapid CSF flow during positional changes.

In conclusion, ASDs in the shunt system played an important role in reducing the incidence of SLV in the treatment of pediatric hydrocephalus, but some work on the use of ASDs for treating tall adolescent patients will still be necessary because of the large hydrostatic pressure involved.

Keywords. Anti-siphon device — Slit-like ventricle — Hydrocephalus — Ventriculoperitoneal shunt — Thermistor

Introduction

Ventriculoperitoneal (VP) shunts have been widely adopted for the surgical treatment of hydrocephalus. Surgical results have been improved by advanced

---

[1] Department of Neurosurgery, Kanagawa Rehabilitation Center, Atsugi, 243-01 Japan

diagnostic procedures and shunt systems. Obstruction and infection, however, are the most frequent complications in shunting for hydrocephalus (Keucher and Mealy 1979), and overdrainage of cerebrospinal fluid (CSF) has been recognized as a third complication. Representative findings of this phenomenon are easily revealed on computerized tomography (CT) as subdural hematoma (SDH) and slit-like ventricles (SLV) or collapsed ventricles.

SLV may lead to an acute shunt obstruction, but the obstruction in most cases with SLV is fortunately intermittent, because the increased intraventricular pressure which follows shunt obstruction dilates the ventricle and reopens the catheter (Salmon 1978). Slit ventricle syndrome (SVS) is therefore infrequent, but is a troublesome and life-threatening condition when it does occur (Epstein et al. 1974; Gruber 1981; Holness et al. 1979; Kiekens et al. 1982; Nakada et al. 1982; Oi 1983; Salmon 1978). Low pressure shunts are used in many neurological centers for the treatment of pediatric hydrocephalus (Salmon 1978), and with the passage of time, ventricles may become slit-like.

This study evaluates the incidence of SLV in relation to the presence or absence of an ASD, the activity of daily living (ADL), and the CSF flow patterns in shunt systems during patients' positional changes.

Clinical Material and Methods

For 12 years, between 1978 and 1989, 64 pediatric and adolescent patients with hypertensive hydrocephalus were treated with CSF shunting; all but two patients had a VP shunt. All the valves inserted were of medium pressure. The patients were divided into three groups: Group A consisted of 27 patients treated with an ASD, group B consisted of 32 patients without an ASD, and group C consisted of 5 bedridden patients without an ASD. Patients in group A and group B had full ADL. The average age of group A was 10.8 years (ranging from 2 to 19 years). The etiology of hydrocephalus in group A was congenital in 20 patients, postmeningitic in 3, and intraventricular hemorrhage in 4. The average age of group B was 12.7 years (ranging from 1 to 19 years). The etiology of hydrocephalus in group B was congenital in 26 patients, postmeningitic in 5, and intraventricular hemorrhage in 1. The average age of group C was 6.9 years (ranging from 1 to 14 years). The etiology of hydrocephalus in Group C was only congenital. The details of each group are presented in Table 1. The ASDs used were manufactured by Heyer Schulte, Inc. and were of the integral type, except for two. In two of the adolescent patients, an ASD was placed 10 cm below the level of the foramen of Monro, for reasons which will be discussed later.

Among the 64 patients, 15 in each of groups A and B, and 5 in group C were studied using the thermosensitive technique (Chiba and Yuda 1980; Chiba et al. 1985) and the shunt flow during positional changes from the supine to a sitting or standing position was examined. Shunt patency was ascertained by shuntography with radionuclide or contrast medium. The thermosensitive method has already been reported in previous papers (Chiba and Yuda 1980;

Table 1. Clinical summary

	Group A	Group B	Group C
Number (cases *n*)	27	32	5
ASD	+	−	−
ADL	Full	Full	Bedridden
Age (years)			
mean	10.8	12.7	6.9
range	2–19	1–19	1–14
Age of initial shunting			
mean	8.1 months	3.5 months	4.1 months
range	26 days–44 months	4 days–15 months	10 days–6 months
Follow-up period (years)			
mean	8.7	9.2	6.7
range	1–8.7	2–18	1–14
Shunt device	Medium pressure Mishler dual chamber or multi-purpose valve	Medium pressure Mishler dual chamber	Medium pressure Mishler dual chamber

ADL, activity of daily living; ASD, anti-siphon device

Chiba et al. 1985), but is summarized as follows: A patient is placed in the supine position and a small thermistor is taped to the skin of the upper chest overlying a catheter 4 cm distal to the cooling area. A second thermistor is taped to the skin beside the catheter, and both thermistors are connected to a recorder. To cool the CSF, a cube of ice in a vinyl covering is applied over the proximal shunt tube for 1 min. During the study, the patient is moved from the supine position to a sitting or standing position. When the two thermistors are balanced at the same temperature, the indicator points to the center of the scale on the recording device. When the measuring thermistor detects a drop in temperature, the indicator is deflected and the recording trace declines. When a temperature difference of more than 0.1°C occurs between the two thermistors, the recording trace swings fully. After the patient has been kept supine, usually for a minute, his position is changed to a sitting and then standing position.

Results

SLVs were evaluated on CT as small or collapsed ventricles. The incidence of SLV was 2 out of 27 cases (7.4%) in group A, 17 out of 32 cases (53.1%) in group B, 1 out of 5 cases (20%) in group C, and 20 out of 64 cases (31.3%) in total. Group A had a significantly lower incidence of SLV than group B (X^2 test, $P < 0.001$). One patient in group B developed slit ventricle syndrome.

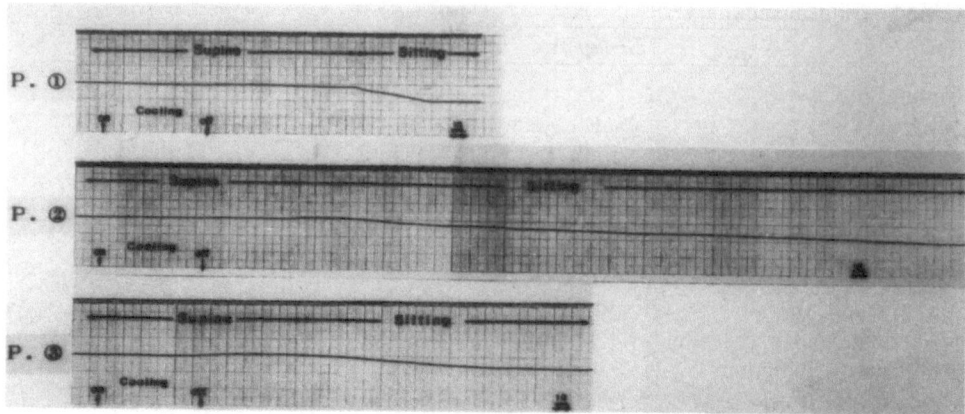

Fig. 1. Recording traces obtained by the thermosensitive method. *P.1*, Steep downward deflection; *P.2*, Gradual downward deflection; *P.3*, Flat-line recording with initial downward deflection

On recording traces using the thermosensitive method, a slight downward deflection was observed in the supine position in most cases. However, a definite downward deflection was observed in the sitting and standing positions. The downward deflection included three different recording traces (Fig. 1): (1) a steep downward deflection, (2) a gradual downward deflection, and (3) a flat-line recording with initial downward deflection. A steep downward deflection indicated exessive CSF drainage and was assumed, for the sake of convenience, to swing down within 100 s on the recording trace. A gradual downward deflection was assumed to swing down slowly over more than 100 s. A flat-line recording with initial downward deflection was thought to be the appropriate function of ASD to prevent overdrainage.

Relationship Between SLV and ASD (Table 2)

In group A, a steep downward deflection was observed in 4 patients, two of whom had SLV. A gradual downward deflection was observed in 5 patients, none of whom had SLV. A flat-line recording with initial downward deflection was observed in 6 patients, none of whom had SLV. The incidence of SLV in group A, on which the thermosensitive technique was conducted, was 2 out of 15 patients. The average time required between beginning the sitting or standing position and the full swing of the recording trace was 113.8 ± 86.0 s in patients with a steep downward or a gradual downward deflection. In group B, in contrast, a steep downward deflection was observed in 11 patients, 10 of whom had SLV. A gradual downward deflection was observed in 4 patients, none of whom had SLV. A flat-line recording with initial downward deflection was not observed at all. The incidence of SLV in group B, on which the thermosensitive technique was conducted, was 10 out of 15 patients. The average time required between beginning the sitting or standing position and

Table 2. Thermosensitive recording patterns and SLV

	No. of cases (n)	No. of SLV
Group A: 15 cases		
Steep downward deflection	4	2
Gradual downward deflection	5	0
Flat-line recording with initial downward deflection	6	0
Group B: 15 cases		
Steep downward deflection	11	10
Gradual downward deflection	4	0
Flat-line recording with initial downward deflection	0	—
Group C: 5 cases		
Steep downward deflection	4	1
Gradual downward deflection	1	0
Flat-line recording with initial downward deflection	0	—

SLV, slit-like ventricle

the full swing of the recording trace was 62.4 ± 40.6 s in patients with a steep downward or a gradual downward deflection. In group C, a steep downward deflection during positional changes was observed in 4 patients, and a gradual downward deflection was observed in 1 patient. SLV, however, was observed only in 1 patient showing a steep downward deflection. The average time required between beginning the sitting or standing position and the full swing of the recording trace was 60.4 ± 51.4 s. The CSF flow in the shunt system during positional changes seemed to be more rapid in groups B and C than in group A, but statistical analysis using Student's t-test did not show significant differences (Table 3).

Discussion

The siphon effect of CSF shunts is well known. Chronic overdrainage is a functional shunt problem in upright patients. A small ventricle or SLV, both of which are chronic overdrainage phenomena, are easily identified by CT scan or ultrasound. In children who remained shunt dependent; it appears that the incidence of SLV was approximately 30% (Nakada et al. 1982; Oi 1983; Tani et al. 1981).

In the present study, the incidence of SLV was 31.3%, which was a standard incidence. The patients who had full ADL and a shunt system with an ASD had a significantly lower incidence of SLV than patients who had full ADL and a shunt system without an ASD. When patients without an ASD were bedridden, the incidence of SLV was low.

It has been recognized that the majority of patients with SLV are asymptomatic, but SLV is a condition to be avoided, because, first of all, some patients with this condition develop SVS. The incidence of SVS is said to be

Table 3. Required time between beginning the sitting or standing position and full swing of the recording trace

	Mean
Group A (9 cases)	113.8 ± 86.0 s
Group B (15 cases)	62.4 ± 40.6 s
Group C (5 cases)	60.4 ± 51.4 s

aproximately 5% of children who remain shunt dependent (Chapman 1990; Kiekens et al. 1982). Patients with SVS may face life-threatening conditions, because the ventricles remain small or slit-like despite shunt malfunction. Secondly, SLV interferes with mental development in younger infants (Oi and Matsumoto 1983); thirdly, SLV can lead to secondary cranio synostosis; and fourthly, SLV is the preliminary condition in shunt malfunction (Tani et al. 1981).

In the present study, it was ascertained that SLV was closely related to the presence or absence of an ASD and to ADL. In fact, a rapid flow in the shunt system was observed in aproximately two-thirds of the patients without an ASD during changes from the supine to the sitting or standing position. In patients without an ASD, SLV appeared frequently, but it was observed in only one-fourth of the bedridden patients without an ASD, despite rapid flow in the shunt system during positional changes.

The ASD was described by Portnoy et al. (1973). It prevents CSF flow through the shunt whenever a negative pressure of 100–200 mmH$_2$O is exerted at the outlet of the device. In the present study, ASDs played an important role in reducing the incidence of SLV. Gruber et al. (1984) also insisted on the importance of the ASD in pediatric hydrocephalus shunt therapy for reducing symptoms and preventing shunt dysfunction due to chronic CSF overdrainage. Adverse effects of ASDs in patent shunt systems, however, have been reported by McCullough (1986), McCullough and Wells (1982), and Seida et al. (1987). Inappropriate CSF flow was thought to have resulted from excessive CSF volume which accumulated before there was sufficient pressure to initiate drainage in the ASD (McCullough and Wells 1982). In the present study, the representative flow pattern of an ASD, characterized by a flat-line recording with initial downward deflection, was observed in only 40% of patients with an ASD and a slow flow was also observed in one third of the patients with an ASD.

It seems that ASDs were not completely successful in the pediatric patients because of the low hydrostatic pressure in these patients, however at the same time we also encountered adverse effects of ASDs in tall adolescent patients. Thus, we tried to reduce ASD function. To this end, based on experimental and clinical experience (Tokoro and Chiba 1989), we placed the ASD 10 cm below the level of the foramen of Monro.

In conclusion, ASDs in the shunt system played an important role in reducing the incidence of SLV in the treatment of pediatric hydrocephalus, but some work on the use of ASDs for treating tall adolescent patients will still be necessary.

References

Chapman PH (1990) Hydrocephalus in childhood. In: Youmans JR (ed) Neurological Surgery, 3rd edn. WB Saunders, Philadelphia, pp 1236–1276

Chiba Y, Yuda K (1980) Thermosensitive determination of CSF shunt patency with a pair of small disc thermistors. J Neurosurg 52: 700–704

Chiba Y, Ishiwata Y, Suzuki N, Muramoto M, Kunimi Y (1985) Thermosensitive determination of obstructed sites in ventriculoperitoneal shunts. J Neurosurg 62: 363–366

Epstein F, Fleischer AS, Hochwald GM, Ransohoff J (1974) Subtemporal craniectomy for recurrent shunt obstruction secondary to small ventricles. J Neurosurg 41: 29–31

Gruber R (1981) The relationship of ventricular shunt complications to the chronic overdrainage syndrome: A follow-up study. Z Kinderchir 34: 346–352

Gruber R, Jenny P, Herzog B (1984) Experiences with the anti-siphon device (ASD) in shunt therapy of pediatric hydrocephalus. J Neurosurg 61: 156–162

Holness RO, Hoffmann HJ, Hendrick EB (1979) Subtemporal decompression for the slit-ventricle syndrome after shunting in hydrocephalic children. Childs Brain 5: 137–144

Keucher TR, Mealy JJ (1979) Long-term results after ventriculoatrial and ventriculoperitoneal shunting for infantile hydrocephalus. J Neurosurg 50: 179–186

Kiekens R, Mortier W, Pothmann R, Bock WJ, Seibert H (1982) The slit ventricle syndrome after shunting in hydrocephalic children. Neuropediatrics 13: 190–194

McCullough DC (1986) Symptomatic progressive ventriculomegaly in hydrocephalics with patent shunts and anti-syphon devices. Neurosurgery 19: 617–621

McCullough DC, Wells M (1982) Complications with antisiphon devices in hydrocephalics with ventriculoperitoneal shunts. In: Epstein F, Raimondi AJ (eds) Concepts in pediatric neurosurgery, vol. 2. Karger, Basel, pp 63–75

Nakada Y, Enomoto T, Maki Y (1982) Clinical and computed tomographical analysis of hydrocephalic children showing slit-like ventricle after shunt operation (in Japanese). Shoni no No-shinkei 7: 59–66

Oi S (1983) Slit-like ventricle and isolation of CSF pathway as complication of shunt procedure in child hydrocephalus (Part-1). The pathophysiology and clinical problems (in Japanese). Shoni no No-shinkei 8: 107–117

Oi S, Matsumoto S (1983) Complications (slit ventricle, isolated fourth ventricle) of shunt procedure in child hydrocephalus (in Japanese). No to Hattatsu 15: 199–209

Portnoy HD, Schulte RR, Fox JL, Croissant PD, Tripp L (1973) Anti-siphon and reversible occlusion valves for shunting in hydrocephalus and preventing post-shunt subdural hematomas. J Neurosurg 38: 729–738

Salmon JH (1978) The collapsed ventricle: management and prevention. Surg Neurol 9: 349–352

Seida M, Ito U, Tomida S, Yamazaki, Inaba Y (1987) Ventriculoperitoneal shunt malfunction with anti-siphon device in normal-pressure hydrocephalus: Report of three cases (in Japanese). Neurol Med Chir (Tokyo) 27: 769–773

Tani S, Kumamura Y, Kusano T, Yamanouchi Y, Matsumura H (1981) Clinical analysis of 13 hydrocephalic children with slit-like ventricles caused by shunt procedures (in Japanese). Shoni no No-shinkei 6: 33–40

Tokoro K, Chiba Y (1989) Effects on shunt flow of position of anti-siphon device and of changes in posture in hydrocephalus (abstract). Ninth International Congress of Neurological Surgery, New Delhi, India, p 100

38 — The Antisiphon Device — its Value in Preventing Excessive Drainage

Robert F.C. Jones, Charles Teo, Bruce Currie[1], Bernard C.T. Kwok[1,2], and Vimala V. Nayanar[3]

Summary. During the period 1978–1988, 340 children with hydrocephalus have been controlled by the Heyer-Schulte valve with antisiphon device (ASD). No children with tumors are included. There were 99 primary insertions; 42 in infants with myelomeningocele. The mean follow up was 7 years. During this time, in the 225 children without myelomeningocele, revision of the ventricular catheter was required on 29 occasions.

In the children with myelomeningocele, 23 of the 25 of those who had a low pressure valve inserted initially required change of their ventricular catheter. Overall, in the 115 children with myelomeningocele, a change of the ventricular catheter was required on 52 occasions.

Six patients showed major problems with intolerance, three adjusted in time, and of the remaining three, two required change of their ventricular catheter and one required lowering of pressure from a high pressure to a medium pressure valve.

Keywords. Antisiphon device — Cerebrospinal fluid drainage shunts

Introduction

Despite the improvements in results following the introduction of the valved shunt (reviewed by Pudenz 1981), overdrainage of the cerebrospinal fluid (CSF) remains a problem. It leads to premature fusion of the cranial sutures, subdural effusions, and collapsed lateral ventricles which predispose to blockage of the ventricular catheter. This has been proposed as the mechanism behind the "slit-ventricle syndrome" (Becker and Nulsen 1968; Holmes et al. 1979). Recently, McLaurin (1989) wrote, "Complications involving the prox-

---

[1] Department of Neurosurgery, Prince of Wales Children's Hospital, Sydney 2031 Australia
[2] Department of Neurosurgery, Institute of Neurological Sciences, Prince Henry Hospital, Sydney 2036 Australia
[3] Department of Radiology, Prince of Wales Hospital, Sydney 2031 Australia.

imal catheter were the most frequent (referring to Forrest and Cooper series, 1968) and this has been true in nearly all reported series."

In an attempt to remedy this problem, Portnoy, Shulte, Fox, Croissant, and Tripp (1973) introduced the antisiphon device (ASD).

As we had also experienced overdrainage we resolved in 1978 to utilise the ASD in all patients in an attempt to alleviate this problem. This has since been done. All of our old patients with other shunt apparatus have been changed to this type and all new patients, with the exception of those undergoing third ventriculostomy, have been fitted with this type of shunt.

Subjects and Methods

Assessment of Stuctural Change

From 1977 to 1980, 37 patients were seen with abnormally small ventricles, as imaged by computerised tomography (CT) or sonography. Some had a premature sutural fusion and some were symptomatic, i.e., they had afternoon headaches which were relieved by lying down.

Initially, an antisiphon device was added but later a medium or high pressure Heyer Schulte pump was used. This apparatus was the standard size burrhole type.

Structural studies done before and afterward were reviewed independently by V.V. Nayanar. The size was judged either to be unchanged or to have increased to normal size or greater than normal size (Fig. 1 and Table 1).

Blockages of the Ventricular Catheter (Table 2)

The numbers of operations and their type that these 37 patients underwent before and after the insertion of this apparatus were analyzed. Although the earlier group is not strictly a control group, the results can usefully be compared.

Assessment of Ventricular Catheter Blockage

This has been carried out in all patients from 1978, since the insertion of this apparatus. All patients with progressive hydrocephalus under our care (RJ) have been treated in a standard fashion with Heyer Schulte valves with an antisiphon device. This has either been inserted as a primary apparatus or patients with other shunt systems have been converted to this one.

We have taken the period of follow up to cease when the patient moves to another service, is lost to follow up, or dies. Patients in whom the period of follow up is less than 2 years have been excluded from this survey. During this period, the operative technique and the operating room conditions were unchanged.

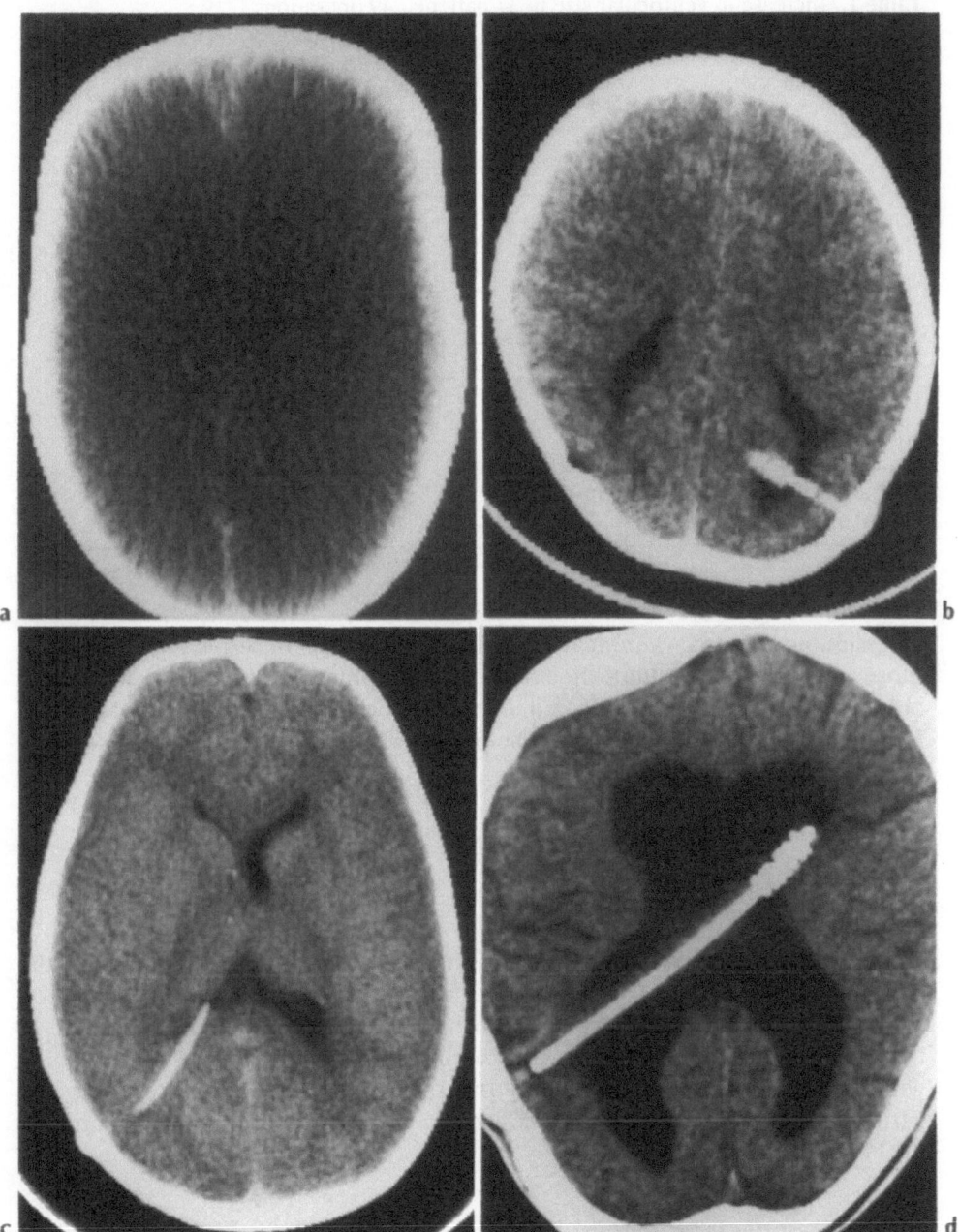

Fig. 1. a Ventricles not visualized, **b** smaller than normal ventricles, in this case collapsed anteriorly, **c** normal size ventricles, **d** larger than normal size ventricles

Table 1. Increase in ventricular size in 37 patients, 49 operations

Apparatus inserted	*Ventricular size*		
	No change	Normal	Larger than normal
ASD only	9	6	3
MP + ASD	3	12	5
HP + ASD	3	8	0

ASD, antisiphon device; MP, medium pressure valve; HP, high pressure valve

Table 2. Shunt operations in 37 patients

Before ASD etc	*After ASD etc*
Ventricular catheter 16 (11 patients)	13 (7 patients)
Distal blockages 58	19
Change of pressure 11	12
Operations for infections 14 (6 infections)	0
Period of observation 5.3 years	Period of observation 6.4 years

Assiduous attempts were made to culture organisms in suspicious cases, as in those who had distal shunt blockages. No prophylactic antibiotics were used either systemically or locally. All infections occurring in shunts at any time following operation were included as postoperative infections.

Results

Structural Changes

In these 37 patients all but 3 showed an increase in ventricular size with the additional apparatus. In some this increased with the addition of the antisiphon device alone but in 9 cases this did not happen. These 9 patients and some of the others who did not change with the insertion of a medium pressure valve with antisiphon device, subsequently had this changed to a high pressure valve with antisiphon device. This accounts for the 49 operations in 37 patients. (Table 1)

Blockage of the Ventricular Catheter

In the 37 patients with lateral ventricles of smaller than normal size there was a decreased rate of ventricular catheter obstruction (Table 2) after conversion. This was required on 11 occasions over 6 years as compared with 16 occasions over 5 years before conversion. When one takes into account the fact that 6 of the 11 ventricular catheter revisions were in one patient whose lateral ventricles were loculated, the improvement is more encouraging.

Table 3. Hydrocephalics without myelomeningocele (225 patients). Primary and secondary insertion of anti siphon device with Heyer Shulte valve

Site of block		Change of pressure	No. of infections	No. of ops. (infection)	Mean follow up (months)
Ventricle	Other				
29	87	43	6	26	88

Two deaths; three subdural hematomas. Infection rate 1.6%

The Ventricular catheter Blockages 1978–1990

In the years 1978–1990, 225 children with hydrocephalus but without myelomeningocele were followed up for a mean time of 7.4 years. Twenty-nine patients required reoperation for blockage of their ventricular catheters (Table 3).

The vast majority either had a medium pressure pump installed or were soon fitted with one. There was no significant difference between the primary and secondary insertion of this apparatus as far as blockage of the ventricular catheter was concerned.

In the group of hydrocephalic children with an associated myelomeningocele (Table 4) there was a group of 25 patients who were initially fitted with a low pressure system. For some reason these children were not promptly converted to a medium pressure system and they suffered, in total, ventricular catheter blockage on 23 occasions. This is quite different from the 17 who were fitted with a medium pressure pump initially and in whom blockage of the ventricular catheter occurred on only four occasions. (Table 4).

The group with myelomeningocele who were converted to this system (Table 5) did not have much trouble from blockage of the ventricular catheter. One of these children suffered from a loculated fourth ventricle and the difficulty associated with the accurate placement of this catheter necessitated 7 revisions of this ventricular catheter; this was in addition to the child mentioned earlier with 6 revisions due to loculated lateral ventricle.

Discussion

Despite the use of Portnoy's (1971) ventricular catheter we continued to be plagued by ventricular catheter obstructions. The incidence was less than Selkar, Moossy, and Guthkelch's (1982) rate of 60% of blockages, but was enough to provoke the adoption of a new shunt system. Initially, we tried increasing the shunt pressure using high pressure Raimondi type catheters or Holter valves, but we failed to achieve Salmon's (1978) success. We have continued to use the relatively high profile Heyer Schulte burrhole type pressure valve plus or minus the antisiphon device and have had no problems with ulceration of the scalp.

Table 4. Hydrocephalus with myelomeningocele in 43 patients. Heyer Shulte valve with antisiphon device used for initial shunt

No. of patients (n)	Valve pressure	Site of block		Change of pressure	No. of infections	No. of ops. (infection)	Follow up (months)
		Ventricle	Other				
25	Low	23	20	12	1	2	74
17	Medium	4	8	2	2	3	90

Infection Rate 2.5%

Table 5. Hydrocephalics with myelomeningocele (72 patients). Secondary insertion of antisiphon device + Heyer Schulte valve

Site of block		Change of pressure	No. of infections	No. of ops.	Misc	Follow up (months)
Ventricle	Other					
26[a]	66	15	3	8	14	117.4[b]

[a] One child with loculated 4th ventricle had 7 revisions. One child with loculated contralateral ventricle had 6 revisions
[b] Two are "stabilized"
Infection rate 1.8%

We also find it useful in that it allows the parents (and patient) to assess the shunt by palpation. We have had some problems associated with retrieval of the ventricular catheter and more importantly, with the tendency of these valves to open at lower pressures after some years. This has been less noticeable lately.

The value of inserting valves with antisiphon devices in infants has been questioned by Hoffman (1982). At that time we were frequently using medium pressure valves with attached antisiphon devices in children. Since then we have tended to use the ASD with a low pressure proximal valve and a distal medium pressure atrial slit valve. This was then increased to a medium pressure valve with ASD at 6–24 months of age.

However, the difference in the rate of blockage of the ventricular catheter is quite striking (Table 4). Although the low pressure pump with antisiphon device should no doubt be used in the premature, we feel that the medium pressure model is probably better in the full term infant, as suggested by Portnoy. (1984)

In addition to the complications listed (Tables 2, 3, 4, and 5) we have encountered problems similar to those described by McCullough (1986). We have seen one patient in whom an antisiphon device was added by a colleague while the patient was in another city. The patient became unconscious and the shunt was reexplored. The ventricular catheter and the distal catheter were both patent to the flow of fluid through the tubing at operation, the device was removed, and the patient woke up. Later we elected to add the antisiphon device. At operation fluid flowed freely from the ventricular catheter. In view of our colleague's previous experience with this child and the knowledge that a patent ventricular catheter is important it was changed, a medium pressure valve with ASD was used, and the patient tolerated the procedure well.

In two other cases with problems persisting beyond 48 h changing the seemingly working ventricular catheter has led to resolution of the problem. In addition, three patients have had incoordination lasting 1–3 months.

However, we must emphasise that the hydrodynamic changes we have carried out have been done in children. They seem to be more tolerant of these stresses than adults — even young adults.

In addition, one should change the pressure slowly — only increase one pressure level at a time and pump the shunt for 24–48 h postoperatively if the headache is worrying or vomiting occurs.

In order to avoid problems associated with sudden changes in intracranial pressure, it is preferable to use this system from the start of treatment (Portnoy 1984). Hyde-Rowan, Rekake, and Nulsen (1982) suggested the use of a higher pressure valve to alleviate the problem. They used an ASD in association with a Holter valve. This certainly increased the ventricular size significantly. However, Portnoy (1984) cautions against using the ASD in such a system as it may increase the intracranial pressure unduly. Our results utilizing the Heyer Schulte valve have produced similar pleasing results.

In one of our patients we have had to change a high pressure valve with ASD to a medium pressure valve. Otherwise, the intracranial pressure as assessed by palpation of the fontanelle or artificial fontanelle or by direct measurement seems normal.

Conclusion

We believe, as do others (Gruber et al. 1984; Hyde-Rowan et al. 1982; Portnoy et al. 1973) that the maintenance of a normal intracranial pressure with larger than normal ventricles diminshes the rate of complications which flow from slit-like ventricles. Our rate of ventricular catheter blockage is less than half that of Keucher and Mealey (1979) who had 30 ventricular catheter blockages in 90 ventriculoperitoneal shunts followed up for 7 years.

In infancy, it would seem advisable to use a medium pressure Heyer Schulte valve with antisiphon device (or its equivalent) to prevent the ventricles from becoming too small. If a lower pressure is used it should be increased earlier rather than later in infancy.

Consideration should be given to increasing the pressure if the ventricles are starting to get unduly small or if the rate of head growth is progressing slowly. It is preferable to do this before the catheter blocks, if possible, while the patient is asymptomatic.

Acknowledgments. We wish to thank Cristina Kew for her accuracy and patience in typing the manuscript and the Department of Medical Illustration, University of New South Wales, for the illustrations.

References

Becker DP, Nulsen FE (1968) Control of hydrocephalus by valve-regulated venous shunt: Avoidance of complications in prolonged shunt maintenance J Neurosurg 28: 215–226

Forrest DM, Cooper DGW (1968) Complications of ventriculo-atrial shunts. A review of 455 cases. J Neurosurg 29: 506–512

Gruber R, Jenny P, Herzog B (1984) Experiences with the antisiphon device (ASD) in shunt therapy of pediatric hydrocephalus. J Neurosurg 61: 156–162

Hoffman HJ (1982) Technical problems in shunts. In: Choux M (ed) Symposium on shunts. Karger, Basel, pp 158–169

Holmes RO, Hoffman HJ, Henrick EB (1979) Subtemporal decompression for the "slit-ventricle-syndrome" after shunting in hydrocephalic children. Childs Brain 5: 137–144

Hyde-Rowan MD, Rekake HL, Nulsen FE (1982) Reexpansion of previously collapsed ventricles: The slit-ventricle syndrome. J Neurosurg 56: 536–539

Keucher TR, Mealey J (1979) Long-term results after ventriculo atrial and ventriculo peritoneal shunting for infantile hydrocephalus. J Neurosurg 50: 179–186

McCullough DC (1986) Symptomatic progressive ventriculomegaly in hydrocephalics with patent shunts and antisiphon devices. Neurosurgery 19: 617–621

McLaurin RL (1989) Ventricular shunts: Complications and results. In: McLaurin RL, Venes JL, Schut L, Epstein F (eds) Pediatric neurosurgery, 2nd edn. WB Saunders, Philadelphia, pp 219–229

Portnoy HD (1971) Ventr. Cath J Neurosurg 34: 702–703

Portnoy HD (1984) Antisiphon devices in shunt therapy (letter). J Neurosurg 61: 1158

Portnoy HD, Schulte RR, Fox JL, Croissant PD, Tripp L (1973) Antisiphon and reversible occlusion valves for shunting in hydrocephalus and preventing post-shunt subdural hematomas. J Neurosurg 38: 729–738

Pudenz RH (1981) Surgical treatment of hydrocephalus: An historical review. Surg Neurol 15: 15–26

Salmon JN (1978) The collapsed ventricle: Management and prevention. Surg Neurol 9: 349–352

Sekhar LN, Moossy J, Guthkelch AN (1982) Malfunctioning ventriculo-peritoneal shunts. J Neurosurg 56: 411–416

39 — Effect of an Anti-Siphon Device on Shunting Procedure: Intraventricular Pressure During Posture Changes

Hiroyuki Abe, Yasuhiro Chiba, and Kazuhiko Tokoro[1]

Summary. Intraventricular pressure (IVP) is closely related to the posture of patients who have had cerebrospinal fluid (CSF) shunting for hydrocephalus. An overdrainage of CSF through the shunt tube sometimes causes low pressure syndrome, and this syndrome sometimes influences the daily activity of the patient (LPS). The anti-siphon device (ASD) was designed to prevent LPS. We investigated IVP in patients with a CSF shunt with or without an ASD during posture changes. In this study, patients were divided into two groups: Group A consisted of patients with shunts with an ASD placed 10 cm below the level of the foramen of Monro (11 cases), and Group B consisted of patients with shunts without an ASD (6 cases). IVP was measured by inserting a 25 G needle attached to a transducer into the dome of the shunt device during changes of the patient's posture (positional IVP monitoring). In the supine position, IVP was significantly lower in Group B than in Group A (Student's t test, $P < 0.05$). In the semi-sitting (head raised 30°) and sitting or standing positions, the differences between Group B and Group A were greater than in the supine position ($P < 0.001$). In conclusion, an ASD was effective in restoring physiological pressure to patients in a sitting or standing position. Nevertheless, LPS was observed in only one patient in Group B (16.7%), and shunt malfunctions due to the adverse effects of an ASD were observed in two patients in Group A (18.2%). Adequate usage of ASDs in shunting must be considered as part of the important effort to prevent LPS.

Keywords. Low pressure syndrome — Anti-siphon device — Shunt function — Positional IVP monitoring

Introduction

The ventriculoperitoneal (VP) shunt is the most common treatment for hydrocephalus. There are two main complications, mechanical and functional.

---

[1] Department of Neurosurgery, Kanagawa Rehabilitation Center, Atsugi, Kanagawa, 243-01 Japan

Mechanical complications are those caused by shunt infection, obstruction, and disconnection. Functional complications are caused by inadequate CSF flow through the shunt system. In the latter case, overdrainage sometimes results in the low pressure syndrome, which frequently influences the daily activity of the patient because it is closely related to the patient's position, especially the erect position.

To prevent this syndrome, an ASD was developed by Portnoy and coworkers (1973). Various reports of the effects of ASDs on shunting have already been published. This study evaluates the effects of an ASD on shunting procedure with regard to IVP dynamics during postural changes as well as with regard to shunt malfunctions due to the adverse effects of an ASD.

Clinical Materials and Methods

From February 1989 to October 1990, 16 patients with 17 shuntings for hydrocephalus were examined by computed tomography (CT) scan, radionuclide shuntography (Rudd et al. 1973), and positional IVP monitoring. The etiology of hydrocephalus was normal pressure hydrocephalus (NPH) due to subarachnoid hemorrhage (SAH) in 12 cases, congenital in 2 cases, head injury in 1 case, and intracerebral hemorrhage in 1 case. None of the patients had mechanical complications, but functional complications were found and shunt revision was performed (case 6). The patients were divided into two groups

Table 1. Summary of cases

Case number (n)	Age	Sex	Etiology of hydrocephalus	Type of shunt device	Pressure	ASD	
1	67	F	SAH	D.C	Low	−10	
2	13	M	Congenital	Sophy	Medium	−10	
3	48	M	SAH	Sophy	Low	−10	
4	67	F	SAH	Sophy	Low	−10	
5	59	M	SAH	Sophy	Low	−10	Group A
6[a]	69	F	SAH	Sophy	Low	− 8	
7	64	M	Brain tumor	Sophy	Low	−10	
8	52	F	SAH	D.C	Low	−10	
9	69	M	SAH	D.C	Low	−10	
10	15	M	Congenital	P	?	−10	
11	58	M	SAH	Sophy	Low	−10	
12[a]	69	F	SAH	Sophy	Low	−	
13	72	F	SAH	D.C	Low	−	
14	67	M	ICH	D.C	Low	−	Group B
15	51	M	SAH	P	?	−	
16	19	M	Trauma	?	?	−	
17	54	F	SAH	?	?	−	

[a] cases 6 and 12 are the same patient; SAH, subarachnoid hemorrhage; D.C, Mishler dual chamber flushing device; P, Pudentz burr hole type flushing device; M.P, Multipurpose device; − 10, insertion of an ASD 10 cm below the level of the foramen of Monro; −, without ASD

according to the presence (Group A:11 cases) or absence (Group B:6 cases) of an ASD. VP shunting was carried out on all patients. We inserted an ASD in a low position in the shunt system, usually 10 cm below the level of the foramen of Monro (Tokoro and Chiba 1989). Low pressure valves were used in 10 cases, but in only 1 case in Group A. This exceptional case developed slit ventricle syndrome and had a high preoperative IVP, so a programmable pressure valve (Sophy valve, SU-8) at medium pressure was used. Many different valves used in Group B were of unknown origin, because some of the patients in this group were not operated on at our hospital. The details for each group are summarized in Table 1. IVP measurement was performed as follows. After the patient had rested in the supine position for more than an hour, a sterile technique was used to insert a 25 G needle attached to a transducer (P 10 EZ, San-Ei Inc., Tokyo, Japan; reliable pressure range from -50 mmHg to $+300$ mmHg) into the dome of the shunt reservoir, which was connected to a polygraph (type 362, San-Ei Inc., Tokyo, Japan). The IVP monitoring consisted of an initial measurement in the supine position, measurements at upper-body elevations of 10°, 30°, 45°, and 90°, and, if possible, a standing measurement. IVP was described as a water column. Student's t test was used for statistical analyses. A P-value of less than 0.05 was considered significant.

Results

1. IVP in the Supine Position (Table 2)

In Group A, the mean IVP in the supine position was 11.1 ± 6.7 cmH$_2$O. The patient (case 2), who had a shunt revision due to shunt obstruction related to a slit-like ventricle had a very high postoperative IVP of 25.8 cmH$_2$O, but no symptoms of increased IVP appeared. In Group B, the mean IVP in the supine position was 3.28 ± 5.13 cmH$_2$O. In case 17, a markedly negative IVP of -6.8 cmH$_2$O appeared in the supine position, but no symptoms of LPS appeared. IVP in the supine position was significantly lower in Group B than in Group A ($P < 0.05$).

2. IVP in the Semi-Sitting (Head Raised 30°) Position (Table 2)

The mean IVP in the semi-sitting position was -1.71 ± 6.23 cmH$_2$O in Group A and -16.22 ± 10.93 cmH$_2$O in Group B. In Group B, IVP immediately fell into a negative range even with the head slightly raised (10°). In Group A, IVP fell into a negative range with the head raised from 30° to 45°. In the semi-sitting position, IVP in Group B was also significantly lower than that in Group A ($P < 0.01$).

3. IVP in the Sitting or Standing Position (Table 2)

In this position, the difference of IVP between Group B and A was greater than that in the other two positions noted above. In Group A IVP was -9.93 ± 6.02 cmH$_2$O and in Group B IVP was -29.17 ± 8.42 cmH$_2$O. There was a

Table 2. IVP in three positions, pressure fall in each group, and references

		IVP (cmH_2O)			
		Supine	30° Head up	Sitting or standing	Pressure fall
With ASD	Group A	11.1 ± 6.71	-1.71 ± 6.23	-9.93 ± 6.02	17.76 ± 11.72
	Portnoy (1973)	2.17 ± 4.48		-3.30 ± 5.2	4.70 ± 2.55
	Chapman[a] (1990)	4.14 ± 4.56		-4.0 ± 6.88	8.14 ± 7.84
Without ASD	Group B	3.28 ± 5.13	-16.2 ± 10.93	-29.2 ± 8.42	32.62 ± 8.41
	Portnoy (1973)	-1.1 ± 5.73		-20.9 ± 12.4	20.4 ± 10.2
	Chapman[a] (1990)	4.78 ± 3.49		-23.8 ± 7.8	27.2 ± 8.43
		B < A (P < 0.05)	B < A (P < 0.01)	B < A (P < 0.001)	B > A (P < 0.05)

[a] Modified from Chapman 1990

Table 3. IVP and CSF flow in cases of shunt malfunction before and after shunt revision

	IVP (cmH₂O)		CSF flow (ml/day)	
	Supine	Standing	Supine	Standing
Before revision (case 6)	10.2	−9.5	0.00	24.2
After revision (case 12)	6.8	−17.7	0.53	554

significant difference between these two groups ($P < 0.001$). Nevertheless, low pressure syndrome was observed in only one patient in Group B (16.7%). This 69-year-old woman was shunted for NPH following SAH. A subdural hematoma developed over the following 4 months. At first, an ASD was placed 8 cm below the level of the foramen of Monro, and a Sophy valve was used at low pressure. In the supine position IVP was 10.2 cmH₂O and in the standing position IVP was −9.5 cmH₂O. CSF flow was 0 ml/day in the supine position and 24.2 ml/day in the standing position. As symptoms of NPH did not disappear and ventriculomegaly remained on the CT scan one month after the initial shunting, a shunt revision was performed and the ASD was removed. After the second shunting, the patient became active and began to walk by herself. After the shunt revision IVP was 6.8 cmH₂O in the supine position and −17.7 cmH₂O in the standing position. CSF flow after the shunt revision was 0.53 ml/day an the supine position and 554 ml/day in the standing position (Table 3).

As she had hemiparesis on her left side, she tended to fall down repeatedly and hit her head. Three months after the shunt revision, she began low level activity and developed a gait disturbance. A CT scan revealed a subdural hematoma at the left parietal convexity. She was kept supine for a week and the Sophy valve was upgraded to a high pressure valve without an ASD. A few days later, she had fully recovered.

In the subjects described by Portnoy et al. in 1973 IVP in an erect position was −3.3 ± 5.2 cmH₂O; in the subjects described by Chapman et al. in 1990 (rearranged from Fig. 3 of their article) it was −4 ± 6.9 cmH₂O.

There were significant differences between the IVPs of our subjects and theirs in an erect position. The position of an ASD causes these differences. Our attempt to insert an ASD in a lower position in the shunting system will suppress the adverse effect of the ASD.

4. Pressure Fall During Full Positional Change (Table 2)

From the supine to the erect position, IVP fell immediately and markedly in each group. The degree of the fall in pressure was 17.76 ± 11.72 cmH₂O in Group A and 32.62 ± 8.41 cmH₂O in Group B. There was a significant difference between Groups A and B in the fall in pressure ($P < 0.05$). It was confirmed that an ASD was effective in restoring physiological pressure to patients in the erect position.

Discussion

The low pressure syndrome in patients with shunting is well known. Its symptoms in adults have been described as headache, nausea, vomiting, visual disturbances, lack of energy, lack of interest, and lethargy (Foltz and Blanks 1988). In infants, sunken fontanel, overriding of cranial bones, and irritability are the signs of this syndrome (Shulman et al. 1965).

Chronic subdural hematoma (SDH) has sometimes been observed on a CT scan. In shunted patients, the incidence of SDH has been reported as 20.8% (Samuelson et al. 1972), 38.5% (Portnoy et al. 1973), and 23% (McCullough and Fox 1974), with a higher risk of SDH in shunts without an ASD. An interesting case of acute subdural hematoma due to overdrainage of CSF through the shunt catheter in a lumboperitoneal (LP) shunt was reported by Ishiwata (1989). In children, CT sometimes reveals slit-like or collapsed ventricles resulting from the low intracranial pressure. These phenomena were the result of overdrainage of CSF through the shunt system and this over-drainage was explained as a siphon effect (Portnoy et al. 1973). It is true that IVP falls to under zero cmH_2O in normal subjects in an erect position. A siphon effect in the normal CSF column and blood flow will induce this phenomenon. Various studies concerning this problem have been made. (Loman et al. 1935; Bradely 1987; Fox et al. (to be published); McCullough and Fox 1974; Magnes 1976; Chapman et al. 1990).

Various attempts have been made to prevent LPS. They can be divided into three groups: The use of a high pressure or high resistance valve (Salmon 1972; Yamada 1982; Saint-Rose et al. 1987; Foltz and Blanks 1988), the insertion of a distal catheter into the venous system (Sharkey 1956; El-Shafei 1985), and the insertion of an ASD into the shunt system (Portnoy et al. 1973; McCullough and Fox 1974; Hyde-Roman et al. 1982; Gruber et al. 1984; Portnoy 1984, 1985; Tokoro and Chiba 1989; Chapman et al. 1990).

On the other hand, the adverse effects of an ASD have been pointed out in some articles (McCullough 1986; Seida et al. 1987). For normal press-ure hydrocephalus patients, we think it most important that IVP has to be sufficiently reduced by CSF shunting. We sometimes experience shunt com-plications of insufficient CSF flow when using an integrated ASD device. Overfunction of the ASD seems to prevent CSF flow in an erect position. For these reasons, we insert the ASD in a low position in the shunt system, usually 10 cm below the level of the foramen of Monro.

In this study, the mean IVP in Group B was significantly low in the supine position. As an ASD does not work in this position, then logically, the IVPs in Groups B and A must be equal. One hour of resting in the supine position prior to measurement was not enough to determine the IVP in each group in order to compare them. IVP in the supine position had to drop to the pressure which was determined by the differential pressure of the valve.

In Group B, IVP became negative even when the patient's head was raised only 10°. In contrast, in Group A, IVP remained in a positive range in this position. In most patients in Group A, IVP became negative when the head was raised between 30° to 45°. This indicated that, in patients without an ASD, IVP was much more influenced by postural changes.

In conclusion, in Group B, it was confirmed that the siphon effect was well observed in patients in the erect position. However, low pressure syndrome was observed in only one of six patients without an ASD. On the other hand, reduced CSF flow due to the adverse effect of an ASD was observed in two of eleven patients with ASDs.

The IVP levels in the erect position varied widely; however, a large number of patients had no symptoms of hydrocephalus or low pressure syndrome. It is therefore difficult to determine the proper IVP level of hydrocephalic patients before shunting. However, as the low pressure syndrome leading to subdural hematoma or the slit ventricle syndrome is a troublesome and sometimes life threatening condition, we must place priority on preventing this syndrome. The insertion of an ASD in a lower position in the shunt system has great possibilities for treating hydrocephalus.

References

Bradely KC (1987) Cerebrospinal fluid pressure. J Neurol Neurosurg Psychiatry 33: 387–397

Chapman PH, Cosman ER, Arnold MA (1990) The relationship between ventricular fluid pressure and body position in normal subjects and subjects with shunts. Neurosurgery 26: 181–189

El-Shafei IL (1985) Ventriculovenous shunt against the direction of blood flow. A new approach for shunting the cerebrospinal fluid to venous circulation. Nerv Syst Child 1: 200–207

Foltz EL, Blanks JP (1988) Symptomatic low intracranial pressure in shunting hydrocephalus. J Neurosurg 68: 401–408

Fox JL, McCullough DC, Green RC (to be published) Effect of CSF-shunts on the intracranial pressure and CSF dynamic. A new technique of pressure measurements, results, and concepts. J Neurol Neurosurg Psychiatry

Gruber R, Jenny P, Herzog B (1984) Experience with the anti-siphon device (ASD) in shunt therapy of pediatric hydrocephalus. J Neurosurg 61: 156–162

Hyde-Roman MD, Rckatc HL, Nulsen FE (1982) Reexpansion of previously collapsed ventricles. J Neurosurg 56: 536–539

Ishiwata Y (1989) Analysis of CSF flow through L-P shunt during change of posture (in Japanese). Neurol Surg 17: 351–358

Loman J, Myerson A, Goldman D (1935) Effect of alterations in posture on the cerebrospinal fluid pressure. Arch Neurol Psychiatry 33: 1279–1295

Magnes B (1976) Body position and cerebrospinal fluid pressure and the hydrostatic indifferent point. J Neurosurg 44: 698–705

McCullough DC (1986) Symptomatic progressive ventriculomegaly in hydrocephalics with patent shunts and antisiphon devices. Neurosurgery 19: 617–621

McCullough DC, Fox JL (1974) Negative intracranial pressure hydrocephalus in adults with shunts and its relationship to the production of subdural hematoma. J Neurosurg 40: 372–375

Portnoy HD (1984) Antisiphon devices in shunt therapy (letter). J Neurosurg 61: 1158

Portnoy HD (1985) Antisiphon device, technical details (letter). J Neurosurg 63

Portnoy HD, Schulte RR, Fox JL, Croissant PD, Tripp L (1973) Antisiphon and reversible occlusion valves for shunting in hydrocephalus and preventing post-shunt subdural hematomas. J Neurosurg 38: 729–738

Rudd TG, Shurtleff DB, Loeser JD, Nelp WP (1973) Radionuclide assessment of cerebrospinal fluid shunt function in children. J Nucl Med 14: 683–686

Saint-Rose C, Hooven MD, Hirsch JF (1987) A new approach in the treatment of hydrocephalus. J Neurosurg 66: 213–226

Salmon JH (1972) The collapsed ventricle: Management and prevention. Surg Neurol 9: 349–352

Samuelson S, Long DM, Chou SN (1972) Subdural hematoma as a complication of shunting procedure for normal pressure hydrocephalus. J Neurosurg 37: 548–551

Seida M, Ito U, Tomita S, Yamazaki S, Inaba Y (1987) Ventriculo-peritoneal shunt malfunction with anti-siphon devices in normal pressure hydrocephalus (in Japanese). Neurol Med Chir (Tokyo) 27: 769–773

Sharkey PC (1956) Ventriculo sagittal-sinus shunt. J Neurosurg 22: 362–367

Shulman K et al. (1965) Workshop in hydrocephalus. University of Pennsylvania, Philadelphia

Tokoro K, Chiba Y (1989) Effects on shunt flow of antisiphon device and of changes in posture in hydrocephalus. Ninth Congress of Neurological Surgery. New Delhi, India, pp 100

Yamada H (1982) A flow-regulation device to control differential pressure in CSF shunt systems. J Neurosurg 57: 570–573

40 — Sophy Shunts in the Treatment of 130 Patients

D. Maitrot, C. A. Valery, P. Boyer, P. Kehrli, and F. Buchheit[1]

Keywords. Hydrocephalus — Shunt system — Hydrodynamics

I. How Does a Shunt Work?

A shunt is a connection between two tanks, as shown in Fig. 1. When the first tank is on a table while the second is on the floor, for example, the water will go from the first tank to the second without any problem. If now the second tank comes to the level of the first, there will be a quick balance between the two tanks. This small experience illustrates the siphon effect, which will become more effective when the height between the two tanks is increased. The valve acts as a small resistance whose effects depend on the level of the opening pressure.

The flow in a shunt can be estimated according to Poiseuille's law:

$$Q = \frac{DP \times \pi R^4}{8\eta L}$$

where Q is the flow,
  R is the radius of the shunt, which is almost the same for most of the shunts,
  η is the viscosity of the CSF,
  L the length of the tube, and
  DP is the differential pressure

According to this equation, the flow in a shunt depends on the differential pressure between the apertures of the valve. This differential pressure is equal to:

$$DP = IVP - IAP + L$$

---

[1] Department of Neurosurgery, CHU Hautepierre, Strasbourg University School of Medicine, Strasbourg, France

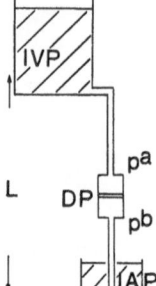

Fig. 1. How a shunt works IVP, intraventricular pressure; IAP, intra abdominal pressure; DP, differential pressure

where IVP is intraventricular pressure
and IAP is intra abdominal pressure

Poiseuille's law can now be written:

$$\overset{\circ}{Q} = \frac{(IVP - IAP + L)\pi R^4}{8\eta L}$$

In this equation, the single factor subject to important variations is the height of the tube, when the patient leaves his bed, for instance.

According to Poiseuille's law and the scheme shown in Fig. 1 we tested various kinds of shunts; the results of the observed flows are illustrated in Figs. 2 and 3.

II. Comments About

The physiological flow,
    The flow of most shunts,
    The fact that low, medium, or high pressure valves don't influence flow, and
    The variations of flow between the supine and the upright positions.

III. Reasons for our Choice of Sophy Shunts and Their Adaptable Opening Pressure Valve

Premature Infants

Supine posture at beginning.
Need of a high flow with small opening pressure.

Children

They begin to walk or sit very often.
Need of less flow, that means higher opening pressure than for premature infants.

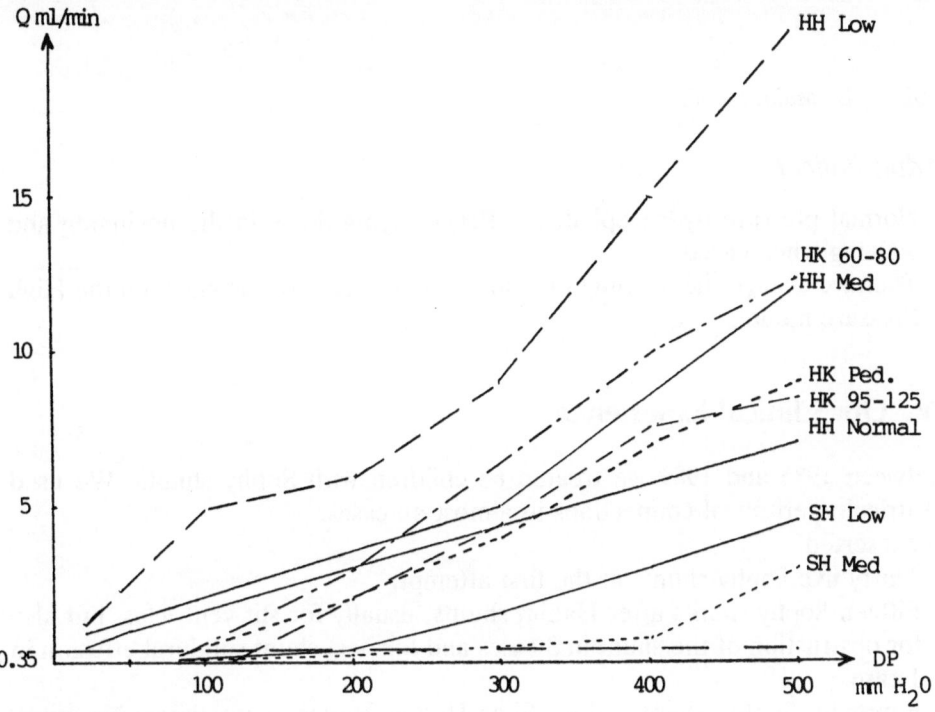

Fig. 2. Shunt flows
HH, Holter-Hausner; HK, Hakim; SH, Spitz-Holter; DP, differential pressure; Q, flow

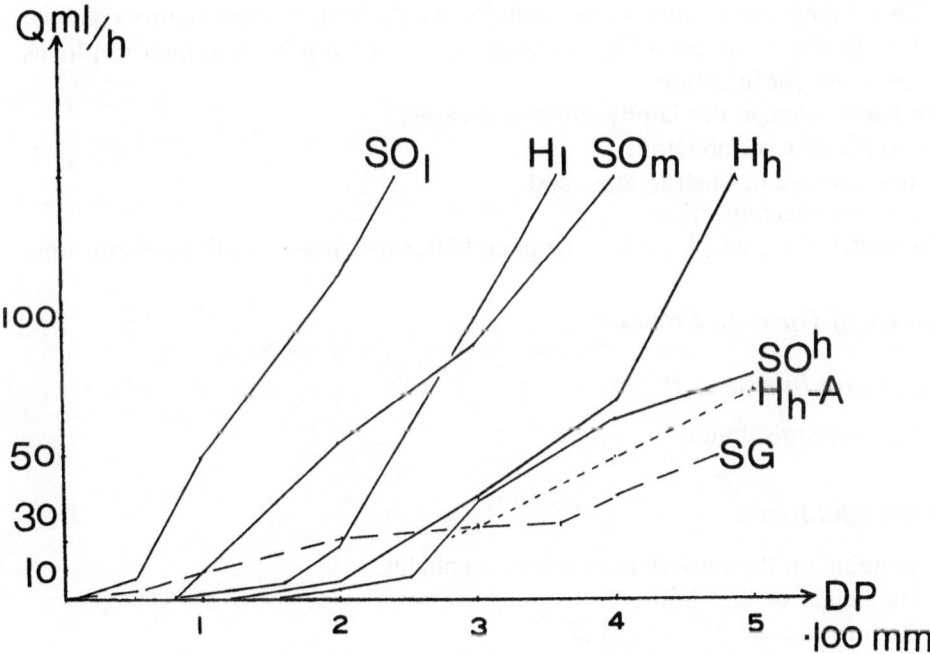

Fig. 3. Shunt flow
SO, Sophy; H, Spitz-Holter; SG, Sigma; H_h-A, Spitz-Holter high with anti-siphon device; DP, differential, pressure; Q, flow; L, low; h, high; m, medium

Adult Patients

Normal pressure hydrocephalus (NPH) → lying down in the beginning and walking when cured.
Then we change the opening pressure, which is set, for instance, on the High Pressure mode.

IV. Our Clinical Experience

Between 1985 and 1989 we treated 68 children with Sophy shunts. We used ventriculo peritoneal connections in almost all cases.
We inserted.
Thirty five Sophy shunts at the first attempt.
Fifteen Sophy shunts after Hakim shunts, usually for slit ventricles, but also for obstruction of the shunt in 3 cases and for post-shunt subdural effusion in 1 case.
Fourteen Sophy shunts after Spitz-Holter shunts, sometimes for over-drainage, in cases where low pressure Spitz-Holter valves were used some-times for persistent hydrocephalus, in cases where high pressure Spitz-Holter valves were used.
Two Sophy shunts after Heyer-Schulte shunts for persistent hydrocephalus.
Two Sophy shunts after Sigma shunts, in 1 case for persistent hydrocephalus, in the other for infection.
We had to change the Sophy shunt in 8 cases,
two because of infections,
four because of obstructions, and
two after deconnections.
The obstructions which we had happened after treatment of subdural effusions.

Choice of Opening Pressure

Premature Infants L.P.

Low pressure shunts

Other Children

Depending on the importance of hydrocephalus.
The height of the children.
The intracranial pressure (ICP).

Change of Opening Pressure

This depended on the results noted on the computed tomography (CT) scan some weeks or months after insertion:

Persistent hydrocephalus: lowering the opening pressure.

Slit ventricles and subdural effusions: increasing the opening pressure.

As the child grows, the opening pressure is increased because the differential pressure (DP) becomes higher.

V. Technical Problems

In cases of small subdural effusions, it's sometimes difficult to fill up the valve. It becomes necessary to fill up the shunt with physiological serum to avoid the presence of air in the valve.

It's also necessary to gently shake the valve before insertion, because the semi-circular spring of the valve sometimes moves too easily.

It's also important to remember that we have to use Sophy catheters. If we do not, the flow will not be the one indicated on the diagrams. If we insert a shunt with a medium or high opening pressure it's necessary to suck CSF into the valve when connecting the ventricular catheter. It's important to remember that the arrow sited on the shunt must be put near the scalp and not against the skull.

Finally, for premature infants, it's sometimes better to insert the shunt on the chest wall. This can also be done in order to avoid artifacts if MRI explorations are expected. However, when premature infants were one year of age we had to change the site of valve insertion.

VI. Adult Hydrocephalus

Sixty four shunts for 61 patients

Fifty nine Ventriculo-cardiac (VC) connections

Why do we use VC connections?

We can fix the height of the connection to 30–32 cm. Under these conditions, the flow of the shunts at high pressure will be near the physiological flow and at medium pressure will be no more than twice the physiological flow. So, we avoid subdural effusions.

We changed the opening pressure 14 times and usually inserted a shunt with high opening pressure. After control with CT scan, we changed the opening pressure, depending on the clinical and CT scan results. We noted three subdural effusions. Two were asymptomatic and disappeared after increasing the opening pressure, and one needed operation and an increase of the opening pressure.

It's interesting to note that this last subdural effusion occured after moving the opening pressure from high to medium because the patient was not completely happy with the results. He was 72 years old and a great bridge player!

VII. Conclusions

All the clinical results can be compared with other series treated with other kinds of shunts, but we noted no more slit ventricles, post-shunt craniostenosis, or subdural effusions.

41 — Pitfalls of the Sophy Programmable Pressure Valve: Is it Really Better than a Conventional Valve and an Anti-Siphon Device?

Kazuhiko Tokoro, Yasuhiro Chiba, and Hiroyuki Abe[1]

Summary. Twelve patients with hydrocephalus were shunted using the Sophy programmable pressure valve (SU-8). Positional shunt flow and intraventricular pressure (IVP) were measured. An anti-siphon device (ASD) was inserted primarily in seven patients. Two of the five patients without an ASD developed subdural hematoma (SDH) and one developed slit ventricle syndrome (SVS). Upgrading the valve resistance failed to control SDH and SVS and required the addition of an ASD to control overdrainage.

In the sitting position, shunt flow was maximal in the low-pressure valve without an ASD (group A1: 1164 ml/day) and least in the medium- and high-pressure valves with an ASD (group B2: 48 ml/day). Intermediate values were found in the medium- and high-pressure valves without an ASD (group A2: 528 ml/day) and in the low-pressure valve with an ASD (group B1: 183 ml/day). For supine shunt flow, there were no significant differences among the four groups (1.1–9.1 ml/day).

In all groups, IVPs in the sitting position were significantly lower than those in the supine position. IVPs in the supine position were the lowest in group A1 (0.7 ± 1.1 cmH$_2$O) and the highest in group B2 (22.0 ± 4.3 cmH$_2$O). Intermediate values were found for groups A2 and B1 (5.9 ± 3.0 and 12.7 ± 5.4 cmH$_2$O, respectively). IVPs in the sitting position were also the lowest in group A1 (-17.5 cmH$_2$O) and the highest in group B2 (0.5 ± 4.0 cmH$_2$O). Intermediate values were found for groups A2 and B1 (-13.0 ± 2.8 and -10.7 ± 9.1 cmH$_2$O, respectively). Even the high-pressure Sophy valve without an ASD showed overdrainage and highly negative IVP in the sitting position. In contrast, overdrainage was well controlled in the shunt systems with an ASD. The experimental shunt flow and the least IVP necessary to initiate shunt flow account well for our clinical experiences.

Upgrading the Sophy valve resistance alone is not sufficient to prevent SDH and SVS. Combined use together with an ASD is essential when patients assume the erect position.

---

[1] Department of Neurosurgery, Kanagawa Rehabilitation Center, Atsugi, 243–01 Japan

Keywords. Pressure-adjustable valve — Anti-siphon device — Ventriculoperitoneal shunt — Slit ventricle syndrome — Subdural hematoma

Introduction

A widely recognized complication associated with the use of cerebrospinal fluid (CSF) shunts for hydrocephalus is excessive negative intracranial pressure (ICP) (See references Abe et al. 1990 – Portnoy et al. 1973 and Sainte-Rose et al. 1987–Tokoro and Chiba [to be published]). This is due to overdrainage of CSF by a siphon effect when patients are erect. Overdrainage contributes to the "slit ventricle syndrome (SVS)" and subdural hematoma (SDH) (Abe et al. 1990; Dietrich et al. 1987; Epstein et al. 1974; Foltz and Blanks 1988; Fuse et al. 1990; Gruber et al. 1984; Kikuch, et al. 1990; Loayza 1987; McCullough and Fox 1974; Portnoy et al. 1973; Tokoro and Chiba [to be published]).

Treatment of CSF overdrainage can be divided into two main approaches: (1) use of a higher resistance valve (Dietrich et al. 1987; Foltz and Blanks 1988; Fuse et al. 1990; Itoh et al. 1989; Kikuchi et al. 1990; Loayza 1987; Sainte-Rose et al. 1987; Schmitt et al. 1989) and (2) use of an anti-siphon device (ASD) (Abe et al. 1990; Chapman et al. 1990; Gruber et al. 1984; Horton and Pollay 1990; McCullough 1986; Portnoy et al. 1973; Seida et al. 1987; Tokoro and Chiba 1989; Tokoro and Chiba [to be published]). The former approach includes the use of a pressure-adjustable valve (PAV).

The Sophy programmable pressure valve was designed to control the overdrainage of CSF shunts. The valve's resistance can be changed non-invasively over the scalp with a magnet. It has been argued that the use of a PAV can prevent SVS and SDH (Dietrich et al. 1987; Fuse et al. 1990; Itoh et al. 1989; Kikuchi et al. 1990; Loayza 1987).

According to our experience with 12 cases, however, upgrading of the valve resistance could not prevent SVS and SDH, which subsided after the addition of an ASD. We would therefore like to discuss both the pitfalls of the PAV and how it can be used effectively.

Clinical Material and Methods

During the period from May 1989 to April 1990, 12 patients with hydrocephalus were shunted using the Sophy programmable pressure valve (SU-8) (Sophysa Inc., Levillier sur Mer, France). The etiology of hydrocephalus was: subarachnoid hemorrhage in seven patients, congenital anomaly in two, cerebellar hemangioblastoma in one, and thalamic hemorrhage in one. Nine patients had normal pressure hydrocephalus (NPH) and three had hypertensive hydrocephalus. There were 11 ventriculoperitoneal (VP) shunts and 1 ventriculoatrial (VA) shunt (case 7). A burr hole was usually made in the right occipitotemporal region. The shunt systems used were a double lumen ventricular catheter, a Foltz reservoir, a Sophy valve, an ASD (American V.

Mueller, Chicago, Ill., USA), and a kink-resistant peritoneal catheter. In the Sophy valve, the three main closing pressure (CP) values were as follows: low pressure was 5 cmH$_2$O; medium, 11 cmH$_2$O; and high, 17 cmH$_2$O. An ASD was inserted primarily at 10 cm below the level of the foramen of Monro in five patients and just distal to the Sophy valve in two. The ASD was later removed from one of these patients (case 9). In five patients an ASD was not used primarily, although subsequently an ASD was added in two of these patients (cases 7 and 8).

The patients were divided into two groups according to the absence (group A) or presence (group B) of an ASD. Each group was divided into two subgroups according to the closing pressure of the valve, as follows:

Group A: Sophy valve without ASD (nine patients)
   Group A1: Low-pressure valve without ASD (three patients)
   Group A2: Medium- and high-pressure valves without ASD (six patients)
Group B: Sophy valve with ASD (nine patients)
   Group B1: Low-pressure valve with ASD (six patients)
   Group B2: Medium- and high-pressure valves with ASD (three patients)

Shunt flow, calculated using radionuclide shuntography in the supine and sitting and/or standing positions, was expressed as ml/day (Rudd et al. 1973; Tokoro and Chiba 1989; Tokoro and Chiba [to be published]). Positional changes of intraventricular pressure (IVP) were monitored through the Foltz reservoir, referenced to the level of the foramen of Monro (Abe et al. 1990; Chapman et al. 1990). Experimental shunt flow in vitro was measured according to the method used by Portnoy et al. (1973). Raising or lowering the proximal water level above the shunt valve produced positive or negative pressures between 10 and −10 cm in 5-cm intervals, while lowering the distal catheter tip 0–60 cm in 10-cm intervals provided negative outlet pressures. The position of the ASD was varied: 0 cm (integral), 10 cm, and 60 cm (theoretically without an ASD) from the shunt valve. Flow was measured at a given inlet pressure for varying outlet pressures.

Shunt flow data were transformed into natural logarithms before analysis. These results were expressed as a geometric mean (antilog of mean of log value) with range (standard deviation) and graphs were drawn on a logarithmic scale. ICP data were expressed as an arithmetic mean with standard deviation. Statistical analyses included the Student t test. A P value of less than 0.05 was considered significant.

Results

The cases are summarized in Table 1.

Shunt Flow and ICPs During Positional Changes (Fig. 1)

The results of the positional shunt flow and ICPs are shown in Table 2 and Fig. 1. In all but group B2, sitting shunt flow was significantly greater than supine

Table 1. Summary of cases

Case number (n)	Age (years)	Etiology of hydrocephalus	Type of hydrocephalus	ASD	Pressure setting	Clinical course
1	48	SAH	NPH	10 cm	L^a	Uneventful
2	67	SAH	NPH	10 cm	L^a	Uneventful
3	55	Ruptured AVM	NPH	10 cm	L^a	Uneventful
4	58	SAH	NPH	(−)	$H^a \rightarrow M^a$	Uneventful
5	64	Cerebellar tumor (hemangioblastoma)	Hypertensive	Below	$M^a \rightarrow L^a$	Good after a low-pressure setting
6	12	Congenital	Hypertensive	10 cm	M^a	Slit ventricle subsided
7	14	Congenital	Hypertensive	(−) → 10 cm	$L \rightarrow H \rightarrow H^a \rightarrow M^a$	SVS subsided after addition of an ASD, Ventriculoatrial shunt
8	49	SAH	NPH	(−) → 10 cm	$L \rightarrow H \rightarrow H^a$	SDH subsided after addition of an ASD
9	68	SAH	NPH	Below → (−)	$L^a \rightarrow L \rightarrow H \rightarrow L$	ASD was removed. SDH subsided after a high-pressure setting, but NPH recurred
10	57	SAH	NPH	(−) → 10 cm	$L \rightarrow M \rightarrow L^b$	Elevated setting pressure, replaced by low-pressure Mishler valve with ASD 10 cm below
11	57	Thalamic hemorrhage ventricular rupture	NPH	(−) → 10 cm	$L \rightarrow L^b$	Elevated setting pressure, replaced by low-pressure Mishler valve with ASD 10 cm below
12	42	SAH	NPH	10 cm	L^a	Sophy valve occlusion ? Revision was not permitted

[a] with ASD

[b] = Mishler valve with ASD 10 cm downstream ASD, anti-siphon device; (−), without ASD; below, placed just below the shunt valve; 10 cm, placed 10 cm downstream; L, low pressure; M, medium pressure; H, high pressure; AVM arteriovenous malformation; NPH, normal pressure hydrocephalus; SAH, subarachnoid hemorrhage due to ruptured aneurysm; SDH, subdural hematoma; SVS, slit ventricle syndrome

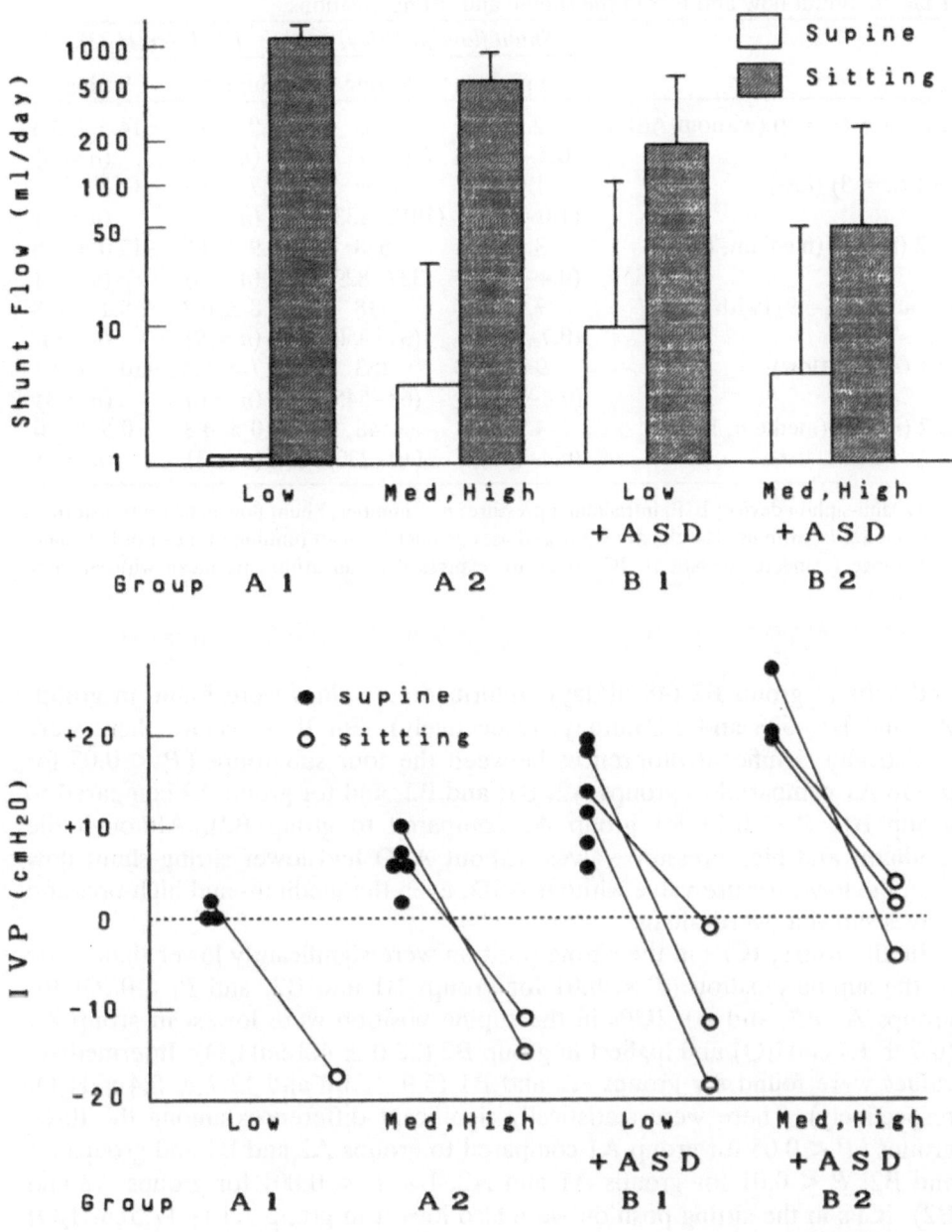

Fig. 1. Shunt flow (*upper*) and intraventricular pressure (*IVP*) (*lower*) during positional changes in the four groups. Med, medium pressure

shunt flow ($P < 0.001$ for groups A, A1, A2, and B; $P < 0.05$ for group B1).

For supine shunt flow, there were no statistically significant differences between these four subgroups (1.1–9.1 ml/day). Conversely, in the sitting position, shunt flow was maximal in group A1 (geometric mean 1164 ml/day)

Table 2. Shunt flow and ICP in the supine and sitting positions

	Shunt flow (ml/day)		I C P (cmH₂O)	
	Supine	Sitting	Supine	Sitting
Group A (n = 9) (without ASD)	2.34	685	3.9 ± 3.6	−14.5 ± 3.3
	(0.4–13.3)	(399–1176)	(n = 8)	(n = 3)
A 1 (n = 3) (low)	1.06	1164	0.7 ± 1.1	−17.5
	(1.0–1.2)	(1012–1339)	(n =3)	(n = 1)
A 2 (n = 6) (medium, high)	3.46	528	5.9 ± 3.0	−13.0 ± 2.8
	(0.4–27.4)	(337–829)	(n = 5)	(n = 2)
Group B (n = 9) (with ASD)	7.03	118	15.8 ± 6.7	−5.1 ± 8.8
	(0.7–71.5)	(31–450)	(n = 9)	(n =6)
B 1 (n = 6) (low)	9.12	183	12.7 ± 5.4	−10.7 ± 9.1
	(0.8–103)	(62–545)	(n = 6)	(n = 3)
B 2 (n = 3) (medium, high)	4.22	48	22.0 ± 4.3	0.5 ± 4.0
	(0.4–51.4)	(10–230)	(n = 3)	(n = 3)

ASD, anti-siphon device; ICP, intracranial pressure; n = number. Shunt flow data are transformed into natural logarithms. Results are expressed as a geometric mean (antilog of mean of log value) with range (standard deviation). ICP data are expressed as an arithmetic mean with standard deviation.

and least in group B2 (48 ml/day). Intermediate values were found in groups A2 and B1 (528 and 183 ml/day, respectively). For these values there were statistically significant differences between the four subgroups ($P < 0.05$ for group A1 compared to groups A2, B1, and B2, and for group A2 compared to group B1; $P < 0.01$ for group A2 compared to group B2). Although the medium- and high-pressure valves without ASD had lower sitting shunt flow than the low-pressure valve without ASD, even the medium- and high-pressure valves showed overdrainage.

In all groups, ICPs in the sitting position were significantly lower than those in the supine position ($P < 0.01$ for groups B1 and B2, and $P < 0.001$ for groups A, A2, and B). ICPs in the supine position were lowest in group A1 (0.7 ± 1.1 cmH₂O) and highest in group B2 (22.0 ± 4.3 cmH₂O). Intermediate values were found for groups A2 and B1 (5.9 ± 3.0 and 12.7 ± 5.4 cmH₂O, respectively). There were statistically significant differences among the three groups ($P < 0.05$ for group A1 compared to groups A2 and B1 and groups B1 and B2; $P < 0.01$ for groups A1 and A2, B2; $P < 0.001$ for groups A2 and B2). ICPs in the sitting position were also lowest in group A1 (-17.5 cmH₂O) and highest in group B2 (0.5 ± 4.0 cmH₂O). Intermediate values were found for groups A1 and B1 (-13.0 ± 2.8 and -10.7 ± 9.1 cmH₂O, respectively). There were statistically significant differences between groups A2 and B2 ($P < 0.05$) and groups A and B2 ($P < 0.01$). The difference in ICP between the supine and sitting positions was 23.7 ± 9.9 cmH₂O in group A and 23.3 ± 7.9 cmH₂O in group B. These differences were not considered statistically significant. Shunt systems without an ASD (group A) resulted in a lower ICP and highe sitting shunt flow than those with an ASD (group B). In shunt

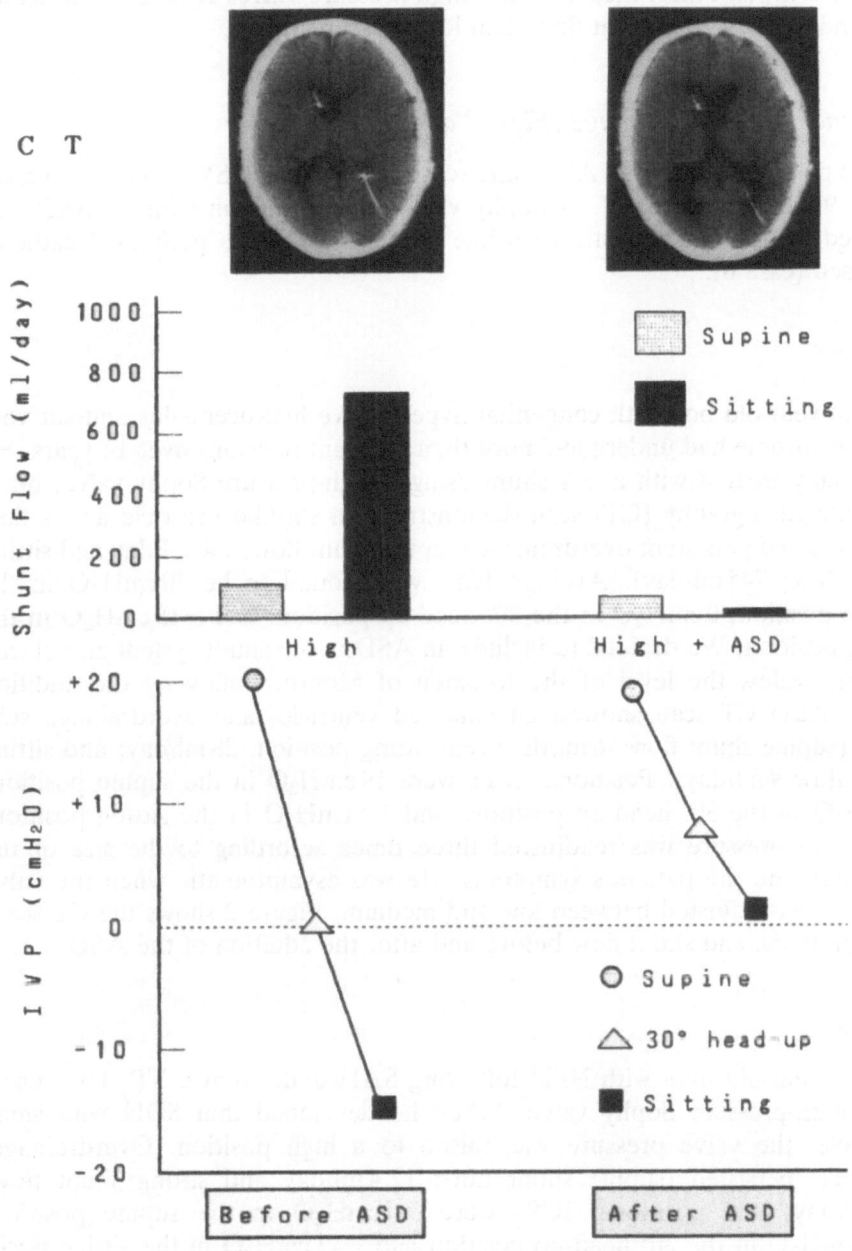

Fig. 2. Case 7, congenital hypertensive hydrocephalus with slit ventricle syndrome (*SVS*). *Top*, CT scan; *middle*, shunt flow; *bottom*, average ICPs before and after the addition of an ASD into a high-pressure Sophy valve. Slit-ventricles, a much lower sitting ICP and overdrainage improved after the addition of the ASD

systems with an ASD, medium- and high-pressure valves resulted in a higher ICP and lower sitting shunt flow than low-pressure valves.

Treatment of Overdrainage (Figs. 2 and 3)

Of the patients without an ASD, one (case 7), developed SVS, and two, (cases 8 and 9), developed SDH. A Sophy valve in combination with an ASD was inserted in one patient with a slit-like ventricle when his peritoneal catheter occluded (case 6).

Case 7

This 14-year-old boy with congenital hypertensive hydrocephalus and slit ventricle syndrome had undergone more than 10 shunt revisions over 14 years. He was finally treated with a VA shunt using a high-pressure Sophy valve, but a compute tomography (CT) scan demonstrated a slit-like ventricle and a flow study showed persistent overdrainage (supine shunt flow; 140 ml/day and sitting shunt flow; 745 ml/day). Average ICPs were found to be 20 cmH$_2$O in the supine position, 0 cmH$_2$O in the 30° head-up position, and -15 cmH$_2$O in the sitting position. We decided to include an ASD in the shunt system and placed it 10 cm below the level of the foramen of Monro. Following the addition of the ASD CT scan showed an enlarged ventricle, and overdrainage subsided (supine shunt flow 76 ml/day; semisitting position, 28 ml/day; and sitting shunt flow 9 ml/day). Positional ICPs were 19 cmH$_2$O in the supine position, 8 cmH$_2$O in the 30° head-up position, and 1.5 cmH$_2$O in the sitting position. The valve pressure was readjusted three times according to the size of the ventricles and the patient's symptoms. He was asymptomatic when the valve pressure was adjusted between low and medium. Figure 2 shows the CT scan, average ICPs, and shunt flow before and after the addition of the ASD.

Case 8

This 49-year-old man with NPH following SAH underwent a VP shunt using a medium-pressure Sophy valve. When he developed thin SDH with small ventricle, the valve pressure was raised to a high position. Overdrainage, however, persisted (supine shunt flow; 12.4 ml/day and sitting shunt flow; 501 ml/day) and positional ICPs were 5.5 cmH$_2$O in the supine position, -1.5 cmH$_2$O in the 30° head-up position and -11 cmH$_2$O in the sitting position. As SDH increased, he underwent a burr hole irrigation of the hematoma and the addition of an ASD 10 cm downstream. Overdrainage and SDH subsided, and ventricular size enlarged without symptoms. Postoperative supine shunt flow was 0 ml/day, and sitting shunt flow was 207 ml/day. Positional ICPs were 20 cmH$_2$O in the supine position, 11 cmH$_2$O in the 30° head-up position and 4 cmH$_2$O in the sitting position. Figure 3 shows the CT scan, average ICPs, and shunt flow before and after the addition of an ASD.

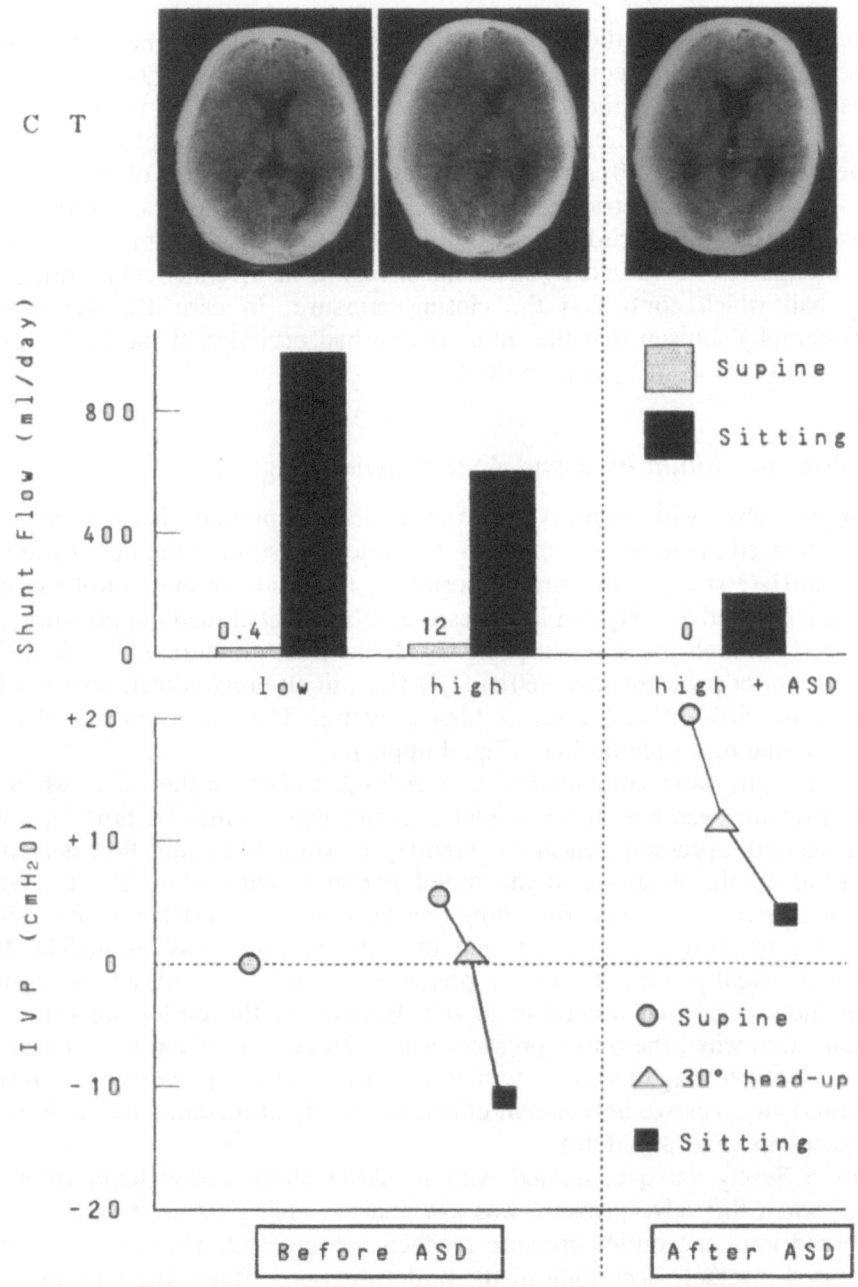

Fig. 3. Case 8, Normal pressure hydrocephalus (*NPH*) with subdural hematoma (*SDH*); *Top*, CT scan; *middle*, shunt flow; bottom, average ICPs before and after the addition of an ASD into the high-pressure Sophy valve. After the addition of the ASD and hematoma irrigation, SDH with small ventricles, a much lower sitting ICP, and over-drainage improved

Elevation of Setting Pressure

Three patients, two without an ASD (cases 10 and 11) and one with an ASD (case 12), showed inadequate shunt flow or shunt occlusion (3/12; 25%). Shunt revision showed both the ASD and the peritoneal catheter to be patent in cases 10 and 11. The Sophy valve was replaced with a low-pressure Mishler valve with an ASD 10 cm below the level of the foramen of Monro, with good results. Manometric tests of the Sophy valve showed an elevated setting pressure: 7.5–11 cmH$_2$O at low pressure (5 cmH$_2$O). This complication was thought to be caused by mechanical failure in a semicircular spring and ruby ball which controlled the closing pressure. In case 12, metrizamide shuntography showed that the shunt system had occluded at the Sophy valve, but shunt revision was not permitted.

Experimental Shunt Flow and ASD Function (Fig. 4)

In Sophy valves without an ASD, even if the inlet pressure became negative, flow increased inversely according to the outlet pressure. If the outlet pressure was 0 cmH$_2$O (i.e., in the supine position), flow did not start until the inlet pressure reached 5 cmH$_2$O at low pressure, 10 cmH$_2$O at medium pressure, and 17 cmH$_2$O at high pressure, respectively. If the inlet pressure was −10 cmH$_2$O and the outlet pressure was −60 cmH$_2$O (i.e., in an erect adult), flow reached 5.7 ml/min (8200 ml/day) even at high pressure. The results indicated overdrainage due to a siphon effect (Fig. 4 upper).

For a Sophy valve combined with an ASD just distal to the valve, when the valve pressure was low and the inlet pressure was 10 cmH$_2$O, flow increased until the outlet pressure reached −30 cmH$_2$O. After that point, flow decreased according to the decrease in the outlet pressure (anti-siphon effect). When the inlet pressure was negative, flow was zero at every outlet pressure. When the valve pressure became high and the inlet pressure was 10 cmH$_2$O, flow increased slightly until the outlet pressure reached −10 cmH$_2$O. After that point, flow decreased according to the decrease in the outlet pressure, and became zero when the outlet pressure was −50 cmH$_2$O. When the inlet pressure was zero or negative, flow was zero at every outlet pressure. The results indicated an excessive anti-siphon effect, especially at medium and high pressure positions (Fig. 4 middle).

For a Sophy valve combined with an ASD 10 cm downstream from the valve, when the valve pressure was low and the inlet pressure was zero, flow increased until the outlet pressure reached −30 cmH$_2$O. However, flow then decreased inversely according to the outlet pressure. When the inlet pressure was −5 cmH$_2$O, flow decreased, but did not reach zero. When the valve pressure was medium, flow decreased compared to when the pressure was low. When the valve pressure was high, flow decreased markedly and was equal to that in patients with an ASD just below the valve. This combination of low- or medium- pressure Sophy valve with an ASD 10 cm downstream provided an appropriate anti-siphon effect (Fig. 4 lower).

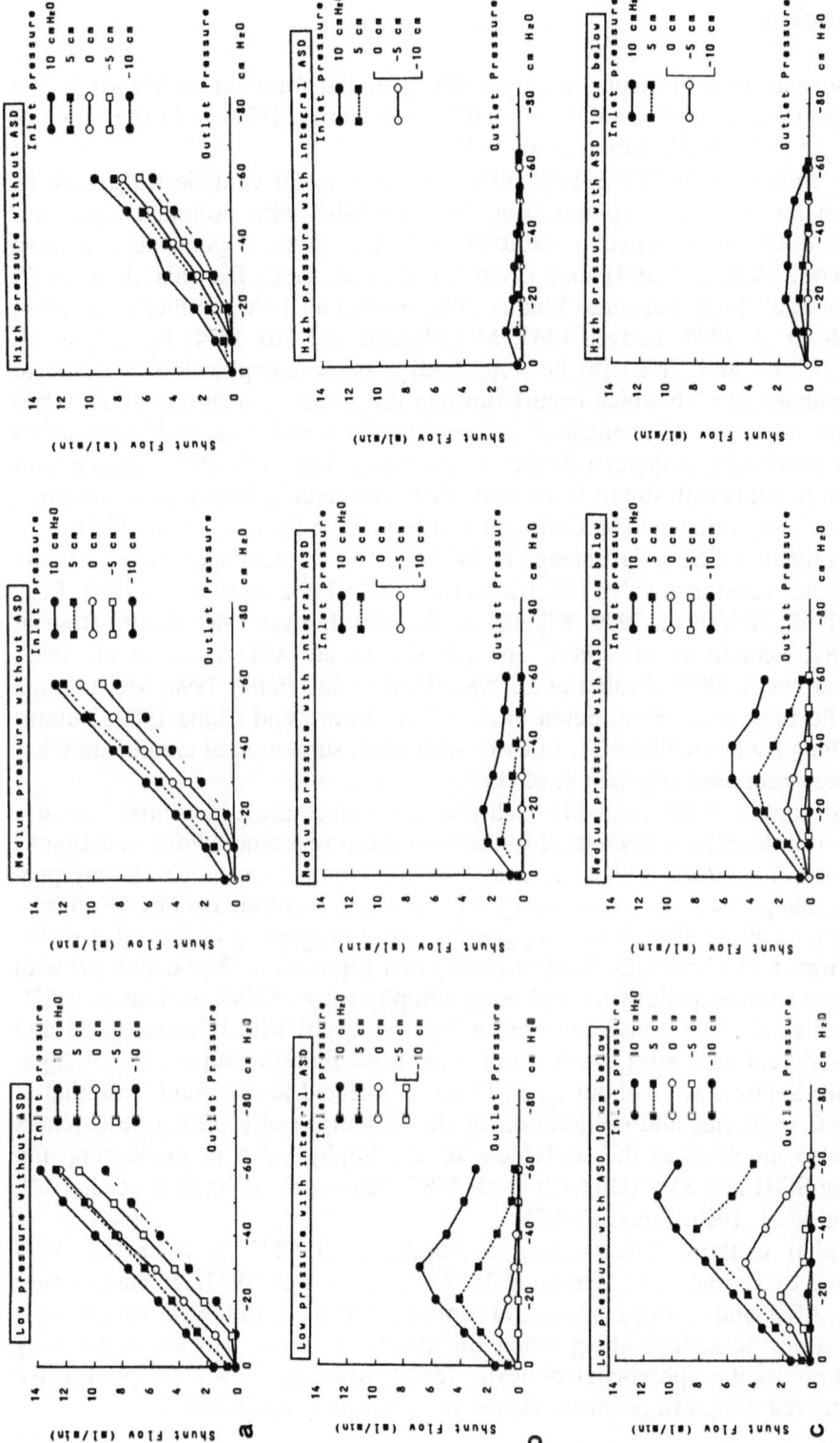

Fig. 4a–c. Changes in experimental shunt flow for various combinations of low-, medium-, and high-pressure Sophy valves with ASDs under the influence of various inlet and outlet pressures, **a** low-, medium-, and high-pressure valves without an ASD, **b** the same valves with an ASD just below the valve, and **c** the same valves with an ASD 10 cm downstream

Discussion

The normal intraventricular pressure (IVP) at the foramen of Monro in the erect position is approximately $-7\,\mathrm{cmH_2O}$ (Fox et al. 1973) or in the range of -5 to $+5\,\mathrm{cmH_2O}$ (Chapman et al. 1990).

CSF shunts lower IVP significantly, and as a result complications such as craniosynostosis, noncommunicating hydrocephalus with occluded aqueduct, occlusion of the ventricular catheter, extreme shunt dependency, chronic headache, SVS, and SDH may occur (Abe et al. 1990; Dietrich et al. 1987; Epstein et al. 1974; Foltz and Blanks 1988; Fuse et al. 1990; Gruber et al. 1984; Kikuchi et al. 1990; Loayza 1987; McCullough and Fox 1974; Portnoy et al. 1973; Tokoro and Chiba [to be published]). These complications are due to overdrainage of CSF which occurs through the shunt by a siphon effect when patients are erect. "Slit ventricle" is thought to be a major cause of obstruction of the ventricular catheter (Gruber et al. 1984). The 10%–20% incidence of SDH in patients with shunts is attributable to intracranial hypotension resulting from CSF overdrainage (McCullough and Fox 1974; Portnoy et al. 1973).

Treatment of CSF overdrainage is divided into two main approaches: (1) use of a higher resistance valve (Dietrich et al. 1987; Foltz and Blanks 1988; Fuse et al. 1990; Itoh et al. 1989; Kikuchi et al. 1990; Loayza 1987; Sainte-Rose et al. 1987; Schmitt et al. 1989), and (2) use of an ASD (Abe et al. 1990; Chapman et al. 1990; Gruber et al. 1984; Horton and Pollay 1990; McCullough 1986; Portnoy et al. 1973; Seida et al. 1987; Tokoro and Chiba 1989; Tokoro and Chiba [to be published]). In cases with SVS, subtemporal craniectomy has also been proposed (Epstein et al. 1974).

Most commercially available high-pressure valves are differential pressure valves and these have been used to increase shunt resistance. Foltz and Blanks (1988) recommended a high-pressure CSF Flo-Control valve. The Sophy programmable pressure valve was designed to control overdrainage of CSF shunts. A simple manipulation allowed upgrading and downgrading of the valve resistance from 5 to $17\,\mathrm{cmH_2O}$. Loayze (1987) first reported a 13-year-old girl with SVS who was successfully treated using a Sophy valve (SU-8) without an ASD. Dietrich et al. (1987) also reported a 7-year-old girl with bilateral SDH and collapsed ventricles after a VA shunt using a medium-pressure valve. A high-pressure Sophy valve without an ASD was connected to the shunt, resulting in enlarged ventricles and obliteration of the subdural space. Other researchers have also emphasized the usefulness of the Sophy valve in preventing and treating SDH and SVS (Dietrich et al. 1987; Fuse et al. 1990; Itoh et al. 1989; Kikuchi et al. 1990; Loayza 1987).

Another method of preventing overdrainage of CSF shunts is the ASD designed by Portnoy and Schulte in 1973 (Portnoy et al. 1973). If the pressure at the ASD outlet drops below atmospheric pressure, the ASD closes, thus eliminating the siphon effect when the patient is erect. Horton and Pollay (1990) reported a siphon-control device (SCD) which is a new anti-siphon valve of improved design (a normally closed vs. a normally open ASD).

Portnoy et al. (1973) examined the IVP of 13 patients with VP or VA shunts with integral ASDs and reversible occlusion valves. In the sitting position, in the same patients, IVP was $-21 \pm 12\,cmH_2O$ without an ASD and $-3 \pm 5\,cmH_2O$ with an integral ASD. Chapman et al. (1990) reported that IVP in the upright position ranged from -15 to $-35\,cmH_2O$ without an ASD, and from -7 to $3\,cmH_2O$ with an ASD, and concluded that the ASD maintains a normal IVP in the upright position. We also reported the IVP of patients in the supine position who had a VP shunt with a low-pressure valve (Mishler dual chamber) (Tokoro and Chiba 1989; Tokoro and Chiba [to be published]). Average supine IVPs were $1.9\,cmH_2O$ without an ASD and $9.4\,cmH_2O$ with an integral ASD. Intermediate values ($5.6\,cmH_2O$) were found for patients with

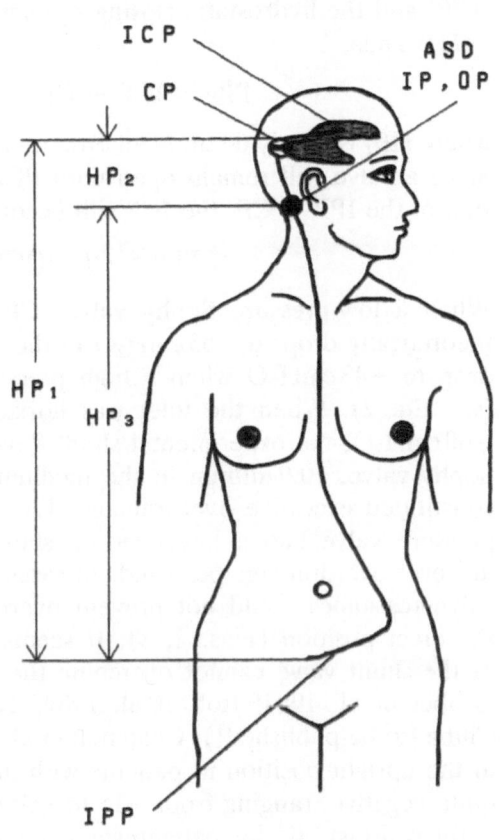

Fig. 5. Various pressure variables that determine the perfusion pressure through a shunt valve (PP_v) and an ASD (PP_{ASD}). Flow continues until PP_v and $PP_{Asd} = 0$. ICP, intracranial pressure (intraventricular pressure); CP, hydrostatic closing pressure of the shunt valve; IPP, intraperitoneal pressure; HP_1, shunt hydrostatic pressure related to vertical height of fluid-filled tubing; HP_2, hydrostatic pressure between the shunt valve and the ASD; IIP_3, hydrostatic pressure between the ASD and the end of the peritoneal catheter; IP, inlet pressure of the ASD; OP, outlet pressure of the ASD; ICP_{ASD}, the least ICP required to open the ASD

$$PP_v = ICP + HP_1 - (CP + IPP) > 0$$

$$PP_{ASD} = 8 \cdot IP - OP > 0$$

$$ICP_{ASD} = -\frac{9}{8} \cdot HP_2 + CP + 7.5$$

an ASD 10 cm downstream. Even with the same low pressure valve, IVP in the supine position was also affected by the presence of an ASD. Shunt systems with ASDs had a higher IVP than those without.

Which is more effective and practical for preventing overdrainage, a PAV or an ASD? We prefer the ASD. We would like to discuss this preference with respect to our experimental and clinical studies.

Does a High-Pressure Valve Really Prevent Overdrainage in the Erect Position? (Figs. 4 and 5)

The perfusion pressure through the shunt valve (PPv) is equal to the ICP plus shunt hydrostatic pressure (HP_1) minus the sum of the intraperitoneal pressure (IPP) and the hydrostatic closing pressure of the shunt valve (CP) (Fox et al. 1973). Thus,

$$PPv = ICP + HP_1 - (CP + IPP) > 0 \qquad \text{(Eq. 1)}$$

where HP_1 is nearly 60 cm in an erect Japanese adult and the IPP tends to zero. Since a valve will remain open until PPv equals zero, when HP_1 exceeds the sum of the IPP + CP, the ICP will become negative.

$$PPv = 60 + (ICP - CP) > 0 \qquad \text{(Eq. 2)}$$

When a low-pressure Sophy valve (CP = $5 \text{cmH}_2\text{O}$) is used, the ICP can theoretically drop to $-55 \text{cmH}_2\text{O}$ in the sitting or standing positions; ICP can drop to $-43 \text{cmH}_2\text{O}$ when a high pressure valve (CP = $17 \text{cmH}_2\text{O}$) is used (see Eq. 2). When the inlet was horizontal ($0 \text{cmH}_2\text{O}$) and the outlet was $-60 \text{cmH}_2\text{O}$, the experimental shunt flow was 12.4 ml/min in the low-pressure Sophy valve, 10.9 ml/min in the medium, and 7.4 ml/min in the high, which constituted excessive overdrainage (Fig. 4 upper). In our patients, the high-pressure valve had a lower sitting shunt flow than the low-pressure valve; however overdrainage persisted. In cases 7 (SVS) and 8 (SDH), increasing the valve resistance could not prevent overdrainage and highly negative IVP in the erect position (Figs. 2, 3). It seems that increasing the closing pressure of the shunt valve cannot overcome the siphon effect (Chapman et al. 1990; Gruber et al. 1984; Itoh et al. 1989; Tokoro and Chiba 1989; Tokoro and Chiba [to be published]). Chapman et al. (1990) also reported that IVPs taken in the upright position in patients with medium- or high-pressure valves were quite negative, ranging from -15 to $-35 \text{cmH}_2\text{O}$.

By contrast, if the patient stays supine, increase in the valve resistance becomes a sizable factor. If the patient is in the supine position, the outlet and HP are horizontal ($0 \text{cmH}_2\text{O}$).

$$PPv = ICP - CP > 0 \qquad \text{(Eq. 3)}$$

Shunt flow never starts until the ICP reaches more than $5 \text{cmH}_2\text{O}$ in the low-pressure Sophy valve, $11 \text{cmH}_2\text{O}$ in the medium, and $17 \text{cmH}_2\text{O}$ in the high (see Eq. 3). When the inlet was $10 \text{cmH}_2\text{O}$ and the outlet was horizontal ($0 \text{cmH}_2\text{O}$), the experimental shunt flow was 1.53 ml/min in the low-pressure

Sophy valve, 0.60 ml/min in the medium, and 0 ml/min in the high. It should be noted that increasing the valve resistance cannot affect the ICP unless the patient stays supine.

Relationship Between the Function and the Position of the ASD

In shunt systems without an ASD, only those factors considered in Equations 1–3 restrict shunt flow, but in shunt systems with an ASD, the opening pressure of the ASD, as well as PPv, must be considered (Tokoro and Chiba 1989; Tokoro and Chiba [to be published]).

The inlet pressure of the ASD (IP) is equal to the sum of the ICP plus the hydrostatic pressure between the shunt valve and the ASD (HP$_2$) minus CP:

$$IP = ICP + HP_2 - CP \qquad \text{(Eq. 4)}$$

The outlet pressure of the ASD (OP) is equal to the hydrostatic pressure between the ASD and the end of the peritoneal catheter (HP$_3$) minus IPP:

$$OP = HP_3 - IPP \qquad \text{(Eq. 5)}$$

where the sum of HP$_2$ plus HP$_3$ is HP$_1$ and is nearly 60 cm in erect Japanese adults.

The perfusion pressure of the ASD (PP$_{ASD}$) in the erect position is defined as follows:

$$PP_{ASD} = 8 \cdot IP - OP > 0 \qquad \text{(Eq. 6)}$$

where the ratio of the area of the diaphragm of the inlet to the outlet of the ASD is 8: 1. The IPP tends to zero. Since the ASD will remain open until PP$_{ASD}$ equals zero, by substituting equations 4 and 5 into equation 6 and rearranging, the equation for the least ICP that can open the ASD (ICP$_{ASD}$, cmH$_2$O) is obtained:

$$ICP_{ASD} = (-9/8) \cdot HP_2 + CP + 7.5 \qquad \text{(Eq. 7)}$$

Equation 7 can be applied to a Sophy valve combined with an ASD in varying positions. Thus the least ICP required to open both the shunt valve and the ASD must be greater than 12.5, 18.5, and 24.5 cmH$_2$O in the low-, medium-, and high-pressure Sophy valves with the ASD just distal to the valve. Since these valves are much higher than the negative ICP in erect adults, it is difficult to initiate shunt flow. The results of the experimental shunt flow also indicated an excessive anti-siphon effect, especially at medium and high pressure (Fig. 4 middle). When a medium- or high-pressure Sophy valve with an ASD just distal to the valve was used, shunt flow could start in neither the supine nor the sitting positions, as was the case with the initial shunt in case 5, where the shunt was patent but functionally occluded.

McCullough (1986) and Seida et al. (1987) have reported on the adverse effects of ASDs. Clinical symptoms and ventriculomegaly improved when the shunt system was replaced by one without an ASD. We reported that the optimum position for an ASD appeared to be 10 cm downstream, because the resulting hydrostatic column helps to initiate flow when the patient assumes the erect position (Tokoro and Chiba 1989; Tokoro and Chiba [to be published]). When an ASD is placed 10 cm below the level of the foramen of Monro, the least ICP required to initiate flow can be reduced to 1.25, 7.25, and 13.25 cmH$_2$O in the low-, medium-, and high-pressure Sophy valves, respectively (see Eq. 7). A low-pressure Sophy valve combined with an ASD 10 cm downstream provides an attainable range of ICP in erect adults. The experimental shunt flow also indicated that this combination of Sophy valve with an ASD placed 10 cm downstream produced an appropriate anti-siphon effect (Fig. 4 lower).

It is evident that a PAV becomes useful only when used with an ASD, when upgrading or downgrading the valve resistance can effect a shunt flow within the physiological range of ICP.

Conclusions

1. Upgrading of PAV resistance alone cannot prevent SDH and SVS. Combined use with an ASD is essential when patients assume the erect position.
2. The combination of a PAV and an ASD is useful for patients with hypertensive hydrocephalus.
3. If an ASD placed 10 cm downstream with a conventional valve is used primarily, there is no need to use the PAV, especially for patients with NPH.

Acknowledgments. We thank Mr. Setsuo Sasaki and Mr. Yoshio Hosonuma for their technical assistance in radionuclide shuntography.

References

Abe H, Chiba Y, Tokoro K (1990) Effect of anti-siphon device in shunting procedure: intraventricular pressure during positional changes (abstract). 1st International Symposium on Hydrocephalus, Kobe, Japan (this volume)

Chapman PH, Cosman ER, Arnold MA (1990) The relationship between ventricular fluid pressure and body position in normal subjects and subjects with shunts: A telemetric study. Neurosurgery 26: 181–189

Dietrich U, Lumenta C, Sprick C, Majewski B (1987) Subdural hematoma in a case of hydrocephalus and macrocrania. Experience with a pressure-adjustable valve. Nerv Syst Child 3: 242–244

Epstein F, Fleischer AS, Hochwald GM, Ransohoff J (1974) Subtemporal craniectomy for recurrent shunt obstruction secondary to small ventricles. J Neurosurg 41: 29–31

Foltz EL, Blanks JP (1988) Symptomatic low intracranial pressure in shunted hydrocephalus. J Neurosurg 68: 401–408

Fox JL, McCullough DC, Green RC (1973) Effect of cerebrospinal fluid shunts on intracranial pressure and on cerebrospinal fluid dynamics. 2. A new technique of pressure measurements: Results and concepts. 3. A concept of hydrocephalus. J Neurol Neurosurg Psychiatry 36: 302–312

Fuse T, Takagi T, Ohno M, Nagai H (1990) Experience with shunting operation using a pressure-adjustable valve (in Japanese). No Shinkei Geka 18: 139–144

Gruber R, Jenny P, Herzog B (1984) Experiences with the anti-siphon device (ASD) in shunt therapy of pediatric hydrocephalus. J Neurosurg 61: 156–162

Horton D, Pollay M (1990) Fluid flow performance of a new siphon-control device for ventricular shunts. J Neurosurg 72: 926–932

Itoh K, Matsumae M, Tsugane R, Sato O (1989) The shunt flow in a programmable pressure valve (in Japanese). Shoni No Noshinkei 14: 143–148

Kikuchi K, Kowada M, Sasaki J, Watanabe K, Sasajima H, Yoneya M (1990) Ventriculoperitoneal shunts with the use of a pressure-adjustable valve in the management of hydrocephalus (in Japanese). No Shinkei Geka 18: 241–246

Loayza P (1987) Válvula de presión variable en el tratamiento de hidrocefalia con ventrículos chicos. Rev Chil Neurochirurg 1: 299–302

McCullough DC (1986) Symptomatic progressive ventriculomegaly in hydrocephalics with patent shunts and antisiphon devices. Neurosurgery 19: 617–621

McCullough DC, Fox JL (1974) Negative intracranial pressure hydrocephalus in adults with shunts and its relationship to the production of subdural hematoma. J Neurosurg 40: 372–375

Portnoy HD, Schulte RR, Fox JL, Croissant PD, Tripp L (1973) Anti-siphon and reversible occlusion valves for shunting in hydrocephalus and preventing post-shunt subdural hematomas. J Neurosurg 38: 729–738

Rudd TG, Shurtleff DB, Loeser JD, Nelp WB (1973) Radionuclide assessment of cerebrospinal fluid shunt function in children. J Nucl Med 14: 683–686

Sainte-Rose C, Hooven MD, Hirsch F (1987) A new approach in the treatment of hydrocephalus. J Neurosurg 66: 213–226

Schmitt J, Sperke N, Spring A (1989) The treatment of idiopathic normal pressure hydrocephalus by magnetic transcutaneous adjustable valves (abstract). Ninth International Congress of Neurological Surgery, New Delhi, India, p 98

Seida M, Ito U, Tomida S, Yamazaki S, Inaba Y (1987) Ventriculo-peritoneal shunt malfunction with an anti-siphon device in normal-pressure hydrocephalus: Report of three cases (in Japanese). Neurol Med Chir (Tokyo) 27: 769–773

Tokoro K, Chiba Y (1989) Effects on shunt flow of position of anti-siphon device and of changes in posture in hydrocephalus (abstract). Ninth International Congress of Neurological Surgery, New Delhi, India, p 100

Tokoro K, Chiba Y (to be published, 1991) Optimum position for an anti-siphon device in a cerebrospinal fluid shunt system? Neurosurgery 29(4)

42 — A New Shunt System with Non-Invasive Flow Rate Regulation and Pressure Measurement

Takuo Hashimoto, Norio Nakamura, Toshinori Kanki,[1]
Hideaki Shimazu,[2] *Ken-ichi Yamakoshi,*[3] *Masakazu Gondoh,*
and Toshiaki Tamai[4]

Summary. We have developed a new non-invasive method for the regulation of cerebrospinal fluid (CSF) flow and the measurement of intracranial pressure (ICP) in ventriculo-peritoneal shunt tubes. This method depends on an implantable regulatory device, containing two titanium balls, which controls CSF flow with four settings: off, low, medium, and high. The titanium balls can be moved non-invasively by a neurosurgeon who can regulate the flow of CSF through the slit valves. The pressure measuring device contains a thin silicone dome reservoir. It is possible to measure ICP percutaneously by a collapsing technique, a modification of the coplanar method. The authors suggest a new method of treating hydrocephalus, which is to control CSF flow within the appropriate physiological ICP range by this new shunt system.

Keywords. Hydrocephalus — Ventriculo-peritoneal shunt — Cerebrospinal fluid — ICP — Differential pressure valve

Introduction

Since the introduction of the Spitz-Holter valve (Nulsen and Spitz 1952) many hydrocephalic patients have been treated with different types of shunting systems. Shunt technology has been advancing over the past three decades. Unfortunately, complications following shunting procedures have been extraordinarily frequent and often the shunt either does not work adequately or it overworks. Therefore, various problems have been encountered in the treatment of hydrocephalus by shunting procedures (Carteri et al. 1980; Engel et al.

[1] Department of Neurosurgery, Jikei University School of Medicine, Minato-ku Tokyo, 105 Japan
[2] Department of Physiology, Kyorin University School of Medicine, Mitaka Tokyo, 181 Japan
[3] Institute of Applied Electricity, Hokkaido University Sapporo, 060 Japan
[4] Japan MDM Ltd., Tokyo, 162, Japan

1979; Epstein et al. 1979; Epstein et al. 1988; Faulhauer and Schmitz 1978; Hakim 1973; Illingworth 1970; Kierkens et al. 1982; Kloss 1968; McCullough and Fox 1974; Portnoy et al. 1976).

Complications due to under- or overdrainage are directly related to the hydrodynamic characteristics of valves and have been extensively studied for many years.

The ideal shunt valve should be non-invasively flow-rate controlled to prevent under- or overdrainage. Such a valve regulation system should not be influenced by MRI examination. Furthermore, non-invasive measurements of pressure in the shunt system are also very important to detect shunt malfunction. Until now there has been no such ideal shunt system.

The authors have developed a new non-invasive method for regulating CSF flow and measuring shunt function and have applied it clinically. The purpose of this paper is to describe the non-invasive flow-rate switching mechanism we used and our method of measuring pressure in the shunt system.

Principles and Methods

The new shunt tube consists mainly of a CSF flow-rate regulation unit and a pressure measurement unit (Fig. 1). The flow-rate regulation unit is implantable and contains two slit valves and two titanium balls. One of the slit valves has a high resistance and the other has a low resistance. The flow rate of CSF is different between the two valves and is regulated through them by changing the location of two titanium balls (Fig. 2); these balls can be moved percutaneously

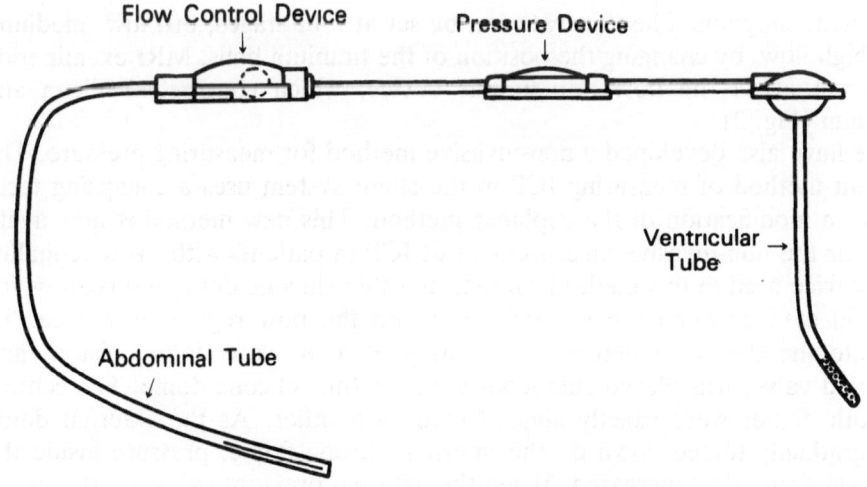

Fig. 1. Multipurpose shunt system

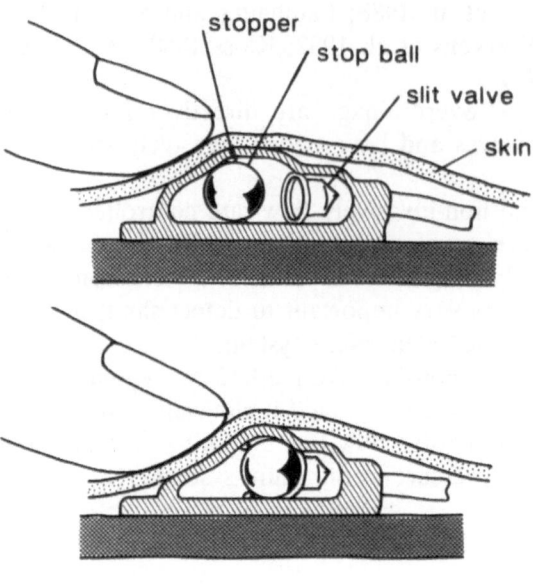

stopper

stop ball

slit valve

skin

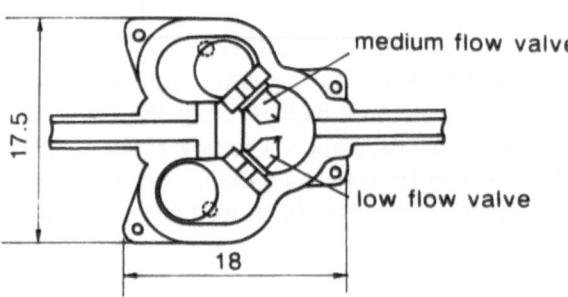

medium flow valve

low flow valve

17.5

18

Fig. 2. Flow control device. Two titanium balls regulate CSF flow through slit valves at four levels: off, low, medium, and high

by a neurosurgeon. The flow rate can be set at four stages, off, low, medium, and high flow, by changing the position of the titanium balls. MRI examination does not affect the flow rate in this device, which consists of silicon and titanium (Fig. 2).

We have also developed a non-invasive method for measuring pressure. The present method of measuring ICP in the shunt system uses a collapsing technique, a modification of the coplanar method. This new method is now available for the non-invasive measurement of ICP in patients with hydrocephalus. The device used in this method consists of a thin silicone dome reservoir which is connected between the ventricle port and the flow regulation device. To operate the device, a detector, consisting of a pressure dome, piston, and solenoid valve, was placed cutaneously on the thin silicone dome. The centers of both domes were exactly aligned with each other. As the external dome was gradually forced down on the internal silicone dome, pressure inside the external dome (Pe) increased. When the external pressure exceeded the pressure inside the internal dome (Pi), a collapse of the internal dome occurred.

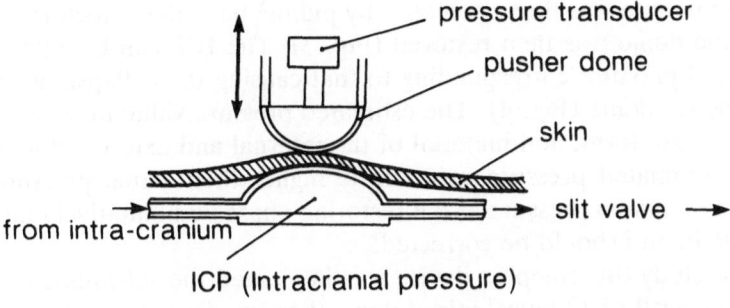

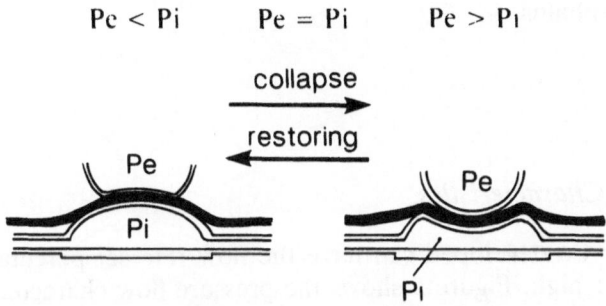

Fig. 3. Indirect non-invasive pressure measurement. Collapse and restoration of the domes occurs through differences in pressure between the internal and the external dome. Pe, external pressure; Pi, internal pressure

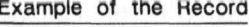

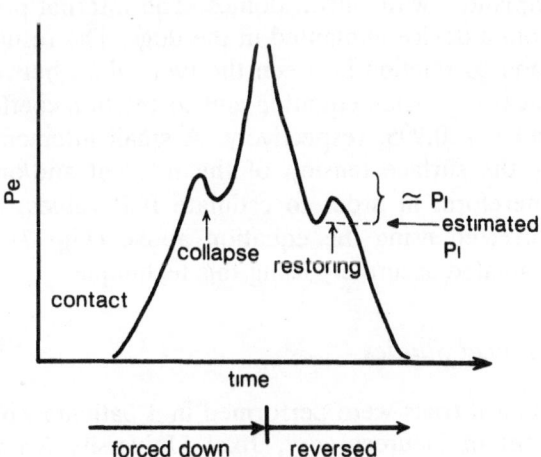

Fig. 4. Pressure transducer recording showing collapse and restoration of the dome. Restoring point indicates intracranial pressure (*ICP*). Pe, external pressure; Pi, internal pressure

External pressure was then decreased by pulling back the detector; the form of the silicone dome was then restored (Fig. 3). The ICP can be evaluated from the external pressure corresponding to that causing the collapse or restoration of the silicone dome (Fig. 4). The estimated pressure value may vary, depending on the size, form, and material of the internal and external domes. Therefore, the estimated pressure was a little higher than actual pressure. In this study, the minimum pressure at the restoring phase was tentatively taken as the indirect ICP, and should be corrected.

For this study this complex device was implanted the subcutaneous tissue of the thoracic wall of 13 anesthetized dogs. Pressure recordings were made over a 6-month period, using the collapsing technique. This device for pressure measurement has been used with a Sophy shunt system and used in the treatment of hydrocephalus.

Results

Pressure-Flow Characteristics

The device that we developed can have the flow rate set percutaneously off, low, medium, or high. Figure 5 shows the pressure-flow characteristics of this device. This flow control system can be applied to different pressures which occur in hydrocephalus (Fig. 5).

Animal Studies

The experiments were performed on 13 dogs. The animals were anesthetized and a pressure dome was placed in the subcutaneous tissue of the thoracic wall of each dog. Pressure measurements in these chronically implanted silicone domes were carried out for up to 6 months. Figure 6 shows typical records of the indirect pressure estimated by the collapsing technique in dogs chronically implanted with silicon domes. The internal pressure was measured constantly from a device implanted in the dogs. The results in this animal study suggest a good correlation between the two values between 0–40 cm H_2O (Fig. 7). The linear regression equation and correlation coefficient were $Y = 1.087X + 2.636$ and $r = 0.995$, respectively. A small intercept which may have been caused by the surface tension of the internal and/or external dome was observed. Therefore, in order to estimate ICP values, the indirect pressure should be corrected using the equation above (Fig. 7). The internal pressure can be evaluated accurately using this technique.

Clinical Studies

Clinical trials were performed in 4 patients with hydrocephalus in the Department of Neurosurgery, Jikei University School of Medicine. The pressure

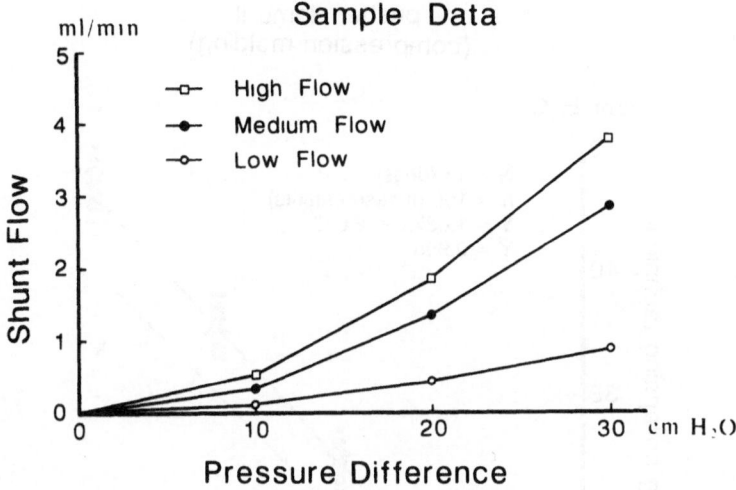

Fig. 5. Pressure flow relationship using the flow control device

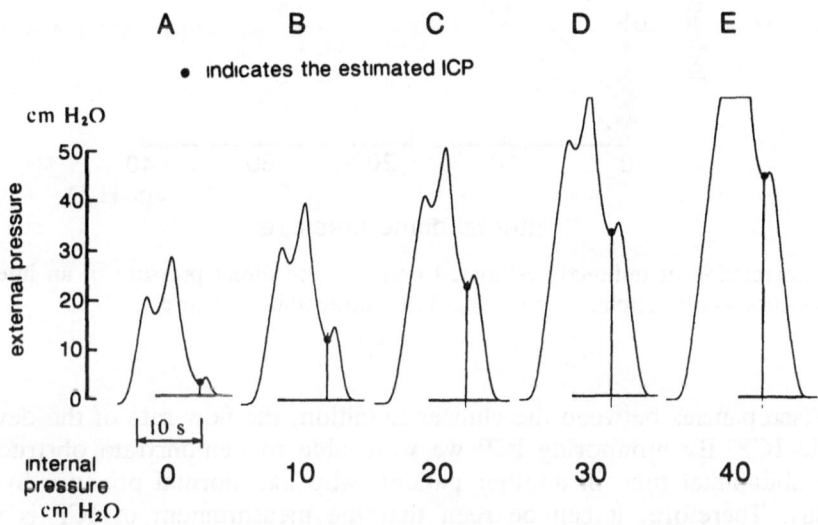

Fig. 6. Recordings of external pressure change during measurement in dogs. ICP, intracranial pressure

device was connected with a Sophy shunt system. Pressure measurements were carried out after shunt operation. In hydrocephalus with Dandy-Walker syndrome, a shunt procedure controlled by a medium pressure Sophy shunt tube showed an ICP of 8.8 cm H_2O. The patient showed signs of increased ICP in spite of decreased ventricle size (observed on CT scan). After change of flow rate in this case ICP dropped to 1.7 cm H_2O and clinical symptoms disappeared (Fig. 8). Studies of ICP measurement in shunt systems suggested that there

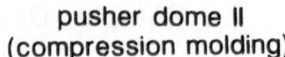

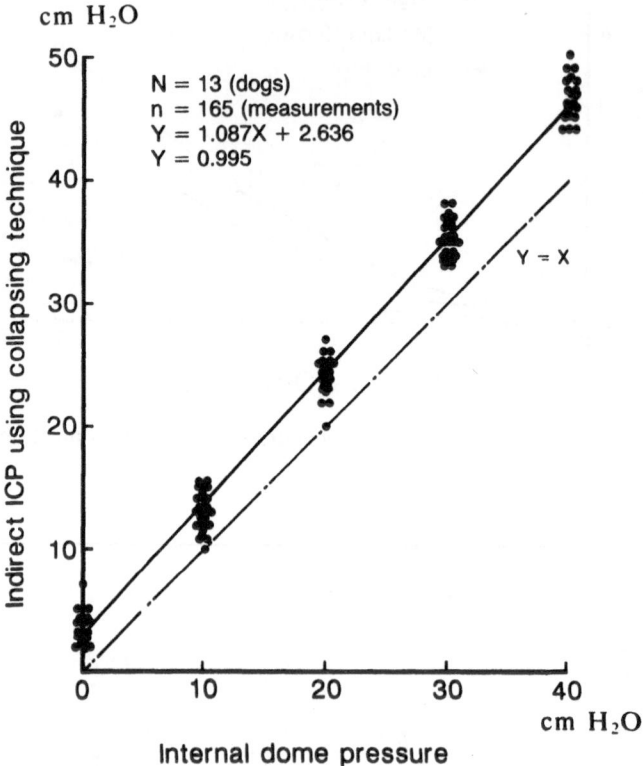

Fig. 7. Correlation of indirectly estimated pressure and direct pressure of an internal dome subcutaneously implanted in a dog. ICP, intracranial pressure

were discrepancies between the clinical condition, the flow rate of the device, and the ICP. By monitoring ICP we were able to demonstrate obstruction of the abdominal tube in another patient, who had normal pressure hydrocephalus. Therefore, it can be seen that the measurement of ICP is very important in the management of hydrocephalus.

Discussion

Ventriculo-peritoneal shunts, which have now been carried out routinely for 30 years, have proven to constitute the most important progress yet made in the treatment of hydrocephalus. Obstruction and infection remain the most common complications in CSF shunting (McLaurin 1989). There are, however, numerous complications involving under- or overdrainage of CSF with collapse of ventricle (Carteri et al. 1980; Engel et al. 1979; Epstein et al. 1979; Epstein

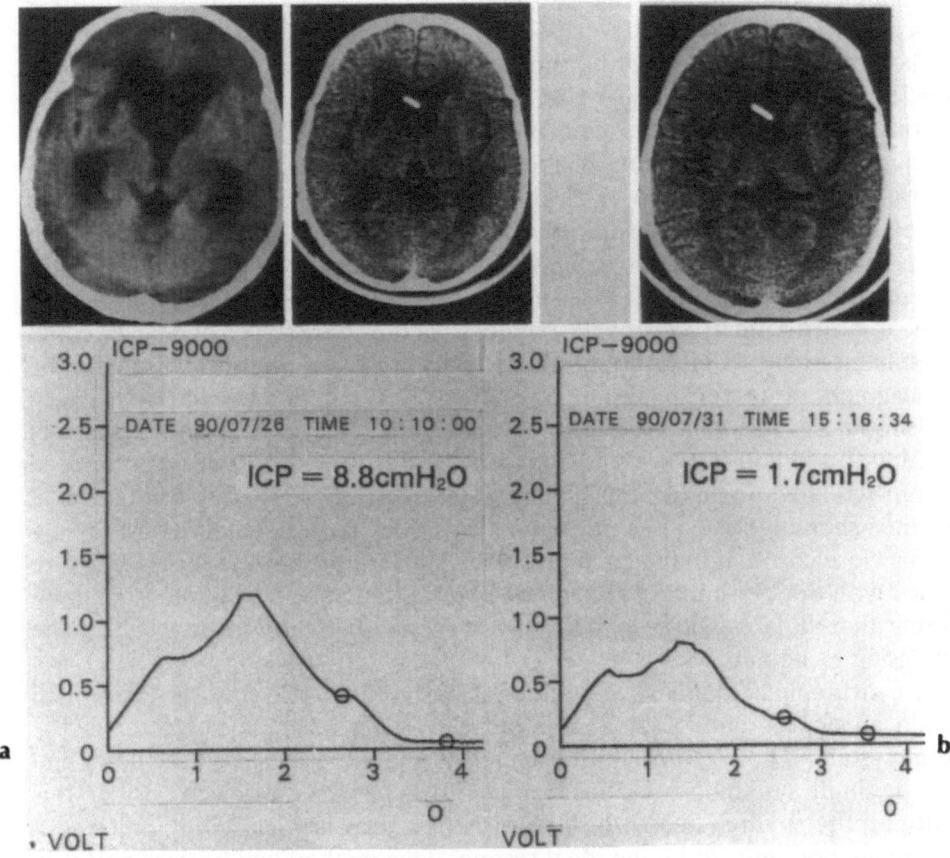

Fig. 8. Postoperative intracranial pressure (*ICP*) recording in a patient with Dandy-Walker syndrome. **a** shows ICP with medium pressure Sophy shunt system, **b** indicates ICP with low pressure Sophy shunt system

et al. 1988; Faulhauer and Schmitz 1978; Kierkens et al. 1982; Matsumoto and Oi 1985), subdural hematoma (Illingworth 1970; McCullough and Fox 1974), and postshunt craniostenosis (Kloss 1968). These complications following shunt procedures are well recognized. When conventional shunt systems are used shunt revision is sometimes required because of under- or overdrainage. Flow through the shunt tube must be controlled in hydrocephalic patients. In recent years, some methods have been developed to prevent these complication in shunt systems (Hakim 1973; Portnoy et al. 1973, 1976; Sainte-Rose et al. 1979; Yamada 1982). Sophy and Cordis shunt systems are available and have been used to prevent these complications. However, in available flow or pressure controlled devices, the flow rate could change after MRI examination and would need to be re-adjusted by the neurosurgeon. In addition to that problem, ICP measurement is not accurate in these shunting systems. The overdrainage phenomenon can also occur in the upright position when these devices are used.

The new device developed by the authors is not affected by MRI examination. Measurements of ICP or CSF flow rate are very valuable in preventing various complications in the shunt tubing. There have been several reports on measurement of the flow rate in the shunt system using the Doppler method (Hara et al. 1983; Numoto et al. 1984), tracer material, and thermography; however, these methods have not been used in clinical cases. There have also been several reports on the quantitative measurement of pressure in shunt systems (Sato et al. 1982). Devices used for measuring pressure are too large to implant in pediatric hydrocephalic patients. And as these types of devices could be influenced by MRI, most of them have not been routinely used in the management of hydrocephalus.

Using the device which we developed, it is possible to measure pressure in the shunt tube non-invasively and moreover, this pressure device can be used in connection with conventional shunt systems. It can be used to estimate ICP in other shunting systems. In the animal studies, the estimated pressure suggests a close correlation to actual pressure. The authors have used this pressure device with Sophy shunting systems in several patients and this study demonstrates that it is possible to clinically measure ICP non-invasively, by the collapsing technique.

In hydrocephalic patients treated by CSF shunting. ICP must be controlled within an appropriate physiological range by an adjustable flow rate in the shunt system. The relationship between neurological changes, CSF flow, and ICP in shunt systems should be studied further. However, we consider this multipurpose shunt system, which consists of a pressure measuring unit and a flow regulation unit, to be the ideal system. This method will be very useful in the management of hydrocephalus.

References

Carteri A, Longatti PL, Gerosa M, et al. (1980) Complications due to incongruous drainage of shunt operations. Adv Neurosurg 8: 199–203

Engel M, Carmel PW, Chutorian AM (1979) Increased intraventricular pressure without ventriculomegaly in children with shunt; "Normal volume" hydrocephalus. Neurosurgery 5: 549–552

Epstein F, Marlin AE, Wald A (1979) Chronic headaches in the shunt-dependent adolescent with nearly normal ventricular volume: Diagnosis and treatment. Neurosurgery 3: 351–355

Epstein F, Lapras C, Wisoff JH (1988) "Slit ventricle syndrome": Etiology and treatment. Pediatr Neurosci 14: 5–10

Faulhauer K, Schmitz P (1978) Overdrainage phenomena in shunt treated hydrocephalus. Acta Neurochir (Wien) 45: 89–101

Hakim S (1973) Hydraulic and mechanical mis-matching of valve shunts used in the treatment of hydrocephalus; the need for a servo-valve shunt. Dev Med Child Neurol 15: 646–653

Hara M, Kadowaki C, Konishi Y, Ogashiwa M, Numoto M, Takeuchi K (1983) A new method for measuring cerebrospinal fluid flow in shunts. J Neurosurg 58: 557–561

Kierkens R, Mortier W, Pothmann R, Bock WJ, Seibert H (1982) The slit ventricle syndrome after shunting in hydrocephalic children. Neuropediatrics 13: 190–194

Kloss JL (1968) Craniostenosis secondary to ventriculoatrial shunt. Am J Dis Child 116: 315–317

Illingworth RD (1970) Subdural hematoma after the treatment of chronic hydrocephalus by ventriculocaval shunts. J. Neurol. Neurosurg. Psychiatry 33: 95–99

Matsumoto S, Oi S (1985) Slit ventricle syndrome. Annu. Rev. Hydroceph. 3: 108–109

McCullough DC, Fox JL (1974) Negative intracranial pressure hydrocephalus in adults with shunts and its relationship to the production of subdural hematoma. J Neurosurg 40: 372–375

McLaurin RL (1989) Ventricular shunts: Complications and results. In: McLaurin RL, Schut L, Venes JL, Epstein F (eds) Pediatric neurosurgery. WB Saunders, Philadelphia, pp 219–229

Nulsen FE, Spitz EB (1952) Treatment of hydrocephalus by direct shunt from ventricle to jugular vein. Surg Forum 2: 239–403

Numoto M, Hara M, Kadowaki C, Takeuchi K (1984) A non-invasive CSF flowmeter. J Med Eng Technol 8: 218–220

Portnoy HD, Schulte, RR, Fox JL, Croissant PD, Tripp L (1973) Anti-siphon and reversible occlusion valve for shunting in hydrocephalus and preventing post-shunt subdural hematomas. J Neurosurg 38: 729–738

Portony HD, Tripp L, Croissant PD (1976) Hydrodynamics of shunt valves. Childs Brain 2: 242–256

Sainte-Rose C, Hooven M, Hirsch JF (1979) A new approach in the treatment of hydrocephalus. J. Neurosurg 66: 213–226

Sato O, Ohya M, Tsugane R, et al. (1982) Quantitative measurement of cerebrospinal fluid shunt flow. Monogr Neural Sci 8: 34–38

Yamada H (1982) A flow regulatory device to control differential pressure in a CSF shunt system technical note. J Neurosurg 57: 570–573

43 — A New Curved Peritoneal Passer for Shunting Operations — Technical Note

Shuzo Sato, Naoki Ishihara, Kazuta Yunoki, Terutoshi Nakamigawa[1], Takayuki Oohira, Hideichi Takayama, and Shigeo Toya[2]

Summary. Various operations have been reported for hydrocephalus. Even if these operations consist of minor surgery, general anesthesia or laparotomy is required. To avoiding this complicated type of procedure, we developed a peritoneal and a long subcutaneous passer. This paper indicates the usefulness of these passers for VP shunt operations.

Local anesthesia was performed at the right occipital, right hypochondrium, and the route of the shunt tube. After ventricular tapping at the right occipital, a 4 mm skin incision was made at the right hypochondrium. A ventricular tube was passed through subcutaneously from head to abdomen without any additional incision, using a long curved subcutaneal passer. An abdominal tap was performed using a peritoneal passer with double lumen. The inner part of the peritoneal passer was pulled out and, after making sure that the tip of the passer was in the upper lateral surface of the liver, a peritoneal tube was inserted to the peritoneal cavity in a manner similar to the Seldinger method. As the outer part of peritoneal passer has a side slit, the passer could be removed easily.

The peritoneal passer was used in 124 cases and when it was used, the average operation time was 10–15 min. CSF shunt was performed under local anesthesia or neuroleptanalgesia (NLA). Because the operation time was decreased, the rates of infection and other complications were minimal.

Keywords. Ventriculoperitoneal shunt — Hydrocephalus — Abdominal tap

Introduction

Hydrocephalus is common after subarachnoid hemorrhage (Planger et al. 1987) or cerebral tumor and a shunting operation is one of the most frequently used neurosurgical procedures for the treatment of this condition.

[1] Institute of Brain and Blood Vessels, Mihara Memorial Hospital, Isesaki, Gunma. 372 Japan
[2] Department of Neurosurgery, Keio University School of Medicine, Shinjuku-ku, Tokyo, 160 Japan

Various operations for hydrocephalus have been reported, e.g., ventriculoperitoneal, lumboperitoneal and ventriculoatrial shunts. Problems and complications following shunt operation have been reported (Dean and Keller 1972; Golladay and Wagner 1990). Frequent complications are infection and obstruction (Niggeman et al. 1990; Oi et al. 1987). The occurrence of infection is partially dependent on the duration of operative time. To avoid possible infection, we developed a curved peritoneal passer and a long subcutaneous passer that can take the peritoneal tube into the peritoneal cavity without laparotomy.

Materials and Methods

The peritoneal passer has two parts, an inner and an outer part (Figs. 1, 2). The outer part is used as a stilet during peritoneal puncture. After peritoneal puncture, the inner part is extubated and the peritoneal tube is inserted to the peritoneal cavity through the outer part of the peritoneal passer. The outer part of the peritoneal passer has a side slit so that the passer can be extubated by placing the peritoneal catheter in the upper lateral part of the liver (Fig. 3).

The length of the long subcutaneous passer is 75 cm and one third of it is curved so as to pass the neck and the supraclavian region easily (Fig. 4). Its tip has a small hole through which to connect the peritoneal tube (Fig. 5).

Use During Operation

The patient was placed in a supine position and the neck was extended to the left so as to pass the long subcutaneous passer directly from abdomen to occipital region. Local anesthesia was performed at right occipital, right hypochondrium, and the route of shunt tube. Prior to the operation, the part of each shunt system was connected to one piece by measuring the cerebral mantle by CT scan and by measuring the distance between head and abdomen. A curved linear incision was made at the right occipital area and a 4 mm skin incision was made at the right hypochondrium. The long subcutaneous passer was then passed through from the hypochondrium to the right occipital region. The peritoneal tube was connected to the tip of the subcutaneous passer and was pulled out from the occipital area to the hypochondrium without any other incision.

Standard burr hole craniectomy was performed at the right occipital area and a ventricular tube was inserted to the right lateral ventricle. After making sure of CSF passage by aspirating from the peritoneal tube, an abdominal tap was performed at the right hypochondrium. When pulling out the inner part of the peritoneal passer, no displacement of its tip on intraperitoneal bleeding was confirmed by the flushing of saline water from its outer part. After the peritoneal tube was inserted into the upper lateral surface of the liver, its outer part was extubated. One small suture was made at the right hypochondrium and the right occipital incision was closed by the layer to layer method.

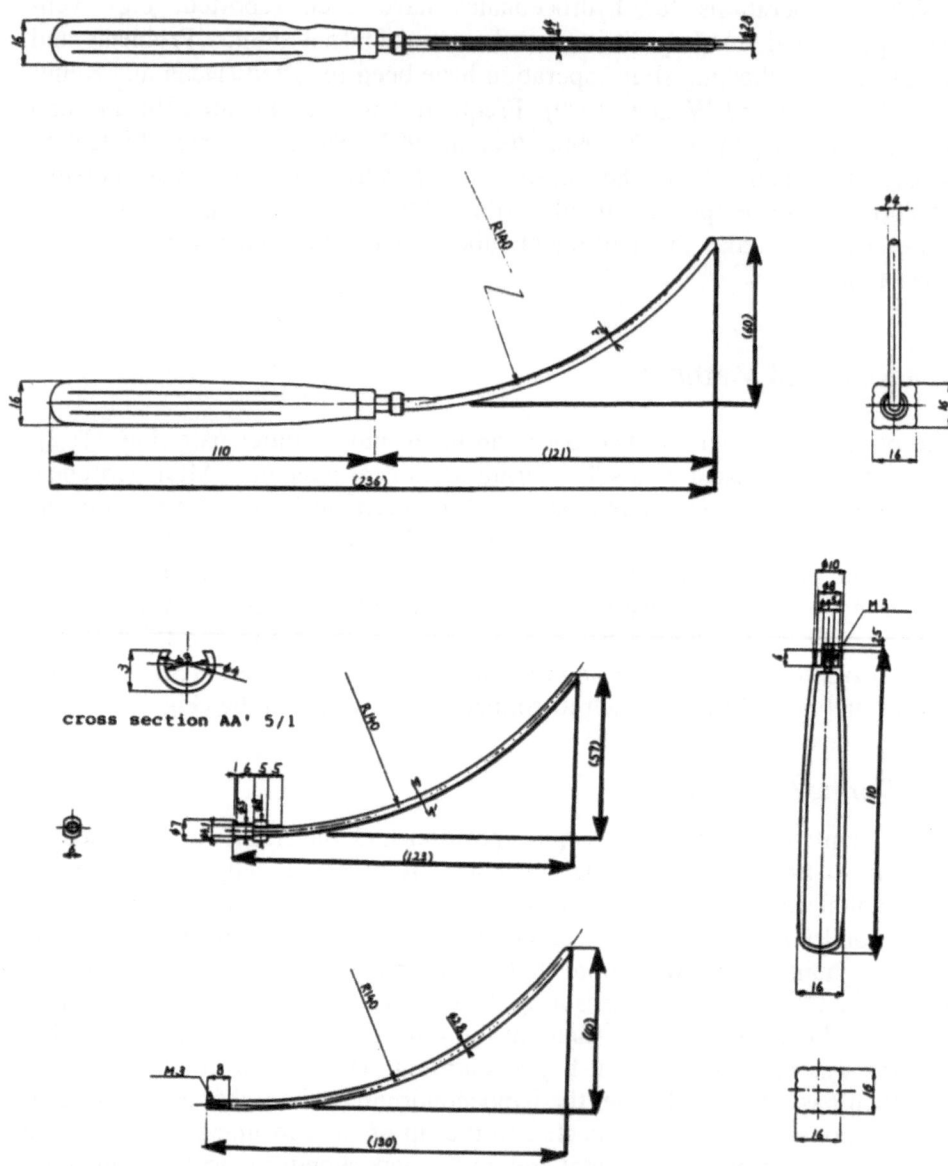

Fig. 1. Curved peritoneal passer; its outer part has a side slit

Results

The combination of long subcutaneous and peritoneal passers was used in 124 cases. This combination reduced operation time to about 10–15 min. The only complications observed were three infections. Because the operation time was decreased, the incidence of infection was minimal. Using the combination of

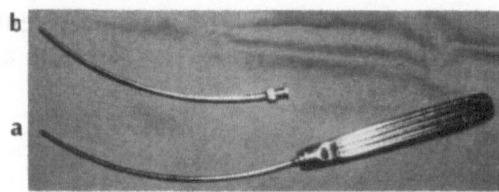

Fig. 2. The peritoneal passer consists of an inner (*a*) and an outer part (*b*)

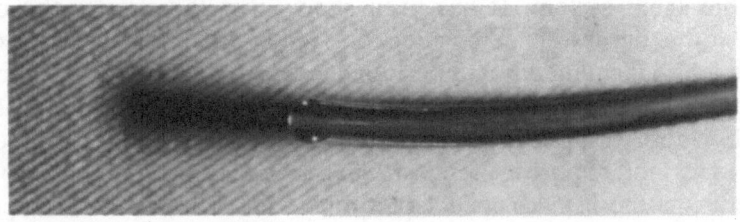

Fig. 3. The outer part of the peritoneal passer has a side slit for placing the peritoneal tube in the abdomen.

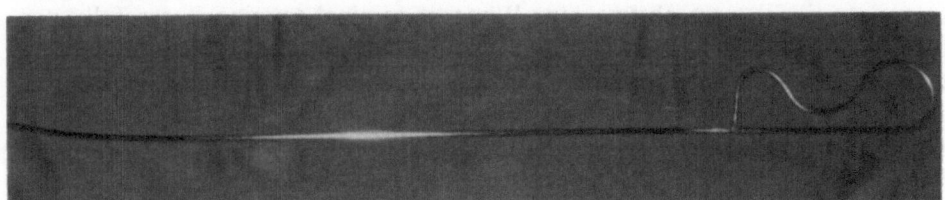

Fig. 4. Long subcutaneous passer; it is 75 cm long and one third of it is curved

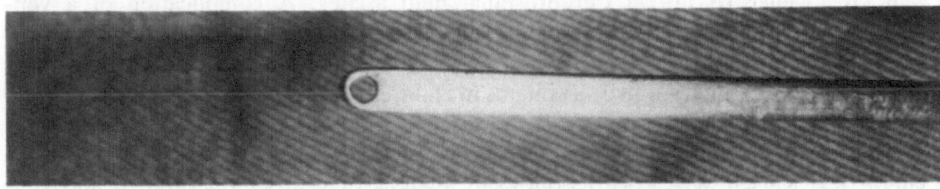

Fig. 5. Tip of the peritoneal passer; a 2 mm-diameter hole for the connection of the peritoneal tube can be observed

these two instruments, laparotomy was not required. Ventriculoperitoneal shunts and CSF shunts could be performed under local anesthesia or by neuroleptanalgesia without general anesthesia.

Discussion

Since ventriculoperitoneal shunting was reported by Scott et al. (1955), numerous complications have been reported (Lgnelze and Kersch 1975; Little et al. 1972; Fernell et al. 1985).; the major ones being infection and obstruction of the shunt system. It has been shown that the shorter the operation time the lower the incidence of infection. When operation time is reduced by using the long subcutaneous and peritoneal passer combination, the occurrence of postoperative meningitis can be decreased. General anesthesia is accompanied by more complications than local anesthesia. Our instrument combination does not require general anesthesia and laparotomy and so the risk of general anesthesia and open laparotomy can be avoided. Intraperitoneal bleeding and puncture of the gastrointestinal tract should be considered during peritoneal puncture. Numerous explorative abdominal taps to detect intraperitoneal bleeding have been performed, but no fatal complications have been reported. The risk of gastrointestinal pauncture is increased, especially in patients with obstructive ileas, but hydrocephalic patients usually do not have gastrointestional tract obstruction. When abdominal tapping is carefully performed intraperitoneal bleeding and puncture of the gastrointestinal tract can be avoided. So far the use of the long subcutaneous and peritoneal passer combination has shown that ventriculoperitoneal shunt operation time can be shortened and that general anesthesia can be avoided, with consistently satisfactory results.

References

Dean DE, Keller IB (1972) Cerebrospinal fluid ascites: A complication of a ventriculoperitoneal shunt. J. Neurol Neurosurg Psychiatry 35: 474–476

Fernell E, Wendt LV, Serlo W, et al. (1985) Ventriculoatrial or ventriculoperitoneal shunts in the treatment of hydrocephalus in children. Z Kinderchir 40(Suppl)1: 12–14

Golladay ES, Wagner CW (1990) Transthoracic complication after previous abdominal surgery: An alternate approach. South Med J 83: 1029–1032

Lgnelze RJ, Kersch WM (1975) Follow-up analysis of ventriculoperitoneal and ventriculoatrial shunts for hydrocephalus. J Neurosurg 42: 679–682

Little JR, Rhoton AL Jr, Mellinger JF (1972) Ventriculoperitoneal and ventriculoatrial shunt for hydrocephalus in children. Mayo Clin Proc 47: 396–401

Niggemann B, Kauerz U, Petersen v, et al. (1990) Massive ascites formation due to unabsorbed cerebrospinal fluid following abdominal surgery in ventriculoperitoneal shunt. A case report. Klin Padiatr 202: 180–182

Oi SZ, Shose Y, Asano N, et al. (1987) Intragastric migration of a ventriculoperitoneal shunt catheter. Neurosurgery 21: 255–257

Plangger C, Twerdy K, Mohsenipour I, et al. (1987) Hydrocephalus following spontaneous subarachnoid hemorrhage. Neurochirurgia (Stattg) 30: 154–157
Scott M, Wycis HT, Murtagh F, et al. (1955) Observations on ventricular and lumbar subarachnoid shunts in hydrocephalus in infants. J Neurosurg 12: 165–175

44 — Hydrogel Ventriculo-Subdural Shunt for the Treatment of Hydrocephalus in Children

Tai-Tong Wong, Liang-Shong Lee[1], Ren-Shyan Liu, Shih-Hwa Yeh[2], Tsuen Chang[3], Donald M. Ho[4], Gregory C.C. Niu, and Yng-Jiin Wang[5]

Summary. We designed a hydrogel ventriculo-subdural shunt and implanted it in eight infants with nontumoral hydrocephalus. Through this shunting procedure, cerebral spinal fluid (CSF) was drained to the subdural space over the cerebral hemisphere and was absorbed there. Computerized tomography (CT) brain scan studies were performed pre- and post-operatively to evaluate the function of the shunt and the change of intracranial CSF spaces after shunt insertion. Most of the infants demonstrated gradual relief of intracranial pressure with diminished head circumference and ventricular size. Postoperative CT scan studies showed no subdural fluid collection in one infant, unilateral subdural CSF collection in four infants, and bilateral subdural CSF collection in two infants. Three infants required no further shunt operation. Four infants required additional extracranial shunt insertions because of disturbance of CSF absorption in the subdural lining. One patient died suddenly at home, during sleep, two months after the ventricular subdural shunt insertion, without evidence of acute or chronic increase of intracranial pressure.

Keywords. Hydrocephalus — Infant — Ventriculo-subdural shunt — Hydrogel — PHEMA

Introduction

The ventriculo-subdural shunt was once one of the various surgical methods of treating hydrocephalus. Through this procedure, ventricular CSF was drained to the surface of the cerebral hemisphere and was absorbed there by the subdural lining. In 1957, Forrest and his colleagues reported a "Forrest disc" made of poly-tetra-fluoro-ethylene, designed for ventriculo-subdural drainage (Forrest et al. 1957b). This shunting procedure has now been abandoned due

[1] Division of Pediatric Neurosurgery, Departments of [2] Nuclear Medicine, [3] Radiology, [4] Pathology, and [5] Institute of Medical Engineering, Veterans General Hospital and National Yang Ming Medical College, Taipei, 11217 Taiwan

to its high failure rate and due to the improvement of other extracranial shunting procedures. This failure might be due to tissue reaction because of material incompatibility. We designed a new ventriculosubdural shunt. This new device consisted of a thin film and a ventricular tube made of crosslinked poly-2-hydroxyethyl methacrylate hydrogel material. With the permission of the Human Experimental Committee at this hospital, we implanted this device in eight infants with nontumoral hydrocephalus. Hydrocephalus with blockage at the level of the arachnoid villi (external hydrocephalus) was excluded. Clinical observations and postoperative CT brain scan studies were used for the evaluation of function and for the evaluation of changes in ventricles and CSF spaces after shunt insertion. We wished to know whether, by improving the biomaterial, the abandoned ventriculo-subdural shunt could be revived as an alternative method for the treatment of hydrocephalus in children.

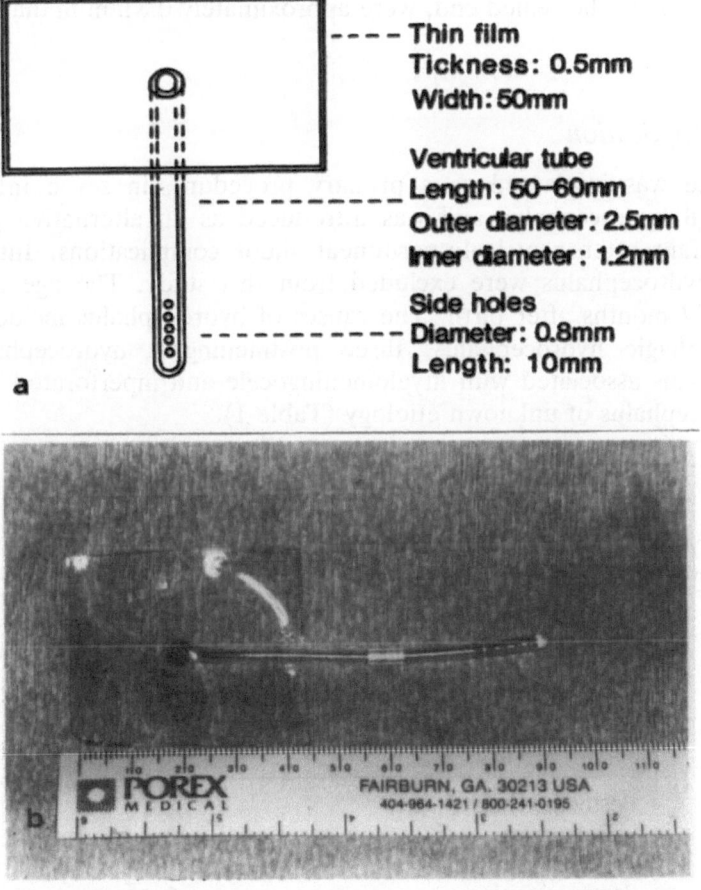

Fig. 1. a Drawing and **b** photograph showing the design and structure of a hydrogel ventriculo-subdural shunt

Material and Methods

Design of Hydrogel Ventriculo-Subdural Shunt

The device was composed entirely of poly-2-hydroxyethyl methacrylate (hereinafter, PHEMA or hydrogel), which is a water-insoluble hydrophilic polymer. It consisted of 20%–80% water when placed into a physiological fluid and could be sterilized by autoclave steam sterilization. The technique for making this shunting device was developed by Niu and his colleagues and the device was produced by Oxlex Taiwan Limited, by the lost-wax casting process (Wang 1986; Chiang 1988). The device was designed to have a thin film laid on the brain surface to hold the ventricular CSF drainage tube. The thin film, 50 mm wide and 0.5 mm thick, was set at the top end of the ventricular tube, with the top hole of the ventricular tube formed at the center of the film. The ventricular tube is 60 mm in length, with an internal diameter of 1.2 mm and an external diameter of 2.5 mm. The side holes, which were placed in the 10 mm-section closest to the sealed end, were approximately 0.8 mm in diameter (Fig. 1a,b).

Clinical Application

The device was implanted as a primary procedure, in seven infants with nontumoral hydrocephalus and was introduced as an alternative procedure in one infant after ventriculo-peritoneal shunt complications. Infants with external hydrocephalus were excluded from this study. The age range was from 1 to 4 months after birth. The causes of hydrocephalus included: three posthemorrhagic hydrocephalus, three postmeningitic hydrocephalus, one hydrocephalus associated with myelomeningocele and inperforated anus, and one hydrocephalus of unknown etiology (Table 1).

Operative Method

The apparatus was implanted through a curved linear incision to expose the lateral angle of the anterior fontanel. The dura was opened with the base

Table 1. Causes of hydrocephalus in eight infants with nontumoral hydrocephalus implanted with hydrogel ventriculo-subdural shunts

Causes of hydrocephalus	No. of cases (n)
Posthemorrhagic	
Premature	2
Perinatal trauma	1
Postmeningitis	3
Myelomeningocele	1
Unknown	1

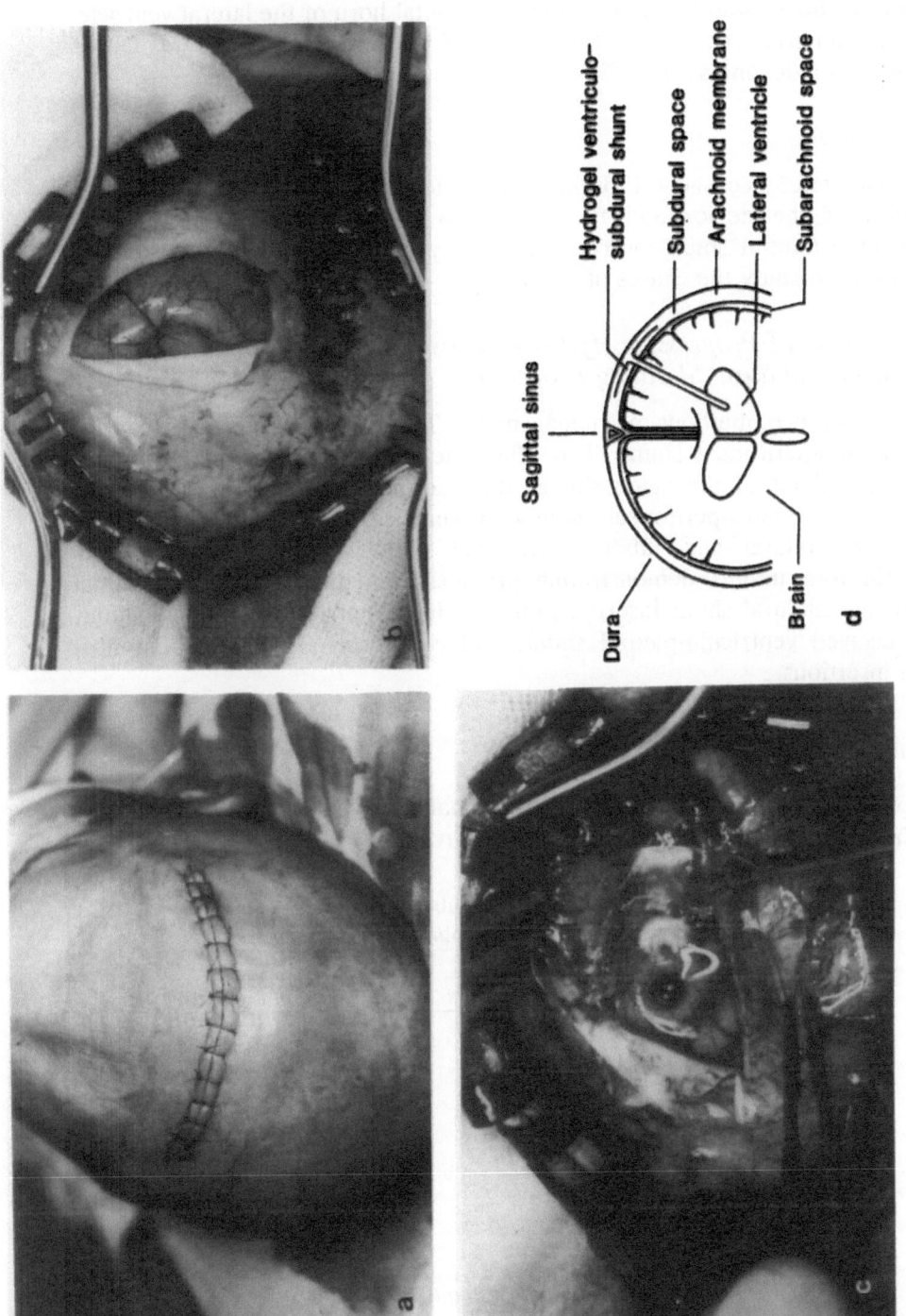

Fig. 2. a Scalp incision, **b** opening of dura, **c** placing of shunt with the film coating on the surface of brain, and **d** location of ventriculo-subdural shunt after implanation

facing the interhemispheric fissure. The thin film was tailored so that the ventricular tube could be inserted into the frontal horn of the lateral ventricle, and the film could be laid on the surface of the brain. The dura was closed tightly with a dexone suture (Fig. 2a–d).

Investigation

Head circumference and CT brain scan studies were used for evaluating the function of the device and the change of intracranial CSF spaces after ventriculo-subdural shunt insertion. A biopsy of the surrounding tissue was performed to study the causes of failure.

Management of Progressive Hydrocephalus After Failure of Hydrogel Ventriculo-Subdural Shunting Procedure

There were two methods of management. The first method was to insert a ventriculo-peritoneal shunt. The other method was to insert a subduro-peritoneal shunt at the same site as the ventriculo-subdural device and to change the subduro-peritoneal shunt to a ventriculo-peritoneal shunt as the ventriculo-subdural and subduro-peritoneal shunt systems failed to function. Of four infants demonstrating progressive hydrocephalus after initial ventriculo-subdural shunt insertion, one received ventriculo-peritoneal shunt, one received ventriculo-pleural shunt, and two received subduro-peritoneal shunt insertions.

Results

In seven infants with nontumoral hydrocephalus, a ventriculo-subdural shunt was inserted as the primary procedure. The result was three cases of arrested

Table 2. Results of hydrogel ventriculo-subdural shunt implantation in eight infants with nontumoral hydrocephalus

As a primary shunt procedure		
Result	Causes of hydrocephalus	No. of cases (n)
Arrest		3
	Posthemorrhagic	
	Premature 2	
	Perinatal trauma 1	
Progressive		4
	Postmeningitis 2	
	Myelomeningocele 1	
	Unknown 1	
As an alternative procedure after other shunt complications		
Result	Causes of hydrocephalus	No. of cases(n)
Death	Postmeningitis	1

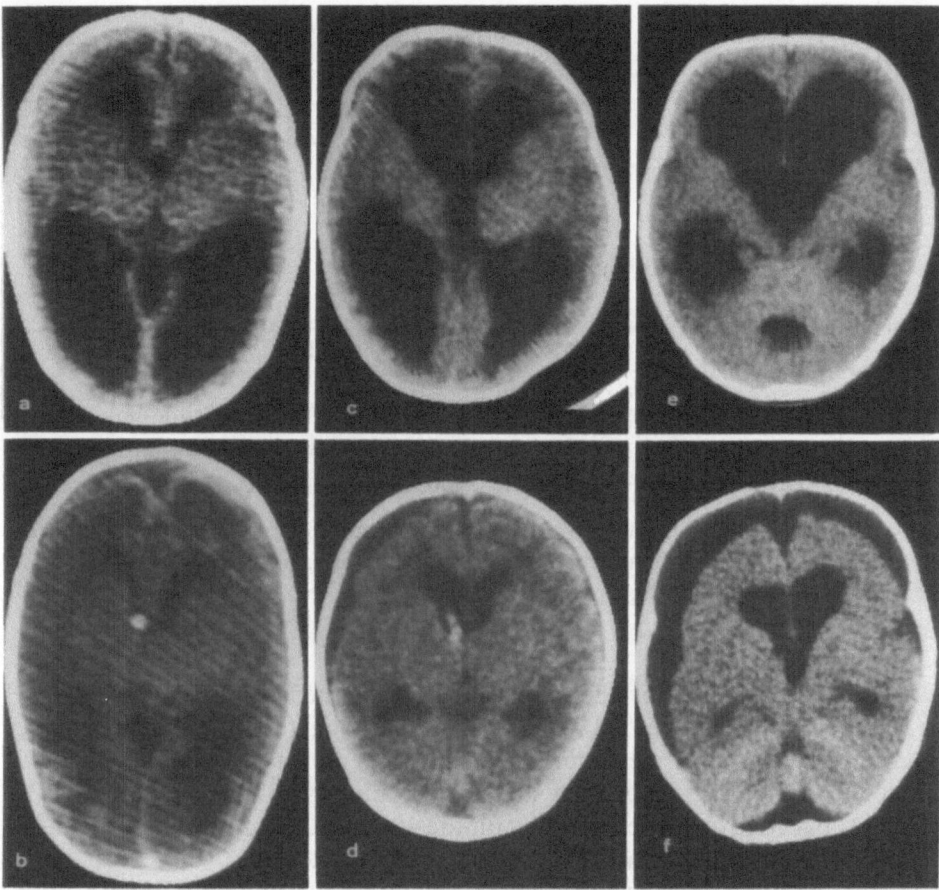

Fig. 3. Follow up CT studies in seven infants after implantation of hydrogel ventriculo-subdural shunt, showing decreased ventricular size with asymmetrical lateral ventricles. **a,b** No subdural fluid collection in one infant; **c,d** unilateral subdural fluid collection in four infants **e,f** bilateral subdural fluid collection in two infants

and four cases of progressive hydrocephalus. There was no shunt infection. Unilateral chronic subdural hematoma occurred in one infant. The ventriculo-subdural shunt was also inserted as an alternative procedure in an infant after chronic ventriculo-peritoneal and ventriculo-pleural shunt infection. This infant died suddenly at home, during sleep, without evidence of acute or chronic increase of intracranial pressure (Table 2).

Follow up CT brain scan studies in seven infants from 1–5 weeks after implantation of the device demonstrated decrease of ventricular size with no subdural fluid collection in one infant, unilateral subdural fluid collection in four infants, and bilateral subdural fluid collection in two infants (Fig. 3a–f).

Arrested hydrocephalus occurred in three infants with posthemorrhagic hydrocephalus. Their head circumferences decreased in the first 15 postopera-

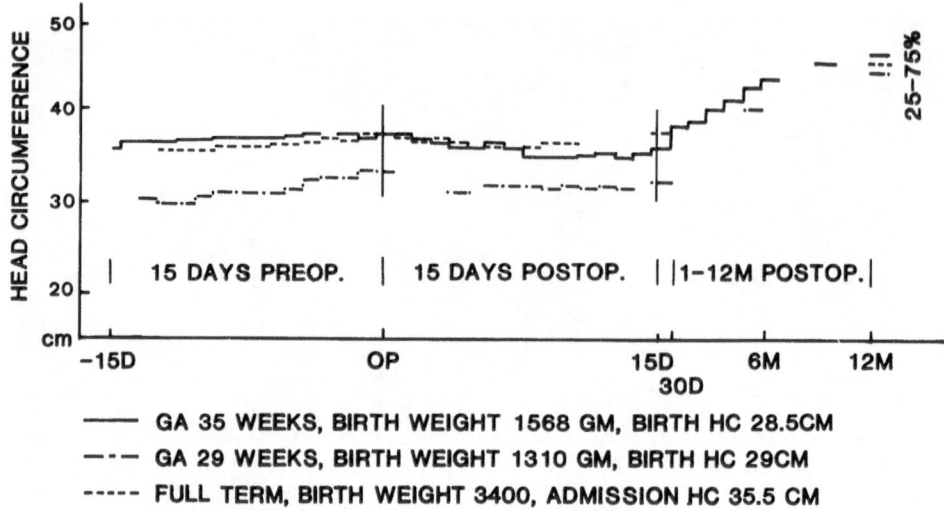

Fig. 4. Change of preoperative and postoperative head circumference (*HC*) in three infants with arrested posthemorrhagic hydrocephalus after ventriculo-subdural shunt operation. GA, gestational age

tive days. At 1 year after their operations, their head circumferences were measured at curves of 25%–75% (Fig. 4). Among them was a premature infant girl with progressive communicating posthemorrhagic hydrocephalus in whom the device was implanted at 56 days after birth. She received I-131 TC-99 DTPA RISA ventriculography on the 10th postoperative day. It demonstrated patency of the ventriculo-subdural shunt; however, there was slow clearance of tracers in the ventricles. Follow up CT brain scan 6 months after operation demonstrated asymmetrical dilatation of ventricles. The lateral ventricle was smaller at the site of the ventriculo-subdural shunt insertion. Her head circumference at 12 and 21 months of age was a curve of 75% and 50%, respectively (Fig. 5a–e).

Progressive hydrocephalus was observed in four infants from 1 week to 3 months after ventriculo-subdural shunt insertion. Their head circumferences decreased initially and then remained unchanged from 4 to 90 days. Additional extracranial shunt procedures were applied in these four infants. A ventriculo-peritoneal shunt was inserted in one infant with hydrocephalus of unknown cause, a ventriculo-pleural shunt was performed in an infant with myelomeningocele and inperforated anus treated by colostomy, and subduro-peritoneal shunts were implanted in two infants with postmeningitic hydrocephalus. However, for these last two infants, ventriculo-peritoneal shunt procedures were finally required, at 6 and 9 months, respectively, after the subduro-peritoneal shunt operations (Fig. 6).

The hydrogel ventriculo-subdural device was removed from one infant after 7 months of implantation. This was the infant who had developed hydrocephalus of unknown cause. The device had been implanted at 3 months. We

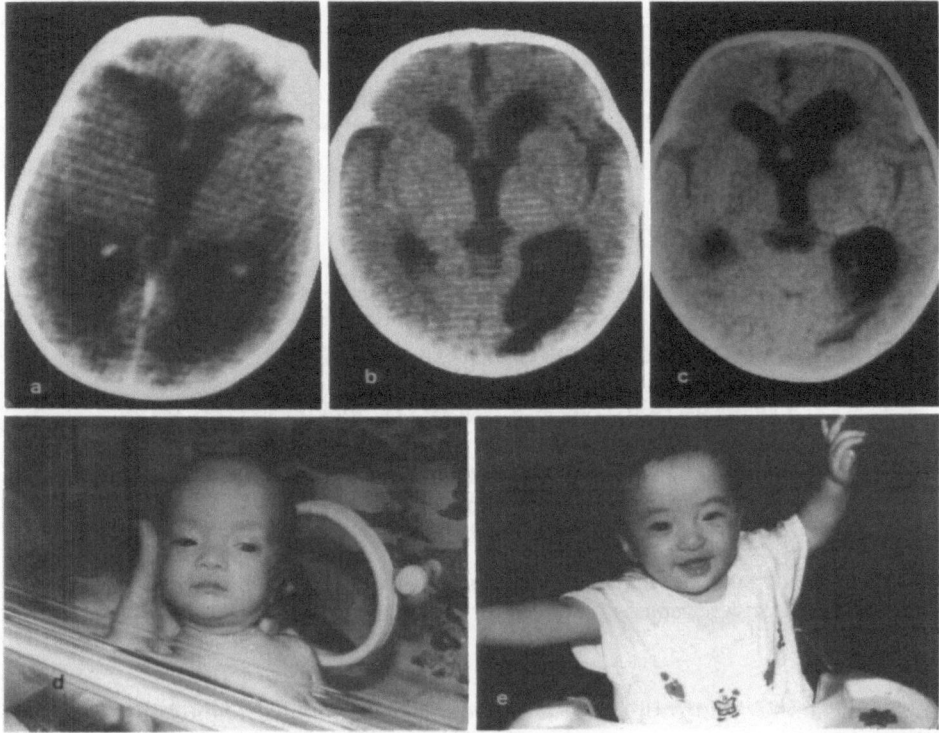

Fig. 5. A premature infant with progressive posthemorrhagic communicating hydro-cephalus; hydrogel ventriculo-subdural shunt was implanted 56 days after birth. CT scan **a** 16 days after birth, **b** 3 months after shunt insertion, and **c** 6 months after shunt insertion. Photograph **d** 31 days after birth, before shunt operation and **e** 8 months after birth

found that there was a subdural membrane covering the film of the ventriculo-subdural device. This subdural membrane spread to the thickened tissue on the cerebral surface beneath the film, enveloping the film and causing disturbance of CSF absorption. However, the device still drained CSF from ventricles. It demonstrated no adhesion to surrounding tissues. Histological study showed mild tissue reaction with subdural fibrous membrane formation. There was also evidence of recent minor hemorrhage, with degenerative blood and fibrous exudate coating the inner surface of the subdural membrane, and degenerative blood and inflammatory exudate on the cerebral surface beneath the film (Fig. 7a–e).

Discussion

Forrest et al. (1975a) designed a dye-study to test the absorptive power of subdural linings. The test was satisfactorily performed in 63 hydrocephalic

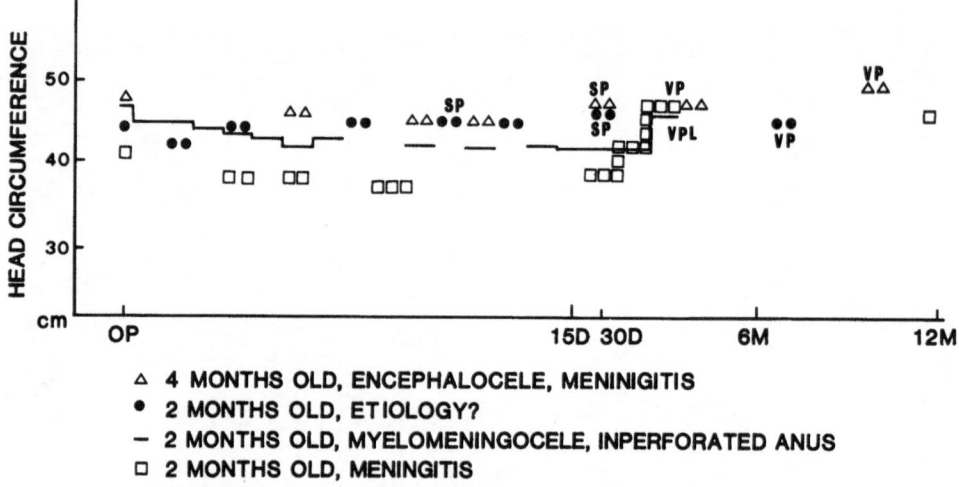

Fig. 6. Change of postoperative head circumference in four infants with progressive hydrocephalus after ventriculo-subdural shunt insertion.

patients by subdural introduction of phenolsulfonphthalein. The total excretion of dye in the first 6 hours varied from a trace to up to 85% of the injected dye. They found that a high excretion rate of the dye from the subdural space (50% or more within 6 hours of injection) indicated that the ventriculo-subdural shunt operation would be successful. For our experimental study, we designed a silicone ventriculo-subarachnoid (actually ventriculo-subdural) shunt and implanted it in an acute hydrocephalic monkey model. The arachnoid membrane near the interhemispheric fissure was torn during the operation. CT brain scan and I-131-RISA ventriculography were performed pre-operatively and at two days and two weeks post-operatively to evaluate the function of the shunt. Radioisotope studies demonstrated that intraventricular CSF was diverted to the subdural space and was absorbed there (Wong et al. 1986). These studies clearly demonstrated the absorption potential of subdural linings in human beings. Also, the arachnoid lining in the subdural space, and the arachnoid villi, especially, played an important role in CSF absorption in the subdural space. This phenomenon was the basis of the ventriculo-subdural shunt for the treatment of hydrocephalus, excepting external hydrocephalus.

The ventriculo-subdural shunt was one of various surgical methods which had been used before, with different materials, to treat hydrocephalus (Pudenz 1981). Forrest and his colleagues (1957b) in England reported the "Forrest disc" made of polythene, nylon, and finally, poly-tetra-fluoro-ethylene for ventriculo-subdural drainage. Forrest and colleagues used this device to treat 36 hydrocephalic babies, resulting in 18 arrested, 1 progressive, and 17 dead. In the failed cases, they usually found that the disc, and sometimes the sub-

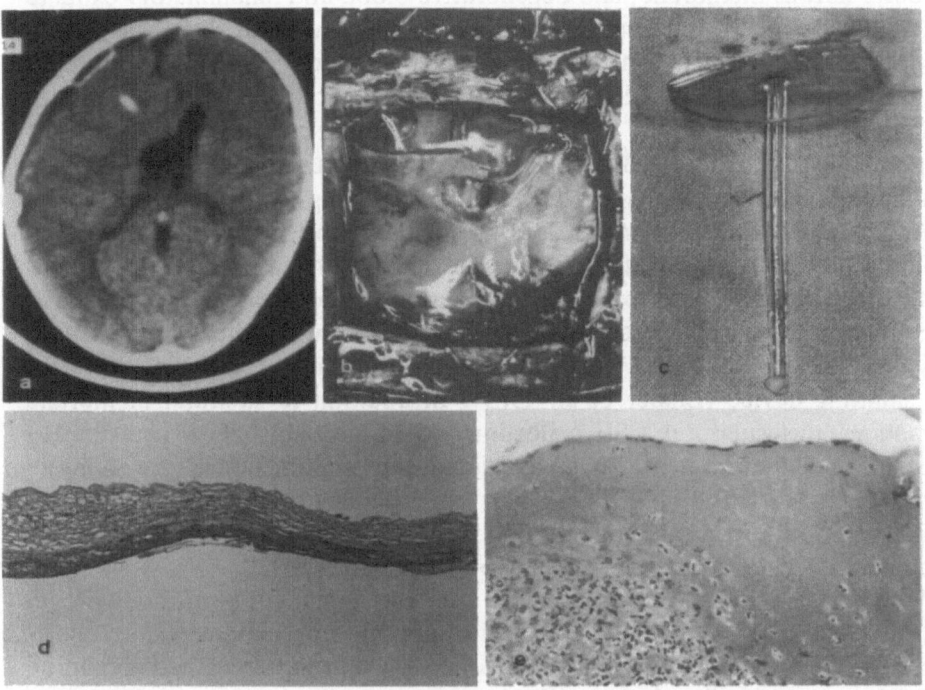

Fig. 7. An infant with ventriculo-subdural shunt implantation carried out at three months of age. Additional subduro-peritoneal shunt insertion was carried out at four months for progressing hydrocephalus. **a** CT scan at ten months of age, after shunt malfunction. **b** Subdural neomembrane formation **c** Apparatus after seven months of implantation **d** Section of subdural membrane **e** Section of tissue beneath film

dural space itself, became occluded by adhesions. More rarely, the disc was patent but the subdural space was lined by a membrane and filled with un-absorbed CSF. We used a hydrogel ventriculo-subdural shunt as a primary shunting procedure to treat seven babies with nontumoral hydrocephalus. The result was three cases of arrested and four cases of progressive hydrocephalus. In one of the failed cases, the device was removed after seven months of implantation. This hydrogel ventriculo-subdural shunt was still transparent and flexible. There was no opacity and the shunt was patent. These findings were different from those on hydrogel sheet implantation in animals. Calcium phosphate deposition in the device was not evaluated in this study (Imai et al. 1982). Histologically, there was evidence of recent minor subdural hemorrhage around and beneath the device film; however, the subdural space around the apparatus film was lined by a fibrous membrane. This fibrous membrane spread and linked with the thickened tissue on the cerebral surface beneath the film, thus encapsulating the device and causing shunt malfunction. Neither active nor old fibrosis was observed in the tissue beneath the film. However, degenerative blood and fibrinous exudate was found coating the inner surface of the subdural fibrous membrane, and degenerative blood and inflammatory exudate were shown beneath the film. These findings suggested that there was a very mild tissue reaction to the hydrogel ventriculo-subdural shunt in the subdural space (McFadden 1972; Imai et al. 1982). The degenerative blood and fibrinous exudate encountered might have been due to recent minor subdural hemorrhage. This hemorrhage would be a result of the rupture of small bridging veins after mild head injury or the result of bleeding from capillaries of the neomembrane formed under the dura. After the hydrogel ventriculo-subdural shunting procedure, most of the infants developed unilateral or bilateral subdural CSF collection with ipsilateral diminution of the lateral ventricular size. This phenomenon was caused by communication between the subdural space and the enlarged ventricles (Koizumi et al. 1987) and the dumping effect of the shunting device (Linder et al. 1981). In addition to subdural membrane formation, this subdural CSF collection would probably be a contributing factor in the subdural hemorrhage and in causing malfunction of the shunting device (Ohno et al. 1987). There was one occurrence of chronic subdural hematoma on the contralateral side following ventriculo-subdural shunt insertion and bilateral subdural fluid collection (Koizumi 1987).

We did experience a high failure rate after the implantation of the hydrogel ventriculo-subdural shunt in babies with nontumoral hydrocephalus. Postoperative symptomatic subdural fluid collection and subdural neomembrane formation with bleeding from capillaries were contributing factors. However, of the seven infants receiving hydrogel ventriculo-subdural shunt implantation as a primary procedure to treat nontumoral hydrocephalus, arrested hydrocephalus occurred in three babies with posthemorrhagic hydrocephalus due to prematurity and perinatal trauma. These three babies presented with progressive hydrocephalus before operation and they did not have the risk of shunt dependency and slit ventricle syndrome. For those infants showing progressive hydrocephalus after implantation of the hydrogel ventriculo-subdural apparatus, additional ventriculo-peritoneal shunt insertion was the best method of management. A subduro-peritoneal shunt applied at the site of the ventriculo-subdural shunt could usually function for a few months.

Hydrogel is an important polymer material for biomedical application, although it appears to be tumorigenic and undergoes calcification at the site of implant and in the surrounding tissue in certain animals (Pedley et al. 1980; Imai 1979; Imai and Masuhara 1982). We designed a hydrogel ventriculo-subdural shunt and implanted it subdurally in dogs. Histological studies in dogs sacrificed at 30 and 120 days showed fibrosis only in the dura and gliosis in the brain at the site of implantation (Wong, 1986). We then applied this apparatus to the treatment of eight infants with nontumoral hydrocephalus, excepting external hydrocephalus. We wished to know whether, by changing the biomaterial, the abandoned ventriculo-subdural shunt could be revived as an alternative method for the management of hydrocephalus in infants and children. From this study, we conclude that the hydrogel subdural implant is very well tolerated. Except for external hydrocephalus, a hydrogel ventriculo-subdural shunt can be tried as the initial shunting procedure in infants with progressive nontumoral hydrocephalus. However, the possibility of this material being tumorigenic is of great concern. Also, it is not an ideal shunt because of its high failure rate and prominent subdural collection in most cases after implantation. In successful cases, complications such as shunt dependence and slit ventricle syndrome, which might occur in ventriculo-peritoneal shunt surgery, could be avoided.

References

Chiang CT (1988) Hydrogels as biomaterial implants for drainage tubes of glaucoma and hydrocephalus. Master's Thesis, Institute of Biomedical Engineering, National Yang-Ming Medical College, Taiwan

Forrest DM, Laurence KM, Macnab GH (1957a) Ventriculo-subdural drainage in infantile hydrocephalus. Lancet II: 827–828

Forrest DM, Laurence KM, Macnab GH (1957b) Ventriculo-subdural drainage in infantile hydrocephalus. Analysis of early results. Lancet II: 1274–1277

Imai, Kojima K, Masuhara E (1979) Tumorigenesis by polymeric materials. Proceedings of the 2nd Meeting of ISAO: 249–252

Imai Y, Masuhara E (1982) Long term in vivo studies of poly (2 hydroxyethyl methacrylate). J Biomed Mater Res 16: 609–617

Koizumi H, Fukamachi A, Nukui H (1987) Postoperative subdural fluid collections in neurosurgery. Surg Neurol 27: 147–153

Linder M, Diehl JT, Sklar FH (1981) Significance of postshunt ventricular asymmetries. J Neurosurg 55: 183–186

McFadden JT (1972) Tissue reactions to standard neurosurgical metallic implants. J Neurosurg 36: 598–603

Onho K, Suzuki, Masaoka H, Matsushima H, Inaba Y, Monma S (1987) Chronic subdural hematoma preceded by persistent traumatic subdural fluid collection. J Neurol Neurosurg Psychiatry 50: 1694–1697

Pedley DG, Skelly PJ, Tighe BJ (1980) Hydrogels in biomedical applications. Br Polym J 12: 99–110

Pudenz RH (1981) The surgical treatment of hydrocephalus — an historical review. Surg Neurol 15: 15–26

Wang YH (1986) Hydrogels as biomaterial-implant devices for correction of glaucoma and hydrocephalus. Master's Thesis, Institute of Biomedical Engineering, National Yaug-Ming Medical College, Taiwan

Wong TT, Lee LS, Shen ALY, Yeh SH, Liu RS, Chang T, Ho DM, Chang KP, Wang YH, Chiang CT, Niu GCC, Wang YJ (1987) Research concerning intracranial ventriculo-subarachnoid (ventriculo-subdural) shunts. NSC 74-0412-B075 National Science Council (ROC) Progress report IV: 1–33

Wong TT, Lee LS, Liu RS, Yeh SH, Chang T, Chou MT (to be published) Ventriculo-subdural shunt: An experimental study for its drainage function and absorption of shunting CSF in the subdural space. Ann Nucl Med Sci 4: 96–102

III. Shunt Complications

45 — Evaluation of Shunt Failures by Compliance Analysis and Inspection of Shunt Valves and Shunt Materials, Using Microscopic or Scanning Electron Microscopic Techniques

Wolfgang F. Schoener, Christian Reparon, Raphaela Verheggen, and Evangelos Markakis[1]

Summary. Shunt dysfunction or malfunction in the treatment of hydrocephalus still causes multiple difficulties in the clinical management of this condition. In this study the results of micro-inspection of explanted shunt valves and tubes by light and scanning electron microscopy are presented. From our findings in 36 patients aged from 1 month to 79 years (mean age 49.03 years) we discovered that 61.1% of the patients had shunt related defects which led to tissue migration into the shunt lumens or to tissue adherence to the tube surface. Calcification and destruction of the silicone-elastomer tubing was found in all cases of shunt tube occlusion (25%). There were shunt fractures in 11.1% of the tubes. Histological analysis verified foreign body tissue reactions on all explanted alloplasts. In five cases (13.8%) migration of chorioid plexus or glial cells to the inner lumen of the ventricular catheter was found. Of 36 patients who underwent compliance (Co), reabsorption resistance (R), and cerebrospinal fluid (CSF) formation rate (F) analysis, one patient required a valve replacement due to significant intracranial content compliance changes after craniostenosis surgery. Furthermore, four of 36 patients had shunt infections, three cases with bacteria *Staphylococcus aureus* (8.3%), and one case with *Candida albicans* (2.8%) hyphae inside the valve lumen. Work-bench valve tests, following the ISO/DIS 7197 protocol (1989), clarified that of seven valves tested, six did not match the CSF-drainage requirements for an individual patient.

Keywords. Shunt-failure — Occlusion of shunts — Cell migration — Material defects — Calcification of shunt tubes

Introduction

Since Nulsen and Spitz (1952) introduced the valve-regulated shunt to ensure unidirectional cerebrospinal fluid (CSF) flow, ventriculo-peritoneal and

---

[1] Department of Neurosurgery, University Hospital and Medical School, Robert Koch Straße 40, 3400 Goettingen, Germany

ventriculo-atrial shunts have been widely accepted for the treatment of hydrocephalus. Many attempts to improve shunt systems and surgical techniques have been made over the last 38 years. However, the line of treatment still is associated with complications. Widely recognized complications are found to be infection, mechanical failure due to tube-fracture or disconnection, and shunt system and valve failure with over- or underdrainage of CSF. Less recognized complications are tissue reactions to the shunt material as a foreign body (Gower et al. 1984) as well as thromboembolic complications due to clotting on the tube surface or to calcium uptake of the silicone-elastomers found primarily in ventriculo-atrial shunts (Emery and Hilton 1961; Talner et al. 1961; Noonan and Ehmke 1963; Nugent et al. 1966; Schmaltz et al. 1980; Olsen and Frykberg 1983; Piatt and Hoffmann 1989).

The primary problem to be addressed in the clinical management of shunt complications is the surgical treatment and the proper selection of the most suitable valve to ensure adequate opening and closing pressures which correspond to the CSF-hydrodynamic parameters of the individual (Buchheit et al. 1972; Fox et al. 1973; Foltz 1984). With our study we tried to complete the "check-list" for the proper selection of ventricular catheters and draining tube materials, where manufacturing quality must be taken into consideration as well.

Clinical Material and Methods

CSF-hydrodynamic parameter analysis was preformed in 34 of 36 patients who underwent surgery for shunt revision because of shunt failure or shunt infection. Two children were excluded from these measurements because of CSF leakage at the insertion site of the ventricular catheter. The parameters calculated were compliance of the intracranial contents (Co), CSF-outflow resistance (R), and CSF-formation rate (F) at baseline pressure (Po) (Marmarou 1984; Portnoy 1984). The individual pressure volume relation could be be derived from an artificial CSF bolus in injection and withdrawal technique via the ventricular catheter (Simon et al. 1984; Blomquist et al. 1986). The effects of volume removal on the pressure compliance relation were plotted on a pressure compliance diagram. Pressure, compliance, and resistance data for a pressure compliance^2 versus compliance and for a compliance versus ln-resistance linear regression were taken from 33 patients (Børgesen et al. 1987). One child with open sutures was excluded from these regression calculations, because of the significant elevation of his compliance compared to individuals with closed sutures.

In vitro evaluation of the explanted shunt valves to test shunt valve characteristics by means of the flow to pressure relation was carried out following the ISO/DIS 7197 standard (1989). Valves presenting obvious tissue-related abnormalities or unreasonable malfunction during surgery were selected for micro-inspection by light or scanning electron microscopy. Fixation was performed in a buffered glutaraldehyde solution. Following the same procedure, all 36 tubes were evaluated by searching for defects and destruction, and by

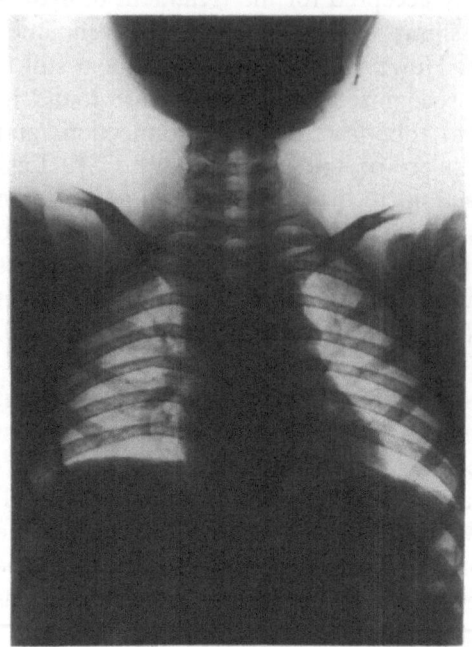

Fig. 1. a Chest radiograph showing pulmonary tree calcification on the *right side* and shunt disconnection at *left retroauricular valve site*, **b** shunt tube ascension and obstruction, and **c** pulmonary catheter embolism

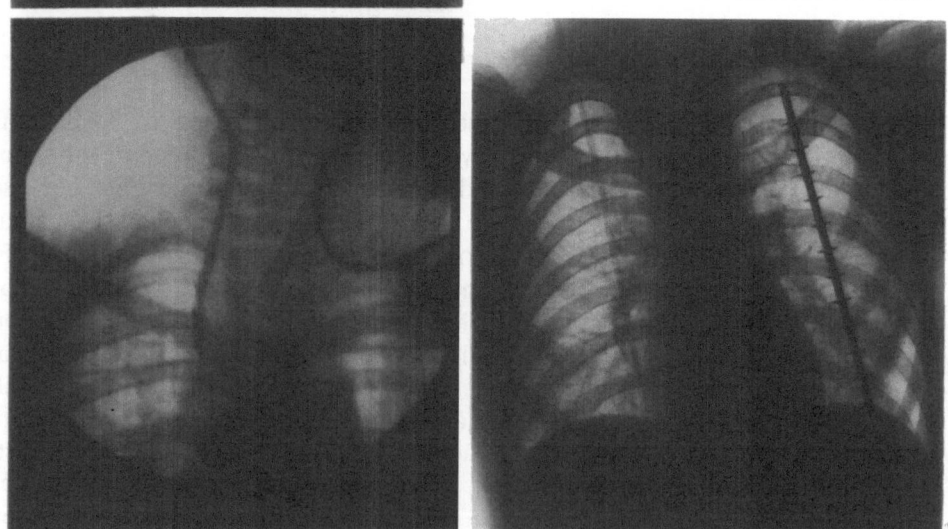

looking for alterations in the surrounding shunt tissues (Wuest and Rosenbauer 1984).

Results

All 36 patients from this series underwent surgery for shunt revision; 17 patients were male and 19 were female (47.2%/52.8%). Of 3 children (2 male,

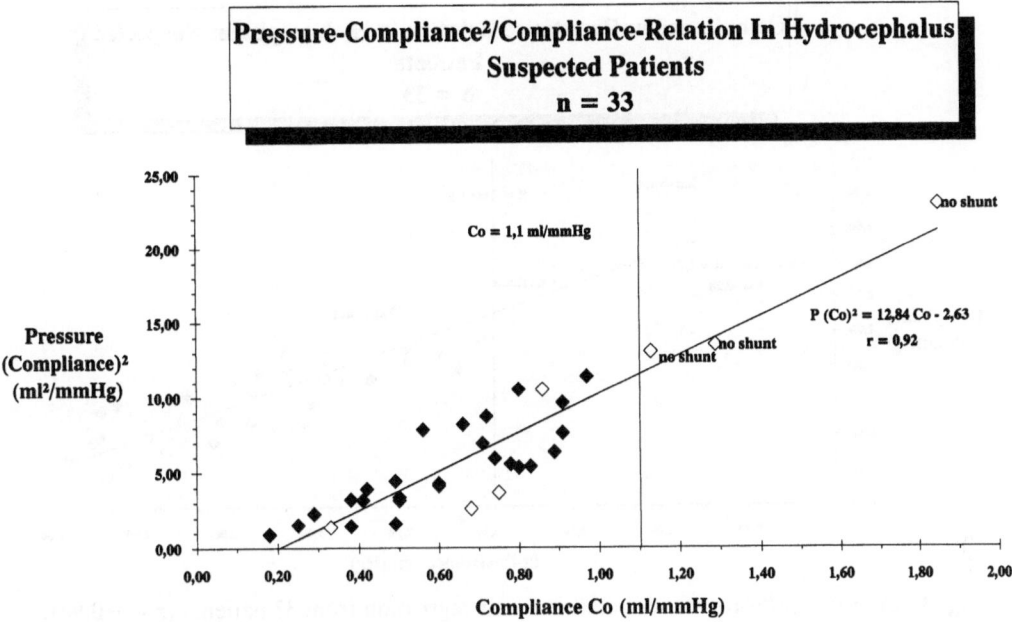

Fig. 2. Pressure-compliance^2/compliance-relation linear regression from 33 patients ($r = 0.92$). Co, compliance at base line pressure Po; lozenge, patients not shunted, and or temporary external CSF drained

1 female) only one could be examined by pressure volume analysis, because of insufficient supply of data during the bolus injection procedure. Another child, a 7-month-old boy, suffered from severe hydrocephalus and craniosynostosis related to the Carpenter Syndrome and at time of shunt revision he had undergone surgery for biparietal and frontal bone flapping; his status was regarded as equal to that of the children with open sutures. Patients's ages ranged from 1 month to 79 years (mean age 49.03 years) and the children's ages ranged from 1 month to 8 months. (mean age 4.67 months).

The indications for shunt revision were derived from a combination of the clinical onset of symptoms correlated to raised intracranial pressure or shunt infection and the course of follow up with cerebral computer tomography or magnetic resonance images indicating shunt or shunt-valve dysfunction (Milhorat 1982; O'Brien 1982; Ojemann and Black 1982). Radiography of the entire shunt pathways verified shunt fractures in four patients (11.1%) and, in two patients (5.6%), disconnection of the draining catheter at the valve outlet site was discovered. Chest radiographs verified atrial catheter embolism and in five patients (13.9%) ascension of the draining catheter and indications of calcifications in the pulmonary arterial tree were found (Fig. 1). Indications of an obstruction of the ventricular catheter in five patients (13.9%) and reduction of distal valve-outflow in nine patients (2%) were found by digital transcutaneous valve-manipulation. Results from 33 patients for the pressure (Po) compliance^2 (Co^2) versus compliance (Co)-relation and the compliance

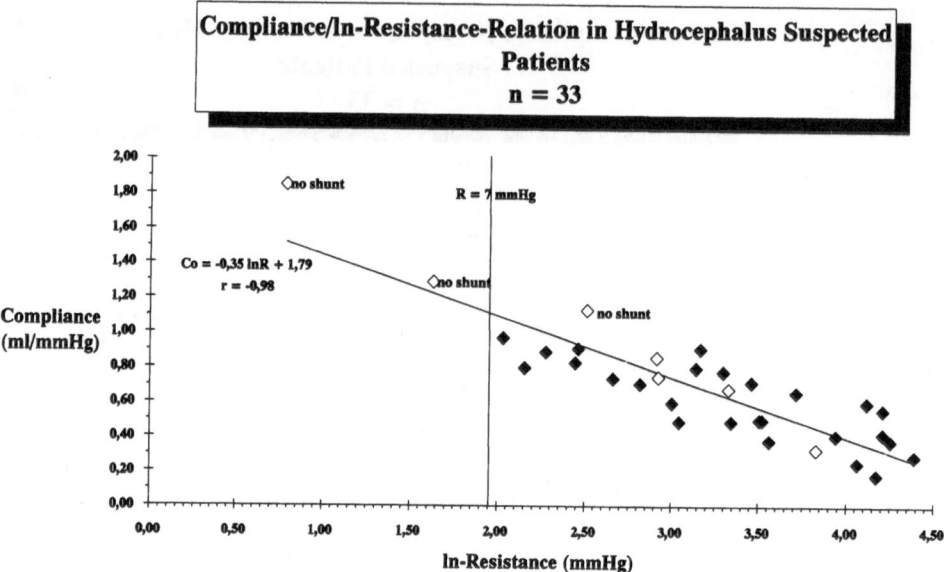

Fig. 3. Compliance/ln-resistance-relation linear regression from 33 patients ($r = -0.98$). R, outflow resistance at Po; lozenge, patients not shunted, and or temporary external CSF drained

(Co) versus ln-CSF-outflow-resistance (ln R)-relation performed by linear regression show that this population with $r = 0.92$ and $r = -0.98$ at a compliance of >1.1 ml/mmHg and a resistance of >7 mmHg/ml/per min carries a low risk of shunt dependancy. Two patients were not re-shunted (indicated by lozenge and "no shunt" in Figs. 2 and 3) and four patients with infections, indicated by lozenge, were externally CSF-drained.

The 7-month-old boy with Carpenter syndrome developed acute onset of decompensating hydrocephalus so that immediate shunt supply was required. CSF-hydrodynamic parameters verified a flow-regulated shunting device, which worked properly until a revision became necessary following biparietal and frontal flapping during craniosynostosis surgery. Compliance had changed so drastically that a valve replacement had to be preformed (Figs. 4 and 5).

Seven explanted valves, four flow regulated and three multistage trancutaneously programmable, were work-bench tested and the pressure-flow characteristics of 6 of these are presented in Figs. 6, 7, and 8.

These test results do not match the limits of pressure-flow characteristics stated by the manufacturers, where six out of seven valves performed outside their stated performance ranges. The valve in Fig. 7 (small dotted line) worked in a manner very close to its designed flow regulation, but failed to drain CSF sufficiently in the case of the boy with Carpenter Syndrome after craniostenosis surgery (Fig. 5).

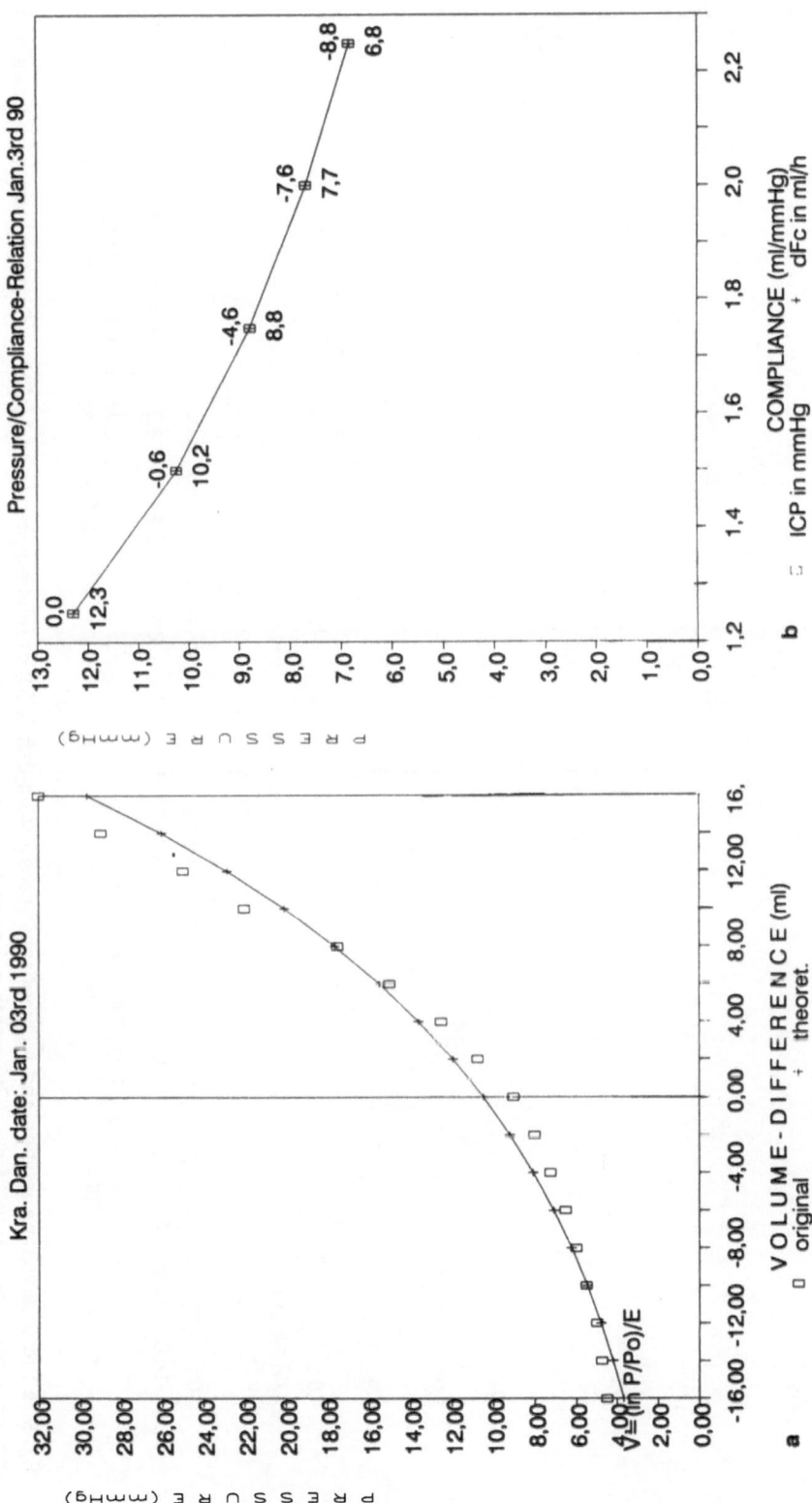

Fig. 4. a Pressure/volume relation and **b** compliance reabsorption deficit (*dFc*) relation; marks and labels indicate volume withdrawal and change of pressure; derived from a 7-month-old patient with carpenter syndrone before shunt insertion

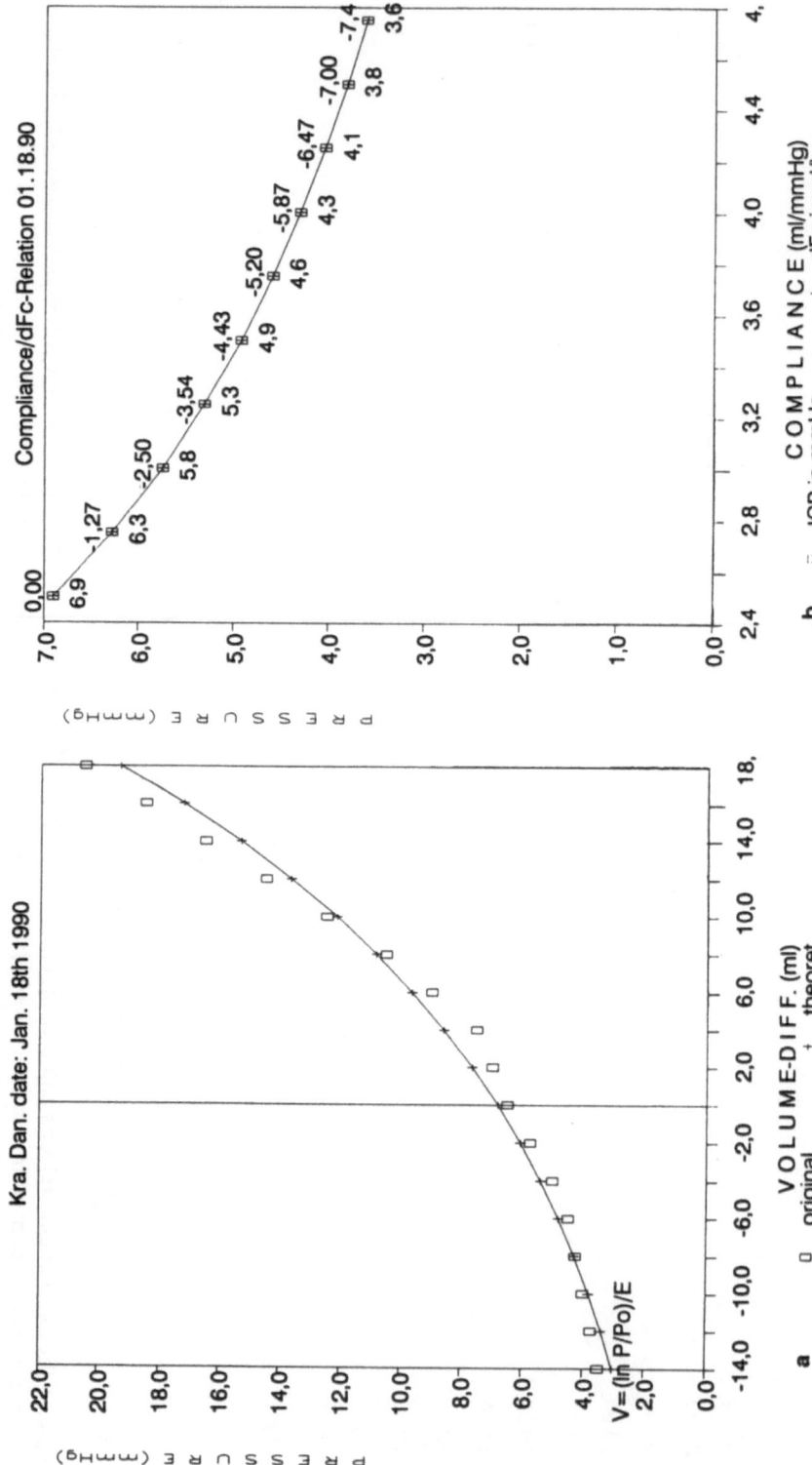

Fig. 5. a Pressure/volume relation and **b** compliance reabsorption-deficit (dFc) relation; *marks* and *labels* indicate volume withdrawal and change of pressure; derived from a 7½-month-old patient during shunt revision

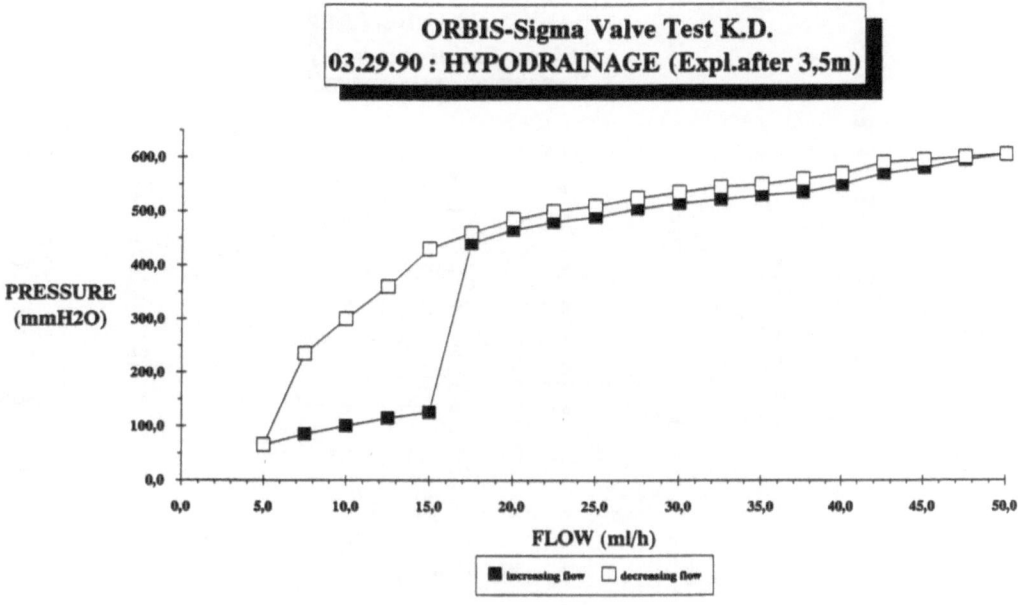

Fig. 6. Pressure/flow condition of an improperly functioning valve (hypodrainage)

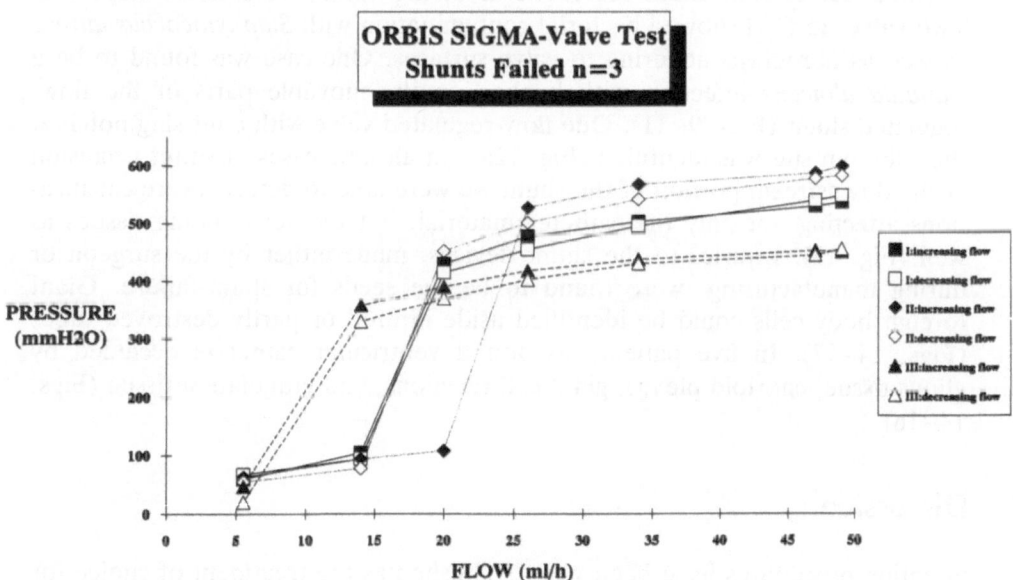

Fig. 7. Test results from three explanted valves; *dotted line* indicates sample which caused hyperdrainage

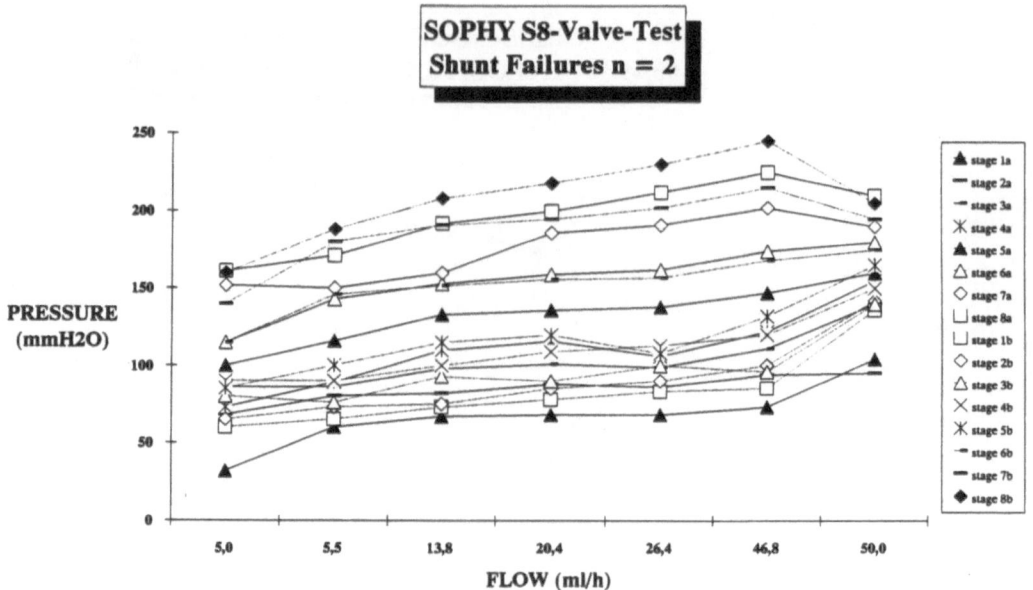

Fig. 8. Test results from two programmable valves explanted because of hypodrainage in stages 1a and 1b

Three out of four shunt infections involving valves were micro-inspected. Two valves (5.6%) showed bacterial contamination with *Staphylococcus aureus* as well as fibroblasts adhering to valve surfaces. One case was found to be a *Candida albicans* infection with hyphae on the movable parts of the flow-regulated shunt (Figs. 9–11). One flow-regulated valve with a missing notch at the ruby-pin site was identified (Fig. 12a). In all nine cases of shunt occlusion at the downstream portion of the shunt we were able to detect severe calcifications affecting not only the catheter material, but the surrounding tissues as well (Fig. 13). Injuries to the shunt devices, made either by the surgeon or during manufacturing, were found to be the seeds for shunt-failure. Giant foreign body cells could be identified aside injured or partly destroyed tubes (Figs. 14–17). In five patients we found ventricular catheters occluded by glious tissue, chorioid plexus, giant cell reactions, and granulation tissue (Figs. 14–16).

Discussion

Shunting procedures have been well established as the treatment of choice for hydrocephalus. However, neurosurgeons are quite often forced to carry out revisions because of complications and shunt malfunctions arising from various causes. The indications for shunt revision in all 36 patients in our study were given by clinical signs of increased CSF pressure or shunt malfunction, and by the results of radiograph, computerized axial tomography (CAT), or magnetic

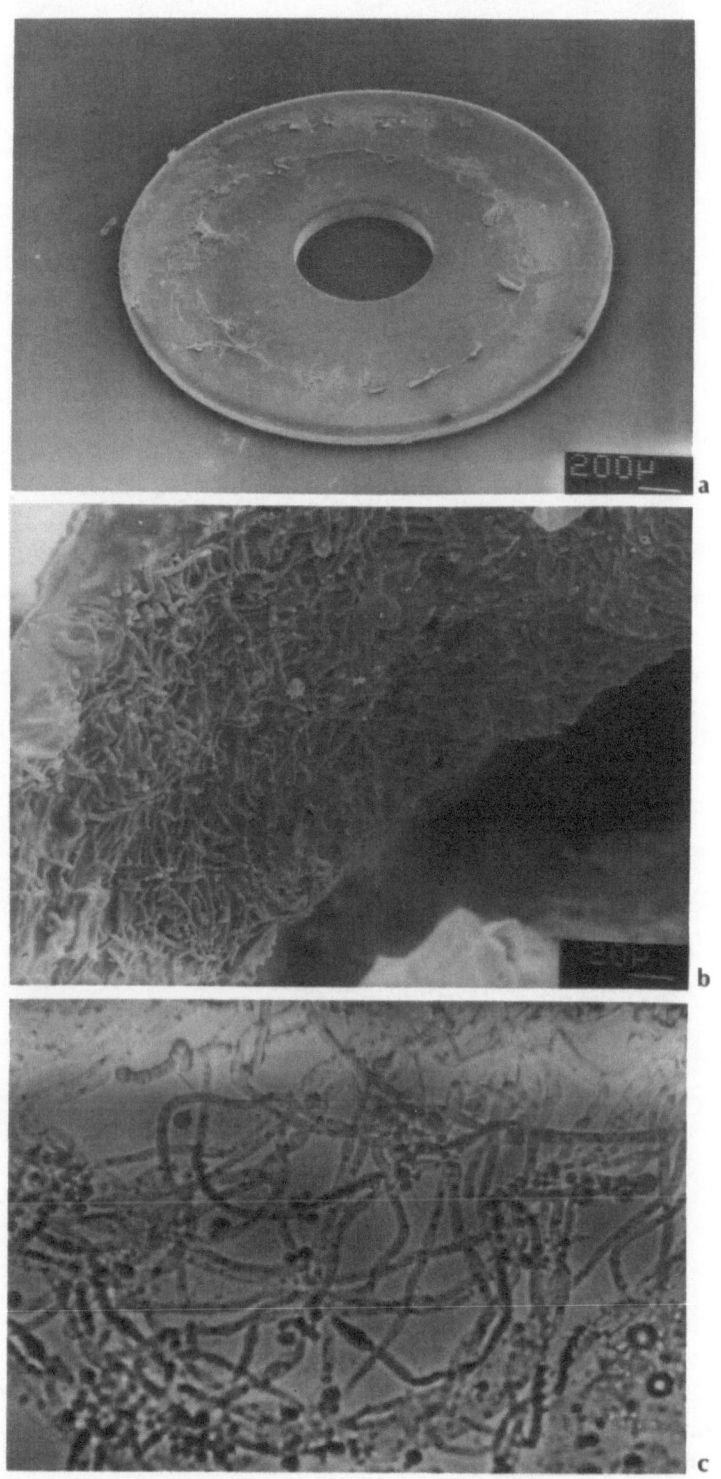

Fig. 9. a Ruby disk with fibroblasts adhering to surface, **b** *Candida* hyphae on disk holding silastic membrane, and **c** *Candida* hyphae

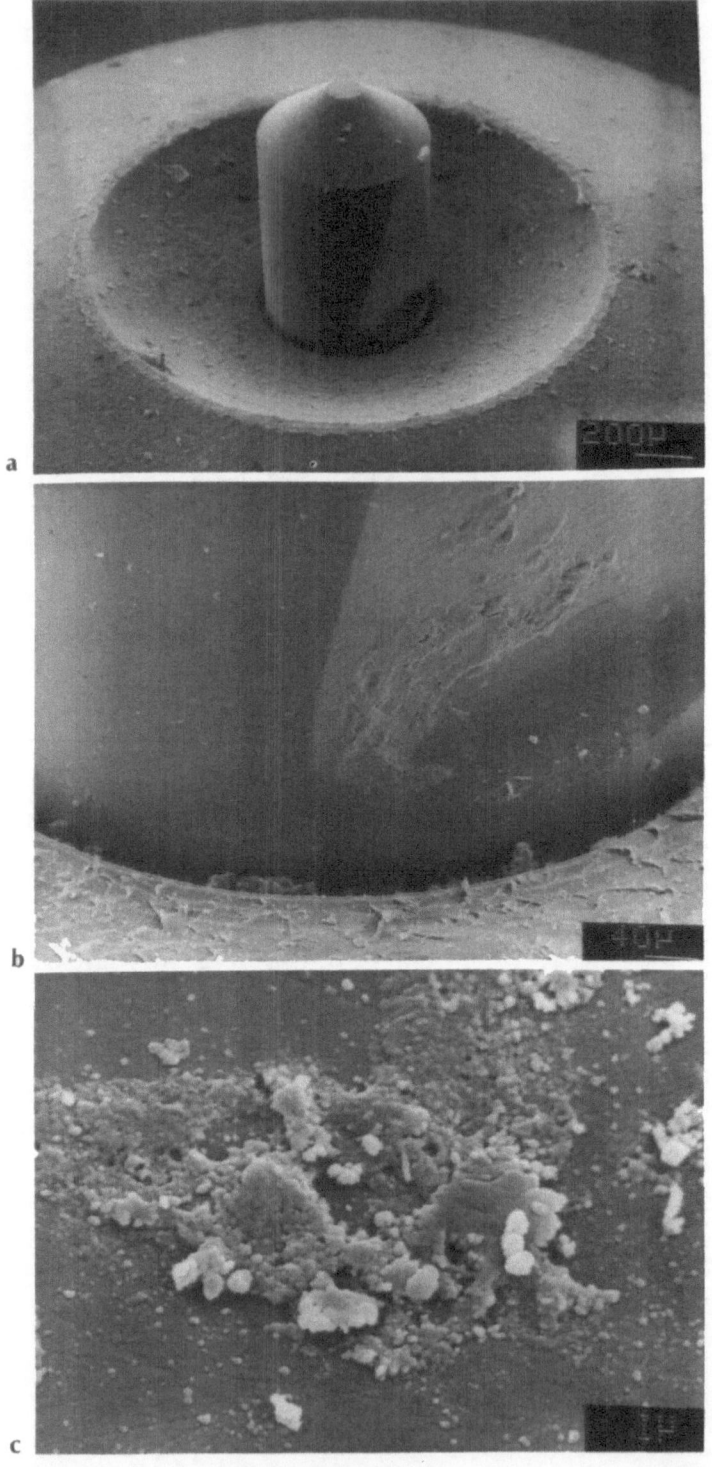

Fig. 10. a Ruby pin of flow-regulated valve, **b** Cutting scratches with surface adherent material at ruby seat, and **c** Bacteria clusters on rough surface

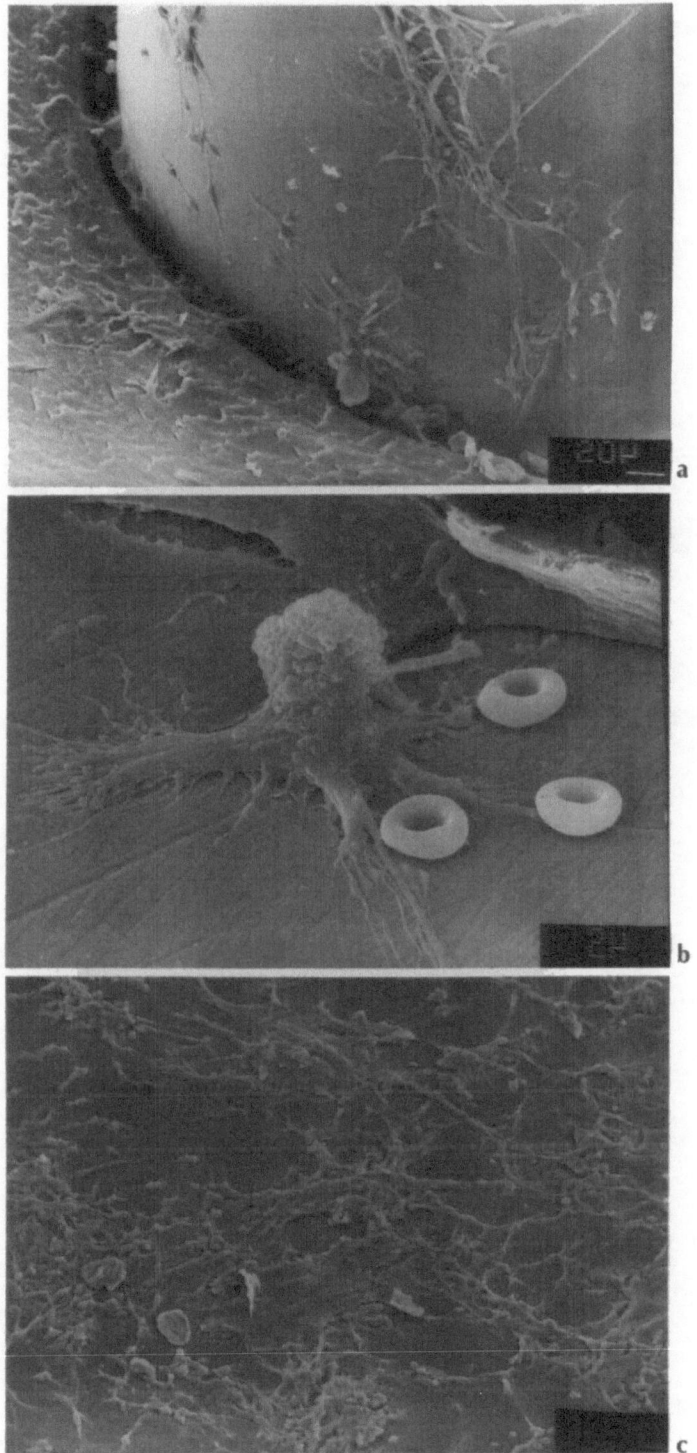

Fig. 11. a Ruby pin with fibroblast net and red blood cells, **b** Surface adherent fibroblast topped by bacteria and red blood cells, and **c** Fibroblast netweok and bacteria on silastic membrane

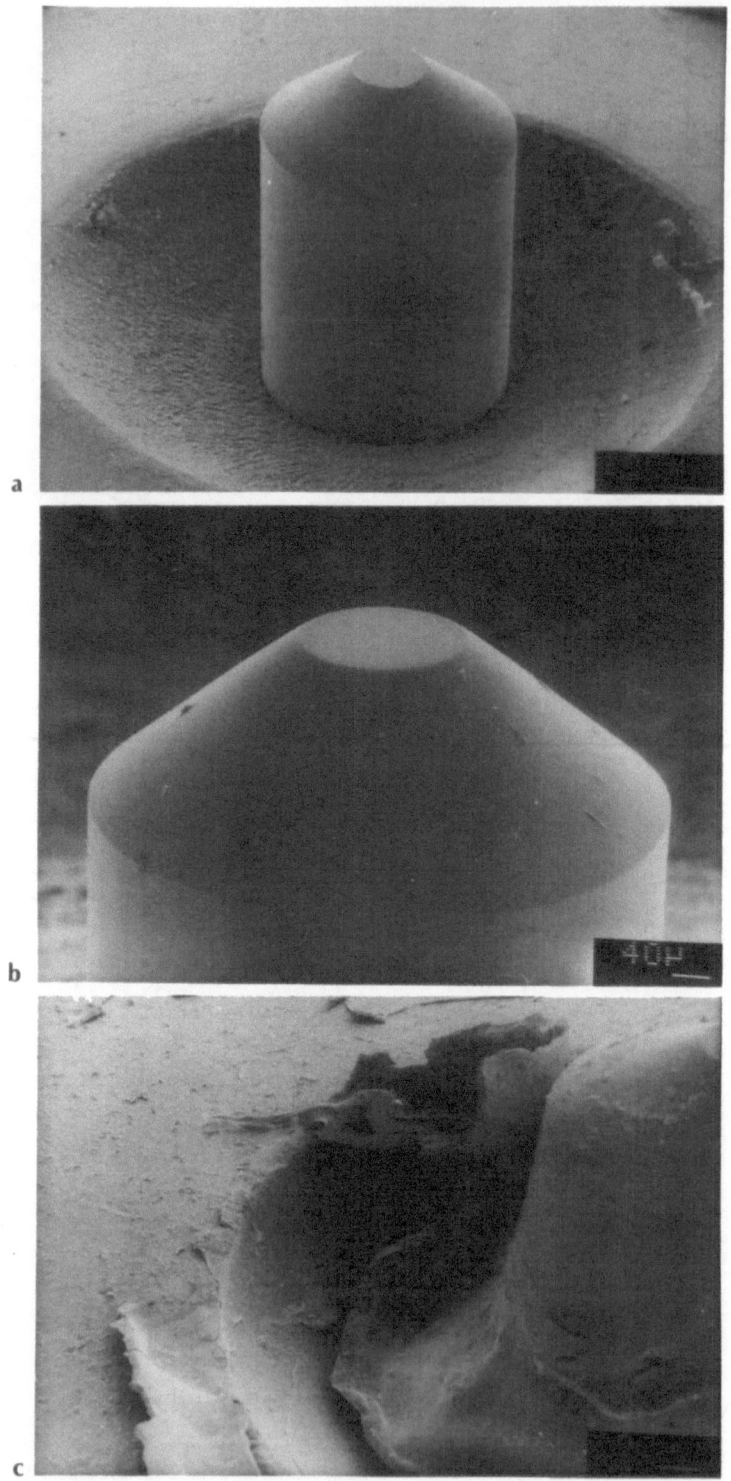

Fig. 12. **a** Ruby pin with missing notch, **b** Tip of ruby pin with adherent fibroblast, and **c** Ruby pin seat with clogging and adhering protein and cell detritus

464

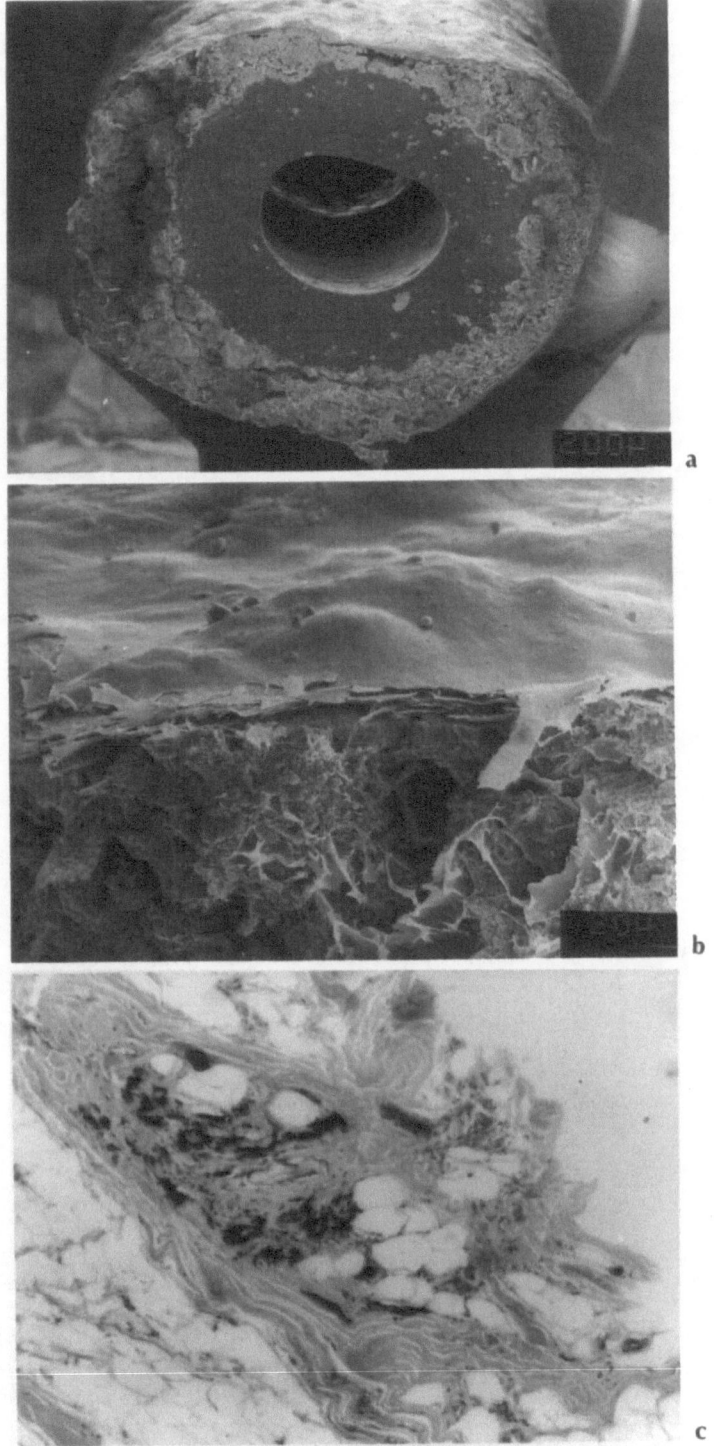

Fig. 13. a Shunt tube calcification and destruction, **b** Calcification caused separation of surface layer from silastic tube body, and **c** Histological preparation showing collagenous fibers surrounding calcification

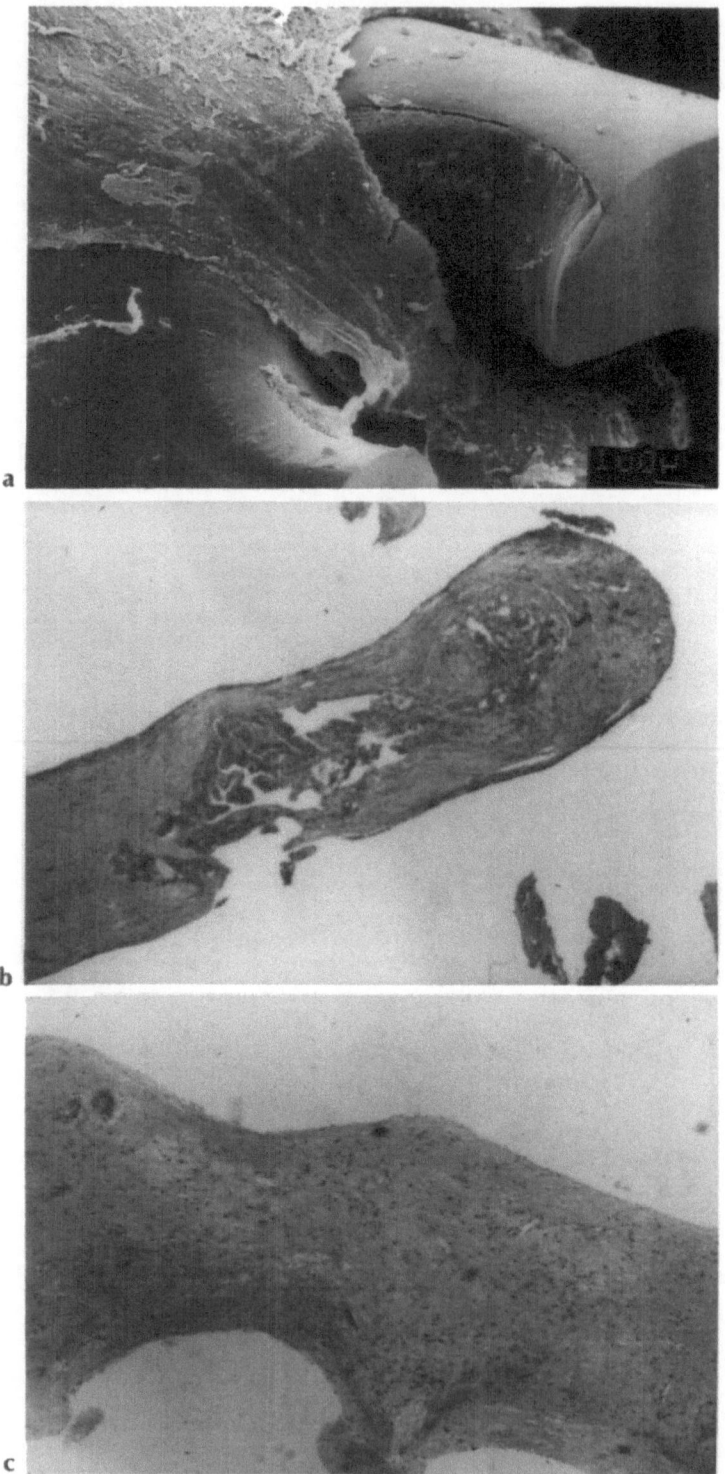

Fig. 14. a Ventricular catheter occluded by cellular migration, **b** Plexus chorioideus preparation from ventricular catheter, and **c** Glious cells from a ventricular catheter

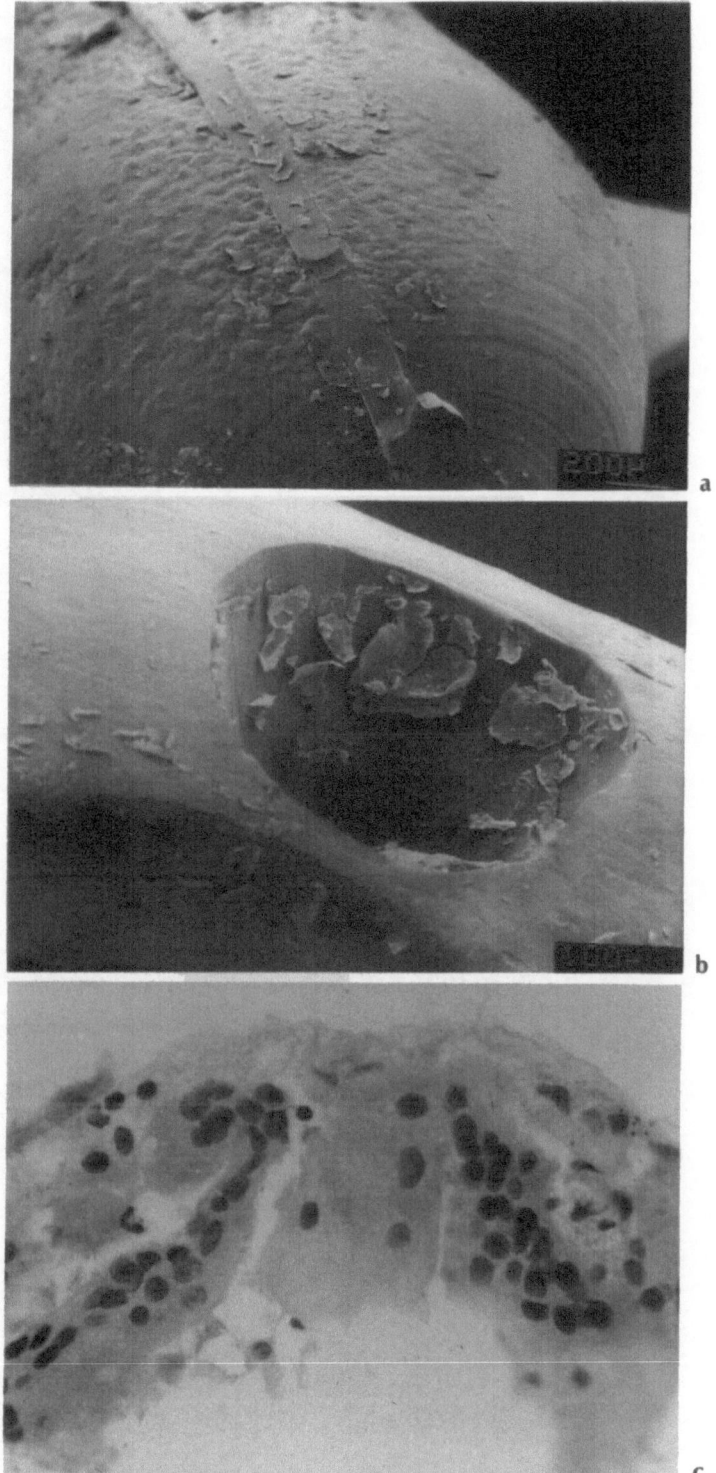

Fig. 15. a Ventricular catheter showing manufacturing fault at tip, **b** Cutting artifact at ventricular catheter holes, and **c** Giant cell (foreign body reaction)

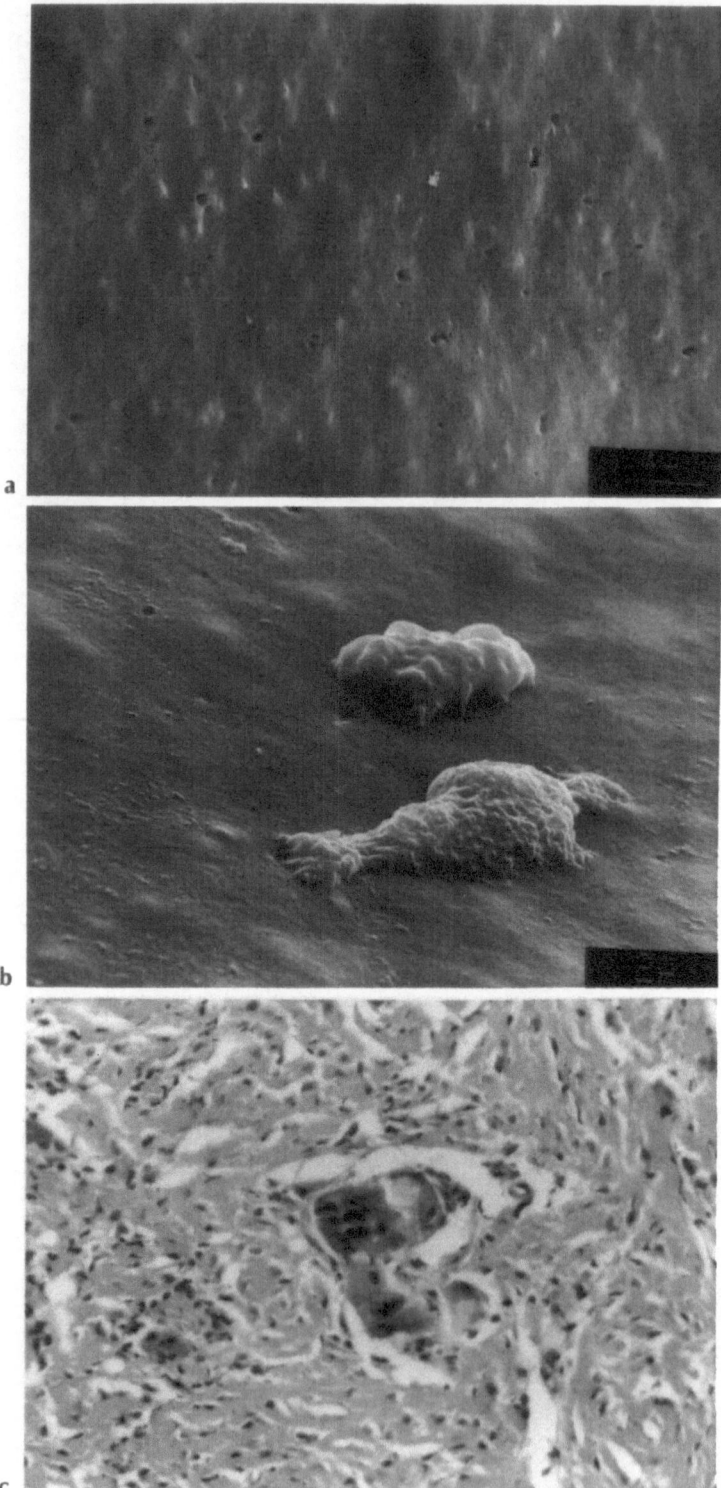

Fig. 16. a Pits in silastic catheter surface, **b** Bacteria adhering to silastic surface of ventricular catheter, and **c** Giant cell (foreign body reaction)

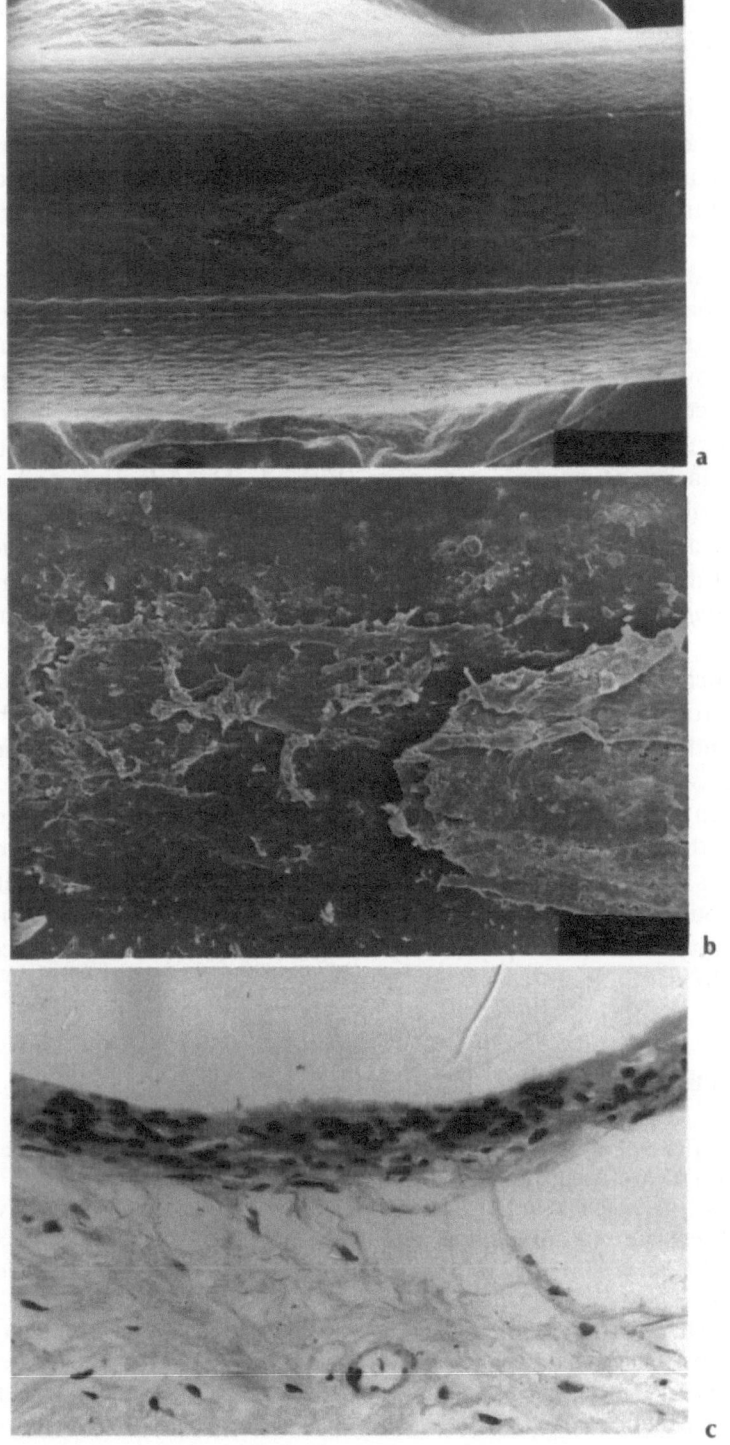

Fig. 17. a Shunt tube injury, **b** Detritus and bacteria adhering to injured tube, and **c** Giant cell reaction from injured tube environment

469

resonance imaging (MRI) examination. The patient's age, sex, and underlying condition appeared not to influence the factors which led to shunt revision, which is contrary to Raimondi's findings (Raimondi et al. 1977). In our study, shunt failure in VA shunts was found to relate more to catheter failure (calcifications, fractures, ascension of the atrial catheter) and catheter embolism than to valve-related problems. CSF-parameter analysis during surgery gave way for the exclusion of three patients (Figs. 2 and 3). This is in contrary to the findings of Hemmer and Boehm (1976). In our series, only four patients were discovered to have no shunting device-related failures. One infant, who required craniosynostosis surgery 1 month after he had not been shunted sufficiently, was found to have such a significantly changed compliance that a valve replacement became necessary (Figs. 4, 5). Adaption and individual selection of valves in respect to valve hydrodynamics (Portnoy et al. 1976; Hakim et al. 1973) is supported by CSF parameter analysis performed during surgery. Infections found in four patients in our series affected the entire shunt system. *Staphylococcus aureus* and *Candida albicans* were found on shunt tubes and on the moving and fixed parts of the valves (Figs. 9–11 and Fig. 13).

We conclude that proper functioning and reliability of a shunt system is not solely a property of its hydrodynamics (Portnoy et al. 1976) but of the quality control and quality assurance of the manufacturer which assumes mirror-like smoothness of all of the surfaces of the system.

Additionally, the finding of a foreign body reaction in 19 of our 36 explanted devices indicates the importance of biocompatibility of the shunt materials. The results of this study, showing 22 out of 36 valve related shunt-failures, are very discouraging. We suggest that further research is necessary to improve biodurability and biocompatibility as well as pressure and flow control in hydrocephalus shunt systems.

References

Blomquist HK, Sundin S, Ekstedt J (1986) Cerebrospinal fluid hydrodynamic studies in children. J Neurol Neurosurg Psychiatry 49: 536–548

Børgesen SE, Gjerris F (1987) Relationship between intracranial pressure, ventricular size and resistance to CSF outflow. J Neurosurg 67: 535–548

Buchheit F, Maitrot D, Healy JL, et al. (1982) How to choose the best valve. Monogr Neural Sci 8: 184–187

Emery JL, Hilton HB (1961) Lung and heart complications of the treatment of hydrocephalus by ventriculoauriculostomy. Surgery 50: 309–314

Foltz EL (1984) Hydrocephalus and CSF pulsatility: Clinical and laboratory studies. In: Shapiro K, Marmarou A, Portnoy H (eds) Hydrocephalus. Raven, New York, pp 337–362

Fox JL, McCullough DC, Green RC (1973) Effect of cerebrospinal fluid shunts on intracranial pressure and on cerebrospinal fluid dynamics. II. A new technique of pressure measurements. III. A concept of hydrocephalus. J Neurol Neurosurg Psychiatry 36: 302–312

Gower DJ, Lewis JK, Kelly DL (1984) Sterile shunt malfunction. J Neurosurg 61: 1079–1114

Hakim S, Duran de la Roche F, Bureton JD (1973) A critical analysis of valve shunts used in the treatment of hydrocephalus. Dev Med Child Neurol 15: 230–255

Hemmer R, Boehm B (1976) Once a shunt, always a shunt? Dev Med Child Neurol 18 (Suppl 37): 69–73

International Organization for Standardization ISO/Draft International Standard DIS (1989) Neurosurgical implants, sterile, single-use hydrocephalic shunts and components. In: 150/TC 150. DIN, Rforzheim, 7197 Annexes B, C pp 7–10

Noonan JA, Ehmke DA (1963) Complications of ventriculovenous shunts for control of hydrocephalus. Report of three cases with thromboemboli to the lungs. N Engl J Med 269: 70–74

Nugent GR, Lucas R, Judy M, Bloor BM, Warden H (1966) Thromboembolic complications of ventriculo-atrial shunts. Angiocardiographic and pathologic correlations. J Neurosurg 24: 34–42

Nulsen FE, Spitz EB (1952) Treatment of hydrocephalus by direct shunt from ventricle to jugular vein. Surg Forum 2: 399–403

Marmarou A (1984) Biomechanics and theoretical model of hydrocephalus: Summary. In: Shapiro K, Marmarou A, Portnoy H (eds) Hydrocephalus. Raven, New York, pp 337–362

Milhorat TS (1982) Hydrocephalus: Historical notes, etiology and clinical diagnosis. In: Section of pediatric neurosurgery of the American Association of Neurological Surgeons (ed) Pediatric neurosurgery of the developing nervous system. Grune and Stratton, New York, pp 197–210

O'Brien MS (1982) Hydrocephalus in children. In: Youmans JR (ed) Neurological surgery, 2nd edn. Saunders, Philadelphia, pp 1381–1422

Ojemann RG, Black PM (1982) Hydrocephalus in adults. In: Youmans JR (ed) Neurological surgery, 2nd edn. Saunders, Philadelphia, pp 1423–1435

Olsen L, Frykberg T (1983) Complications in the treatment of hydrocephalus in children. A comparison of ventriculoatrial and ventriculoperitoneal shunts in a 20-year period Acta Paediatr Scand 72: 385–390

Piatt JH Jr, Hoffmann HJ (1989) Cor pulmonale: A lethal complication of ventriculoatrial CSF diversion. Nerv Syst Child 5: 29–31

Portnoy H (1984) CSF hydrodynamics and physiology: Summary. In: Shapiro K, Marmarou A, Portnoy H (eds) Hydrocephalus. Raven, New York, pp 135–140

Portnoy HD, Tripp L, Croissant PD (1976) Hydrodynamics of shunt valves. Childs Brain 2: 242–256

Raimondi AJ, Robinson JS, Kuwamura K (1977) Complications of ventriculoperitoneal shunting and a critical comparison of three-piece and one-piece systems. Childs Brain 3: 321–342

Schmaltz AA, Huegens R, Heil RP (1980) Thrombosis and embolism complicating ventriculoatrial shunt for hydrocephalus: echo cardiographic findings. Br Heart J 43(2): 241–243

Simon RH, Lehmann RAW, O'Connor J (1984) A comparasion of pressure-volume models in hydrocephalus. Neurosurgery 15: 649–699

Talner NS, Liu H-Y, Oberman HA, Schmidt RW (1961) Thromboembolism complicating Holter valve shunt. A clinico-pathologic study of four patients treated with this procedure for hydrocephalus. Am J Dis Child 101: 602–609

Wuest HJ, Rosenbauer KA (1984) Rasterelektonenmikroskopische Befunde an Epidural kathetern. In: Wuest HJ, Stanton-Hicks d'Arcy M, Zindler M (eds) Neue Aspecte in der Regionalanaesthesie 3. Springer, Berlin Heidelberg New York Tokyo, pp 134–140

46 — Shuntography for Functional Evaluation of Ventriculo-Peritoneal Shunt in Children

S. Yoshioka, M. Kochi, S. Nagahiro, and Y. Ushio[1]

Summary. The usefulness of shuntography in cases of shunt malfunction was evaluated. Metrizamide (1–4 ml) was injected into the flushing device 55 times in 40 children who developed malfunction of ventriculo-peritoneal shunts for hydrocephalus. A flushing device manometric test was performed at the same time. Shunt revision was performed 50 times in 38 children; shuntography findings were evaluated and classified into six types and intra-operative findings were classified into five groups. Shuntogram and intra-operative findings were then compared. Shuntography indicated the location and the cause of malfunction; operative findings could be anticipated using shuntography evaluations.

Shuntography and the manometric test proved to be simple, safe, and useful preoperative examinations in cases of shunt malfunction.

Keywords. Shuntography — Hydrocephalus — Ventriculo-peritoneal shunt — Shunt function

Introduction

Shunt surgery, now performed widely, has markedly improved the prognosis of some hydrocephalic children. Shunt dysfunction, however, remains a major problem and its prevention is most important. Early and accurate diagnosis of dysfunction is essential for management in the long term. Acute or complete shunt dysfunction is diagnosed easily, but chronic or partial dysfunction is often diagnosed with difficulty. Several methods of evaluating shunt function were studied. Valvography, introduced by Amador et al. (1969), yields much information and offers essential safety.

In the past 8 years, we performed shuntography 55 times (in 40 cases), as a preoperative examination before shunt revision, when shunt dysfunction was

[1] Department of Neurosurgery, Kumamoto University School of Medicine, Kumamoto, 860 Japan

suspected clinically. Shunt revision was performed 50 times after shuntography and shuntography findings were compared with operative findings. The diagnostic features and usefulness of shuntography are discussed.

Patients and Methods

Patients

During the 8-year period of this study, 55 shuntographies (40 cases) were performed. The patients ranged in age from 1 month to 19 years, with a mean of 5 years. The diagnoses of the 40 patients were: congenital hydrocephalus (7), meningomyelocele (7), arachnoid cyst (7), hydrocephalus after meningitis (7), intraventricular hemorrhage (4), brain tumor (4), encephalocele (2), holoprosencephaly (1), and hemihydroanencephaly (1). The valves examined in 37 cases were the Pudenz standard type; in two cases they were Foitz flushing valves and in one case, a multipurpose flushing valve.

Procedure

First, the type of flushing valve was verified via the relevant operation report. After a skin area 4 cm in diameter over the valve was shaved and prepared, the area was protected with sterile cloth. The valve was then punctured, not too deeply, with a 25-gauge wing needle. Intraventricular pressure was measured, if necessary, via connection with a vinyl tube. If cerebrospinal fluid (CSF) did not flow out of the valve, slight negative pressure was carefully applied for aspiration. After the CSF sample was obtained, the vinyl tube was filled with CSF or physiological saline solution. In cases of normal patency of the distal catheter, the fluid pressure slowly dropped to 50–150 mmH$_2$O. The closing pressure of the distal catheter was measured.

A small amount of contrast medium (metrizamide, 170 mgI/ml, 1–4 ml) was then injected into the flushing valve, under image intensification fluoroscopic control, and spot films were taken. If no blockage was noted, spot film was taken of the region where the contrast medium flowed into the peritoneal cavity from the catheter end. Clearance of contrast medium in the valve, shunt tube, and peritoneal cavity was examined by spot film 5, 10, and 15 min after injection of the contrast medium. Change in clearance of the contrast medium was examined, if necessary, with digital "pumping" of the valve or alteration of patient position.

Indications for Shuntography

We consider that shuntography is indicated if shunt dysfunction is suspected on the basis of clinical signs or CT scan findings, and that it should be performed as a preoperative examination just before shunt revision.

Results

1. At puncture of the shunt valve, CSF was obtained in 47 instances (85%), complete obstruction of the ventricular catheter was revealed in 7 instances, and partial obstruction of the ventricular catheter in 1 instance. Intraventricular CSF pressure, measured 46 times, ranged from 60 to 750 (mean 285) mmH$_2$O. In one case, meningitis was revealed by CSF examination. Reflux of the contrast medium into the ventricle was recognized nine times. In those cases the distal catheter had an abnormality; complete obstruction was seen 7 times and partial obstruction was seen twice. In such cases we stopped further injection of the contrast medium into the valve.

2. Normal shuntograms of the distal side were obtained five times. Abnormal findings in the distal shuntogram were seen 40 times and the type showing absolutely no filling (complete obstruction on the distal side) was seen 10 times. Abnormal findings on the shuntogram in the distal catheter were classified into six types:

Type a, peri-catheter contrast (very thin double contrast line along the peritoneal catheter) (Fig.1)
Type b, sheath contrast (large and irregularly shaped) (Fig. 2)
Type c, discontinuance of catheter contrast (Fig. 3)
Type d, localized perfusion of contrast medium in the peritoneal cavity (Fig. 4)
Type e, kinking of distal catheter at the cervical region (Fig. 5)
Type f, absolutely no filling in distal catheter.

Surgery (shunt revision) was performed 50 times after shuntography. Patients who did not need shunt revision were those with meningitis (one case), normal shuntogram (two cases), and symptom improvement after shuntography (two cases).

3. At shunt revision, the operative findings in the distal catheter were:

Group P, shunt malfunction in the peritoneal cavity
Group P1, shunt catheter was normal when catheter was pulled out
Group P2, tip of distal catheter contained debris when catheter was pulled out
Group Q, disconnection of distal catheter
Group R, extraction of distal catheter
Group S, kinking of distal catheter.

4. Shuntography findings were compared with the those of revision surgery (Operative findings) (Shuntography findings)

Group P1	Type a 81%
	Type f 19%
Group P2	Type a 37.5%
	Type d 37.5%
	Type f 25%
Group Q	Type b 73%
	Type c 27%

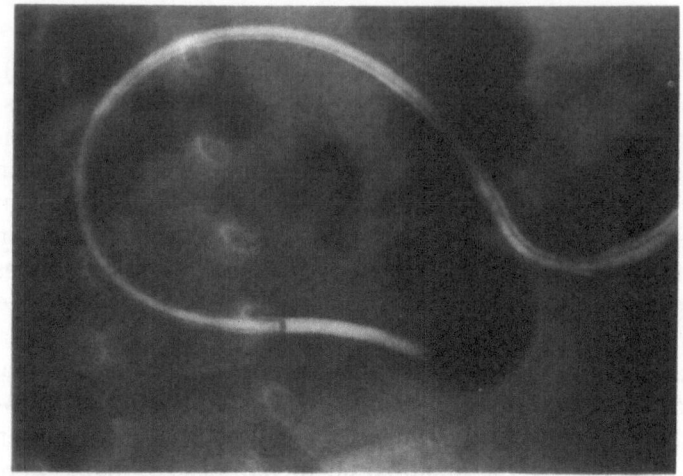

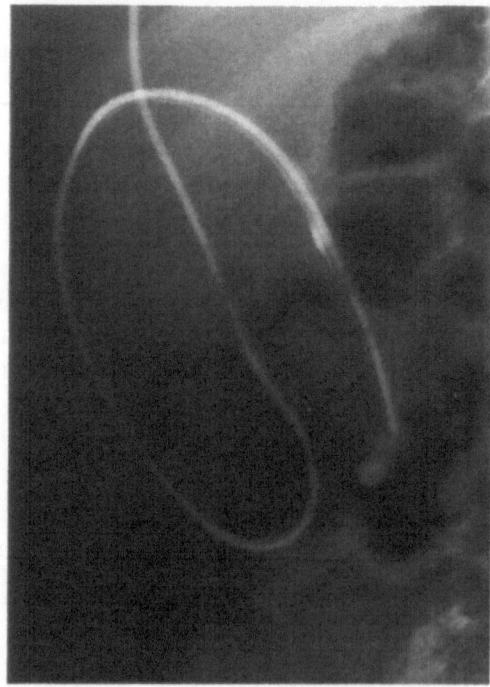

Fig. 1. a "Peri-catheter contrast" of the distal catheter when partially obstructed in the peritoneal cavity. **b** "Peri-catheter contrast" of the distal catheter. Contrast medium passes through the distal catheter, but returns through the peri-catheter space

Group R   Type f 50%
              Type b 25%
              Type c 25%
Group S   Type e 100%

(Shuntography findings) (Cause of shunt malfunction)

Type a: In all cases the cause of malfunction was found to be in the peritoneal cavity.

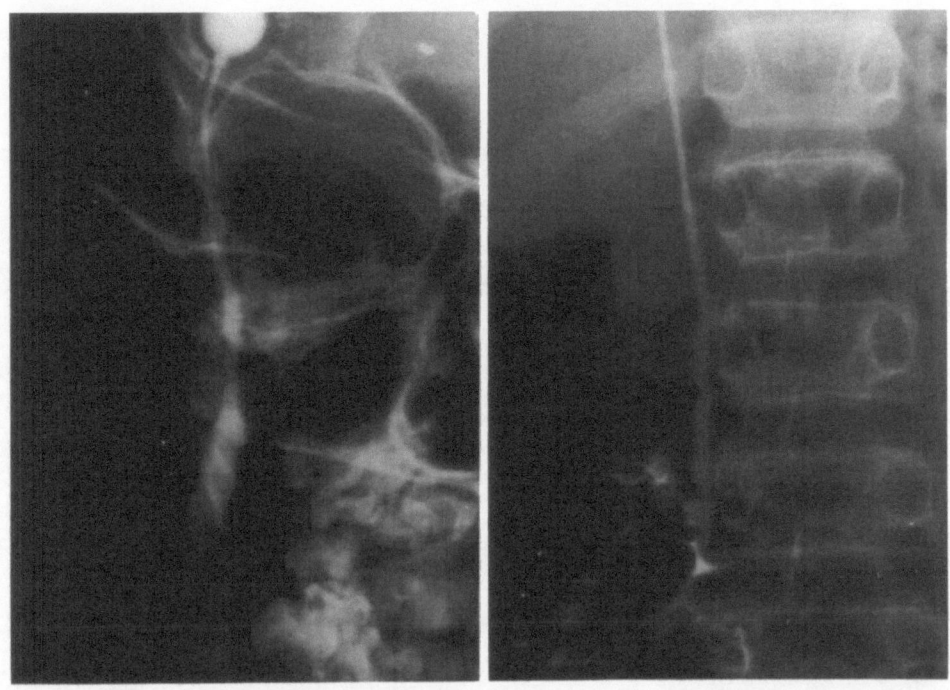

a   b

Fig. 2. a Distal catheter breakage in the subcutaneous region. Contrast medium fills the subcutaneous sheath of the catheter. **b** Distal catheter disconnection from the connector. Contrast medium fills the subcutaneous sheath and extravasates into the subcutaneous space

          Group P1 85%
          Group P2 15%
Type b: Group Q 80%
          Group R 20%
Type c: Group Q 50%
          Group R 50%
Type d: Group P2 100%
Type e: Gruop S 100%
Type f: Group P1 40%
          Group R 40%
          Group P2 20%

We were able to anticipate the operative findings using the shuntography evaluations.

5. No complications such as infection, CSF fistula, rupture of the valve chamber or allergic reactions occurred. In two cases small amounts of contrast medium were inadvertently injected into the subcutaneous region without any observed adverse effects.

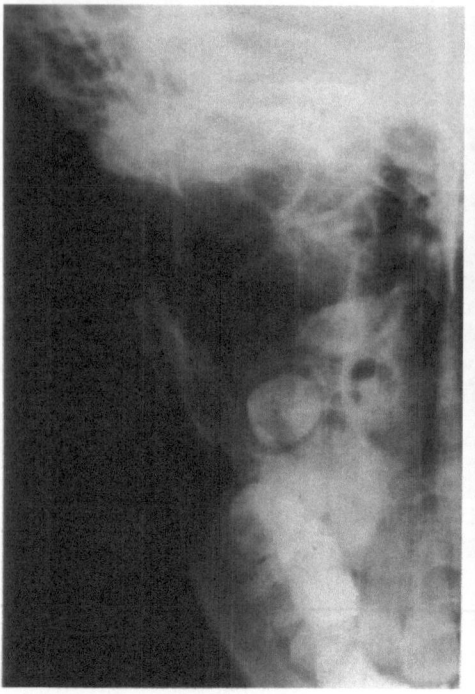

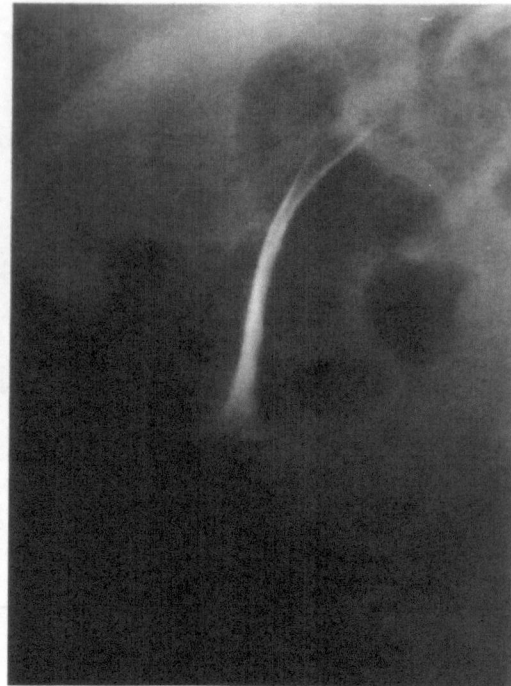

Fig. 3.

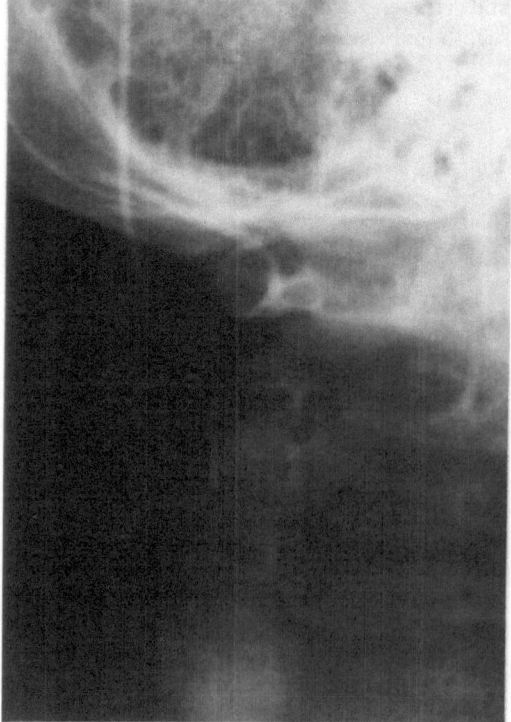

Fig. 5.

Fig. 3. Discontinuance of contrast medium in the distal catheter

Fig. 4. Localized perfusion of contrast medium into the peritoneal cavity

Fig. 5. Kinking of the distal catheter in the cervical region

The procedure took from 5 to 25 min, without general anesthesia, in all cases. We used sodiumtrichlorethyl phosphate (po), or chloral hydrate (pa) in some cases.

6. Information obtained from shuntography (and manometric test):
a. CSF findings, absence or presence of meningitis
b. Intraventricular CSF pressure
c. Presence and degree of obstruction in the proximal catheter
d. Presence and degree of obstruction in the distal catheter
e. Closing pressure of distal catheter
f. Location and cause of obstruction in the distal catheter
g. Lesion in the peritoneal cavity
h. Positional effect on shunt function

Discussion

Examination of shunt function is required when shunt malfunction is suspected clinically and the need for revision surgery must be confirmed. Shuntography and the manometric test are useful because of their simplicity and information yield (Evans 1976, Yamada 1977, Seppanen 1987). In our study, malfunction (especially partial obstruction) of the distal catheter was the most common cause of shunt malfunction and was diagnosed with difficulty via clinical signs, CT findings, and other examinations. In the case of partial obstruction, various shuntography findings were obtained according to the location and cause of malfunction. Shuntography was most useful in choosing the method of revision surgery. According to the shuntography findings, we were able to perform the least revision necessary. The formation of a fibrin-like membrane around the distal catheter in the peritoneal cavity was suspected of causing partial obstruction of this catheter. In such cases, shuntography revealed peri-catheter contrast (type a) and intraoperative findings indicated distal catheter integrity. In these cases, the distal catheter had to be introduced at a different area in the peritoneal region. In cases of distal catheter extraction or disconnection, shuntography revealed three types of problem, depending on the period between accident and shuntography: when the period was short irregular shape sheath contrast (type b) was revealed in the subcutaneous region; with longer periods shuntography revealed discontinuance (type c) or no filling (type f).

Conclusion

Shuntography and manometric testing are simple, safe, and useful in the diagnosis of shunt malfunction.

References

Amador LV, Jara O, Porras CL (1969) Valvulography, a test for patency of Holter Valve Shunts. Am J Dis Child 117: 190–193

Evans RC, Thomas MD, Williams LA (1976) Shunt blockage in hydrocephalic children, the use of the valvogram. Clin Radiol 27: 489–495

Seppanen U, Serlo W, Saukkonen AL (1987) Valvography in the assessment of hydrocephalus shunt function in children. Neuroradiology 29:53–57

Yamada H, Tajima M, Kageyama N, Nakamura S (1977) Shuntography and flushing device manometric test for functional evaluation of ventriculo-peritoneal shunts. Neurol Med Chir (Tokyo) 17: 253–260

47 — Measurement of CSF Shunt Flow with MR Phase Imaging

James M. Drake[1], Alastair J. Martin[2], and R. Mark Henkleman[3]

Summary. The cerebrospinal fluid (CSF) flow rates in 12 patients with symptoms suggestive of CSF shunt obstruction were measured with magnetic resonance (MR) phase imaging. The shunts were imaged over the skull, just distal to any reservoir, using a curved surface coil. Images perpendicular to the direction of flow were made on a 1.5 Tesla clinical unit using a flow-sensitive pulse sequence. The patients' ages ranged between 2 months and 28 years. All patients had ancillary investigations to determine the functional status of the shunt. No flow was detected in seven patients with blocked shunts. Flow rates between 3 and 40 cc/h were found in three patients with functioning shunts. Two patients, one with a blocked shunt and one with a functioning shunt, could not be imaged due to motion artefact. MR phase imaging is a promising technique in the determination of CSF shunt obstruction.

Keywords. Hydrocephalus — Cerebrospinal fluid shunts — Cerebral spinal fluid flow dynamics — Nuclear magnetic resonance

Introduction

The determination of the functional status of an implanted CSF shunt is often difficult. Despite the use of plain X-rays, computed tomography (CT), standard MR images, and palpation of the shunt reservoir, there is frequently some uncertainty as to whether the shunt is functioning. Traditionally, neurosurgeons have resorted to more invasive tests such as injection of radioisotope (Brendel et al. 1983; Chervu et al. 1984; French and Swanson 1981; Harbert et al. 1974; Hayden et al. 1980; Howman-Giles et al. 1984; Matsumae et al. 1989) or contrast material (Dewey et al. 1976; Seppanen et al. 1987) to determine shunt function. Besides the exposure to radiation, these tests present a risk of

[1] Division of Neurosurgery, Hospital For Sick Children, [2] Department of Medical Biophysics, Ontario Cancer Institute, and [3] Sunnybrook Health Science Centre, University of Toronto, Toronto, Ontario, M5G 1X8, Canada

infecting or otherwise damaging the shunt. MR avoids these risks, as well as providing an accurate measurement of shunt flow rate. In a previous report we outlined the technical aspects of CSF shunt flow measurement with MR phase imaging (Martin et al. 1989). In this report we describe our initial experience with this technique in the determination of shunt obstruction in symptomatic patients who had other confirmatory tests.

Methods

This study was approved by the Human Subjects Review Committee of the Hospital for Sick Children, Toronto, Ontario. All patients and/or their families were given a thorough explanation of the study and only those who agreed to participate underwent MR imaging. The patients were all admitted to hospital because of symptoms suggestive of shunt obstruction. Their investigations and treatment proceeded in the normal fashion except that in addition they underwent a MR flow study of their shunts. The MR flow study was performed prior to surgery. The individual analyzing the phase images, (A.M.), had no knowledge of the results of any preoperative tests or postoperative results.

The MR images were generated on a 1.5 Tesla imaging system (GE Medical Systems, Milwaukee) as previously described (Martin et al. 1989). Briefly, the patients were positioned so that the part of the shunt to be imaged (usually the peritoneal catheter just distal to any reservoir) was near the center of the magnet. The long axis of the shunt (direction of flow) was oriented along the bore of the magnet. The patient's head was immobilized with foam cushions and the curved surfaced coil placed over the shunt (Fig. 1.) Small infants and uncooperative patients were sedated. Following two localizing images, using

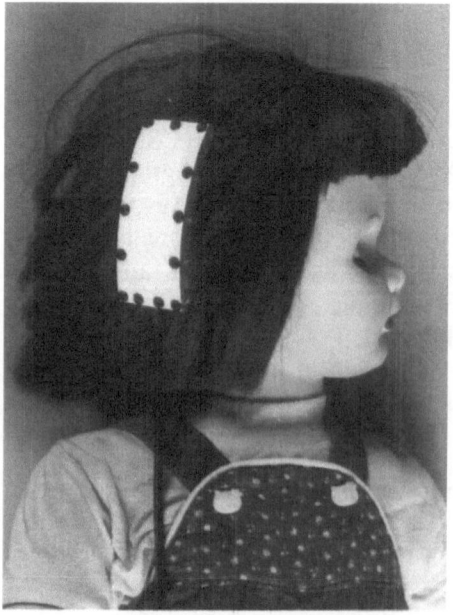

Fig. 1. Shunt flow imaging surface coil. The coil is placed with its center just distal to any shunt reservoir along the course of the shunt. This is a typical location for an occipitally placed shunt, shown here on a mannequin

standard clinical protocols, a flow-sensitive sequence was employed with the image plane perpendicular to the long axis of the shunt. This sequence had a 4 × 4 cm field of view (256 × 256 resolution), TR = 500 ms, TE = 80 ms, with additional flow encoding gradients along the slice selection direction. The flow sequence took 8 min to complete. Magnitude and phase images of the shunt were then displayed (Figs. 2, 3). Flow information was extracted from the phase image after it was processed to remove background phase inhomogeneity and random phase fluctuations due to noise in voxels with low signal intensity (Fig. 4). The peak phase advance within the shunt was then converted to an average flow rate from a calibration curve.

Results

The clinical features and the results of the investigations and treatment of the 12 patients who underwent MR phase imaging of their shunts are shown in Table 1. Their ages ranged from 2 months to 28 years. One patient had a ventriculo-pleural shunt, the rest had ventriculo-peritoneal shunts. One patient had undergone no previous shunt revisions. In the others, revisions had been

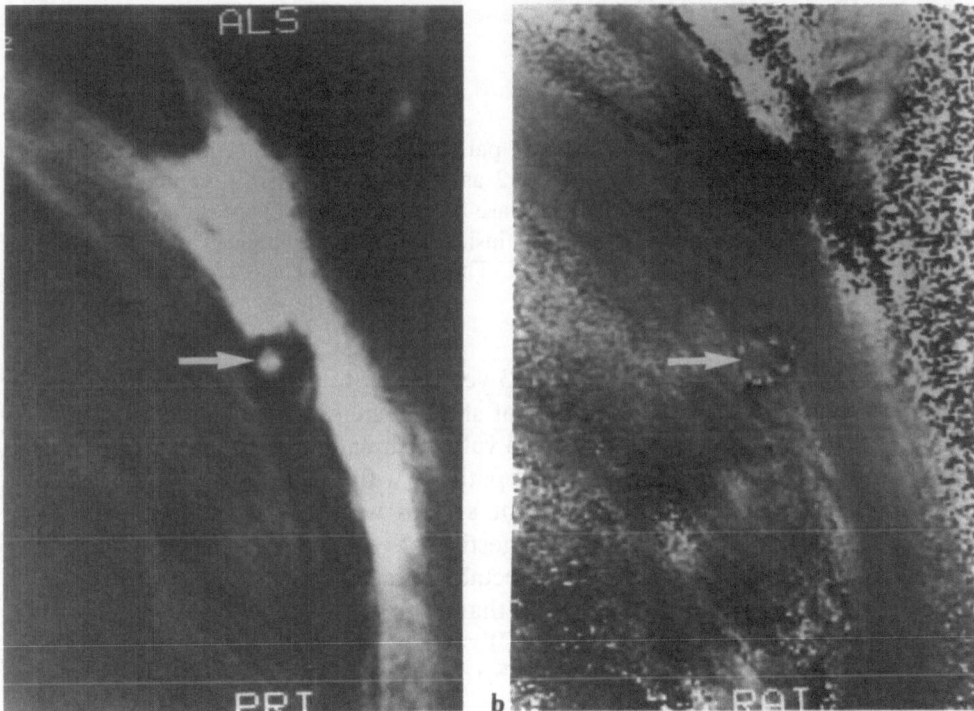

Fig. 2. a Magnitude and **b** phase images in patient no. 2 with a partially obstructed shunt. Shunt lumen (*arrows*) appears as an area of increased signal intensity on the magnitude image. On the phase image there is no obvious increase in phase across the lumen of the shunt, compared to the phase background. Post hoc analysis following correction for phase inhomogeneities revealed no evidence of flow

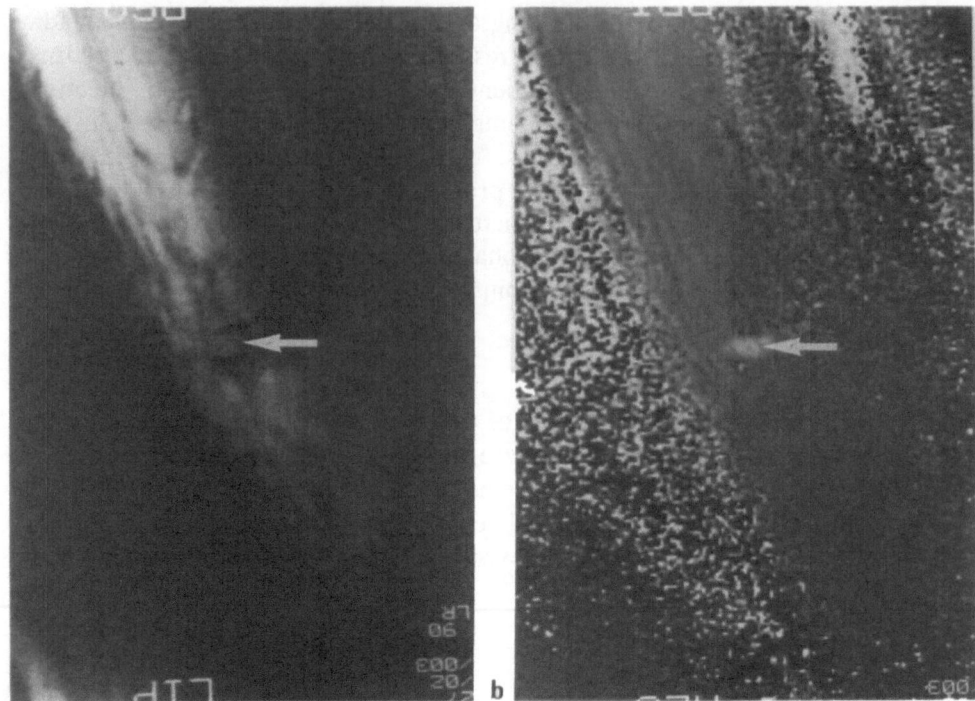

Fig. 3. a Magnitude and **b** phase images in patients no. 3 with a functional shunt. The images are of poorer quality than in Fig. 2 as the image slice is off center from the surface coil. Nevertheless, an increase in phase across the lumen of the shunt (*arrows*) is evident on the phase image. The phase inside the shunt is higher (and therefore brighter) than the surrounding background. The three dimensional phase map for the study is shown in Fig. 4

carried out anywhere from 12 days to 13 years prior to admission. The patients had been treated with a large variety of shunt systems — unishunts, multiple component systems, proximal and distal valves. In patients who had undergone shunt surgery at other institutions, and patients with many revisions, the exact details of the components of the shunt system were not always completely known. All patients had symptoms suggestive of possible shunt malfunction.

MR images of a shunt with no detectable flow are shown in Fig. 2. This patient (no. 2) remained drowsy and lethargic following a shunt revision, and the ventricles remained enlarged on CT. Very slow flow was demonstrated on an isotope flow study. A partial obstruction of the proximal ventricular catheter was found at reoperation.

MR images of a patient (no. 3) with a functioning shunt are shown in Fig. 3. The phase map produced from the phase image of the shunt is shown in Fig. 4.

The results of plain X-rays, CT scans, isotope studies, and surgery demonstrated that the shunt was non-functional in eight patients. No flow was measured on MR in seven patients and one MR study could not be performed due to motion artefact. In four patients, all investigations demonstrated a

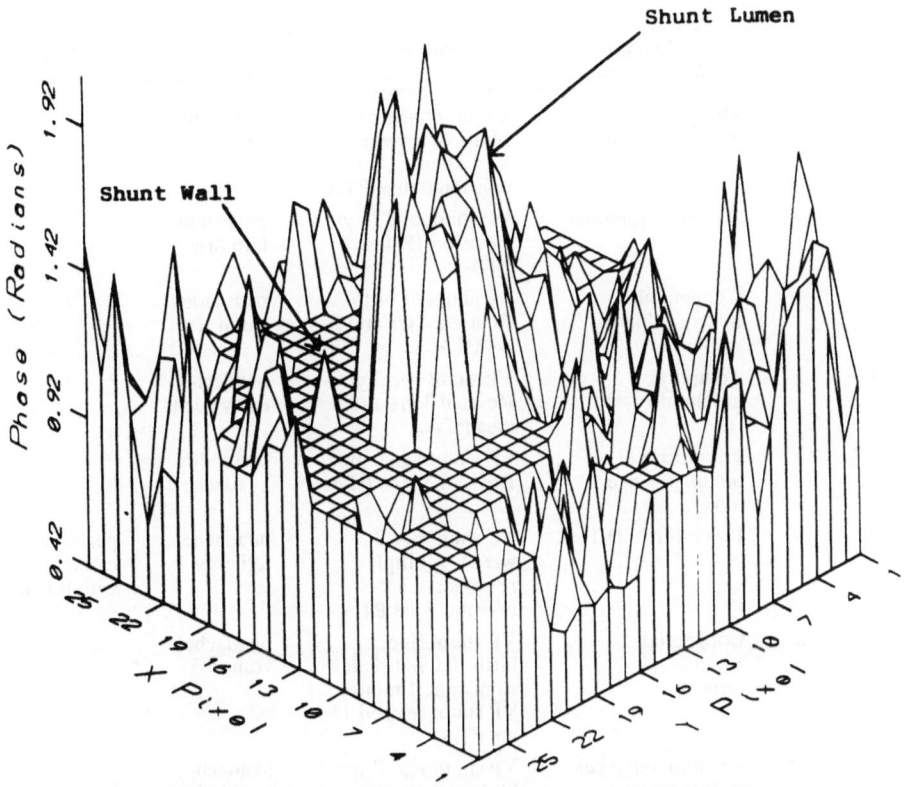

Fig. 4. Three dimensional phase map of shunt lumen, wall, and surrounding tissue of patient no. 3. Moving CSF appears as a parabolic elevation on the phase landscape; height (phase angle) is directly proportional to velocity. Average flow rate can be calculated from a calibration curve.

functioning system. Flow rates of 5, 3, and > 40 cc/h were measured on MR in three patients and one MR study could not be performed due to motion and metal artefact.

In one patient (no. 9) the MR studies initially seemed at variance with the other investigations. This patient had persistent headache and vomiting two weeks following a shunt revision. An isotope flow study showed rapid flow along the shunt. There was some extravasation of isotope around the injected reservoir, thought to be due to leakage around the injecting needle or perhaps a disconnected system. The MR flow study was performed 7 days later and showed no flow. Because of persistent symptoms, the isotope flow study was repeated three days following the MR study and no flow was demonstrated. At operation a disconnected peritoneal catheter was found.

Discussion

The difficulty in determining whether an implanted CSF shunt is functioning properly is an all too familiar problem to most neurosurgeons. In many cases

Table 1.

Pat	Age	Sex	Etiology hydrocephalus	Clinical history	Clinical presentation	Plain X-rays
1.	16	M	Occipital encephalocele	VP shunt age 3 mos. Multiple revisions to VPL shunt. Last revision 6 mos PTA.	headache, drowsy	
2.	28	M	Pineal germinoma	VP shunt age 25 yrs. Revision 12 days PTA.	persistent leth-argy	
3.	11	F	Congenital hydrocephalus	VP shunt at birth. Revised 7 yrs and 2 yrs PTA.	pain along shunt tract	
4.	17	F	Temporal arachnoid cyst	VP shunt age 3 yrs. Revised 3 yrs and 6 mos PTA.	headache, dizzy spells	
5.	2	M	Pnumococcal meningitis age 9 mos	VP shunt age 9 mos. Revised 3 mos PTA.	irritability, headache	
6.	8	M	Prematurity IVH	VP shunt age 2 weeks. Multiple revisions. Last revision 7 yrs PTA.	headache, lethargy	peritoneal cathter withdrawn
7.	16	F	Congenital aqueductal stenosis	VP shunt since birth. III ventriculo-stomy age 1 month. VP shunt revised 13 yrs PTA.	headache, vomiting	
8.	5	M	Myelomeningocele hydrocephalus	VP shunt age 2 mos. Multiple revisions. Last revision 10 mos PTA.	headache, papilledema	
9.	6	F	Congenital hydrocephalus	VP shunt since birth. Multiple revisions, last 2 wks PTA.	headache, vomiting irritability	
10.	6	F	Prematurity IVH	VP shunt age 1 mo.	headache, vomiting	peritoneal cathter withdrawn
11.	11	F	Myelomeningocele hydrocephalus	VP shunt since birth. Slit ventricle syndrome age 4. Multiple revisions.	chronic papill-edema	intact system
12.	2 mo	F	Prematurity IVH	VP shunt age 1 mo. Revision for infection 1 mo PTA	increasing head size, fever	
13.	16	F	Congenital hydrocephalus	VP shunt age 1 yr.	headache, drowsy	

CT	Isotope study	MRI flow study	Surgical findings	Surgical treatment
increased ventricular size		motion artefact	obstructed ventricular catheter	revision ventricular catheter
persistent enlarged ventricles	very slow flow ? partial obstruction	no flow	partial obstruction ventricular catheter	revision ventricular catheter
ventricules unchanged	patent system	5 cc/hr		
ventricles unchanged	patent system	3 cc/hr		
enlarge ventricles no interval change	flow to peritoneum when sitting	>40 cc/hr		
increased ventricular size		no flow	peritoneal catherter extraperitoneal	revision peritoneal catheter
increased ventricular size		no flow	calcified reservoir fracture distal to reservoir	revision peritoneal catheter
increased ventricular size		no flow	obstructed ventricular catheter	revision ventricular catheter
minimal increase ventricle size	1 wk PT MRI patent ? disconnect 3 days after MRI-blocked	no flow	disconnected distal catheter	reconnection peritoneal catheter
increased ventricular size		no flow	ventricular and peritoneal catheter obstruction	shunt removed, new shunt
slit ventricles	patent system	motion metal artefact	patent shunt system	valve changed to Cordis Orbis-Sigma
increased ventricular size, porencephaly		no flow	blocked and infected	interval EVD, shunt replacement
increased ventricular size, slight		no flow		

(and there are several examples in Table 1) it is quite obvious that the shunt is blocked — the ventricles have enlarged from a previous study, or plain X-rays have demonstrated that the shunt has pulled out of the peritoneum or has fractured. However, in many cases it is not initially obvious whether or not the shunt is functioning — the ventricles are large and there is no recent CT when the shunt is functioning, the ventricles are small but the patient is symptomatic, the patient has slit ventricle syndrome, etc. In this setting, neurosurgeons are naturally reluctant to explore the shunt, with all its attendant discomfort and risk, without more convincing evidence that the shunt is indeed blocked.

For this reason a number of different techniques have been developed to measure CSF shunt flow. The most widely used have been the injection of either radioisotope (Brendel et al, 1983; Chervu et al. 1984; French et al. 1981; Harbert et al. 1974; Hayden et al. 1980; Howman-Giles et al. 1984; Matsumae et al. 1989) or contrast material (Dewey et al. 1976; Seppanen et al. 1987) into the shunt reservoir. The progress of the injected material is then followed with serial images. The effects of postural changes or pumping the reservoir can also be ascertained. Reflux into the ventricle, or collection within an abdominal pseudocyst, can assist with determining which end is blocked and the possible etiology. Additional tests, such as CSF pressure, CSF culture, and resistance to distal run off, can also be performed when the reservoir is punctured. A measurement of CSF flow rate can be obtained by the injection of radioisotope if the external detector is calibrated for that particular valve design (Brendel et al. 1983; Chervu et al. 1984; Harbert et al. 1974; Matsumae et al. 1989).

The disadvantages of these techniques are that they are invasive, there is a small risk of infection, and one can damage either the reservoir or the contained valve.

Other ingenious methods for measuring shunt flow have also been developed. Hara implanted an electrolysis unit as part of the shunt and measured the velocity of the generated bubble in the shunt tubing with either Doppler or impedance monitoring (Hara et al. 1983; Numoto et al. 1984). This is a very complex shunt apparatus and the bubble itself may have effects on shunt flow. Chiba cooled the skin over the shunt tubing with ice and detected the downstream cooled CSF with a thermistor (Chiba and Yuda 1980). While an index of the presence of shunt flow, efforts to quantify the flow may be affected by such variables as skin thickness. Flitter examined the characteristics of the Doppler flow in shunts when pumping the reservoir and found a good correlation with the presence or absence of shunt obstruction (Flitter et al. 1975), but made no attempt to measure the flow rate.

MR has the advantage that it is noninvasive and can produce accurate flow measurements. That MR is sensitive to the flow of CSF is evident from the appearance of a signal void in the cerebral aqueduct or 4th ventricle on MR images (Bradley et al. 1986; Citrin et al. 1986). Imaging the flow in a shunt, however, poses several distinct problems: achieving a high enough resolution image to visualize the lumen of the shunt while maintaining acceptable signal to noise, obtaining an image perpendicular to the shunt lumen, and being able to detect flows on the order of 5 mm/s. These problems were addressed by the use of a curved surface coil placed over the shunt, oblique 4 × 4 cm field of view images perpendicular to the shunt, and a phase map produced by a pulse sequence with additional flow encoding gradients along the direction of flow (Martin et al. 1989). The phase angle accumulated by spins moving in the direction of flow is linearly related to their velocity (Bryant et al. 1984; Constantinesco et al. 1984). The correlation of the peak phase advance in the lumen of the shunt to the flow rate is very good for flow rates as low as 2 cc/h. For flow rates less than 2 cc/h, the phase advance becomes difficult to detect from background noise. However, by increasing the strength of the flow encoding gradients, the sensitivity to lower flow rates can be increased.

This is the first report of a comparison of MR measurement of CSF shunt flow rates to standard techniques in the detection of shunt obstruction. A flow void in a functioning shunt (Savader et al. 1988) and confirmation of the utility of MR in measuring shunt flow in phantoms (Frank et al. 1989) has also been reported. The correlation in this small group of patients was very good. MR detected flow in all patients who were documented to have a functioning shunt, and no flow in all patients who were documented as having a non-functional shunt.

However, this group also illustrates the problems in determining what is the gold standard test to which MR should be compared. Patient no. 2 had a partially obstructed shunt which had some evidence of flow on isotope studies. It is possible that the flow rate was below the sensitivity of the MR technique, although his shunt was clinically non-functional. Patient no. 9 had a disconnected shunt system with evidence of flow on isotope study 1 week prior to the MR study (which showed no flow), but no flow on isotope study 3 days after the MR study. Again, this shunt was clinically non-functional.

All the confirmatory tests in this study were separated in time from the MR study. Shunt flow rate is known to vary from minute to minute according to patient activity, posture, or even perhaps circadian rhythm (Hara et al. 1983; Harbert et al. 1974; Matsumae et al. 1979). A confirmatory measurement of MR flow would have to be carried out concurrently. It is difficult, given the restrictions of the MR environment, to imagine how this could be carried out with either radioisotope, shunt cooling, or an implanted electrolysis unit. A comparison of MR to the standard clinical tests appears to be the most reasonable approach.

MR imaging of CSF shunt flow has the distinct advantage of producing accurate measurements of shunt flow non-invasively. It requires an MR compatible shunt, a cooperative or sedated patient, a specialized pulse sequence, surface coil, and off line data analysis. While information on the site or etiology of the obstruction, which may be provided by more invasive tests, is not available, the initial comparison between this technique and standard tests is very good.

Acknowledgment. This work was supported by the Appugliesi Fund, University Research Incentive Fund (Ontario) and GE Medical Systems Canada. A.J.M. was supported by a Natural Sciences and Engineering Research Council (Canada) studentship. Acknowledgment is given to Lily Capin for technical assistance.

References

Bradley WG, Kortman KE, Burgoyne B (1986) Flowing cerebrospinal fluid in normal and hydrocephalic states: Appearance on MR images. Radiology 159: 611–616

Brendel AJ, Wynchank S, Caster JP, Barat JL, Leccia F, Ducassou D (1983) Cerebrospinal shunt flow in adults: Radionuclide quantitation with emphasis on patient position. Radiology 149: 815–818

Bryant DJ, Payne JA, Firmin DN, Longmore DB (1984) Measurement of flow with NMR imaging using a gradient pulse and phase difference technique. J Comput Assist Tomogr 8: 588–593

Chervu S, Chervu LR, Vallabhajosyula B, Milstein DM, Shapiro KM, Shulman K, Blaufox MD (1984) Quantitative evaluation of cerebrospinal fluid shunt flow. J Nucl Med 25: 91–95

Chiba Y, Yuda K (1980) Thermosensitive determination of CSF shunt patency with a pair of small disc thermistors. J Neurosurg 52: 700–704

Citrin CM, Sherman JL, Gangarosa RE, Scanlon D (1986) Physiology of the CSF flow-void sign: Modification by caridac gating. AJNR 7: 1021–1024

Constantinesco A, Mallet JJ, Bonmartin A, Lallot C, Briguet A (1984) Spatial or flow velocity phase encoding gradients in NMR imaging. Magn Reson Imaging 2: 335–340

Dewey RC, Kosnik EJ, Sayers MP (1976) A simple test of shunt function: The shuntogram. J Neurosurg 44: 121–126

Flitter MA, Bucheit WA, Murtagh F, Lapayowker MS (1975) Ultrasound determination of cerebrospinal fluid shunt patency. J Neurosurg 42: 728–730

Frank EH, Buonocore M, Hein LJ (1989) Use of magnetic resonance imaging to evaluate cerebrospinal fluid shunt function in a model system (abstract). Nerv Syst Child 5: 255

French BN, Swanson M (1981) Radionuclide-imaging shuntography for the evaluation of shunt patency. Surg Neurol 16: 173–182

Hara M, Kadowaki C, Konishi Y, Ogashiwa M, Numoto M, Takeuchi K (1983) A new method for measuring cerebrospinal fluid flow in shunts. J Neurosurg 58: 557–561

Harbert J, Haddad D, McCullough D (1974) Quantitation of cerebrospinal fluid shunt flow. Radiology 112: 379–387

Hayden PW, Rudd TG, Shurtleff DB (1980) Combined pressureradionuclide evaluation of suspected cerebrospinal fluid shunt malfunction: A seven-year clinical experience. Pediatrics 66: 679–684

Howman-Giles R, McLaughlin A, Johnston I, Whittle I (1984) A radionuclide method of evaluating shunt function and CSF circulation in hydrocephalus, technical note. J Neurosurg 61: 604–605

Martin AJ, Drake JM, Lemaire C, Henkelman RM (1989) MR measurement of CSF shunt flow. Radiology 173: 243–247

Matsumae M, Sato O, Itoh K, Fukuda T, Suzuki Y (1989) Quantification of cerebrospinal fluid shunt flow rates. Nerv Syst Child 5: 356–360

Numoto M, Hara M, Tatsuo S, Kadowaki C, Takeuchi K (1984) A noninvasive CSF flowmeter. J Med Eng Technol 8: 218–220

Savader SJ, Savader BL, Murtagh FR, Clark LP, Silbiger ML (1988) MR evaluation of flow in a ventricular shunt phantom with in vivo correlation. J Comput Asist Tomogr 12: 765–769

Seppanen U, Serlo W, Saukkonen AL (1987) Valvography in the assessment of hydrocephalus shunt function in children. Neuroradiology 29: 53–57

48 — A Trial for the Evaluation of CSF Shunt Function Using MR Imaging

Masatake Hamasaki[1], Takayuki Shirakuni, Norihiko Tamaki, and Satoshi Matsumoto[2]

Summary. Dysfunction of the ventriculo-peritoneal shunt tube is a common phenomenon. Various diagnostic methods for evaluating shunt flow rate have been devised, but a satisfactory one has not yet been established.

We have applied the "time of flight" effect, which is a characteristic of flow in magnetic resonance imaging (MRI), to evaluate shunt flow. Both "flow related enhancement" and "high velocity signal loss" are "time of flight" effects. In standard multi-slice, spin echo images, when fluid flow was perpendicular to the image plane, in the first slice the signal intensity of the fluid was affected by "flow related enhancement" and "high velocity signal loss", but in other slices the signal intensity of the fluid was affected by "high velocity signal loss" only. The flow rate was measured on the basis of the ratio of the signal intensity of the first slice to that of the other slices.

In the fundamental and clinical studies, we used a 1.5 Tesla superconducting whole body MR system. A simple flow phantom consisting of a Pudenz peritoneal tube was used to determine the signal intensity ratio at different flow rates. In clinical cases, it was possible to determine flow rates using the signal intensity ratio obtained from the phantom studies.

Keywords. Hydrocephalus — Ventriculo-peritoneal shunt — Shunt dysfunction — Shunt flow — Magnetic resonance imaging

Introduction

Hydrocephalus is a common disease in neurosurgery and the ventriculo-peritoneal shunt is an established treatment for it. However, shunt tube dysfunction is common. Various diagnostic methods have been devised for evaluating the shunt flow rate, but a satisfactory one which is accurate, non-invasive, and practical has not yet been established. We have applied the "time

[1] Department of Neurosurgery, Shin-Suma Hospital, Kobe, 654 Japan
[2] Department of Neurosurgery, Kobe University School of Medicine, Kobe, 650 Japan

tube1 tube2

tube3 tube4

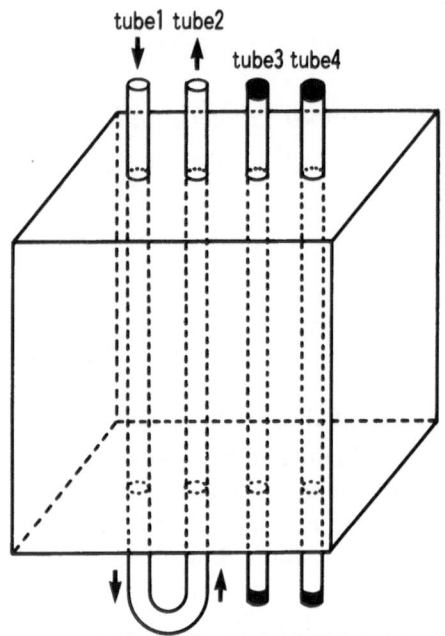

Fig. 1. The flow phantom consisted of four Pudenz peritoneal tubes: *tube 1*, flow of physiological saline was in the same direction as slice order in MR imaging; *tube 2*, flow direction opposite to that in *tube 1*; *tube 3*, stationary physiological saline; *tube 4*, stationary air

of flight" effect which is a characteristic of the flow in MRI (Bradley and Waluch 1985; Moran et al. 1985; Tamaki et al. 1989), to evaluate shunt flow. The purpose of this paper is to report the results of shunt flow investigations, conducted by phantom experiments, and to describe their clinical application.

Materials and Methods

A 1.5 Tesla superconducting whole body imager (VISTA MR, Picker International Inc.) and a Pudenz peritoneal tube of 1.3 mm inner diameter were used in the fundamental and clinical studies. A multi-echo, multi-slice spin echo protocol (repetition time, 2000 ms; echo time, 50,100, and 150 ms; matrix, 256 × 256; two excitations; field of view, 15 cm, 6 slices) was selected and radio frequency (RF) excitation was performed in slice order with no gap placed between slices. In other words, one flow block was divided into six contiguous sub-divisions. In this method, the effects of "flow related enhancement" and "high velocity signal loss", called "time of flight" effects, appeared clearly in each slice.

In phantom experiments, a simple flow phantom (Fig. 1) consisting of four peritonal tubes was used to measure the signal intensity of fluid in the image (Fig. 2). In "tube 1", the flow direction is the same as the slice order and in "tube 2" the flow direction is opposite to the slice order. "Tube 3" contains stationary saline and "tube 4" contains stationary air.

In the clinical analysis, using the same MRI pulse sequence as the phantom study, the signal intensities of CSF in the shunt tubes of hydrocephalic patients

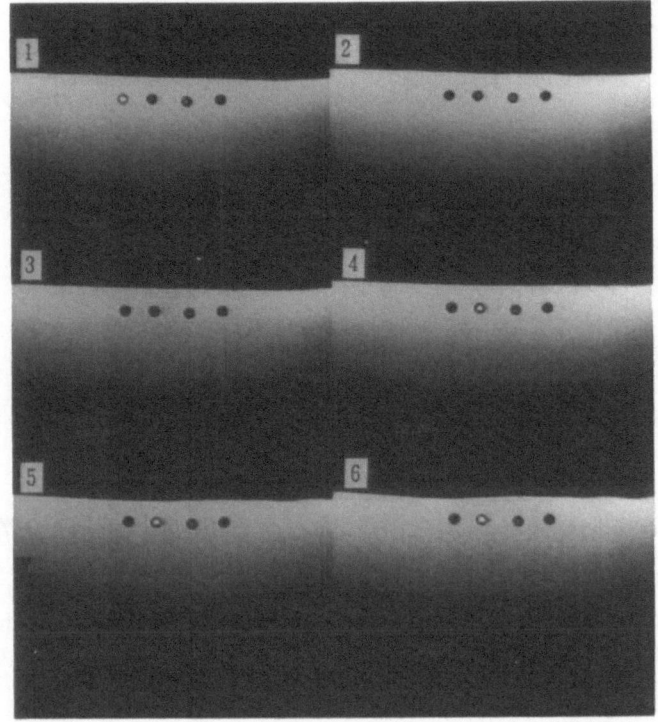

Fig. 2. MR image of flow phantom. Multi slice (6 slices) spin echo image. TR: 2000, TE: 100, flow rate: 20 ml/h

were measured. The shunt flow rates were estimated using the flow rate curve obtained from the phantom study.

Results

Phantom Experiment

For a constant flow rate of 20 ml/h, the signal intensities of each tube corresponding to each slice were noted (Fig. 3). In "tube 1," "flow related enhancement" was recognized as high signal intensity in the first slice only. So, in considering "tube 1," the correlation between signal intensity and flow rate was examined in the first slice (Fig. 4). As the flow rate increased, signal intensity first increased but then decreased. This showed that the effects of both "flow related enhancement" and "high velocity signal loss" were apparent in the first slice in "tube 1." The correlation between the average signal intensities and flow rates from the second through to the sixth slice was examined (Fig. 5). The signal intensity was affected by "high velocity signal loss" only, and as flow rate increased, the signal intensity decreased.

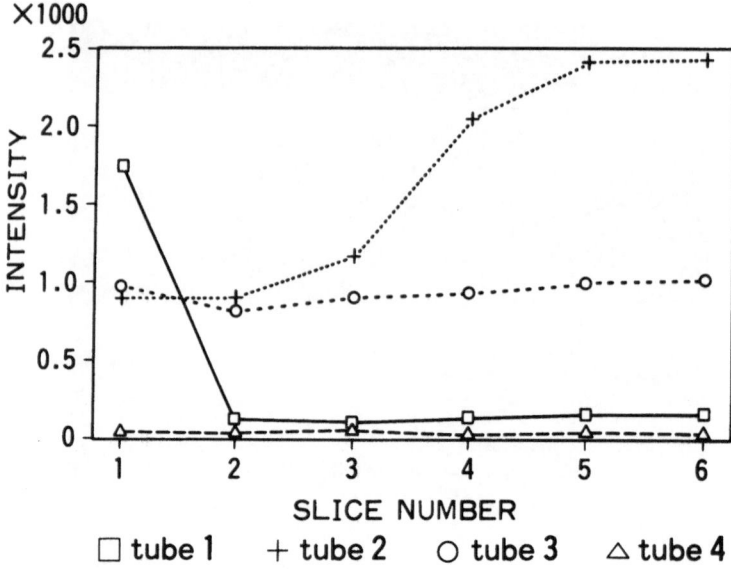

Fig. 3. Change of signal intensity in each image plane. The signal intensity of "tube 1" is higher in the first slice than in other slices, affected by "flow related enhancement". Intensity, signal intensity of saline in the shunt tube; slice number, number of each slice

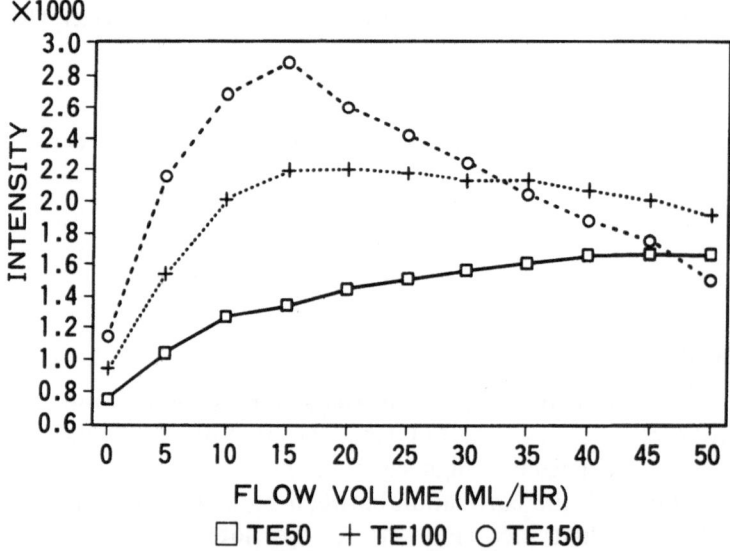

Fig. 4. Change of signal intensity in "tube 1" in the first slice at each flow rate. The signal intensity first increased and then decreased as the flow rate increased, affected by both "flow related enhancement" and "high velocity signal loss." Intensity, signal intensity of saline in the shunt tube; flow volume, flow rate of saline in the shunt tube

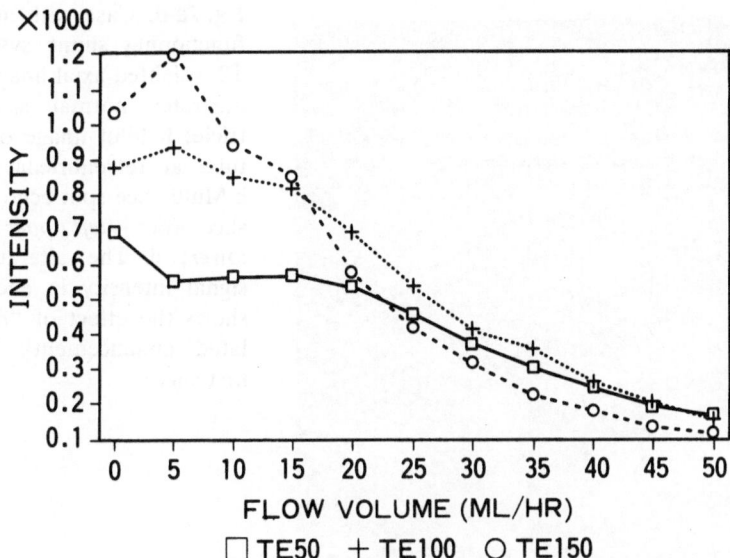

Fig. 5. Change of the average of signal intensities from second slice through to sixth slice in "tube 1" at each flow rate. The average signal intensity decreased as the flow rate increased, affected by "high velocity signal loss" only. Intensity, average of signal intensities from second slice to sixth slice; flow volume, flow rate of saline in the shunt tube

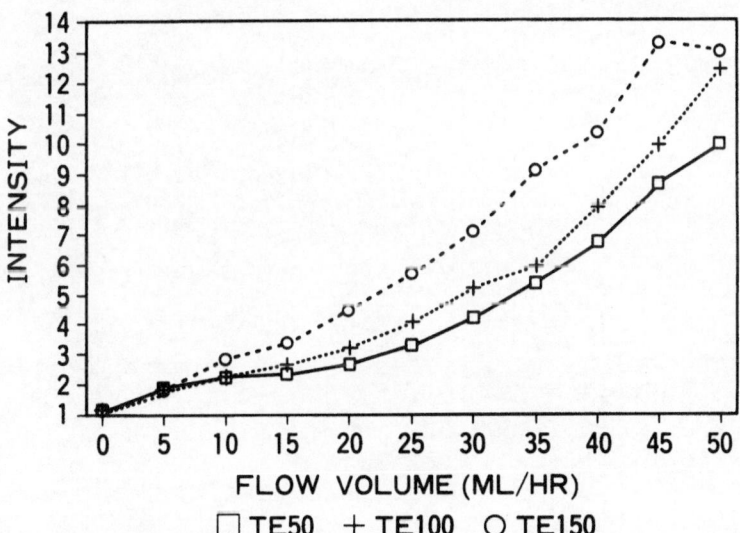

Fig. 6. Signal intensity ratio — flow rate curve. Intensity, ratio of the signal intensity of the first slice to the average of signal intensities from the second through to the sixth slices; flow volume, flow rate of saline in the shunt tube

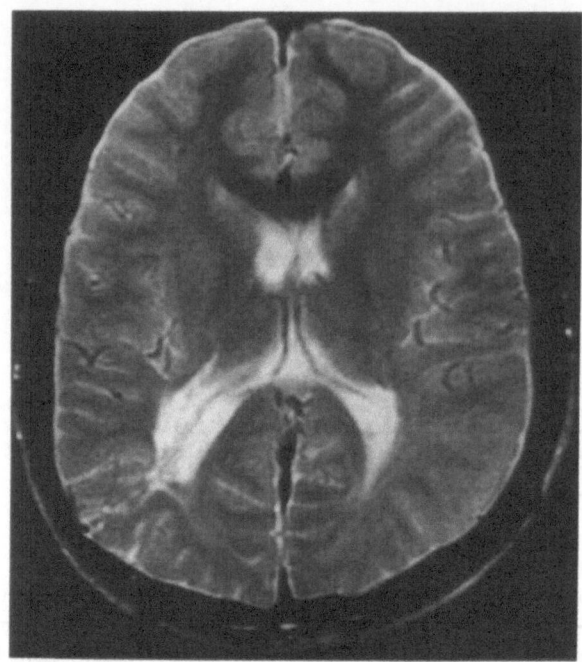

a

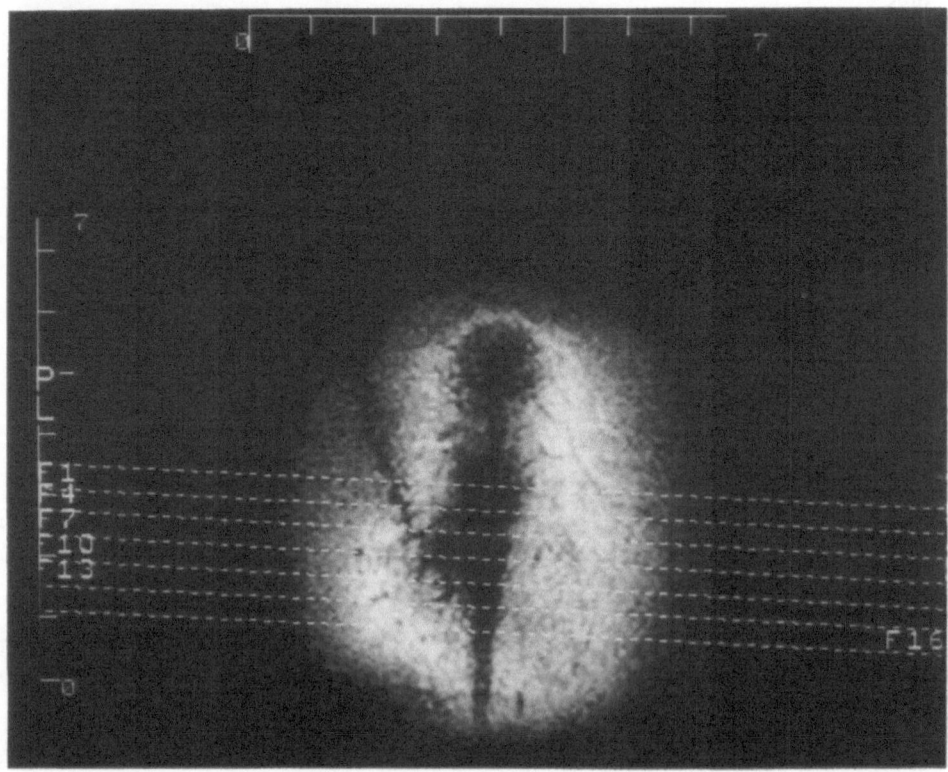

b

Fig. 7a-d. Case with normally functioning shunt system. **a** T2 weighted axial image demonstrates normal size ventricle; **b** Pilot image of shunt tube at retroauricilar space; **c** Multi slice spin echo image; slice order is *left upper to right lower*; **d** The alteration of signal intensity in each slice shows the effect of "flow related enhancement" in the first slice

-10.0mm
F5 -6.0mm
F8 -2.0mm
2.0mm
F14 6.0mm
F17 10.0mm

c

×1000
INTENSITY
SLICE NUMBER
□ TE50 + TE100 ○ TE150

d

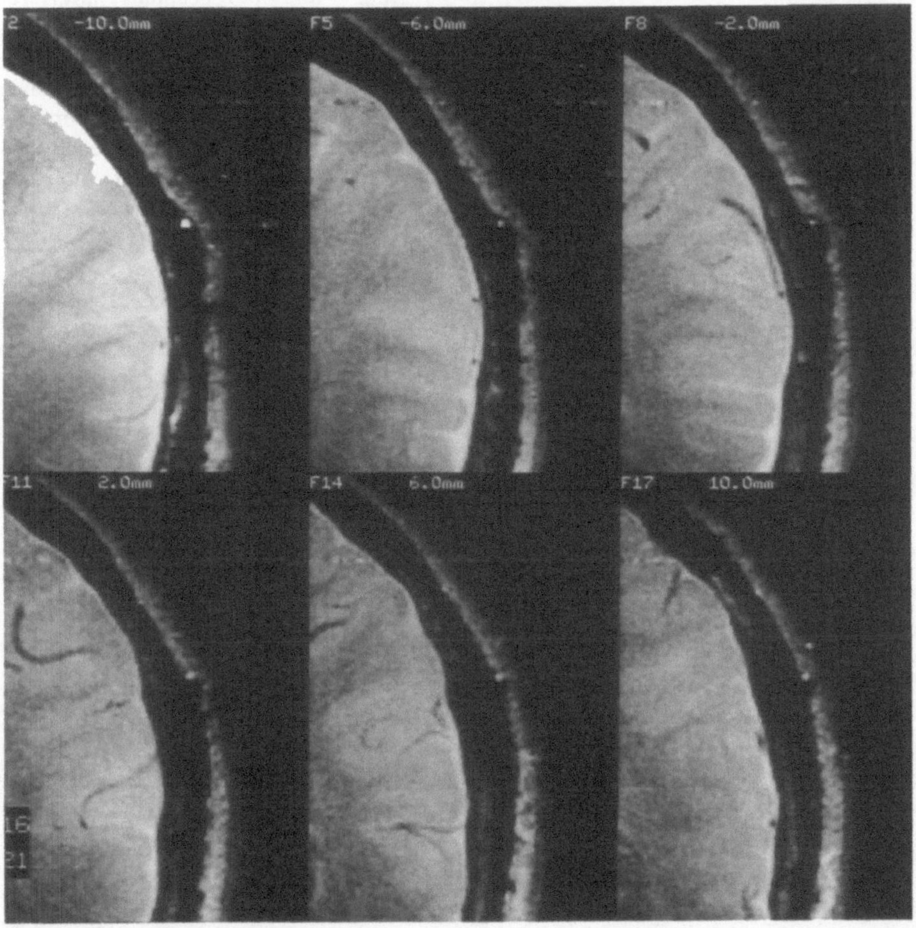

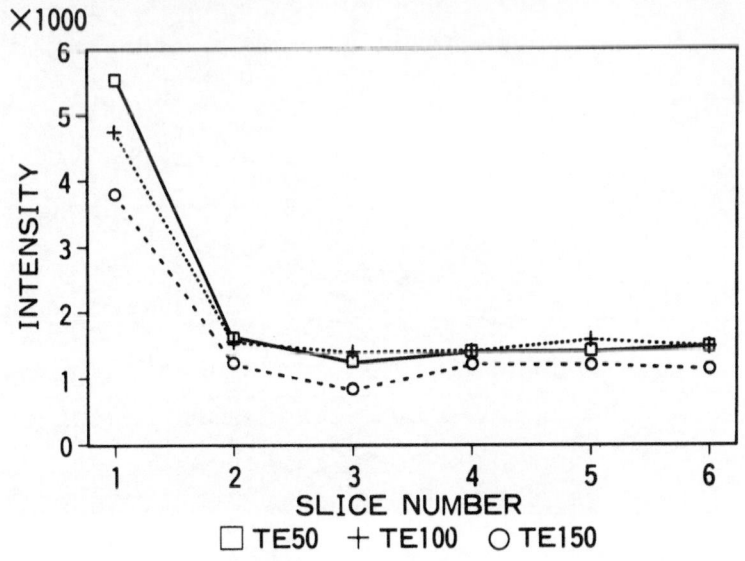

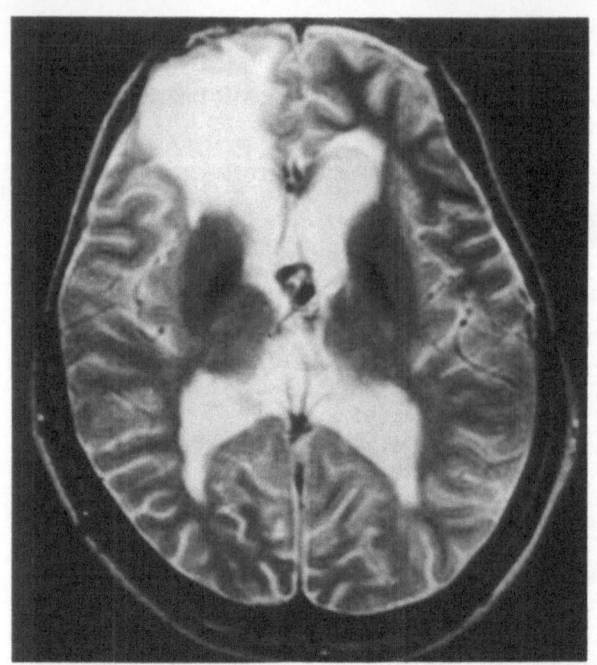

Fig. 8a-d. Case with malfunctioning shunt system. **a** T2 weighted axial image demonstrates mild ventriculomegaly and porencephaly after removal of brain tumor; **b** Pilot image of shunt tube at retroauricular space; **c** Multi slice spin echo image; **d** Alteration of signal intensity in each slice shows no effect of "flow related enhancement"

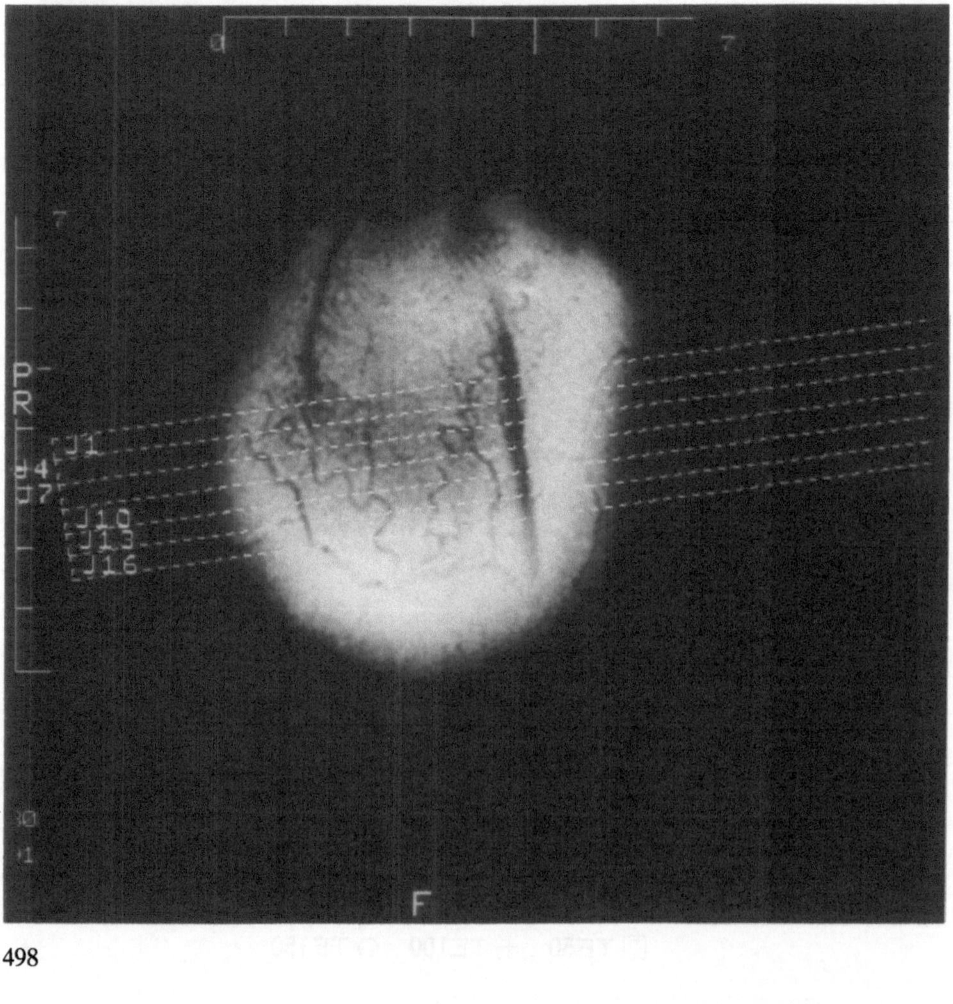

J2 -10.0mm
J5 -6.0mm
J8 -2.0mm
J11 2.0mm
J14 6.0mm
J17 10.0mm

c

INTENSITY
900
800
700
600
500
400
300
200
100
1
2
3
4
5
6
SLICE NUMBER
□ TE50 + TE100 ○ TE150

d

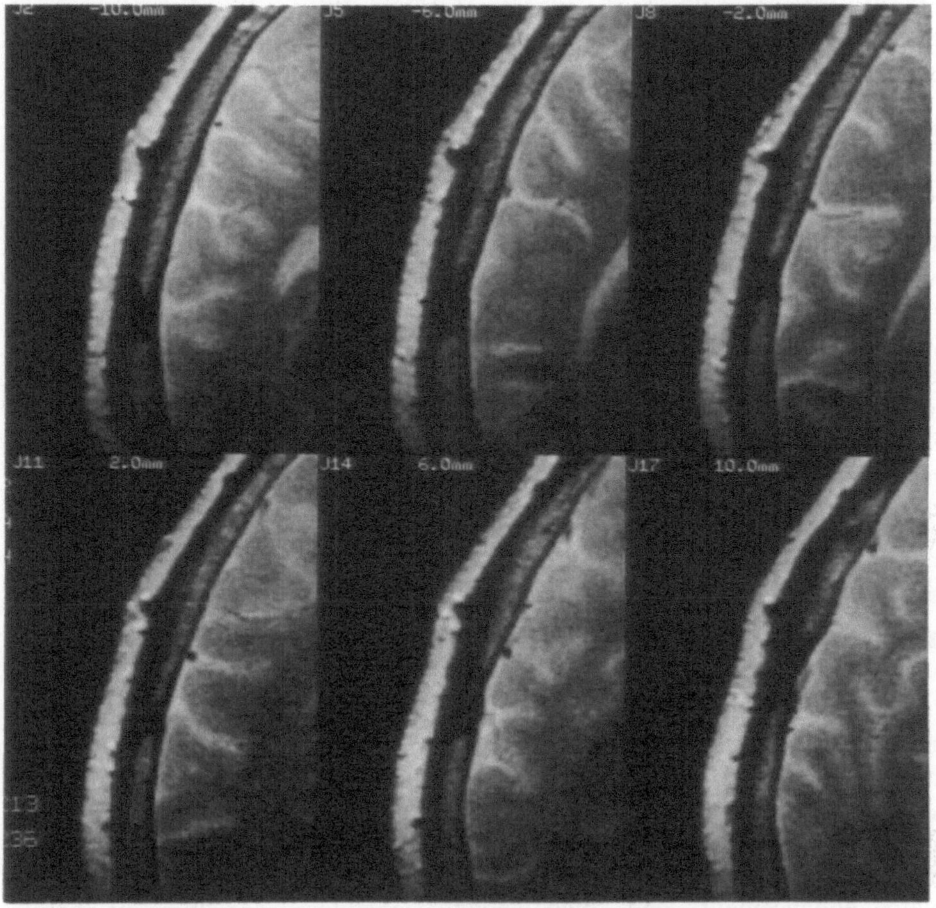

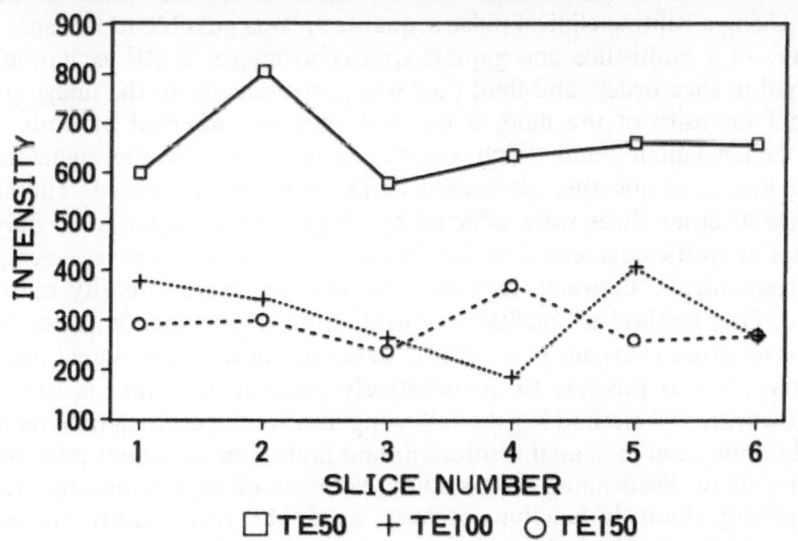

As signal intensities in MRI are relative values, the ratio of the signal intensity of the first slice to the average of the signal intensities from the second through to the sixth slices (signal intensity ratio) was obtained. Flow rates were estimated using the flow rate — signal intensity ratio curve (Fig. 6).

Clinical Analysis

The first patient was diagnosed clinically as having normal pressure hydrocephalus and, on the basis of neurologic status, shunt function was evaluated as normal (Fig. 7a). The MR image of the shunt tube was obtained with a surface coil of 10 cm inner diameter at the retroauricular space (Fig. 7b); the shunt tube was observed beneath the scalp (Fig. 7c). The change of signal intensity in each image plane showed "flow related enhancement" as high signal intensity in the first slice (Fig. 7d). The signal intensity ratio was 3.2 and the flow rate was calculated to be 20 ml/h. In the next patient, in whom clinical diagnosis was non-communicating hydrocephalus with a brainstem tumor, the flow rate was calculated to be 0 ml/h (Fig. 8a-d). The mean shunt flow rate in six hydrocephalic patients with normally functioning shunts was 15 ml/h.

Discussion

Various diagnostic methods have been devised for evaluating shunt flow rate; one such method used a radio isotope clearance curve (Matsumae et al. 1987) and another method used two thermisters (Fujita et al. 1982). However, a satisfactory method which is accurate, non-invasive, and simple to handle has not yet been established. We have applied the "time of flight" effects, which are characteristic of the flow in MRI, to evaluate shunt flow rate. Both "flow related enhancement" and "high velocity signal loss" are "time of flight" effects. Using a routine clinical pulse sequence, it was possible to measure CSF flow rate. In a multi-slice and gapless spin echo image, if RF excitation was performed in slice order, and fluid flow was perpendicular to the image plane, the signal intensity of the fluid in the first slice was affected by both "flow related enhancement" and "high velocity signal loss," so the signal intensity first increased and then decreased as the flow rate increased. The signal intensities of other slices were affected by "high velocity signal loss" only, so the signal intensities decreased as the flow rate increased. A curve which gives the correspondence between the flow rate and the signal intensity ratio was obtained. One method of qualitatively evaluating shunt function, using MRI, has been reported (Savader et al. 1988). Using our flow rate — signal intensity ratio curve, it was possible to quantitatively evaluate flow rate in the shunt tube. However, this method has the following disadvantages: long time required for study, limitation in spatial resolution, and limitation in patient positioning.

Despite these disadvantages, this study has resulted in a promising method for diagnosing shunt dysfunction, because, no doubt, these disadvantages will be resolved by technological developments in the near future.

References

Bradley WG, Waluch V (1985) Blood flow: Magnetic resonance image. Radiology 154: 443–450

Fujita K, Tamaki N, Matsumoto S (1982) Thermosensitive measurement of shunt flow using two thermisters. Surg Neurol 10: 1085–1090

Matsumae M, Murakami T, Ueda M (1987) Dynamics change of cerebrospinal fluid in patient daily life. Nerv Syst Child 3: 30–34

Moran PR, Moran RA, Karstaed N (1985) Verification and evaluation of internal flow and motion. Radiology 154: 433–441

Savader SJ, Savader BL, Mutagh FR, Clerk LP, Silbiger ML (1988) MR evaluation of flow in a ventricular shunt phantom with in vivo correlation. J Comput Assist Tomogr 12: 765–769

Tamaki N, Shirakuni T, Kojima S, Okuda H, Maeda F (1989) Flow and MRI. In: Tamaki N, Matsumoto S (eds) MRI diagnosis of neurological disease. Asakura, Tokyo, pp 56–65

49 — An Evaluation of the Use of Perioperative Antibiotics in CSF Shunts

Fernando Rueda-Franco[1], Irene Maulén-Radován, and
Beatriz Llamosas-Gallardo[2]

Summary. The authors analyzed complications due to infection in a group of selected shunted patients during the year 1987, in order to assess the effectiveness of perioperative antibiotics. Sixty three patients were studied and such variables as sex, age, etiology of hydrocephalus, germs involved, antibiotics used, and mortality were analyzed. Differences of sex and age were not statistically significant. Arnold-Chiari and other congenital problems accounted for 47 cases (69.8%). Fourteen patients (22%) developed infection, nine of them (14.7%) during the first 2 months after the shunt procedure, and two patients died. *Staphylococcus epidermidis* infections were found in three cases (21.4%), gram negatives infections in six cases (42.8%), and *Staphylococcus aureus* infections in two cases.

There were two antibiotic prophylactic groups: Dicloxacillin only and dicloxacillin — amikacin; six patients did not received any antibiotic.

There were no statistical differences between the frequency of neuroinfection in the two antibiotic groups.

We conclude that it is necessary to perform a prospective study with a more representative number of patients, using other antimicrobial agents, both perioperatively and for a more prolonged period.

Keywords. Hydrocephalus — Meningomyelocele — Congenital hydrocephalus — Cerebrospinal fluid — Shunt — Infection

Introduction

In spite of improvements in surgical techniques and shunt devices and the availability of new and stronger antibiotics, infection is still one of the most frequent and serious complications in cerebrospinal fluid (CSF) diversions; mortality for shunt infections can be as high as 30%–40% (Klein 1983, 1990; George et al. 1979).

[1] Departments of Neurosurgery, [2] Emergencies, Instituto Nacional de Pediatria, Mexico, DF 04530, Mexico

The reported frequency of infection varies from 5% to 30% in different studies (Walters et al. 1984; McClone et al. 1982; Odio et al. 1984; Schoenbaum et al. 1975; McCullough et al. 1980; Venes 1976; Frame and McLaurin 1984). CSF infection has devastating effects on brain parenchyma, mostly in children under 1 year of age, with a very high percentage of mortality and morbidity. Another high-risk group of patients are those with Arnold-Chiari syndrome (Gurtin 1987). *Staphylococcus epidermidis* is the germ most frequently implicated in the production of this kind of infection, followed by *Staphylococcus aureus*, gram negative bacteria and enterococcus. Usually the infection of a ventriculo — peritoneal (VP) shunt is caused by the skin flora (George et al. 1979; Odio et al. 1984; Schoenbaum et al. 1975; McCullough et al. 1980; McLaurin 1989; McLaurin and Frame 1987), but such shunts can also be infected hematogenously or via contiguous infection or by direct exposure of the hardware; it has also been suggested that contamination can be caused by the patient's nasopharyngeal germs or can result from the operating room environment (Klein 1983, 1990; Shapiro et al. 1988; Bayston and Lari 1974; Henderson 1967). The clinical picture of a VP shunt infection includes: fever, vomiting, irritability, seizures, meningeal signs, and in some cases, signs of peritoneal infection. Other patients only show signs of local infection under the skin where the VP shunt was placed. Once a VP shunt infection is diagnosed, there are two avenues to follow: remove the CSF shunt and give antibiotics or treat the patient with antibiotics without removing the shunt, unless the infection does not respond to the antibiotics.

There is an abundant literature on the use of so-called prophylactic antibiotics in VP shunts (McCullough et al. 1980; Venes 1976; O'Brien and Parent 1979). Some authors chiefly emphasize a very rigid protocol in the operating room as one of the most important preventive measures for shunt infections. Several reports, however, point out the fact that the use of perioperative antibiotics reduces the incidence of infection to 2%–5% (Venes 1976; O'Brien and Parent 1979; Luthardt 1970); with the combination of oxacillin and a topical antibiotic, the incidence was reduced to 1.2% (Klein 1990).

In our Institution roughly 80% of the patients who are shunted receive prophylactic antibiotics, which include dicloxacillin and amikacin. Nevertheless, the incidence of shunt infection remains high. Therefore the authors decided to carry out a retrospective evaluation of the problem in a group of patients who were shunted in a 1-year period: January 1, 1987 through December 31, 1987.

Patients and Methods

The study included those patients who fitted the following criteria: (1) Shunted for the first time, (2) normal CSF at the time of shunt procedure, and (3) a follow-up of at least 12 months after the initial operation. Patients shunted because of TB meningitis were excluded.

Table 1. Age and sex distribution in 63 VP shunted patients

Age	Male	Female	Total
0–3 Months	10	8	18
3–6 Months	7	7	14
6 Months–1 Year	8	5	13
> 1 Year	10	8	18
Total	35	28	63

$X = 0.363$, $P > 0.05$. X, $X^2(gl\text{-}3) = 0.363$

In addition to the clinical picture, infections of the shunt derivation were diagnosed when we found an increase of cell content in the CSF, consisting mostly of neutrophils and when we found elevation of protein content and decrease in glucose.

The following variables were analyzed: Age, sex, etiology of hydrocephalus, incidence of infection, germ or germs involved, type of antibacterial agents (when used), and other non infectious complications.

Patients were divided into two groups: Those with infection in the CSF diverstions and those without it and different variables were compared.

Results

Of 89 patients shunted in this 1-year period, 63 were included for analysis in this study. Age and sex distribution is shown in Table 1, which also shows the statistical analysis that demonstrated no significance in these two variables. The etiology of hydrocephalus in this group of patients was varied and included myelomenigocele (Arnold-Chiari) 42.8%, other congenital hydrocephalic conditions 26.9%, tumoral 11.1%, postinfection 6.3%, posthemorrhagic 6.3%, and neurocysticercosis 4.7%. All 63 patients had a normal CSF and negative

Table 2. Incidence of infection in different etiological groups

Etiology of hydrocephalus	Without infection	With infection	Total
Myelomeningocele	21	6	27
Cong. hydrocephalus	14	3	17
Tumoral	5	2	7
Post-hemorrhagic	4	0	4
Post-infections	1	3	4
Neurocysticercosis	3	0	3
Cong. hydrocephalus + intracranial hemorrhage	1	0	1
Total	49	14	63

culture, at the time of the shunt operation. Table 2 shows the incidence of infection in the different etiological groups.

Fourteen patients (22%) developed meningitis after VP shunting, over periods ranging from 2 to 266 days; in six patients the infection occurred during the 1st post-operative month and in nine (14.3%) the infection was seen during the first 2 months after surgery. Table 3 lists the different germs that were identified in the CSF cultures of patients with infections. Two patients (14.2%), both under 6 months of age, died as a result of the CSF infection.

Six patients did not receive any antibiotic and one of them developed VP shunt infection. In 43 children, antibiotics were prescribed after the shunt procedure; 25 received dicloxacillin and 18 received dicloxacillin plus amikacin for at least 5 days (Table 4). No statistically significant difference was found between the incidence of neuroinfection in the group of patients that received one antibiotic and the incidence in the group that received two antibiotics, as seen in Table 5. It is important to note that infections caused by enteropathogens were seen in patients who did not receive amikacin, whereas infection by *Staphylococcus aureus* or *Staphylococcus epidermidis* occurred in spite of the use of dicloxacillin.

Table 6 shows a comparison of patients with and without neuroinfection in relation to age. The statistical significance is $P < 0.05$, so the younger the patient the greater the incidence of infection. The therapy and outcome in the

Table 3. Germs identified in VP shunt infections

Germs	Surgical	Total	%
Staphylococcus epidermidis	3	3	21.4
Staphylococcus aureus	1	2[a]	14.2
Klebsiella pneumoniae	1	2	14.2
Klebsiella azagnac	1	1	7.1
Hemophilus influenzae	0	1	7.1
Salmonella D	0	1	7.1
Bacillus megaterlum	0	1[a]	7.1
Negative cultures	3	4	28.5

[a] One patient infected with two germs

Table 4. Type of perioperative antibiotic

Antibiotic	Without neuroinfection		With neuroinfection	
	n	%	n	%
Dicloxacillin	25	51	8	57.1
Dicloxacillin + amikacin	18	36.7	5	35.7
None	6	12.2	1	7.1
Total	49	100	14	100

Table 5. Frequency of shunt infection among patients who received antibiotics

Antibiotic	Without neuroinfection	With neuroinfection	Total
Dicloxacillin	25	8	33
Dicloxacillin + amikacin	18	5	23
Total	43	13	56

Fisher exact test = 0.53

Table 6. Age-related comparison of patients with and without neuroinfection

Age	With neuroinfection	Without neuroinfection
Mean age	6 months	2 years 8 months
SD	4.75 months	1 year 1 month

$t = 2.01$, $P < 0.05$

Table 7. Therapeutic approach and outcome in 14 patients with shunt infection

Type of therapy	Number of cases (n)	2nd. neuroinfection	Deceased
Antibiotics only	6	1	0
Antibiotics and shunt replacement	8	2	2

14 infected patients is illustrated in Table 7. Although we had only a small number of patients in this series, it is important to note that in the group only receiving antibiotic we saw only one recurrence of CSF infection, whereas of the eight children in whom the shunt was removed and replaced, two developed a new infection and another two died while the infection was current.

Discussion

Infection remains a frequent and serious complication of CSF diversions. Although the problem has produced a large number of important reports, the different results of prophylaxis and treatment leave many clinical uncertainties. The outcome of these patients depends upon a number of variables that must be controlled to achieve consistent results. Among the most important variables are: Age, etiology of hydrocephalus, immunologic status of the patient, shunt derivation, and surgical techniques. Up to 1970 the rate of shunt infection ranged from 7% to 29% (Luthardt 1970); by 1980 the rate had decreased to 10%–15% (Frame and McLaurin 1984). Reports from the late 1980s coming from neurosurgical centers in industrialized nations, have a rate of 2%–5% (Klein 1983; McCullough et al. 1980; Shapiro et al. 1988; Chapman and Borges 1984; Haines 1985; Shurtleff et al. 1985; Walters et al. 1984). The rate of shunt infection in developing countries is still very high; 14.3% post-operative infections and an overall 22% infection rate in the present series.

Up to the present time no standard protocol for the prevention and treatment of shunt infections has been accepted world-wide.

It has been postulated that the skin flora is the main contaminant of VP shunts; however when Bayston and Lari (1974) performed preoperative skin and intraoperative wound cultures in 100 shunt operations, 58% of these patients showed wound contamination by the end of the procedure, but only 55% of these contained organisms that were present on the patient's skin before surgery. Shapiro et al. (1988) compared the results of skin cultures obtained from the operative sites in 413 pediatric shunt diversions to cultures obtained from 20 subsequent shunt infections in these patients. Only four (20%), showed organisms identical to those originally grown from the skin in the same patient. The authors suggest that many shunt infections may occur as a result of contamination from the patient's nasopharynx, or from operative personnel, or from the hospital environment.

In our series 14 patients (22%) developed shunt infection during the 12-month follow up period. Nine (14.3%) of them presented with the infection during the first 2 months after the operation (surgical infection). In three of this latter group *Staphylococcus epidermidis* was the germ identified; in three there were negative cultures; two patients were infected by a gram negative germ (*Klebsiella*) and in one patient *Staphylococcus aureus* was cultured. These results are similar to other reported results (Odio et al. 1984; Shapiro et al. 1988). It is important to emphasize that all these nine patients received antibiotics; seven receiving only dicloxacillin and two receiving dicloxacillin and amikacin, but this was of no avail in preventing the infection.

Considering the whole group of 14 patients, in 6 (42.8%) the infection was produced by a gram negative germ, a rather high figure in comparison with other reports.

As shown in the results, we did not find any statistically significant difference between the use of dicloxacillin alone or its use with the addition of amikacin. In the literature there are several reports dealing with different kinds of so-called prophylactic antibiotics, e.g., Sulfamethoxazole and triemethoprim vs placebo (Wang et al. 1984), oxacillin vs placebo (Weiss and Raskind 1970), gentamicin–cloxacillin or placebo (Bayston 1975), and methicillin vs placebo (Haines and Taylor 1982).

All of these authors concluded that there were no statistically significant differences in results when these antibioties were used "prophylactically." In addition, the infections that are acquired several months after shunt placement cannot be prevented with any of the above-mentioned protocols. With all of these data we think that in patients with high risk of infection and or bacteremia (e.g., urinary infection in myelomeningocele cases) any infection source must be carefully treated. Therefore we consider it appropriate to carry out preventive administration of antimicrobial agents in these patients in the same fashion as is now done for patients with, for example, cardiac prostheses.

Other important facts to be considered in our population are: loss to follow-up, malnourishment, and carelessness in the care of handicapped children.

Conclusion

Shunt infections are still a severe and frequent complication, in spite of better surgical techniques, improvements in shunt devices, and the availability of strong antimicrobial agents.

In our Institute the infection rate in the group studied was 22% over a follow-up period of 1 year, but the "surgical infection" was 14.3%. *Staphylococcus epidermidis* was the most frequent germ involved in the so-called surgical infections; but enteric gram negative bacteria accounted for 42.8% of the infections in the group as a whole. There were no statistically significant difference between the group treated with dicloxacillin, the group treated with dicloxacillin plus amikacin, and, surprisingly, the group who did not receive any antibiotic.

We consider the use of aminoglycosides mandatory in our patients, because of the high incidence of gram negative infections. It is very important to keep in mind the presence of any infectious process (e.g., urinary) when taking preventive measures in patients with VP shunts.

It is necessary to make a concerted effort to prevent shunt infections in a prospective way which must include a sample size that can permit a real approach to the population sample.

References

Bayston R (1975) Antibiotic prophylaxis in shunt surgery. Dev Med Child Neurol 17 (Suppl 35): 99–103

Bayston R, Lari J (1974) A study of the sources of infection in colonized shunts. Dev Med Child Neurol (Suppl 32): 16–22

Chapman PH, Borges LF (1984) Shunt infections: Prevention and treatment. Clin Neurosurg 32: 652–664

Frame PT, Mc Laurin RL (1984) Treatment of CSF shunt infections with intrashunt plus oral antibiotic therapy. J Neurosurg 60: 354

George R, Leibrock L, Epstein M (1979) Long term analysis of cerebrospinal fluid shunt infections. A 25 year experience. J. Neurosurg 51: 804–811

Gurtin S (1987) Fistulas para liquido cefalorraquideo. Evaluacion, complicaciones y control de crisis. Clin Ped North Am 1: 225

Haines SJ (1985) Antibiotic prophylaxis in neurosurgery. Clin Neurosurg 33: 633–642

Haines SJ, Taylor F (1982) Prophylactic methicillin for shunt operations: Effects on incidence of shunt malfunction and infection. Child's Brain 9: 10–22

Henderson RJ (1967) Staphylococcal infection of surgical wounds: The source of infection. Br J Surg 54: 756–760

Klein DM (1983) Comparison of antibiotic methods in the prophylaxis of operative shunt infections. Concepts Pediat Neurosurg 4: 131–141

Klein DM, (1990) Shunt infections in hydrocephalus. In: RM Scott (ed) Concepts in neurosurgery vol 3. Congress of Neurological Surgeons

Luthardt T (1970) Bacterial infections in ventriculo — auricular shunt sistems. Dev Med Child Neurol 12 (Suppl 22): 105–109

McCullough DC, Kane J, Presper J, Wells M (1980) Antibiotic prophylaxis in ventricular shunt surgery. Child's Brain 7: 182–189

McLaurin RL (1989) Ventricular shunts: Complications and results. In: Section of Pediatric Neurosurgery of the American Association of Neurological Surgeons (ed) Pediatric neurosurgery. Surgery of the developing nervous system, 2nd Ed. WB Saunders, Philadelphia, pp 219–229

McLaurin RL, Frame PT (1987) Treatment of infections of cerebrospinal fluid shunts. Rev Infect Dis (3): 595–603

McLone DG, Czyzewshi D, Raimondi AJ, et al. (1982) Central nervous system infections as a limiting factor in the intelligence of children with myelomeningocele. Pediatrics 70: 338–342

O'Brien M, Parent A (1979) Management of ventricular shunt infections. Child's Brain 5: 304–309

Odio C, Mc Cracken G, Nelson J (1984) CSF shunt infections in pediatrics. Am J Dis Child 138: 110–1108

Schoenbaum S, Gardner P, Shillito J (1975) Infections of cerebrospinal fluid shunts: Epidemology, clinical manifestations, and therapy. J Infect Dis 131(5): 543–552

Shapiro S, Boaz J, et al. (1988) Origin of organisms infecting ventricular shunts. Neurosurgery 22: 868–872

Shurtleff DB, Stuntz JT, Hayden PW (1985) Experience with 1201 cerebrospinal fluid shunt procedures. Pediatr Neurosci 12: 49–57

Venes J (1976) Control of shunt infection. Report of 150 consecutive cases. J Neurosurg 45: 311–314

Walters BC, Hoffman HJ, Hendrick EB, et al. (1984) Cerebrospinal fluid shunt infections: Influences on initial management and subsequent outcome. J Neurosurg 60: 1014–1021

Wang EEL, Prober CG, Hendrick EB, et al. (1984) Prophylactic sulfamethoxazole and trimethoprim in ventriculoperitoneal shunt surgery. JAMA 251: 1174–1177

Weiss SR, Paskind R (1970) Further experience with the ventriculoperitoneal shunt: Prophylactic antibiotics. Int Surg 53: 300–303

50 — A Concerted Effort to Prevent Shunt Infection

Harold J. Hoffman, Donald Soloniuk, Robin P. Humphreys, James M. Drake, and E. Bruce Hendrick[1]

Introduction

Cerebral spinal fluid (CSF) shunt infections affect as many as 27% of patients treated for hydrocephalus with the CSF diversionary shunt (Schoenbaum et al. 1975). Shunt infection is the major cause of morbidity and mortality among patients with CSF shunts. Intellectual and neurologic deficits and massive expenditures in health care funds are the results of these infections.

In a review of shunt infections carried out at the Hospital for Sick Children, out of a total series of 1477 patients treated over a 20-year period, 222 patients developed a shunt infection (Walters et al. 1984). Among these 222 patients, 1450 revisions (6.6 revisions per patient) were required, as compared to 2252 revisions among 1255 patients (1.8 revisions per patient) who did not have a shunt infection. Frykberg and Olsen (1983) stressed that overt or occult shunt infection was the primary cause of early peritoneal catheter obstructions in patients with venticuloperitoneal shunts.

There are many factors that influence the rate of shunt infection. George et al. (1979), in a series from Johns Hopkins University, found that the surgeon was the largest single factor in the incidence of shunt infection. The duration of surgery has been found to influence the rate of shunt infection to the extent that Forrest and Cooper (1968) reported a 16% infection rate in patients whose shunt operations averaged 1 hour compared to 8% when the operating time was under 30 min.

Staphylococcus epidermidis is responsible for the majority of shunt infections, accounting for anywhere between 60% and 75% of such infections (Yoger 1985). These particular organisms produce lectins or other adhesins which give them the capacity to adhere to surfaces (Guevara et al. 1987; Quie and Bellani 1987). Furthermore, these organisms produce a surface slime material that protects them from phagocytosis and from the actions of antimicrobial agents (Quie and Bellani 1987). Moreover, the irregularities

[1] Division of Neurosurgery, The Hospital for Sick Children, University of Toronto, 555 University Avenue, Toronto, Ontario, M5G 1X8 Canada

found on shunt tubing helped to anchor and hide bacterial micro colonies (Guevara et al. 1987).

Borges (1982) found that white blood cells fail to adhere in normal numbers to catheters and therefore failed to ingest fully a bacterial innoculum on the surface of a shunt catheter. Duhaime et al. on the basis of their studies, concluded that bacteria most often associated with shunt infections are airborne in the operating room and are distributed in highest concentration near the surgical team (Duhaime et al. [to be published]). They advocated maintaining a designated operating room in which traffic is limited, with strict adherence to covering skin surfaces of the operating room personnel in order to reduce shunt infection rates.

Hirsch et al. (1978) were able to reduce shunt infections from 19.7% to 7.4% by utilizing a surgical isolator which allowed the shunt procedure to be done in a sterile environment remote from the skin, hair, and air passages of the operating room personnel. Connolly et al. (1987) were able to reduce their shunt infection rate from 6% to 2.4% by utilizing a meticulous surgical technique.

Over a 1-year period (July 1987 to June 1988) the shunt infection rate at the Hospital for Sick Children, Toronto, rose to 12.9% in a series of 581 shunt operations performed. We felt that a radical change in our shunt procedure technique should be introduced to deal with this undesirable shunt infection rate. Choux had advocated a protocol which reduced his shunt infection rate to near zero percent (M. Choux, personal communication). We, therefore, instituted a protocol similar to that advocated by Choux.

Keywords. Shunt infection — Shunt revision

Method

The protocol consisted of carrying out shunt procedures at the beginning of the operating day when the air organism count is lowest. The patients who were to undergo shunt surgery were to have a shampoo and body wash carried out twice before being sent to the operating room. Anesthesia was to be induced in the induction room, where hair was to be clipped and shaved. The instruments in the operating room were to remain under cover until after the patient had been transferred into the operating room, placed on the table, and the transfer stretcher taken out of the operating room.

The operating room personnel were to be kept at a minimum. No visitors would be allowed. No one could come into or leave the operating room during a shunt operation. The staff neurosurgeon or the clinical fellow in neurosurgery would be part of the surgical team.

The patient was to be given cloxacillin 100 mg per kilogram intravenously at the beginning of the case.

The operative sites were to be carefully cleansed with a fat solvent and then appropriately prepared with soap and antiseptic solution. The operative site was to be draped with an adherent plastic drape.

Shunt equipment would be opened only when required. Until used this shunt equipment would be kept in a bath of bacitracin solution.

We used Younger et al.'s (1987) definition of shunt infection which required that there be two or more positive cultures of cerebrospinal fluid or shunt tubing or one positive culture combined with one positive gram stain.

Results

During the period July 1st, 1988, to June 30th, 1989, 576 shunt procedures were undertaken on the neurosurgical service at the Hospital for Sick Children. Twenty two of these operations resulted in a shunt infection, providing an infection rate of 3.8%. These 22 infections occurred in 20 patients. The organisms in these infections consisted of *staphylococcus epidermidis* in 13 (59.1%) and *staphylococcus aureus* in six (27.3%); two patients had infections with multiple enteric organisms (9.1%) and one patient had an *E. Coli* infection (4.5%). The duration of stay for these 20 patients with infection varied between 10 and 216 days, with a mean period of stay of 49.1 days. Nine of these 22 infections were discovered during the period of hospitalization.

Ten of the 22 infections were heralded with fever and shunt malfunction (45.5%). Six had shunt malfunction (27.3%). Three had abdominal pain (13.6%). Two had only fever (9.1%) and one had an abdominal pseudocyst (4.5%). Five developed fever within 96 h of the operative procedure (22.7%).

When we compared the 22 procedures with infection to the 554 procedures without infection we found that of the 22 infected patients, 16 had received antibiotics (81.8%), whereas among the 554 patients without infection, 506 had received antibiotics (91.3%). Nine of the infected patients had their surgery before noon (40.9%). Three hundred and two of the non-infected patients had their surgery before noon (54.5%). Thirteen of the infected patients had their surgery after noon (59.1%) and 252 of the non-infected patients had their surgery after noon (45.5%).

The infection risk in before noon surgery was 9 out of 311 patients or 2.9%. The infection risk for surgery carried out after noon was 13 out of 265 patients or 4.9%.

Seven of the 22 patients with infection (31.8%) had their surgery performed in less than 1 hour. Four hundred and sixty-five of the 554 patients without shunt infection (83.9%) had their surgery done in less than 1 hour. Fifteen of the infected patients (68.2%) had their surgery done in 1–3 h. Eighty-nine of the non-infected patients (16.1%) had their surgery done in 1–3 h.

The mean age of the 22 patients whose procedure ended in infection was 3 years and 4 months and the mean age of the 554 patients without infection was 2 years 8 months. Among the 576 operative procedures there were 224 insertions with nine infections (4%) and 352 revisions with 13 infections (3.7%).

Discussion

Our protocol has not lowered our infection rate to zero, but it has reduced the infection rate from 12.9% to 3.8%. However, we have not been as rigorous as we should have been in following our protocol. Consequently, many of our shunts are still done later in the day when the infection rate significantly increases.

Despite insisting on experts being present for all shunt procedures, many of our shunts were done over periods as long as 3 hours with a consequently higher infection rate in those patients whose shunt procedures took more than 1 hour. Not all of our patients received their antibiotics; this played a noticeable but not statistically significant role in increasing our infections.

Finally, despite our protocol, there were frequently as many as three nurses and two anesthetists in the operating room. The presumed result of all these breaks in our protocol still leaves us with a lingering infection rate of 3.8%.

Conclusion

CSF Shunt infection is costly to the patient, the institution, and to society. The vast majority of shunt infections are introduced in the operating room and probably come from the skin and air passages of the OR personnel. Careful adherence to a protocol which will reduce this risk of contamination of the shunt apparatus has reduced our shunt infection rate from 12.9% to 3.8%, a reduction of 70.5%. Furthermore, in looking at the infected cases it became obvious that there were breaks in the protocol in this group of patients, which made them more susceptible to shunt infection. We feel, therefore, that a stricter adherence to our protocol will lead to an even more substantial reduction in shunt infection and, possibly, will do away with this dreaded complication.

References

Borges LF (1982) Cerebrospinal fluid shunts interfere with host defenses. J Neurosurg 10: 55–60

Connolly B, Guiney EJ, Fitzgerald RJ (1987) CSF/shunt infections — the bane of our lives. Z Kinderchir 42: (Suppl I): 13–14

Duhaime A, Bonner K, McGowan KH, Schut L, Sutton LN, Platlain S (to be published) Distribution of bacteria in the operating room environment and its relation to ventricular shunt infections: A prospective study.

Forrest DM, Cooper DGW (1968) Complications of ventriculoatrial shunts. A review of 455 cases. J Neurosurg 29: 506–512

Frykberg T, Olsen L (1983) Infection as a cause of peritoneal catheter dysfunction in ventriculo-peritoneal shunting in children. Z Kinderchir 38 (Suppl II): 84–86

George R, Leibrock L, Epstein M (1979) Long-term analysis of cerebrospinal fluid shunt infections. J Neurosurg 51: 804–811

Guevara JA, Zuccaro G, Trevisan A, Denoya CD (1987) Bacterial adhesion to cerebrospinal fluid shunts. J Neurosurg 67: 438–445

Hirsch JF, Renier D, Pierre-Kahn A (1978) Influence of the use of a surgical isolator on the rate of infection in the treatment of hydrocephalus. Childs Brain 4: 137–150

Quie PG, Belani KK (1989) Coagulase — negative staphylococcal adherence and persistence. J Infect Dis 156: 543–547

Schoenbaum SC, Gardner P, Shillito J Jr (1975) Infections of cerebrospinal fluid shunts: Epidemiology, clinical manifestations, and therapy. J Infect Dis 131: 543–552

Walters BC, Hoffman HJ, Hendrick EB, Humphreys RP (1984) Cerebrospinal fluid shunt infections: Influences on initial management and subsequent outcome. J Neurosurg 60: 1014–1024

Yogev R (1985) Cerebrospinal fluid shunt infections: a personal view. Pediatr Infect Dis 4: 113–118

Younger JJ, Christensen GD, Bartley DL, Simmon JCH, Barrett FF (1987) Coagulase-nagative staphylococci isolated from cerebrospinal fluid shunts: Importance of slime production, species identification and shunt removal to clinical outcome. J Infect Dis 156: 548–554

51 — Post-Shunt Isolated Compartments in Hydrocephalus: Proposal for a New Classification and Experimental Proof of the Pathophysiology

Shizuo Oi, Hiroshi Yamada, Hiroshi Kudo, Akihiro Ijichi,
Yasuhiro Okuda, Shigekuni Kim, Seiji Hamano, Yoshiteru Shose,
Seishiro Urui, Minoru Saito, Michio Yamaguchi, Norihiko Tamaki,
and Satoshi Matsumoto[1]

Summary. The clinical features and pathophysiology of specific forms of post-shunt isolated compartments were analyzed. The possible pathogenesis of the individual clinical entity was discussed on the basis of various experimental studies, which included morphological evaluation and pressure monitoring in a canine slit-ventricle model a silicon ventricular system simulation model for post-shunt ICP dynamics analysis, and so forth. A clinically applicable classification was used to evaluate the progression of hydrocephalus (Stage I-IV), and to define the compartment isolation after shunting in previously communicating cerebral ventricles and the central canal of the spinal cord (Type I-IV).

The present study also indicates that the pathophysiology of hydromyelia is closely related to the associated hydrocephalus in some cases. A new concept of the development of an isolated compartment after shunting is proposed to explain the progression of hydromyelia in these cases (hydromyelic hydrocephalus).

Keywords. Post-shunt isolated compartment — Isolated unilateral hydrocephalus — Isolated fourth ventricle — Isolated rhombencephalic ventricle — Isolated central canal dilation

Introduction

It has recently been recognized that overdrainage of cerebrospinal fluid (CSF) is often associated with some harmful, occasionally life-threatening events for children with shunted hydrocephalus. We have previously analyzed the pathophysiology of this clinical entity in 164 patients with pediatric hydrocephalus treated with ventriculoperitoneal shunts. In some cases, the overdrainage was felt to be a causative factor of post-shunt isolated ventricles, such as isolated IV ventricle and isolated unilateral hydrocephalus, as well as being a causative

---

[1] Department of Neurosurgery, Kobe University School of Medicine, Kobe, 650 Japan

Table 1. Proposal for a new classification of hydrocephalus stages and types of post-shunt isolated compartments

Hydrocephalic stages in communicating holo-neural canal

Stage I—Supratentorial hydrocephalus involving lateral ventricle (*STH-1*)
Stage II—Supratentorial hydrocephalus involving III ventricle (*STH-2*)
Stage III—Disproportionately large IV ventricle (*DLFV*)
Stage IV—Holo-neural canal dilatation (*HNCD*)

Post-shunt isolated compartments
Type I—Isolated unilateral hydrocephalus (*IUH*)
Type II—Isolated IV ventricle (*IFV*)
Type III—Isolated rhombencephalic ventricle (*IFCV*)
Type IV—Isolated central canal dilatation (*ICCD*)

factor in a severe form of slit-ventricle syndrome (Oi and Matsumoto 1985a,b, 1986a,b,c, 1987; Oi et al. 1991).

The purpose of this paper is to propose a new classification of post-shunt isolated compartments and to discuss their possible pathophysiology on the basis of various experimental studies.

Proposal for a New Classification of Hydrocephalic Stages and Post-Shunt Isolated Compartments in Communicating Holo-Neural Canal (Oi et al. 1991) (Table 1)

Hydrocephalic Stage in Communicating Holo-Neural Canal

In communicating holo-neural canal, the intracranial ventricular system and the central canal of the spinal cord communicate freely. The lateral ventricles dilate first in cases with internal hydrocephalus (Stage I = supratenorial hydro-cephalus − 1: STH1). When hydrocephalus progresses, the third ventricle also becomes dilated (Stage II = supratentorial hydrocephalus − 2: STH$_2$). In more advanced cases, especially if the outlets of the fourth ventricle to the cistern are obliterated, the whole ventricular system expands, including the fourth ventricle (Stage III = disproportionately large fourth ventricle: DLFV). Futhermore, the central canal of the spinal cord may also be involved (Stage IV = holo-neural canal dilatation: HNCD).

Type of Post-Shunt Isolated Compartment in Communicating Holo-Neural Canal

Various forms of ventricular system isolation may develop along with over-drainage of CSF via the shunt. Functional occlusion of the foramen of Monro may result in progressive unilateral delatation of the lateral ventricle (Type I = isolated unilateral hydrocephalus: IUH). If the aqueduct of Sylvius is involved in cases with obstruction of the fourth ventricular outlets to the cistern, isolation and expansion of the fourth ventricle will occur (Type II = isolated fourth ventricle: IFV). In more advanced cases, dilatation of both the fourth ventricle and the central canal of the spinal cord can develop, forming an expanded primary rhombencephalic ventricle including the metencephalon and myelencephalon (Type III = isolated rhombencephalic ventricle: IRCV). This type, however, may involve only the central canal of the spinal cord without dilating the fourth ventricle (Type IV = isolated central canal dilatation: ICCD).

Individual Form of Hydrocephalic Stages and Post-Shunt Isolated Compartments (Oi et al. 1991)

Hydrocephalic Stage III (Disproportionately Large Fourth Ventricle: DLFV) and Hydrocephalic Stage IV (Holo-Neural Canal Dilatation: HNCD)

(a) Clinical entity
In an adult case of hydrocephalus of unknown etiology and progressive tetraparesis, magnetic resonance (MR T_1-weighted sagittal image) demonstrated markedly dilated third and fourth ventricles with a significant flow void sign in the dilated central canal. Metrizamide computed tomography (CT) cisternography revealed no communication between the subarachnoid space and ventricles. CSF dynamics studies in this case indicated that a hydrocephalic dynamic force was responsible for the spinal symptoms.

This progression is likely in the transitional period from stage III to IV. The more advanced hydrocephalic stage in this condition is the "holo-neural canal dilatation". Our patient, a 17-year-old boy, underwent initial ventriculoperitoneal shunt at 13 years of age for progressive ventriculomegaly. The patient continued to have progressive tetraparesis and gait disturbance. Repeated CT revealed no significant changes of the ventricular size. Metrizamide CT ventriculography revealed a huge hydromyelic cavity communicating with the dilated ventricular system and extending down to the T_4 vertebral level.

At operation, the previous shunt was found to be occluded at the distal end. It was removed and a new shunt system with a multipurpose device was inserted. No surgical procedure was performed for the hydromyelia. Postoperatively, the muscle weakness and gait disturbance improved dramatically and the sensory deficits gradually lessened.

(b) Experimental proof
Fetal hydrocephalic models were developed by induction of 6-AN (6 aminonicotinamide, a niacinamide antimetabolite) to pregnant rats on day 13 of gestation (Yamada et al. [to be published])

In this model, ventricular dilatation together with central canal dilatation was evident after day 17. CSF dynamics were investigated by India-ink injection into the lateral ventricle. The outlets of the fourth ventricle were not patent but the dilated central canal was communicating with the ventricular system. This model mimics the CSF dynamics of stage IV hydrocephalus.

Post-Shunt Isolated Compartment Type I
(Isolated Unilateral Hydrocephalus: IUH)

(a) Clinical entity
Isolated unilateral hydrocephalus (Oi and Matsumoto 1985b) is defined as:

1. Shunt complication which occurrs in an initially bilaterally expanded communicating lateral ventricle.
2. Reexpansion of the contralateral ventricle after a unilateral shunt placement.
3. Progressive hydrocephalus with no evidence of a primary destructive lesion, e.g., porencephaly.

All of our cases were shunted in the neonatal period or in early infancy. The symptoms of isolated unilateral hydrocephalus which appeared as unilateral cranial expansion with or without contralateral hemiparesis were nystagmus, conjugate deviation, or other eye symptoms. The follow-up CTs demonstrated a progressively reexpanding contralateral lateral ventricle, while the shunted side became slit-like with the overdraining well-functioning shunt in place.

Analysis of the CSF dynamics by metrizamide or pneumo-ventriculography/cisternography suggested the existence of a one-way ball valve action at the foramen of Monro.

Continuous and simultaneous bilateral intraventricular pressure monitoring of patients' pulse pressure and compliance revealed independent patterns of pressure gradient.

The pathophysiology of isolated unilateral hydrocephalus demonstrated in this study can be classified into the following two categories:
(i) Permanent isolated unilateral hydrocephalus
(ii) Reversible isolated unilateral hydrocephalus.
Treatment should be based on the pathophysiology of occlusion of the foramen of Monro.

(b) Experimental proof (Oi and Matsumoto 1986d)
Kaolin-induced (20 mg/kg) hydrocephalus in dogs was treated 3 weeks after initiation by overdainage ($-200 \, mmH_2O$) of cerebrospinal fluid (CSF) from one lateral ventricle. An appreciably unbalanced ventricular system, with unilateral slit ventricle, was thereby created. The cerebral mantles of both hemispheres were compared by light microscopy.

Macroscopically, the horizontally cut section showed a slit-like change in the ventricle which had been drained and moderate expansion in the other lateral ventricle. Reconstitution of the brain mantle was caused mainly by re-expanded white matter. Microscopically, interrupted ependymal lining, spongi-form swelling, or expanded extracellular space in the subependymal or adjacent white matter were observed in the cerebral hemisphere with the expanded lateral ventricle, whereas reduction of the findings of CSF edema and gliotic scar changes were seen in the side that had been drained.

In a second experimental model, rapid overdrainage of CSF was performed under bilateral, simultaneous intraventricular pressure (IVP) monitoring, and the possible clinical use of an anti-slit ventricular catheter (ASVC) was determined. This experimental study was repeated in the silicon ventricular system simulation model.

One of us (S.M.) has developed a ventricular catheter with a double lumen and a very flexible soft outer tube to preserve intraventricular pulse pressure within the ventricle. This design is based on the fact that (1) the pulse pressure is an important factor in ventricular enlargement and (2) the intraventricular pulse pressure after shunt placement in hydrocephalus is always lower in the ventricle which is being drained.

The pulse pressure produced in an experimental mode was much less than that achieved using a regular ventricular catheter (0.39–0.59 to 1.00) into the 60 cm-long abdominal tube end. In experimental hydrocephalus, bilateral IVP recordings showed good preservation of the pulse pressure on both sides with the use of this catheter, but using a normal catheter there was early disappearance of the pulse pressure on the side being drained.

In the silicon ventricular system simulation model, early and more significant reduction of the pulse pressure in the shunted side was again observed and this effect was much less if ASVC was used.

This experimental work suggested the possibility of clinical use of this ASVC, which may overcome the complications caused by dynamic changes in IVP after shunt placement.

Regarding pathophysiology, we have reported the extremely high incidence of slit-like ventricles occurring after ventriculo-peritoneal (V-P) shunt insertion in younger infants and we concluded that the main causative factors were probably high intracranial compliance and overdrainage of CSF by the shunt (Oi and Matsumoto 1985b). Bering (1955) clearly showed evidence of pulse pressure as a generator of the force for ventricular enlargement as well as for CSF flow. Kaufman et al. (1973) found that the pulse pressure on the side of shunt placement was always lower than that of the other lateral ventricle. Diminished pulse wave caused by shunt placement should be considered one of the important causative factors in slit-like ventricle and related morphological changes after V-P shunt placement.

Post-Shunt Isolated Compartment Type II
(Isolated Fourth Ventricle: IFV)

Clinical entity

Symptomatic isolation of the fourth ventricle appeared in our eight patients, with as long an interval as 6 years and 7 months on average after the initial shunt.

Although the pathogenesis of isolated fourth ventricle, especially of secondary aqueductal obstruction, remains unclear, our study strongly suggested that there are two different mechanisms operating in the completion of fourth ventricle isolation. One mechanism is "functional obstruction", which is created by shunt overfunction in the lateral ventricle, resulting in supratentorial low intraventricular pressure, pulse pressure, and compliance. The other mechanism is "morphological obstruction" of the aqueduct, which is the consequence of an inflammatory reaction, peri-aqueductal edema, gliosis, and other secondary factors which occur with or without the influence of the shunt procedure.

The choice of treatment method for isolated fourth ventricle should be based on the pathophysiology of the mechanism of isolation and varies from case to case. Methods include veil excision, aqueductal canalization, fourth ventricle shunt, reopening of the associated slit-like ventricle of the lateral ventricles, etc.

Isolation of the fourth ventricle requires an associated secondary aqueductal occlusion, a point which was not described prior to 1969, when Raimondi et al. (1969) first reported it. They considered this phenomenon to be the result of the difference in pressure between the supra- and infra-tentorial compartments. In their opinion a shunt placed in the lateral cerebral ventricle created an unexpectedly low supra-tentorial intraventricular pressure by overdraining CSF. Consequently, they emphasized that this condition could be reversed by decreasing the pressure in the infra-tentorial compartment, which then causes the reopening of the aqueduct. In 1983, Oi and Matsumoto (1986a) described the phenomenon of reopening the aqueduct in cases of isolated fourth ventricle by enlarging the slit-like lateral cerebral ventricle with an upgrading shunt pressure and an anti-siphon valve. De Feo et al. (1975) reported a case of "double compartment hydrocephalus" with cysticercosis meningitis, and considered the mechanism of the secondary aqueductal obstruction to be the result of upward cerebellar veil displacement caused by increased infra-tentorial pressure. Zimmerman et al. (1978) interpreted their cases by postulating a "twisting of the aqueduct" mechanism which occurred as a result of compression exerted from above and below by the supra- and infra-tentorial compartments under pressure.

Post-Shunt Isolated Compartment Type III (Isolated Rhombencephalic Ventricle: IRCV) and Type IV (Isolated Central Canal Dilatation: ICCD)

Our patient, a 4-year-old girl, who had previously undergone repair of myeloschisis and insertion of a V-P shunt for associated hydrocephalus at birth, developed quadriparesis, and a somewhat decreased level of consciousness.

A repeat CT demonstrated massive reexpansion of the fourth ventricle, with slit-like lateral ventricles. MRI demonstrated a hydromyelic cavity extending the length of the spinal cord, together with a reexpanded fourth ventricle and central canal.

At the time of insertion of the fourth ventricule shunt tube, 3 ml of isotonic metrizamide was injected into the fourth ventricle. A spinal CT was performed immediately after the operation, and communication between the dilated fourth ventricle and the hydromyelic cavity was confirmed. (Isolated rhombencephalic ventricle (IRCV)).

Repeat MRI showed a collapsed fourth ventricle with the shunt in place and a normalized central canal. The radiological investigations in this case suggested that the dynamic force from the post-shunt isolated fourth ventricle had caused dilatation of the central canal. Also, in this case, the foramina of Luschka and Majendie were not patent.

Six months later, the patient developed some episodes, repeat MR revealed enlargement of both fourth ventricle and central canal and also slit-like lateral ventricles with the shunt in place. A fourth ventriculo-peritoneal shunt revision was performed and the patient improved just mildly at this time. Repeat MR then revealed a collapsed fourth ventricle as well as lateral ventricles with independently placed shunts, which seemed to be functioning, likely overdraining CSF. However, the MR demonstrated reexpanded central canal and the previously patent obex collapsed together with the slit-like fourth ventricle. (Isolated central canal dilatation: ICCD).

A central canal-subarachnoid shunt was performed and immediate post-operative MR revealed that the central canal had collapsed again; the patient improved as before.

Discussion

The etiology, pathogenesis, and pathophysiology of hydromyelia remain unknown. There have been several different hypotheses proposed regarding this controversial condition. Gardner (1965; Gardner and Angel 1959) hypothesized that arterial pulsations of the CSF are transmitted to the cervical cord in hydromyelia because of impaired outflow from the fourth ventricle. In the previously reported cases in which stage IV hydrocephalus with communicating holo-neural canal dilatation (HNCD) was apparently present, V-P or ventriculo-atrial shunting was generally the first treatment choice (Conway 1967; Krayenbuhl 1974; Krayenbuhl and Benini 1971; Schlesinger et al. 1981; Sullivan et al. 1988). However, not all patients were improved by ventricular shunting alone in this particular form of hydromyelia (communicating holo-neural canal dilatation) (Krayenbuhl 1974).

We have previously reported that excess drainage of CSF via a ventricular shunt system will cause morphological changes in the CSF pathway (Oi and Matsumoto 1986c) and will possibly lead to the isolation of compartments (Oi and Matsumoto 1985a,b, 1986a,b,c,d, 1987). These phenomena produce slit-like ventricle, most commonly in young infants, (Oi and Matsumoto 1987, 1989), and occasionally lead to the slit ventricle syndrome (Oi and Matsumoto 1987). The mechanism of development of an isolated ventricle after shunting is closely related to the presence of slit-like ventricle (Oi and Matsumoto 1985a). The mechanism of obstruction at the foramen of Monro in isolated unilateral hydrocephalus (Oi and Matsumoto 1985b, 1987) and the mechanism of aqueductal obstruction in isolated fourth ventricle (Oi and Matsumoto 1986a) occurring after shunt placement are essentially the same. Both occur in a previously communicating ventricular system and reduction of the size of all ventricles is seen initially after shunting in both cases (Oi and Matsumoto 1985b, 1986a). Then isolation gradually develops and re-enlargement of the

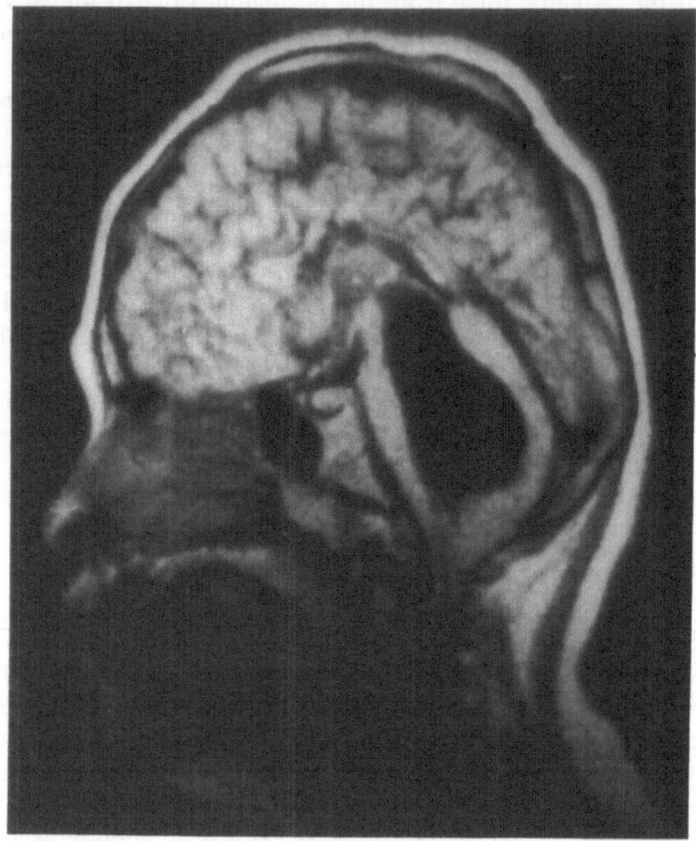

Fig. 1. Post-shunt isolated compartment Type III: isolated rhombencephalic ventricle (*IRCD*). A 7-year-old male with progressive scoliosis and upper extremity weakness occurring over the last several years after V-P shunt placement for communicating hydrocephalus. Note the dilated fourth ventricle and central canal on MRI sagittal section (T_1 weighted image). The lateral ventricles are slit-like with a V-P shunt in place

isolated compartment is observed. CSF dynamic studies using metrizamide CT ventriculography have confirmed the presence of a one-way valve either at the foramen of Monro (Oi and Matsumoto 1985b) or the aqueduct (Oi and Matsumoto 1986a), and pressure gradients between the compartments have also been recorded (Oi and Matsumoto 1985b, 1986a,b). We suggest that similar isolation may occur after placement of a shunt in the lateral ventricle in cases of communicating holo-neural canal dilatation (HNCD, stage IV hydrocephalic stage). Various types of isolation (I to IV) may then develop, depending upon the site of occlusion. (Fig.1)

Acknowledgments. The authors gratefully acknowledge the secretarial assistance of Ms. Sonoe Tsukumo. This study was supported by Grant No.3

(Intractable Hydrocephalus: Chairman Professor Haruhiko Kikuchi) from the Ministry of Health and Welfare, Japan.

References

Bering EA Jr (1955) Choroid plexus and arterial pulsation of cerebrospinal fluid; demonstration of the choroid plexuses as a cerebrospinal pump. Arch Neurol Psychiatry 73: 165–172

Conway LW (1967) Hydrodynamic studies in syringomyelia. J Neurosurg 27: 501–514

De Feo DR, Foltz FL, Hamilton AE (1975) Double compartment hydrocephalus in a patient with cysticercosis meningitis. Surg Neurol 4: 247–251

Gardner WJ (1965) Hydrodynamic mechanism of syringomyelia: its relationship to myelocele. J Neurosurg Psychiatry 28: 247–259

Gardner, WJ, Angel J (1959) The mechanism of syringomyelia and its surgical correction. Clin Neurosurg 6: 131–140

Kaufman B, Weiss MH, Young HF, Nulsen FE (1973) Effects of prolonged cerebrospinal fluid shunting on the skull and brain. J Neurosurg 38: 288–297

Krayenbuhl H (1974) Evaluation of different surgical approaches in the treatment of syringomyelia. Clin Neurol Neurosurg 77: 110–128

Krayenbuhl H, Benini A (1971) A new surgical approach in the treatment of hydromyelia and syringomyelia: The embryological basis and the first results. J Coll Surg Edinb 16: 147–161

Oi S, Matsumoto S (1985a) Slit ventricles as a cause of isolated ventricles after shunting. Nerv Syst Child 1: 189–193

Oi S, Matsumoto S (1985b) Pathophysiology of nonneoplastic obstruction of the foramen of Monro and progressive unilateral hydrocephalus. Neurosurgery 17: 891–896

Oi S, Matsumoto S (1986a) Pathophysiology of aqueductal obstruction in isolated IV ventricle after shunting. Nerv Syst Child 2: 282–286

Oi S, Matsumoto S (1986b) Isolated fourth ventricle. J Pediatr Neurosci 2: 125–133

Oi S, Matsumoto S (1986c) Morphological findings of post-shunt slit ventricle in experimental canine hydrocephalus. Aspects of causative factors of isolated ventricles and slit ventricle syndrome. Nerv Syst Child 2: 179–184

Oi S, Matsumoto S (1986d) Dynamic change in intracranial pressure in slit-like ventricles and isolated ventricles in childhood hydrocephalus after shunt placement. In: Ishii S (ed) Hydrocephalus. Excerpta Medica, pp. 135–147

Oi S, Matsumoto S (1987) Infantile hydrocephalus and slit ventricle syndome in early infancy. Nerv Syst Child 3: 145–150

Oi S, Matsumoto S (1989) Hydrocephalus in premature infants — Characteristics and therapeutic problems. Nerv Syst Child 5: 76–82

Oi S, Matsumoto S, Kudo H, et al. (1991) Hydromyelic hydrocephalus — Correlation of hydromyelia with various stages of hydrocephalus in post-shunt isolated hydrocephalus. J Neurosurg 74(3): 371–379

Raimondi AJ, Samuelson G, Yarzagaray L, Norton T (1969) Atresia of the foramina of Luschka and Magendie: The Dandy-Walker cyst. J Neurosurg 31: 202–216

Schlesinger EB, Antunes JL, Michelsen WJ, Louis KM (1981) Hydromyelia: Clinical presentation and comparison of modalities of treatment. Neurosurgery 9: 356–365

Sullivan, LP, Stears, JC, Ringel, SP (1988) Resolution of syringomyelia and Chiari I malformation by ventriculoatrial shunting in a patient with pseudotumor cerebri and a lumboperitoneal shunt. Neurosurgery 22: 744–747

Yamada H, Oi S, Tamaki N, Matsumoto S, Taomoto K (to be published) Embryo-pathoetiology of congenital hydorcephalus in experimental models — Comparative morphological study of different models

Zimmerman RA, Bilaniuk LT, Gallo E (1978) Computed tomography of the trapped fourth ventricle. AJR 130: 503–506

IV. Neonatal and Childhood Hydrocephalus

52 — Epidemiological Survey of the Management of Fetal Hydrocephalus in the Kansai District of Japan

Kouzo Moritake, Mikio Takaya[1], Haruhiko Kikuchi, Kunio Yamamura[2], Norimasa Sagawa, Takahide Mori[3], and Takehiko Okuno[4]

Summary. In order to carry out an epidemiological survey on the management of fetal hydrocephalus, a questionnaire was sent to 179 major hospitals belonging to the Kinki District Obstetrical Gynecological Society. The authors studied the clinical state at discharge from the obstetrical institute and the follow-up results in 38 cases of fetal hydrocephalus identified in this survey. Of 28 infants delivered alive, 19 were shunted. Most shunts were placed within two weeks postnatally. Of 19 infants shunted, 9 experienced shunt complications and subsequently underwent shunt revision. Postnatal clinical outcome was classified into three grades according to the developmental quotient (DQ) of the infants. Of 20 infants born alive, 8 were normal, 5 were slightly disturbed, and 4 were severely disturbed. The clinical outcome in infants with hydrocephalus caused by aqueductal stenosis was better than that reported by other authors. The clinical outcome in infants with early shunt was better than in those without it. Early ventricular shunting following early induction of delivery was performed in nine infants. Infants treated this way had a better outcome than those not so treated. At the last assessment, the degree of both ventricular dilatation and brain atrophy found on imaging studies correlated well with the degree of neurological disturbance.

Keywords. Fetal hydrocephalus — Hydrocephalus — Shunt — Epidemiology

Introduction

The introduction of high resolution ultrasonography has allowed the diagnosis of intrauterine CNS anomalies (Johnson, et al. 1983 & 1985, Chervenak, et al. 1989, Morimoto, et al. 1989, Oi, et al. 1985). Recently, we have been consulted concerning the diagnosis and management of various fetal anomalies revealed by ultrasonography. In our clinical practice with these cases, we faced

[1] Department of Neurosurgery, Shimane Medical University, Izumo,
Departments of [2] Neurosurgery, [3] Gynecology and Obstetrics, and [4] Pediatrics, Kyoto University Medical School, Kyoto, Japan

many problems; to help resolve these we felt it necessary to have some practical guidelines on the management of intrauterine hydrocephalus. In order to investigate current management of fetal hydrocephalus in Japan, the authors conducted an epidemiological investigation in the Kansai District.

Materials and Methods

As a first step, questionnaires were sent to 179 major obstetric institutes which belong to the Kinki District Obstetrical Gynecological Society. The hospitals investigated in this survey were divided into four groups: university hospitals, national hospitals, public hospitals, and others.

As the second step, we sent individual questionnaires regarding the clinical events of 57 cases of fetal hydrocephalus which had been picked up by the first survey. The clinical state at discharge from the obstetrical institute and the follow-up results were studied.

Results

For each hospital group, the rate of valid replies to the first questionnaire was about 70%.

Table 1 shows the number of institutes which replied, the number of institutes with hydrocephalic fetuses, the total number of deliveries, and the number of hydrocephalic fetuses in each hospital group. The number of institutes which returned valid replies was 125. Of these, 35 (28%), had experienced hydrocephalic fetuses. Hydrocephalus was found more frequently in males than in females. The overall prevalence rate of hydrocephalus per 1000 deliveries was 0.278. This rate was much higher in the university hospital group than in the other groups.

Table 1. Details of the epidemilological survey of fetal hydrocephalus in four hospital groups

Hospital groups	No. of institutes which replied	No. of institutes with hydrocephalic fetuses	No. of total deliveries in 3 years	No. of hydrocephalic fetuses		
				Male	Female	Total
University hospitals	12	10	16725	13	8	21
National hospitals	9	2	17220	1	1	2
Public hospitals	53	11	85748	9	6	15
Others	51	12	85289	9	10	19
Total	125	35	204982	32	25	57

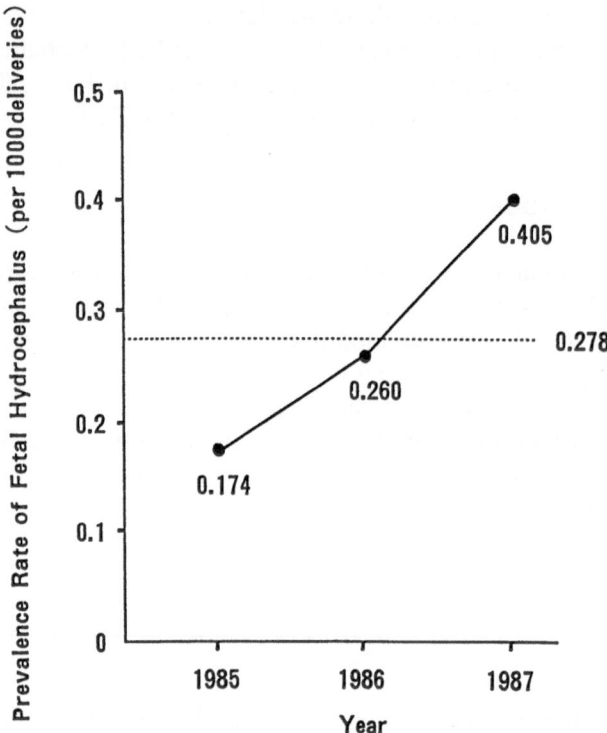

Fig. 1. Yearly changes in the prevalence rate of fetal hydrocephalus during the 3 years surveyed

Yearly changes in the prevalence rate of fetal hydrocephalus from 1985 to 1987 are shown in Fig. 1. The fetal hydrocephalus rate showed a yearly increase of approximately 1.5-fold in the 3 years of the study.

In 24 (63%) of 37 cases of fetal hydrocephalus, ultrasonographic study had been undertaken as a screening measure. In almost all cases the first diagnosis of hydrocephalus was made after the 24th week of pregnancy.

Thirty eight valid replies were obtained from the individual questionnaires. These showed that two fetuses were aborted and eight were still-born. Seven of 28 (73.6%) infants alive at delivery died within 7 days after birth. The early mortality rate, therefore, was 45%. Encephalocentesis was performed in two fetuses in the late gestational stage; both of these babies died soon after delivery. In no case was a ventriculo-amniotic shunt placed.

Of 28 infants delivered alive, 19 (68%) were shunted. Most shunts were placed within two weeks postnatally. Of 19 infants shunted, 9 (47%) experienced shunt complications and subsequently underwent shunt revision. The causes of shunt revision were shunt malfunction in six cases, shunt overfunction in four, and infection in two.

Postnatal clinical outcome was classified into three grades according to the developmental quotient (DQ) of infants. Of 20 infants born alive, 8 (40%) were normal, 5 (25%) were slightly disturbed, and 4 (20%) were severely disturbed.

Table 2. Causative and accompanying lesions of fetal hydrocephalus and clinical outcome

	Alive				Dead	Total
	Normal range	Slightly disturbed	Severely disturbed	Not described		
Primary Simple	1	1	2	0	4	8
Aqueduct stenosis	3	2	0	0	0	5
Arnold-Chiari Type II	1	2	1	2	1	7
Atresia of foramen of Monro	0	0	0	0	1	1
Agenesis of corpus callosum	0	0	0	0	2	2
Dandy-Walker syndrome	0	0	0	1	1	2
Holoporencephaly	0	0	0	0	3	3
Porencephaly	0	0	1	0	0	1
Hydranencephaly	0	0	0	0	1	1
Clover-leaf skull syndrome	0	0	0	0	1	1
Secondary Intracranial hemorrhage	1	0	0	0	2	3
Infection	1	0	0	0	0	1
Brain tumor	1	0	0	0	0	1
Unknown	0	0	0	0	2	2
Total	8	5	4	3	18	38

Table 3. Relationship between CSF shunting and clinical outcome

| | Time of placement (postnatal age) | Alive | | | | | |
		Normal range	Slightly disturbed	Severely disturbed	Unknown	Dead	Total
Ventricular shunting	≤ 1 Week	5	3	2	0	1	11
	1 Week < ≤ 1 Month	1	1	1	1	0	4
	1 Month <	1	0	1	1	1	4
Not shunted		1	1	0	1	5	8
Unknown		0	0	0	0	1	1

Table 4. Early induced delivery for early ventricular shunting and clinical outcome

| | Alive | | | | | |
	Normal range	Slightly disturbed	Severely disturbed	Not described	Dead	Total
Performed	3	0	1	0	5	9
Not performed	3	4	3	3	13	26
Not described	2	1	0	0	0	3

Table 5. Relationship between degree of ventricular dilatation and brain atrophy and clinical outcome

| Last assessment | | Clinical outcome | | |
		Normal range	Slightly disturbed	Severely disturbed
Ventricular dilatation	Normal/slight	5	2	1[a]
	Moderate	1	1	0
	Severe	0	1	2
Brain atrophy*	Normal/slight	4	1	0
	Moderate	0	1	0
	Severe	0	0	3

[a] multiple shunt revisions; * $P < 0.05$

Table 2 shows the classification of fetal hydrocephalus by cause. Thirty one cases were classified as primary hydrocephalus and 5 as secondary. Approximately half of all cases were accompanied by other serious central nervous system anomalies. The clinical outcome in infants with secondary hydrocephalus was much better than in those with primary hydrocephalus. Clinical outcome in all infants with Dandy-Walker syndrome, holoprosencephaly, porencephaly, or hydranencephaly was poor. However, the clinical outcome in infants with hydrocephalus caused by aqueductal stenosis was relatively good.

Table 3 shows the relationship between CSF shunting and clinical outcome. The clinical outcome in infants with early shunt was better than in those without it, although the difference was not statistically significant. Early ventricular shunting following early induction of delivery was performed in nine infants. Table 4 shows the effect of early induced delivery for early ventricular shunting on clinical outcome. Infants treated this way had a better outcome than those not so treated, although the difference was not statistically significant.

Table 5 shows the relationship between degree of ventricular dilatation and brain atrophy and clinical outcome at the last assessment, undertaken 18.2 months (mean) postnatally. The degree of both ventricular dilatation and brain atrophy found on imaging studies such as X-CT, ultrasonography, and MRI, correlated well with the degree of neurological disturbance. The relationship between brain atrophy and neurological disturbance was statistically significant ($P < 0.05$).

Discussion

The high rate of reply to questionnaires in this epidemiological survey reflects the great interest of obstetricians in fetal hydrocephalus. The yearly increase in the prevalence rate of fetal hydrocephalus also suggests the spread of intrauterine ultrasonograpy and the increasing interest of obstetricians in the diagnosis of fetal hydrocephalus.

Of the four hospital groups, the prevalence rate of fetal hydrocephalus was overwhelmingly highest in the university hospital group. The high incidence in this group can be attributed not only to their high-grade diagnostic techniques, but also to the fact that most suspected cases of intrauterine hydrocephalus are referred to them.

In more than half of the infants, ultrasonography was carried out as a screening measure. These cases could not have been diagnosed before the advent of ultrasonography. In almost all cases, however, hydrocephalus was first diagnosed after the 24th week of gestation. This suggests that intrauterine ultrasonograpy has not yet been popularized.

In no case where intrauterine surgery had been performed was the fetus born alive. There was no evidence that fetal surgery was effective in the better prognosis of fetal hydrocephalus (Chervenak, et al. 1985, Cochrane, et al. 1982). Postnatal clinical outcome correlated most with the causative and/or accompanying lesions of fetal hydrocephalus. Clinical outcome was very poor in cases of primary hydrocephalus complicated by other serious cental nervous system anomalies. On the other hand, clinical outcome in cases of simple hydrocephalus or secondary hydrocephalus was relatively good. These results are in accordance with those of other authors (Cochrane, et al. 1982, Oi, et al. 1985). The reason for the relatively good clinical outcome in infants with hydrocephalus caused by aqueductal stenosis seems to be due to improvements in both shunt systems and shunting techniques.

The better clinical outcome in infants with early shunt than in those without it suggests the effectiveness of this treatment for fetal hydrocephalus. The last assessment findings, which showed a correlation between the degree of both ventricular dilatation and brain atrophy on imaging studies and the degree of neurological disturbance, also support the effectiveness of early shunt treatment.

On the basis of the results of this epidemiological survey, the authors propose a tentative guideline for the management of fetal hydrocephalus. If intrauterine ultrasonography reveals hydrocephalus without serious anomalies or complications, we recommend that the fetus be born by elective Cesarean section at the time of pulmonary maturity, and that early ventricular shunting be carried out to minimize nervous system trauma resulting from hydrocephalus and the birth process.

Acknowledgments. This work was supported by a Japanese Ministry of Health and Welfare grant in aid for scientific research into "Intractable Hydrocephalus"

References

Chervenak FA, Berkowitz RL, Tortora M, Hobbins JC (1985). The management of fetal hydrocephalus Am J Obstet Gynecol 151: 933–942

Chervenak FA (1989) Current perspectives on the diagnosis, prognosis, and management of fetal hydrocephalus. In: Hill A, Volpe JJ (eds) Fetal Neurology. Raven, New York, pp 231–251

Cochrane DD, Myles ST (1982) Management of intrauterine hydrocephalus. J Neurosurg 57: 590–596

Johnson ML, Pretorius DH (1985) Ultrasonic diagnosis of fetal and neonatal hydrocephalus. Clin Neurosurg 32: 574–592

Johnson ML, Pretorius D, Clewell WH, Meier PR, Manchester D (1983) Fetal hydrocephalus: Diagnosis and management. Semin Perinatol 7: 83–89

Morimoto K, Yoshimine T, Hayakawa T, Mogami H, Sugita N, Tasaka K, Tanizawa O, Suehara N, Takeuchi T, Seino Y, Minaki T (1989) Antenatal detection of developing nervous system abnormalities and perinatal surgical management. Neurol Surg 17: 965–971

Oi S, Yamada H, Sasaki K, Matsumoto S (1985) Diagnosis and treatment of fetal hydrocephalus. Problems in evolution of the hydrocephalic state and selection for intrauterine shunt procedure. Neurol Med Chir (Tokyo) 25: 195–202

53 — Congenital Central Nervous System Malformations Associated with Hydrocephalus

Mirko Mircevski, Danica Mircevska, Roza Baševska, and Branka Stanković

Summary. We observed and operated on 1124 patients with hydrocephalus. Of these, 642 children had congenital malformation of the brain and spinal cord, except for such congenital malformations of the vessels as angiomas and aneurysms, accompanying the hydrocephalus.

From our 20 years of personal experience (1969–1989) we can rightfully say that with early diagnosis of the malformation and the hydrocephalus and their early surgical treatment, we can achieve satisfactory results with rehabilitation and socialization of the children within their own living environment.

Keywords. Hydrocephalus — CVS malformation — Dysraphism — Spina bifida

Introduction

Malformations of the central nervous system frequently occur in our region of Yugoslavia. Of a population of 4 million, we are confronted with a malformation rate of 1.2%, which means that out of every 1000 newborn children we have 12 born with malformations. Of these malformations, 20% are anomalies of the central nervous system, individually, or are associated with other malformations. Of this number 60% are complicated with hydrocephalus.

In comparison with other parts of Yugoslavia and the other Balkan countries we have a higher rate of accompanied and isolated hydrocephalus; this is due, in our view, to high rotality and to the inadequately organized control of pre- and postnatal medical care.

Birth control, adequate pre-natal care, and, in many cases, the application of sonography in pregnant woman, can reduce the birth of malformed children.

During the study of our material we ascertained that a great number of

[1] Department of Neurosurgery, Medical Faculty, University of "Cyril and Methodij," Skopje, Macedonia, Yugoslavia
[2] Hospital of Neurology and Psychiatry, Medical Faculty, University of Belgrade, Belgrade, Serbia, Yugoslavia

Table 1. Distribution in age group order

Age	No. of children (n)
0–1 month	132
1–6 months	425
6–12 months	58
1–4 years	27
Total	642

Table.2. Localization of malformation associated with hydrocephalus

Type of anomaly	No. of children (n)
Intracranial	198
Extracranial-cranial	444
Total	642

children have one or more central nervous system malformations associated with hydrocephalus. This commits us to early diagnosis of the anomalies and the hydrocephalus and to early surgical treatment of the two manifest pathological conditions.

Clinical Material

During the last 20 years (1969–1989), we observed and operated on 1124 patients who had hydrocephalus. In the 0–4 year age group 642 cases were associated with congenital anomalies. Analysis of our material shows that it concerns children, mostly newborn or during the first 4 years after birth (Table 1).

We divided the children into the following two groups, in accordance with the type of central nervous system and spinal cord malformation: Intracranial-cranial and extracranial (Table 2).

Included in intracranial malformations of the brain were: Agenesis corporis callosum, variable stenosis of aqueductus sylvi, arachnoidal cysts in the III ventricle, suprasellar region or anywhere else in the endocranium, Dandy-Walker and Arnold Chiari Syndromes, arteriovenous malformation (AVM), congenital tumors and tumors of the choroid plexus (Table 3).

Extracranial-cranial malformations associated with hydrocephalus included encephalocele, meningomyelocele, craniosynostosis and platibasia (Table 4).

Malformations of the lower parts of the spinal cord such as spina bifida cystica in the lumbosacral region, were frequently associated with hydrocephalus (Table 5).

The children were admitted directly from the obstetric and children's hospitals where they were born and from their homes. Most of them were

Table.3. Intracranial anomalies associated with hydrocephalus

Malformation	No. of children (n)
Agenesis corporis callosi	14
Stenosis aqueductus Sylvi	75
Benign intracranial cysts	64
Dandy-Walker syndrome	18
Arnold-Chiari malformation	11
Cerebrospinal fluid fistula	8
Tumor of the choroid plexus	8
Total	198

Table 4. Extracranial anomalies associated with hydrocephalus

Malformation	No. of children (n)
Cranium bifidum	139
Dysraphic anomalies:	
Spina bifida occulta	273
Craniosynostosis	28
Platibasia	4
Total	444

Table 5. Dysraphic anomalies: Cranium bifidum and spina bifida associated with hydrocephalus, as in Percentages

Malformation	No. of children (n)	% Hydrocephalus
Encephalocele occipitalis	64	92
Encephalocele parietalis	16	16
Encephalocele frontalis	3	60
Encephalocele syncipitalis	56	12
Total	139	

weak and had been inadequately treated. Because of this we had problems concerning diagnosis of the pathological process and preparation of surgical treatment.

We made our diagnosis on the basis of the clinical manifestation of anamnesis, X-rays of the head and spinal cord, EEG, sonography (pre- and postnatal), computed tomography (CT) scan, gamma cisternography, myelography and magnetic resonance imaging (MRI).

Surgical Treatment

All of the 1124 patients observed and diagnosed with hydrocephalus were operated. Of them, 642 had CNS anomalies. Children who had congenital

Table 6. Complications after operation on hydrocephalus

	No. of children (n)	%
Skin infection	64	10
Liquid fistula	38	6
Shunt malfunction	24	3.7
Total	126	

malformations of the central nervous system and spinal cord were operated immediately after the diagnosis of these anomalies and hydrocephalus.

Firstly, we treated the hydrocephalus with a shunt operation and later we treated the malformation or we treated both together.

We used two shunt operations: Ventriculo-auricu-lostomy and ventriculo-peritoneostomy. Drainage systems used were: Hayer-Pudenz, Spitz-Holter, Hakim-Cordis, and Raimondi.

All 642 children underwent surgical treatment as follows: ventriculo-auriculostomy in 528 children (82%), ventriculo-peritoneostomy in 114 children (18%), and revision of shunt in 71 children (11%).

After the operation we had complications consisting of early and later shunt malfunction, cerebrospinal liquid fistula, infection of the operated wound, and various obstructions of the drainage system (Table 6).

Hospital mortality of the 642 operated children was 4.8%.

Discussion

Intracranial and extracranial malformations of the central nervous system are commonly united with hydrocephalus. Agenesis of the corpus callosum, and partial or total stenosis of the aqueductus Sylvi cause the early manifestation of the most difficult forms of obstructive hydrocephalus which are known clinically as hydranencephalus.

When congenital obstruction occurs on the level of the foramina of Magendie and Luschka a cyst is manifested on the level of the IV ventricle and hydrocephalus ensues. The Arnold-Chiari syndrom with all five variations also causes the appearance of hydrocephalus immediately after birth.

Arachnoidal, porencephalic, cortical, IIIrd ventricular or and endocranial malformations cause the early appearance of hydrocephalus.

Dysraphic anomalies of the spina bifida type, which can be associated with Arnold-Chiari, early obstruction on the level of the posterior cranial fossa or obstruction through latent infection (which causes arachnoiditis and interference in subarachnoidal absorption and circulation of the cerebral spinal fluid) can be causes of latent communicating hydrocephalus which is manifested at a later time.

The percentage of hydrocephalus prevalent in these intracranial and extracranial indigenous defects is high; its rate being from 12% to 92% in some malformations on the level of the brain or in meningomyelocele.

Table 7. Early and later results of surgical treatment

	No. of children (n)	%
Hospital post operation mortality	31	4.8
Follow up: Excellent	98	13.6
Good	231	36.3
Fair	185	31
Unchanged	97	13.5
Total	642	

Early diagnosis of inborn malformation and hydrocephalus is imperative for early surgical treatment. We have used many treatment methods, which consist of removal of the malformation and shunting of the hydrocephalus.

Surgical success depended on how soon the surgical treatment of the malformation and hydrocephalus took place. All of the 642 children observed were in need of surgical treatment, once or twice depending on the malformation and the hydrocephalus; all of them survived the operation.

During hospitalization and the control period we revised the shunts of 71 children (11%). In the postoperative period 31 (4.8%) children died. The reason for the deaths was previous weakening in children with many malformations. Most of these children had heart problems, infection, and shunt malfunction.

For follow up we placed the children into four groups: Excellent, good, improved, and unchanged (Table 7).

In the first three groups the rehabilitation and socialization of the children was satisfactory and they adjusted to normal life. Some of the operated children were lost due to other illnesses and they became part of the generally quite high mortality rate of small children in our region of Yugoslavia.

Early diagnosis of the pathological process and early surgical intervention enables recovery and allows these children to live a normal life.

References

Andeweg J (1976) The cause of hydrocephalus. Bronder-Offset, Rotterdam, pp 249–274

Di Rocco C, Caldarelli M, Trapani D (1981) Infratentorial arachnoid cysts in children. Childs Brain 8: 119–133

Lapras C, Dechaume JP, Fischer G (1968) La malformation D'Arnold-Chiari. Cah Méd Lyonnais 44: 3359

Lepoire J, Lapras C (1967) Traitement de l'hdrocéphalie non tumoral du nourisson par la dérivation ventriculo-atriale. Neurochirurgie 13: 209–342

Matson D (1969) Neurosurgery of infancy and childhood, 2nd edn. Charles C. Thomas, Springfield

Matsumoto S (ed) (1986) Annual review of hydrocephalus, Vol. 4

Mazza C, Pasqualin A, Da Pian R (1980) Results of treatment with ventriculoatrial and ventriculoperitoneal shunt in infantile nontumoral hydrocephalus. Childs Brain 7: No 1

Milhorat HT (1978) Pediatric neurosurgery. FA Devis, Philadelphia

Mircevski M, Mircevska D, Basevska R, Mikolova T, Bojadziev I, Jovkovski S (1977a) Surgical treatment of encephalocele complicated by Hydrocephalus. Mod Probl Paediat 18: 146–148

Mircevski M, Nikolova T, Bojadziev I, Basevska R, Dolgova V, Brezovska K (1977b) Gamma-cysternography in the diagnosis of primary and secondary hydrocephalus, associated with other congenital malformations (abstract). Sixth International Congress of Neurological Surgery, Sao Paulo, Brazil, 1977. Excerpta Medica, p 487

Raimondi AJ, Robinson JS, Kuwamura K (1977) Complications of ventriculo-peritoneal shunting and a critical comparison of the three-piece and one-piece systems. Childs Brain 3: 321–342

Till K (1975) Paediatric Neurosurgery for paediatricians and neurosurgeons. Blackwell Scientific, London

54 — Ventriculo-Peritoneal Shunt as an Initial Treatment Modality for Premature Infants with Hydrocephalus

Susumu Wakai, Kunihiko Watanabe, Youji Andoh, Masakatsu Nagai,[1] *and Goro Tanaka*[2]

Summary. The use of a ventriculo-peritoneal (V-P) shunt as an initial treatment modality in premature infants with hydrocephalus is still controversial. During a 3-year period, we treated seven infants (four males and three females), using a V-P shunt without prior placement of external ventricular drainage or a subcutaneous reservoir. The gestational age at birth ranged from 24 to 34 weeks (mean, 27.6 weeks). The weight at surgery ranged from 1060 to 2340 g (mean, 1580 g). Four infants had severe respiratory distress syndrome (RDS). Hemorrhage was revealed in two while there was no ultra-sonographic or computed tomography (CT) evidence of hemorrhage in the other two. The cause of hydrocephalus or an associated disorder in the remaining three infants was meningitis, aqueductal stenosis and myelomeningocele, respectively. The timing of shunt placement was 1–121 days (mean, 49.8 days) after birth. A pediatric Hakim ball valve was used in five infants and a Mini-LPV (diaphragm valve) was used in one infant. No valve was connected in the remaining infant. Shunt revision was not needed in three infants. Infection occurred in only one case; the infant with postmeningitic hydrocephalus. The other six developed neither infection nor skin erosion. Psychomotor development was rated as normal in five, retarded in one (postmeningitic) and disabled in one (posthemorrhagic). The present results suggest that a V-P shunt can be used as the surgical procedure of first choice in treating premature infants with hydrocephalus without serious complications.

Keywords. Hydrocephalus — Premature infants — V-P shunt

Introduction

The use of a ventriculo-peritoneal (V-P) shunt as an initial treatment modality in premature infants with hydrocephalus, particularly posthemorrhagic hydrocephalus, has been and still is controversial (James et al. 1984; Pezzotta et al.

---

[1] Department of Neurosurgery and [2] 2nd Department of Pediatrics, Dokkyo University School of Medicine, Tochigi, 321–02 Japan

Table 1. Summary of seven premature infants with hydrocephalus treated with a V-P shunt

Case no (n)	Sex	Gestational age (weeks)	Body weight at birth and at surgery (g)		Timing of V-P shunt (days)[a]	Shunt system	Shunt revision	Causes of hydrocephalus	Outcome
1	M	27	1300	1060	17	No valve	0	SEH/IVH (Gr3)	Normal
2	M	29	1250	1100	14	Hakim	1	SEH/IVH (Gr4)	Disabled
3	F	24	790	1810	110	Hakim	0	RDS-related	Normal
4	F	25	735	1200	70	Hakim, bil	3	Meningitis	Retarded
5	M	24	855	2340	121	Hakim	3	RDS-related	Normal
6	M	30	1645	1320	16	Mini-LPV	2	Myelomeningocele	Normal
7	F	35	2255	2255	1	Hakim	0	Aqued. stenosis	Normal

[a] Days after birth

SEH/IVH, subependymal and/or intraventricular hemorrhage; Gr, Papile's grading of SEH/IVH (1978); RDS, respiratory distress syndrome; Hakim, pediatric type (Cordis Corp.); Mini-LPV, mini low profile valve (Heyer-Schulte Corp.)

1987; Hislop et al. 1988; Oi and Matsumoto 1989). As alternative treatments, external ventricular drainage (EVD) (Kreusser et al. 1984; Rhodes et al. 1987; Weniger et al. 1988) or intermittent CSF withdrawal via a subcutaneous reservoir (McComb et al. 1983; Gaskill et al. 1988) have been widely utilized. During a three-year period, we treated seven infants, using a V-P shunt without prior placement of EVD or a subcutaneous reservoir. This report concerns the results of V-P shunt placement in these seven premature infants. Some problems of various CSF diversion methods are also discussed.

Patients and Methods

Of the seven infants we treated in this study four were male and three were female. Their gestational age at birth ranged from 24 to 34 weeks (mean, 27.6 weeks). Their weights at birth and at surgery ranged from 735 to 2255 g (mean, 1260 g) and from 1060 to 2340 g (mean, 1580 g), respectively (Table 1).

Four infants had severe respiratory distress syndrome (RDS). Subependymal and/or intraventricular hemorrhage (SEH/IVH) was demonstrated on CT before surgery in two of these infants. Hemorrhage was not apparent on ultrasonography in the other two infants and hydrocephalus only was seen on their CTs before surgery. Since there were no other underlying disorders leading to hydrocephalus in these two infants, the cause of their hydrocephalus was considered to be related to RDS and is called RDS-related in this paper, although there is a possibility that a small SEH/IVH was missed by ultrasonography. Thus, the cause of hydrocephalus was hemorrhage (SEH/IVH) in two cases, RDS-related in two, meningitis in one, and aqueductal stenosis in one. The remaining infant had an associated myelomeningocele (Table 2). The latter two infants were intentionally delivered before term for surgical treatment at 30 and 35 weeks of gestation, respectively (Table 2).

The timing of the first shunt placement was 1–121 days after birth (mean, 49.8 days). A Hakim low pressure valve, pediatric type (21–62 mmH$_2$O, Cordis Corp.) was used in four infants, a Hakim medium pressure valve, pediatric type (113 mmH$_2$O) in one and a Mini-LPV medium pressure valve

Table 2. Causes of hydrocephalus in seven premature infants treated with V-P shunt

Congenital		2
Myelomeningocele	1	
Aqueductal stenosis	1	
RDS-related		4
SEH/IVH	2	
No hemorrhage	2	
Meningitis		$\frac{1}{7}$

SEH/IVH, subependymal and/or intraventricular hemorrhage; RDS, respiratory distress syndrome

Table 3. Reasons for shunt revision

Proximal obstruction	2
Distal obstruction	2
Disconnection	1
Undershunting	1
Infection (case 4)	
Removal	2
Skin erosion	1

(51–110 mmH$_2$O, Heyer-Schulte Corp.) in one. No valve was connected in the remaining infant. In Case 4 (postmeningitic hydrocephalus), the shunt system was initially placed on both sides because of asymmetric dilatation of the lateral ventricles (Table 1).

A ventricular catheter was implanted via a burr hole placed in the right, if unilateral, posterior parietal region. A peritoneal counterpart was inserted towards a Douglass pouch through a small vertical incision lateral to the navel. No relay point was made between the proximal and distal incisions. Before implantation all catheters and valve devices were soaked in a solution containing 60 mg of gentamycin in 500 ml of normal saline. The wound was also flushed with the same solution before its closure. Anti-staphylococcal antibiotics were administered intravenously for 7–10 days after surgery.

Results

During the 6–41 month follow-up period shunt revision was not needed in three infants, whereas it had to be carried out in four (total, nine revisions). The reasons for shunt revision were: Obstruction of ventricular (2) or peritoneal catheter (2), disconnection of the catheter (1), undershunting (1), and infection (3). Infection occurred in only one infant (case 4); the infant with postmeningitic hydrocephalus (Table 3). In this case both ventricular catheters were replaced by new ones because of the relapse of meningitis. Thereafter the whole shunt system was removed because of skin erosion which followed the placement of EVD on both sides. Finally, a Hakim low pressure valve, pediatric type, was placed on the left side only. The other six infants developed neither infection nor skin erosion.

Psychomotor development was rated as normal at 6–41 months after birth in five infants, retarded (mild) at 15 months after birth in one (postmeningitic), and disabled at 28 months after birth in one (posthemorrhagic). This last poor result was related to severe asphyxia at delivery as well as to associated parenchymal hemorrhage (case 2, Papile's grade 4) (Papile et al. 1978). This patient still has large ventricles with marked brain atrophy. In the other six patients, the ventricles became small or normalized and the cortical mantle appeared prominent on CT at two months to three years after the last shunt insertion (Figs. 1 and 2).

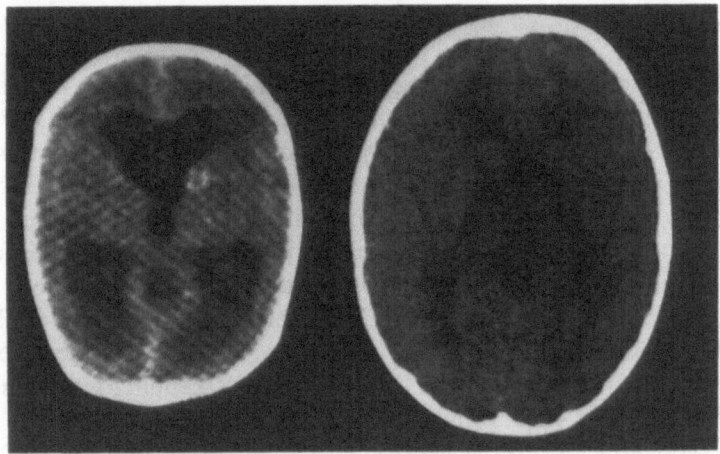

Fig. 1. Computerized tomography scans of case 1 (posthemorrhagic hydrocephalus) taken before surgery (*left*) and 2.5 years after surgery (*right*). *Left*, moderate degree of ventriculomegaly and subependymal hemorrhage are seen. Although no hemorrhage is noted in the ventricle on this CT slice, mild ventricular hemorrhage was seen on other slices. *Right*, the ventricular size is normalized without parenchymal lesions. Psychomotor development of this child is normal at 41 months after birth

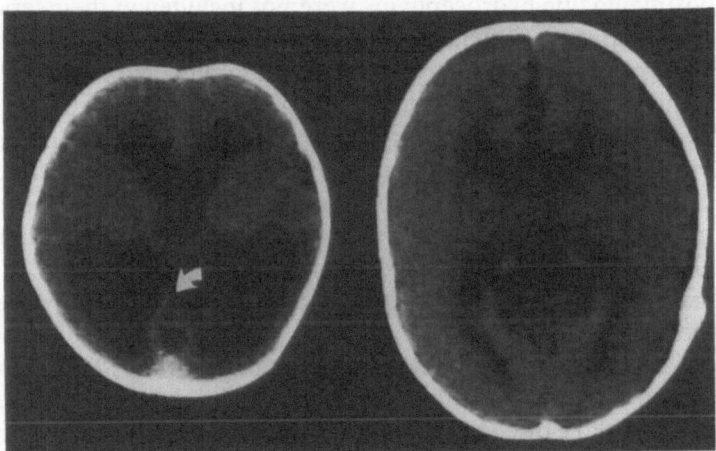

Fig. 2. Computerized tomography scans of case 7 (aqueductal stenosis) taken on the day of birth (*left*) and two months after surgery (*right*). *Left*, marked degree of hydrocephalus is noted, with a small ventricular diverticulum protruding from the medial wall of the right trigone (*arrow*). *Right*, the ventricular size has been normalized. Agenesis of corpus callosum has become apparent. Psychomotor development of this infant is normal at six months after birth

Discussion

There are various methods of CSF diversion in the treatment of premature infants with hydrocephalus. There is no doubt that the placement of a V-P or a ventriculo-atrial (V-A) shunt is the best way of controlling intracranial pressure (ICP) and thus of protecting the cortical mantle (Etches et al. 1987). Because of the high infection rate in early shunt placement, which was as high as 50% (James et al. 1984), and because of the generally poor condition of the infants, however, several management options were introduced. The placement of a ventricular catheter to allow prolonged EVD has been used successfully in premature infants (Kreusser et al. 1984; Rhodes et al. 1987; Weniger et al. 1988). Disadvantages of this technique are the risk of ascending infection and electrolyte disturbances. An alternative approach has been to place a subcutaneous reservoir attached to the ventricular catheter (McComb et al. 1983; Gaskill et al. 1988). Though there are no such disadvantages in this method, control of ICP is intermittent, resulting in possible ill effects upon the developing brain. Medical means such as acetazolamide or lumbar puncture taps may be valuable in allowing the general condition of the baby to improve. Those measures are, however, only employed temporarily (Anwar et al. 1985; Kreusser et al. 1985; Shinner et al. 1985).

Oi and Matsumoto (1989) reported only one infection (4.6%) out of 22 shunt procedures in treating premature infants with hydrocephalus of various causes. Patients with postmeningitic hydrocephalus were not included in their series. In the present series, only one infant with postmeningitic hydrocephalus developed infection after shunt placement. Up till now the outcome is encouraging although the number of infants so treated is small. Oi and Matsumoto's (1989) results and ours suggest that a V-P shunt can be used as the surgical procedure of first choice in treating premature infants with hydrocephalus due to SEH/IVH, as well as hydrocephalus due to congenital causes without serious complications. A prospective comparative study in large patient populations is, however, needed to discover which treatment option (e.g., shunt vs subcutaneous reservoir) really decreases infections and revisions and improves the neurodevelopmental outcome.

In this series, two babies with fetal hydrocephalus who were delivered intentionally before term underwent shunt surgery 16 days (case 6) and 1 day (case 7) after birth. Both babies have been developing normally so far, although case 7 had a ventricular diverticulum, which is said to be a sign of severe hydrocephalus (Fig. 2) (Naidich et al. 1982; Wakai and Nagai 1984).

Acknowledgment. Many thanks are extended to the doctors and the nursing staff at the Neonatal Intensive Care Unit for their painstaking efforts in treating these premature babies; babies who could not have done well without their meticulous care.

References

Anwar M, Kadom S, Hiatt IM, Heygi T (1985) Serial lumbar punctures in prevention of post-hemorrhagic hydrocephalus in preterm infants. J Pediatr 107: 446–450

Etches PC, Chir B, Ward TF, Bhui PS, Peters KL, Robertson CM (1987) Outcome of shunted posthemorrhagic hydrocephalus in premature infants. Pediatr Neurol 3: 136–140

Gaskill SJ, Marlin AE, Rivera S (1988) The subcutaneous ventricular reservoir: An effective treatment for posthemorrhagic hydrocephalus. Nerv Syst Child 4: 291–295

Hislop JE, Dubowitz LMS, Kaiser AM, Singh MP, Whitelaw AGL (1988) Outcome of infants shunted for post-haemorrhagic ventricular dilatation. Dev Med Child Neurol 30: 451–456

James HE, Bejar R, Merritt A, Gluck L, Coen R, Mannino F (1984) Management of hydrocephalus secondary to intracranial hemorrhage in the high risk newborn. Neurosurgery 14: 612–618

Kreusser KL, Tarby TJ, Taylor D, Kovnar E, Hill A, Conry JA, Volpe JJ (1984) Rapidly progressive post-hemorrhagic hydrocephalus: Treatment with external ventricular drainage. Am J Dis Child 138: 633–637

Kreusser KL, Tarby TJ, Kovnar E, Taylor D, Hill A, Volpe JJ (1985) Serial lumbar punctures for at least temporary amelioration of neonatal posthemorrhagic hydrocephalus. Pediatrics 75: 719–724

McComb JG, Ramos AD, Platzker ACG, Henderson DJ, Segall HD (1983) Management of hydrocephalus secondary to intraventricular hemorrhage in the preterm infant with a subcutaneous ventricular catheter reservoir. Neurosurgery 13: 295–300

Naidich TP, McLone DG, Hahn YS, Hanaway J (1982) Atrial diverticula in severe hydrocephalus. AJNR 3: 257–266

Oi S, Matsumoto S (1989) Hydrocephalus in premature infants. Characteristics and therapeutic problems. Nerv Syst Child 5: 76–82

Papile LA, Burnstein J, Burstein R, Koffler H (1978) Incidence and evolution of subependymal and intraventricular hemorrhage: A study of infants with birth weights less than 1500 gm. J Pediatr 92: 529–534

Pezzotta S, Locatelli D, Bonfanti N, Sfogliarini R, Bruschi L, Rondini G (1987) Shunt in high-risk newborns. Nerv Syst Child 3: 114–116

Rhodes TT, Edwards WH, Saunders RL, Harbaugh RE, Little CLC, Morgan LJ, Sargent SK (1987) External ventricular drainage for initial treatment of neonatal posthemorrhagic hydrocephalus: Surgical and neurodevelopmental outcome. Pediatr Neurosci 13: 255–262

Shinner S, Gammon K, Bergman EW, Epstein M, Freeman J (1985) Management of hydrocephalus in infancy: use of acetazolamide and furosemide to avoid cerebrospinal fluid shunts. J Pediatr 107: 31–37

Wakai S, Nagai M (1984) Ventricular diverticulum. J Neurol Neurosurg Psychiatry 47: 514–517

Weniger M, Simbruner G, Salzer HR, Rosenkranz M, Lesigang C (1988) Externe Ventrikeldrainage bei Neugeborenen mit rasch wachsendem posthämorrhagischem Hydrozephalus. Wien Klin Wochenschr 100: 561–564

55 — Surgical Outcome of Neonatal Hydrocephalus

Concezio Di Rocco, Antonello Ceddia, Aldo Iannelli, and Liverana Lauretti[1]

Summary. Two hundred and eight patients with non-tumoral congenital hydrocephalus underwent CSF shunting during their first month of life. Ultrasonograpy was the most frequently utilized tool; hydrocephalus was recognized during pregnancy in 52% of the cases. Hydrocephalus was associated with myelomeningocele in 97 infants; in 38 subjects the ventricular dilation was secondary to aqueductal stenosis. Post-hemorrhagic and post-infective hydrocephalus accounted for only 20 and 13 cases, respectively. At follow-up observations, normal psychomotor development was recorded in only a fourth of the infants; however, a high survival rate was observed in our series (91.8%). CSF infection was the most common cause of death, followed by the natural evolution of congenital associated malformations. Shunt revision did not significantly influence morbidity and mortality. On the other hand, CSF infections appeared to have a hegative influence on prognosis. In our experience, the prognosis for hydrocephalus operated on in the first month of life does not differ from that for hydrocephalus operated on later in life.

Keywords. Congenital hydrocephalus — Prenatal diagnosis — Early surgery — Mortality — Late outcome

Introduction

The possibility of recognizing hydrocephalus in utero, at the end of the fourth month of pregnancy (Williamson et al. 1984), has stressed the current lack of reliable prognostic factors to predict the outcome of this pathological condition. Attempts to treat the hydrocephalus in utero have proved to be of no practical value in the majority of cases. Thus, at the present time, the main interest of the neurosurgeon has again shifted to evaluating, after having reached the correct diagnosis and demonstrated the progression of ventricular dilation, the possible advantages of early surgical treatment, to be performed

---

[1] Section of Pediatric Neurosurgery, Catholic University Medical School, 00168 Rome, Italy

Table 1. Etiology of hydrocephalus

Etiology	No. of cases (n)
Associated with MM	97
Secondary to aqueductal stenosis	38
Post-hemorrhagic	20
Post-infective	13
Communicating	12
Associated with holoprosencephaly	10
Associated with arachnoid cyst	9
Associated with Dandy-Walker cyst	5
Associated with encephalomeningocele	4

MM, myelomeningocele

during the first weeks of postnatal life. There is general agreement on the rationale of an operation carried out soon after birth, based mainly on the diminished time during which the immature brain is exposed to an abnormally elevated intracranial pressure. However, such a theoretical advantage must be weighed against the risk of surgical procedure performed in the very young infant. In the present report we evaluate the mortality observed in a series of 208 infants with congenital hydrocephalus who were surgically treated during the first month of life.

Patients and Methods

During the period January 1975–January 1989, in the Neurosurgical Department of the Catholic University Medical School, Rome, 208 unselected hydrocephalic newborns underwent a CSF shunting procedure before the end of their first month of life. These patients were followed from the operation for a minimum period of 1 year to a maximum of 15 years (mean follow-up period: 6 years). One hundred and fifteen subjects were male and 93 were female. The etiology of the hydrocephalus is shown in Table 1.

In 108 cases the diagnosis of hydrocephalus was reached during pregnancy, by means of ultrasonography, and was confirmed after birth by computed tomography (CT) scan. In the remaining cases, the diagnosis was made after birth, by means of ultrasound, CT scan, and magnetic resonance (MR) imaging techniques; cerebral angiography and fractioned encephalography were utilized in the first patients of the series. All investigations were carried out in patients whose head circumference at birth was >2 standard deviations above the mean both for gestational age and for birth length, or when the occurrence of malformations of the CNS, such as, for instance, myelomeningocele suggested the presence of an associated ventricular dilation. In nine infants the surgical procedure consisted of a ventriculo-atrial CSF shunt, using a Pudenz valve system. The remaining 199 newborns underwent a ventriculo-peritoneal CSF diversion procedure. The Raimondi Unishunt system was utilized in 120 cases,

Table 2. Surgical results

	No. of patients (n)
Normal	50
Mild neurological deficit[a] (socially independent)	90
Mild to severe neurological deficit (socially dependent)	40
Dead	17
Lost to follow-up	11

[a]including 64 patients with myelomeningocele (*MM*)

Table 3. Causes of death (17 cases)

Causes		No. of cases (n)
CSF infection	7	(Within first 2 years p.o.)
Postoperative	2	(Within first month p.o.)
Chiari malformation	3	(Within first 3 years p.o.)
Renal insufficiency	1	(After 6 years p.o.)
Evolution of the disease (holoprosencephaly)	1	(After 2 years p.o.)
Prematurity	1	(Within first month p.o.)
Accidental head injury	1	(After 8 years p.o.)
Pulmonary infection		
(unrelated to the Hy and/or its treatment)	1	(After 3 years p.o.)

the Heyer-Schulte Unishunt in 74 cases, and a multipiece CSF shunt system with a medium pressure opening valve was implanted in five patients.

The total number of surgical procedures was 347, including 53 procedures of elective lengthening of the CSF shunt system; the procedure/patient ratio was 1.6. Two hundred and forty five children with hydrocephalus, operated on after the first month of life during the same period were the "controls".

Results

Of the 208 hydrocephalic newborns here considered, 50 had normal psychomotor development. A further 90 subjects presented a satisfactory mental development, although with varying degrees of motor impairment. Sixty-four patients with myelomeningocele were included in this group. Forty subjects were affected by severe psychomotor retardation (Table 2). Seventeen patients died at different time intervals after surgery: nine of these deaths were due to complications related, or probably related, to the surgical procedure (Table 3). Only in two cases born at term, as well as in one premature infant, did death depend on poor general clinical condition.

Four children died because of late complications due to associated myelomeningocele (MM) (three cases of symptomatic Chiari type II malformation and one case of renal insufficiency). In one case, the exitus depended on the natural evolution of the congenital cerebral malformation (holoprosencephaly).

Table 4. Etiology of hydrocephalus in infants who died (17 cases)

Etiology	No. of cases (n)
MM	6
Aqueductal stenosis	4
Holoprosencephaly	3
Post-hemorrhagic	2
Post-infective	1
Dandy-Walker	1

MM, myelomeningocele

Table 5. Results

No. of revisions	No. of patients (n)	Normal	Mild def.	Severe def.	Died
0	60	14	27	9	10
1	71	20	33	14	4
2	40	8	20	10	2
3	11	2	5	4	—
4	9	3	5	1	—
5	3	2	—	1	—
6	1	—	—	—	1
7	1	—	—	1	—
9	1	1	—	—	—
Lost to follow up	11				
	208	50	90	40	17

Among the 17 patients who died, 6 had hydrocephalus associated with MM, 4 had hydrocephalus secondary to aqueductal stenosis, and 3 had hydrocephalus associated with holoprosencephaly; in two cases the ventricular dilation followed an intracranial hemorrhage and in one case it followed an intracranial infection. Finally, in the last deceased subject, the hydrocephalus was part of a Dandy-Walker syndrome (Table 4). It is worth noting that more than half of the deaths were recorded in patients who had undergone only one surgical procedure (Table 5).

The overall survival rate in the series here considered was 91.8%, which did not statistically differ from that observed in the control group (245 cases of infantile hydrocephalus treated after the first month of life with an overall survival rate of 91.4%).

Discussion

The prognosis of congenital hydrocephalus has been believed to be generally poor, though the heterogeneity of its etiology actually prevents a reliable evaluation. The presence of associated malformations of the CNS plays an essential role, both in mortality and in late outcome (Di Rocco 1987). In a series of 47 infants with hydrocephalus overt at birth, evaluated by Fernell and co-workers (1987b), 37% of those with maldevelopment of the CNS and/or other organs died before 2 years of age and 86% had neurological sequelae. The corresponding figures for infants with "uncomplicated" hydrocephalus was 20% and 44%, respectively. The overall mortality in the same series was 21%, versus a 7% mortality recorded in children born at term who had developed signs of hydrocephalus later in life (Fernell et al. 1987a).

Renier and co-workers (1989), by analyzing a series of 108 infants with congenital hydrocephalus, reported an actuarial survival of 71% at 5 years and 62% at 10 years. These figures were considerably lower than those for hydrocephalus which developed later in life, where the actuarial survival at 10 years was 88%. When associated with other malformations, the survival at 10 years of infants with overt hydrocephalus at birth was 54% of the survivalrate of uncomplicated hydrocephalus. Ten of the 17 deaths recorded in our 208 hydrocephalic patients operated on in the first month of life were observed in patients with CNS associated malformations (six cases of MM, three cases of holoprosencephaly, and one case of Dandy-Walker cyst). CSF infections accounted for five deaths in the series. As already observed (Di Rocco 1987) the number of surgical procedures did not correlate with the death rate. However, the mortality we observed in infants with congenital hydrocephalus was consistently lower than that reported by other authors (Fernell et al. 1987b; Renier et al. 1989), even though the overall mortality of our patients with hydrocephalus (9.6%) did not differ significantly from that described in the literature. Actually, in spite of the fact that we also included in our series 97 cases of hydrocephalus associated with MM, which bears a relatively poor prognosis, we did not observe any difference in mortality among 208 infants treated during the first month of life and 245 children operated on later in life. Even though differences in the etiology of the hydrocephalus, as well as in the obstetric policy eventually adopted, may account for the low mortality rate we observed, it is possible that the early insertion of the CSF shunt device was the main factor responsible for the decreased death rate. About one-third of patients with congenital hydrocephalus are expected to have normal psychomotor development (Renier et al. 1989; Mealey et al. 1982); in our series this result was obtained in only a fourth of the cases. This result could also be directly related to the higher survival rate in our patients, possibly due to early operation. However, without considering the motor deficit associated with spina bifida, a satisfactory outcome, i.e., normal mental development, was observed in 67.3% of the subjects.

Conclusions

Even though hydrocephalus overt at birth is believed to carry a bad prognosis, a series of observations reported in the literature demonstrates that more than one-third of these patients may develop normally and that the majority of them may reach a normal level of mental development. In our experience, the insertion of a CSF shunt device in the first month of life did not seem to increase the mortality rate. In fact, most of the deaths we recorded in infants operated on soon after birth were due to complications related to associated malformations or to progression of the disease responsible for the hydrocephalus. The precocious insertion of the CSF shunt device may be responsible for the higher survival rate recorded in our series. However, this high survival does not correspond to better outcomes, as only one-fourth of our patients achieved normal psychomotor development.

References

Di Rocco C (1987) The treatment of infantile hydrocephalus, Vol. 2. CRC, Boca Raton, pp 1-11

Fernell E, Hagberg B, Hagberg G, von Wendt L (1987a) Epidemiology of infantile hydrocephalus in Sweden. II. Origin in infants born at term. Acta Paediatr Scand 76: 411-417

Fernell E, Uvebrant P, von Wendt L (1987b) Overt hydrocephalus at birth. Origin and outcome. Nerv Syst Child 3: 350-353

Mealey J, Coilmar RL, Bubb MP (1982) The prognosis of hydrocephalus overt at birth. J Neurosurg 57: 378-383

Renier D, Sainte-Rose C, Pierre-Kahn A, Hirsch JF (1989) Prognostic des hydrocephalies antenatales. Presse Med 8: 168-172

Williamson RA, Shanberger CW, Varner MW, Aschenbreber CA (1984) Heterogeneity of prenatal onset hydrocephalus: Management and counseling implications. Am J Med Genet 17: 497-508

56 — Reduction Cranioplasty for Congenital Hydrocephalus

Keizo Sakamoto, Norio Kobayashi, and Yukihiro Kamijo[1]

Summary. Reduction cranioplasty for congenital hydrocephalus with enormous head size was performed in four patients. We employed two techniques. One was reduction cranioplasty with subdural hematoma membrane excision. The other was reduction cranioplasty and V-P shunt performed in one stage to prevent the occurrence of subdural hematoma in neonates and young infants. The operative techniques used are described in detail. To prevent subdural hematoma as a postoperative sequel of V-P shunt we recommend the latter technique for the treatment of congenital hydrocephalus with enormous head size.

Keywords. Reduction cranioplasty — Subdural hematoma — Congenital hydrocephalus

Introduction

In patients with enormous head circumference due to congenital hydrocephalus, surgical implantation of a shunting device results in subdural fluid collection or hematoma and in craniocerebral disproportion as postoperative sequelae.

The aim of this paper is to describe the operative techniques and results of a patient treated by reduction cranioplasty with excision of the hematoma membrane following ventriculoperitoneal shunt (V-P shunt) and to similarly describe three other patients treated by reduction cranioplasty with simultaneous V-P shunt during the operative procedure to prevent occurrence of subdural fluid collection or hematoma in the early stage of life.

Patients

Our Patients were four children with enormous head size. All patients were admitted to our neurosurgical department. One patient (Case 1) had previously

---

[1] Department of Neurosurgery, Kobe Children's Hospital, Kobe, 650 Japan

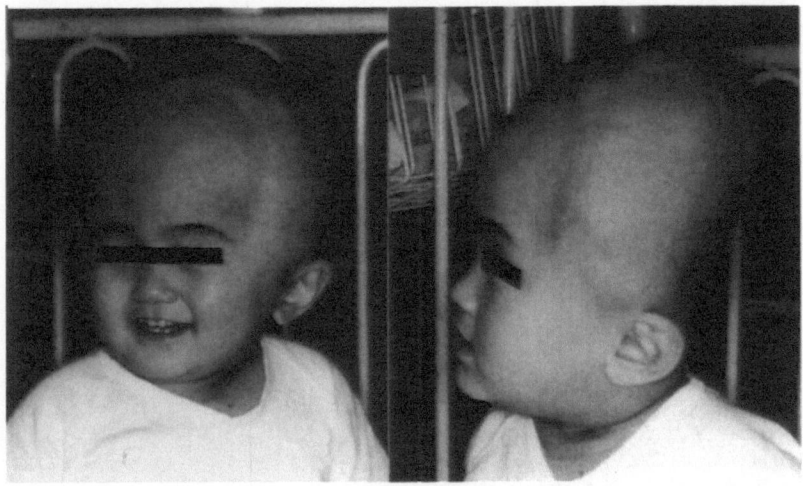

Fig. 1. Patient with large deformed scallop-shaped head, at the age of three years and one month, just before surgery

been treated with a V-P shunt as a neonate. Subdural hematoma, with a large deformed scallop-like head developed as a consequence of the V-P shunt, required reduction cranioplasty at the age of three, because of the child's inability to sit up unaided from the supine position and because other movement was also restricted (Fig. 1). The three other patients (one male, three female) underwent preventive reduction cranioplasty and V-P shunt, performed in one stage, at the ages of 13 days, 25 days and 3 months, respectively. Regarding the etiology of the enormous head size, the lobar type of holoprosencephaly described by DeMyer (DeMyer and Zeman 1963) was the cause in three cases. One of these (Case 3) had a dorsal cyst malformation of the type described by Yokota. (Yokota et al. 1984a,b) and one patient had a semilobar type of holoprosencephaly with Dandy-Walker cyst (Table 1).

Operative Technique

We employed two techniques. One (type I) was to reduce the head size with a hematoma membrane excision; this technique was used in the older child who had a V-P shunt as a neonate. The second technique (type II) was a preventive reduction of head size performed together with a V-P shunt in one stage, without dural opening, in neonates or young infants (Fig. 2).

For either procedure, the patient was placed in the supine position with the head flexed at about 35°–40°. General anesthesia was employed. A bicoronal skin incision was made and the skin flaps were everted upwards and downwards to permit the total exposure of the cranial vaults. The shunt was not removed in the type I technique, but in the type II procedure the V-P shunt was placed at the right side of the anterior fontanel, to drain out cerebrospinal

Table 1. Summary of Clinical Deta of Reduction Cranioplasty for Congenital Hydrocephalus

Case	Sex	Age & Purpose of Operation	Type of Hydrocephalus	Head Circumference before & after Op.	Outcome	Present Age
1. K.M.	female	3 years Hematoma	Holoprosencephaly (lobar type)	60.5–55.5 cm	IQ : 71 (9 y 5 m)	12 y 8 m
2. T.Y.	female	3 months Prevention	Holoprosencephaly (lobar type)	56.5–46.8 cm	DQ : 16 (6 y 7 m)	10 y 1 m
3. Hi.N.	female	13 days Prevention	Holoprosencephaly (lobar type)	44.6–36.0 cm	DQ : 67 (4y)	4 y 3 m
4. Ha.N.	male	25 days Prevention	Holoprosencephaly (semi-lobar type) & Dandy Walker cyst	51.0–43.1 cm	DQ : 8 (3y)	3 y 5 m

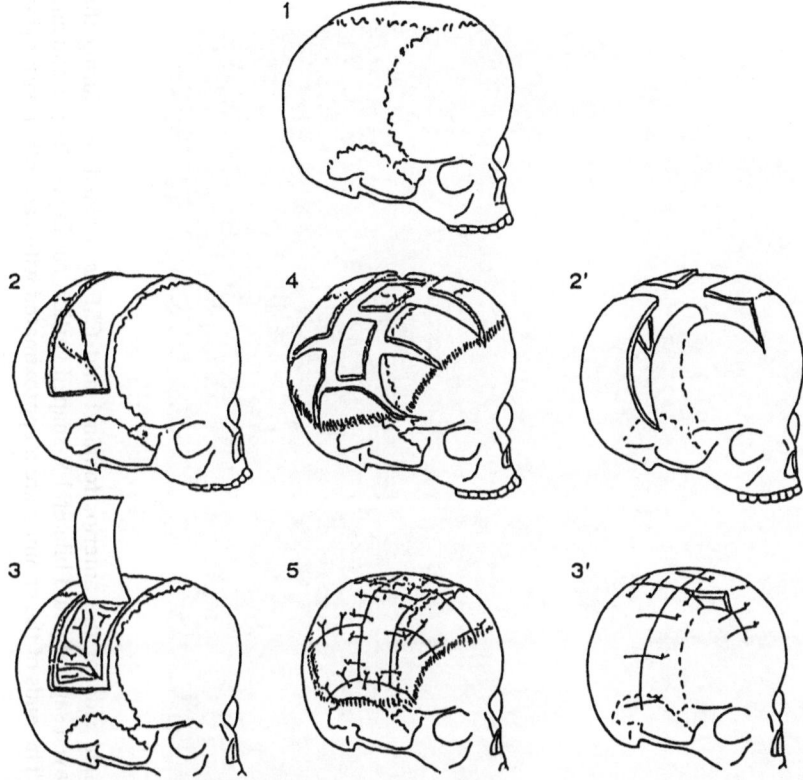

Fig. 2. Operative techniques. Reduction cranioplasty for hematoma (type I); 1,2,3,4,5. Preventive reduction cranioplasty and V-P shunt in one stage (type II): 1,2′,3′

fluid during the procedure for the reduction cranioplasty (Fig. 3a). The Type I technique for craniotomy involved the removal of the bilateral parietal bone flap in rectangular form (Fig. 2.2), together with off vertically V-shaped cutting to the frontal, temporal, and occipital bone (Fig. 2,4). The type II technique for craniotomy involved the removal of the bilateral parietal bone along the sagittal suture sagitally, with bilateral V-shaped cutting to the parietal and temporal bone off coronary. (Fig. 2,2', Fig. 3b). Dural opening for the excision of the subdural hematoma membrane on both sides and diminution of the subdural space by suturing the dura was performed in the type I procedure (Fig. 2,3). However, no attempt at dural opening was made in the type II procedure. In the type I procedure, before reshaping the cranium, the removed parietal bone was cut down to an adequately fitting size (Fig. 2,4) and approximated to the surrounding skull with nylon after making a greenstick fracture inward along the line of the connections at the base of the V-shaped cutting (Fig. 2,5). For reshaping the cranium in the type II procedure, the remaining portions of the cranium in the front and rear and on the right and left were approximated tightly each other with nylon (Fig. 2,3', Fig. 3c). During the approximation in the type II procedure, dural plication was created naturally

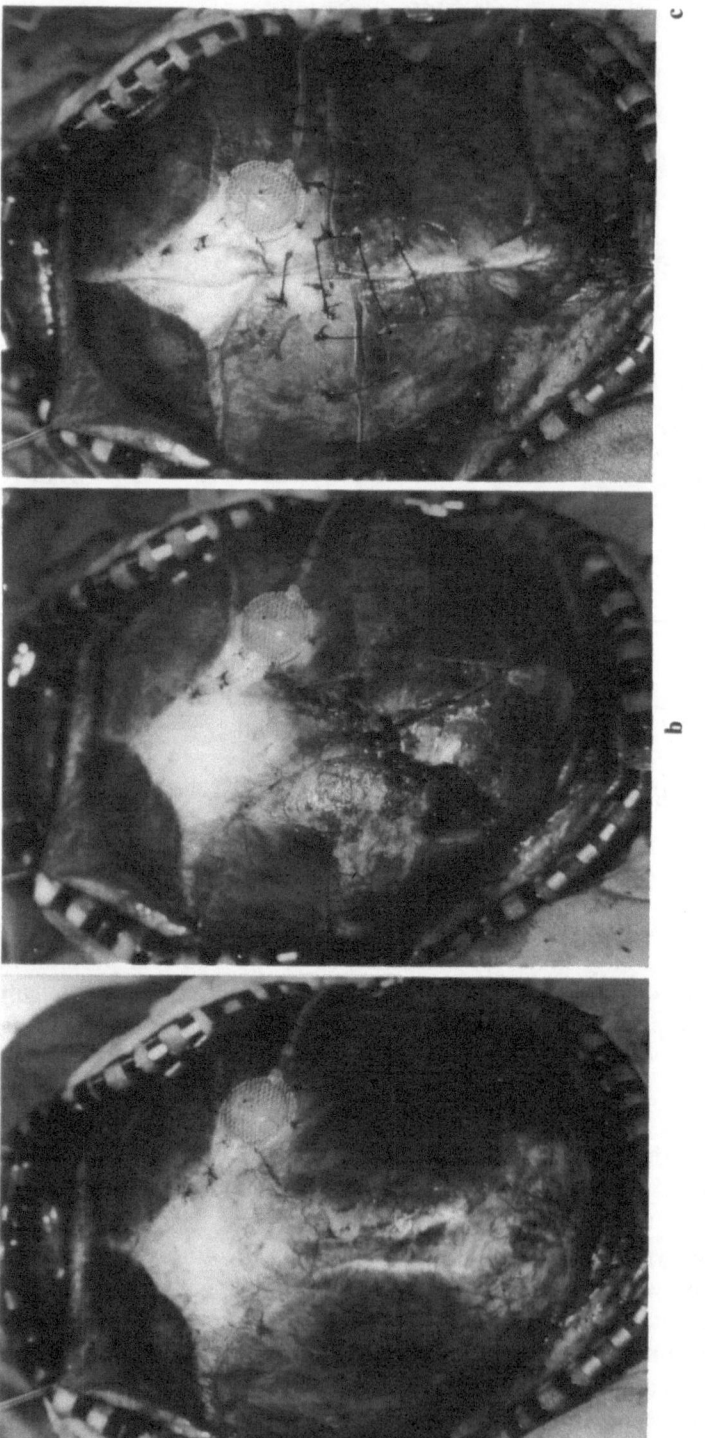

Fig. 3a-c. Operative photograph. **a** V-P shunt is placed at the right side of the anterior fontanel and CSF is drained out during the procedure. **b** Bilateral parietal bone along the sagittal suture is removed sagittally and bilateral V-shaped vertical cutting to the parietal and temporal bone follows, to obtain a reduction of skull dimensions. **c** The ends of the cranium are a approximated with each other with nylon sutures in place

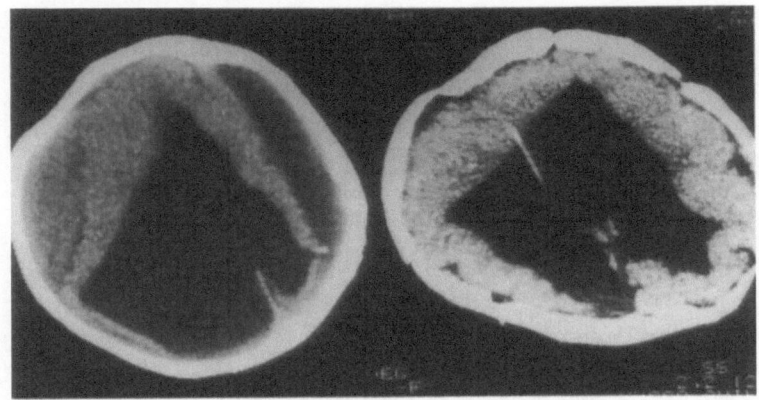

Fig. 4. CT scan before (3 years 1 month) and after (9 years 5 months) operation in (case 1)

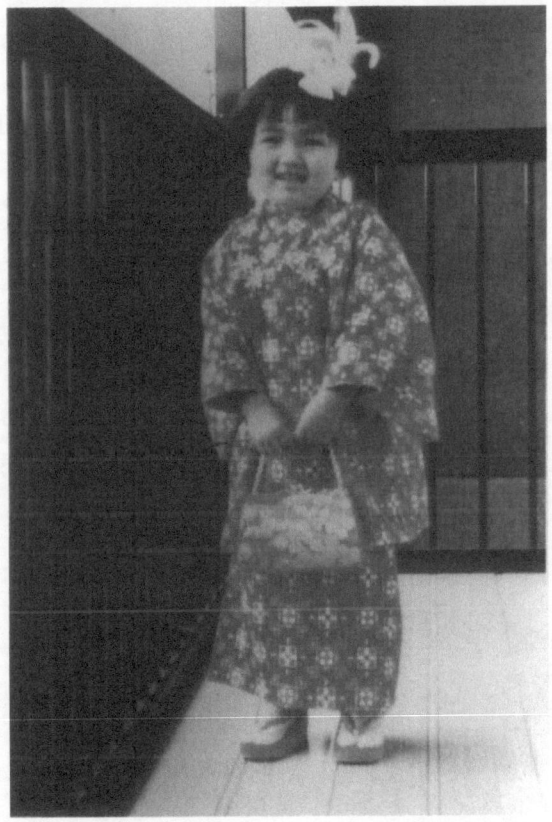

Fig. 5. Photograph of patient (case 1) taken at six years of age

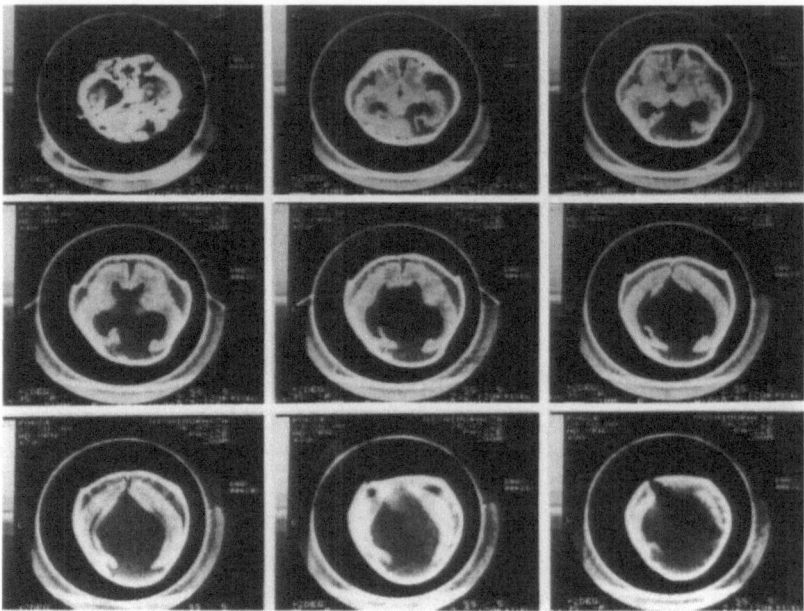

Fig. 6. CT scan showing subdural fluid collection and invagination of the coronal suture bilaterally following a ventricular tapping at 3 days after birth

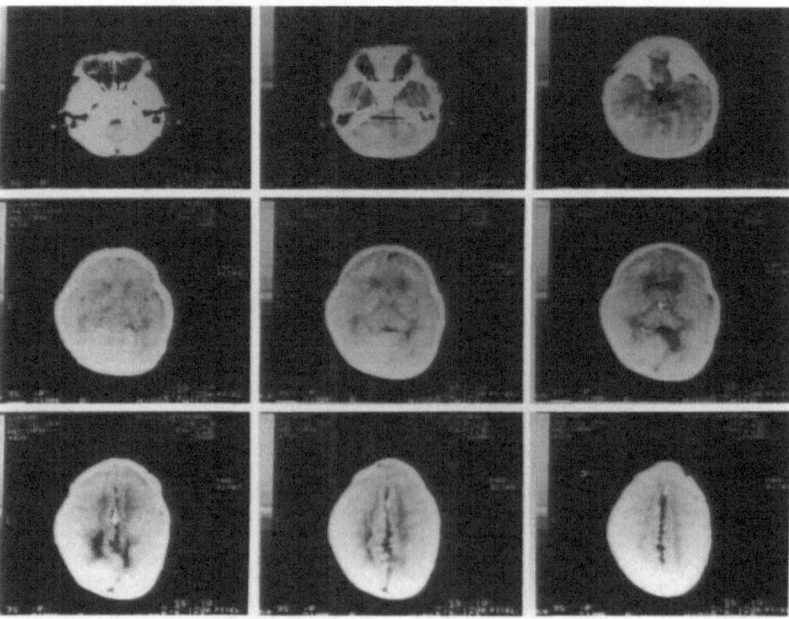

Fig. 7. CT scan showing nearly normal 13 months after 1st op. 4 months after 2nd op. ventricular size

without any dural suture. Furthermore, no evidence of occlusion of the superior sagittal sinus was observed.

Results

No major operative or postoperative complications, or deaths were experienced in our series. However, an additional operative procedure was required in two patients after the initial preventive reduction craniotomy and V-P shunt was performed in one stage. In one patient (case 2) subdural hematoma developed 2 weeks after the initial surgery and reduction craniotomy was repeated. The other patient (case 3), in whom secondary trigonocephaly had occurred, underwent bilateral canthal advancement with frontal bone reshaping at 9 months of age.

The head sizes of the patients before and after surgery decreased from 60.5 to 55.5 cm, 56.5 cm to 46.8 cm, 44.6 to 36.0 cm, and 51.0 to 43.1 cm in cases 1, 2, 3, and 4, respectively (Table 1). Outcomes for these patients are shown in Table I. The daily life of these patients at present can be described thus: The patient described as case 1, is now 12 years and 8 months old, has nearly normal motor function and is able to care for her own basic needs with minimal aid from her parents (CT scan before and after operation is shown in Fig. 4). Figure 5 shows this patient at 6 years of age. The patient described as case 2, now 10 years and 1 month old, is severely mentally retarded, but she was interested in reading the Chinese characters of the name of one of the authors, Sakamoto, on the name plate. The patient described as case 3, now 4 years and 3 months old, is able to walk by herself and to put words together in short phrases (CT scan before and after operation is shown in Figs. 6 and 7). Figure 8 shows this patient before and after cranial reduction. The patient described as case 4, now 3 years and 6 months old, is severely retarded, mentally and physically.

Head circumference curves for all cases are shown in Fig. 9.

Discussion

To our knowledge, reduction cranioplasty in the treatment for hydrocephalus with enormous head size has been the subject of only seven reports (Ehni 1982; Kimura et al. 1985; Park et al. 1985; Sayers and Duran 1964; Thompson and Hoffman 1975; Ventureyra and DaSilva 1981; Vries and Habal 1979) in the literature. However, preventive reduction cranioplasty and V-P shunt performed in one stage has not been presented except in our previous paper.

Although our operative procedure treated hydrocephalus successfully, the following has to be considered from a therapeutic point of view:

1. Deciding the head sizes for which this procedure is indicated.
2. Estimating the reduction of cranial capacity and the desired head shape.
3. Minimizing operative invasion.

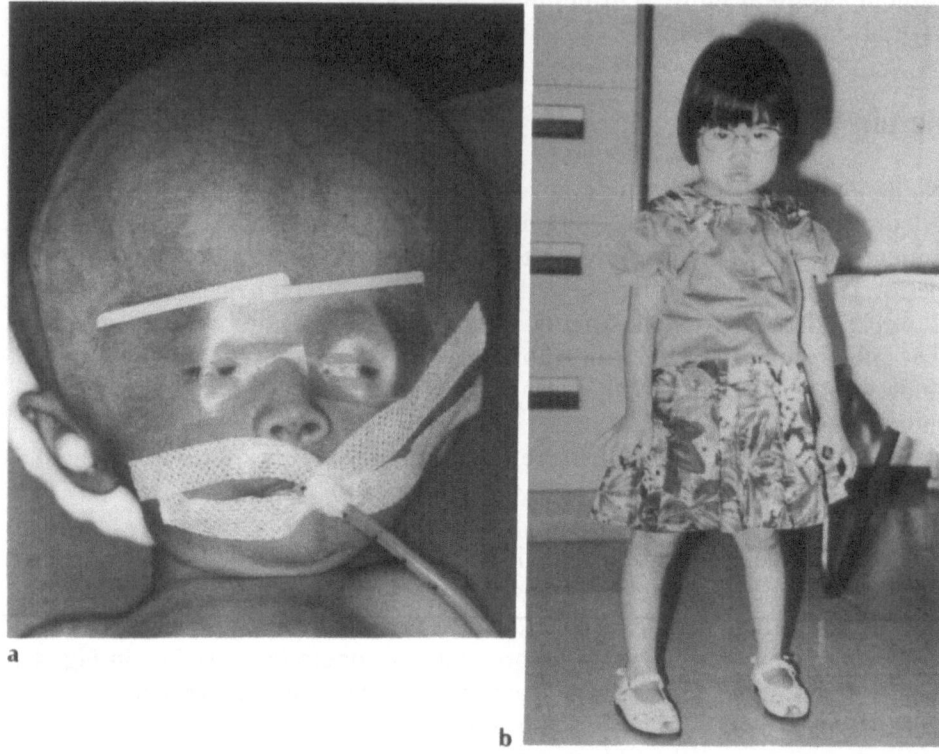

Fig. 8. Preoperative photograph **a** at 13 days after birth and **b** at 4 years of age

Decisions on indications for the procedure are reached by calculating the difference between head and chest circumference. In a normal child under 2 years of age, these measurements are usually the same or the difference is less than 2.5 cm. So if a patient with hydrocephalus has a difference of 10 cm or more, this procedure is indicated. The differences at birth in our cases were 16.5 cm, 14.7 cm, 15 cm, and 20.3 cm in cases 1,2,3, and 4, respectively.

Measurement of the chest circumference is useful for estimation of reduction of cranial capacity, because the required head size is similar to chest circumference in the first two years of life.

Minimizing operative invasion means reducing blood loss and reducing operation time. During the procedure for craniotomy, the pericranium should not be stripped (Ehni 1982). After an occurrence of subdural hematoma, removal of the hematoma membrane should not be attempted because of the large blood loss (Ehni 1982). The procedure should then be confined to irrigating the subdural space with saline. For minimizing operative invasion, our procedure of performing preventive reduction cranioplasty together with V-P shunt in one stage is ecxellent.

In case 3, operation time was 2 ½ h, with 25 g of blood loss and the operative

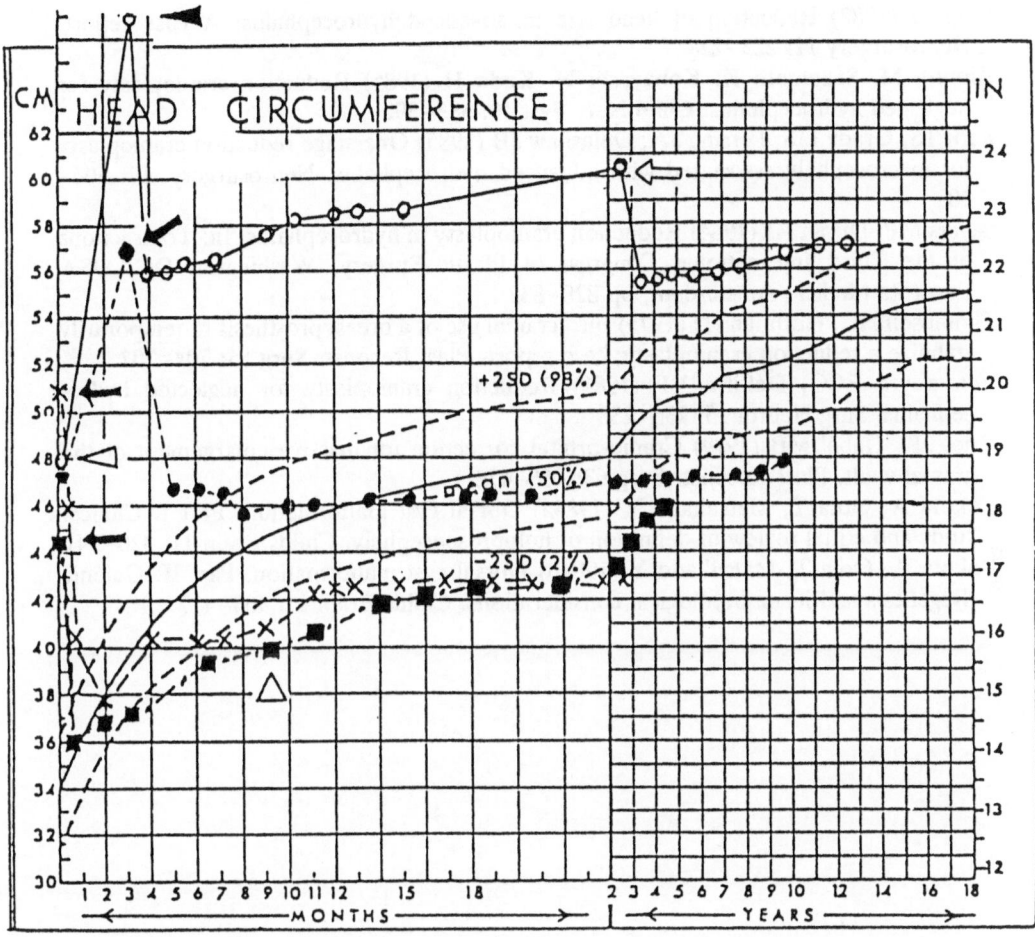

Fig. 9. Changes of head circumference before and after reduction craniotomy. ○—○; Case 1, ●---●; Case 2, ■·—·■; Case 3, x---x; Case 4, ◁; V-P shunt ◀; V-P shunt revision ◀—; Preventive reduction cranioplasty and V-P shunt ◊; Reduction craniplasty ◁; Operation for trigonocephaly

and postoperative courses were uneventful. In case 1, by contrast, operation time was 9 ¼ h, with 430 g of blood loss; the postoperative course was complicated by the development of subgaleal fluid accumulation.

References

DeMyer W, Zeman W (1963) Alobar holoprosencephaly (arhinencephaly) with median cleft lip and plate: Clinical electroencephalographic and nosologic considerations. Confina Neurol 23: 1–36

Ehni G (1982) Reduction of head size in advanced hydrocephalus: A case report. Neurosurgery 11: 223–228

Kimura M, Sakamoto K, Kobayashi N, Kudo H (1985) Reduction cranioplasty for neglected hydrocephalus. Child Nerv Syst 10: 385–392

Park TS, Grady MS, Persing JA, Delashaw JB (1985) One-stage reduction cranioplasty for macrocephaly associated with advanced hydrocephalus. Neurosurgery. 17: 506–509

Sayers MP, Duran RJ (1964) Reduction cranioplasty in hydrocephalus. In: Transactions of the Third International Congress of Plastic Surgery, Washington DC, USA Excerpta Medica, Amsterdam, pp 828–832

Thompson HG, Hoffman HJ (1975) Intracranial use of a breast prosthesis to temporarily stabilize a reduction cranioplasty; case report. Plast Reconstr Surg 55: 704–707

Ventureyra ECG, DaSilva VF (1981) Reduction cranioplasty for neglected hydrocephalus. Surg Neurol 15: 236–238

Vries JK, Habal MB (1979) Cranio-orbital correction for massive enlargement of the cranial vault. Plast Reconstr Surg 63: 466–472

Yokota A, Oota T, Matsukado Y (1984a) Dorsal cyst malformation, Part I. Clinical study and critial review of definition of holoprosencephaly. Childs Brain 11: 320–341

Yokota A, Oota T, Matsukado Y (1984b) Dorsal cyst malformation, Part II. Galenic dysgenesis and its embryological considerations. Childs Brain 11: 403–417

57 — Effect of Ventricular Size on Intellectual Development in Children with Myelomeningocele

Masato Nagasaka and Yuh Tanaka[1]

Summary. Since hydrocephalus is considered to have an unfavorable effect on the intelligence of children with myelomeningocele, we examined the relationship between intelligence quotient (IQ) and ventricular size. Between 1970 and 1989, 130 myelodysplastic infants were admitted to our hospital. Of these infants, 125 received back closure operations, hydrocephalus was observed in 112 (86%), and 94 (72%) were shunted. These 130 infants were followed-up until May 1990. By this time, 9 children were lost to follow-up and 34 children had died. Of the remaining 87 children, those who were 5 years of age or older were the subjects of this study. Ventricular size was graded by Evans' ratio on initial (preshunting) computed tomography (CT) and follow-up CT. IQ was assessed using the Tanaka-Binet test. Both IQ and initial CT were available in 32 patients, and both IQ and follow-up CT were obtained in 55 children. There seemed to be an inverse relationship between IQ and ventricular size on the initial CT in the neonatal period, but there was no correlation between IQ and ventricular size on the follow-up CT. Considering these results, prompt shunting might not be necessary for some myelodysplastic infants with mild to moderate ventriculomegaly.

Keywords. Myelomeningocele — Hydrocephalus — Shunt — Evans' ratio on CT — Intelligence quotient

Introduction

Hydrocephalus is a common concomitant of children with myelomeningocele (Ames and Schut 1972; Laurence 1964; McLone et al. 1982; McLone and Naidich 1989; Nagasaka et al. 1989; Storrs 1988), affecting between 70% and 95% of these patients. Its presence is considered to have an unfavorable effect on the intellectual development (Mapstone et al. 1984; McLone and Naidich 1989; Nagasaka et al. 1989; Soare and Raimondi 1977) of these children.

[1]Department of Neurosurgery, Central Hospital, Aichi Prefectural Colony, Kasugai, Aichi, 480–03 Japan

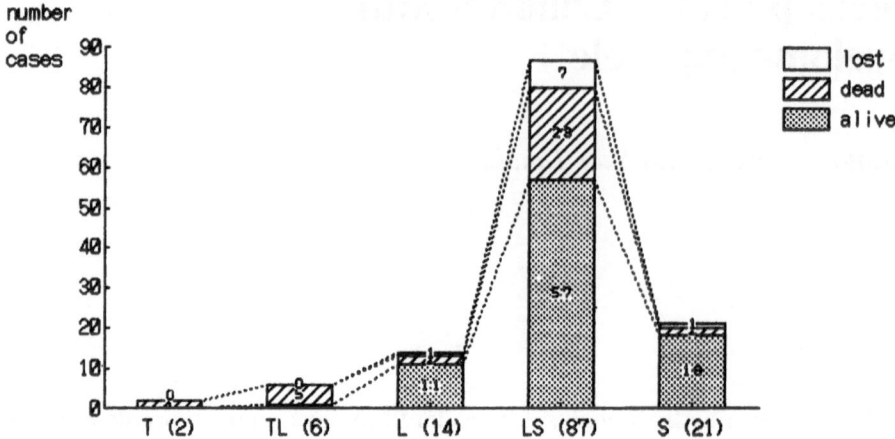

Fig. 1. Sites of myelomeningocele in 130 infants. T, thoracic; TL, thoracolumbar; L, lumbar; LS, lumbosacral; S, sacral

Therefore, it is important for neurosurgeons to minimize the brain damage caused by hydrocephalus and its management. With respect to intellectual development, many authors have investigated (Hunt and Holmes 1975; Kojima et al. 1988; Laurence 1964; Mapstone et al. 1984; McLone et al. 1982; Nagasaka et al. 1989; Raimondi and Soare 1974; Soare and Raimondi 1977; Storrs 1988) the relationship between intelligence quotient (IQ) and many variables such as the presence of hydrocephalus, the sensory level of the lesion, central nervous system (CNS) infection, CNS anomaly, age at first shunt, socioeconomic level, and so forth. The purpose of the present study is, first, to answer the question whether there are any relationships between intellectual development and ventricular size, and, second, to determine the ventricular size which is most suitable for children with myelomeningocele.

Patients and Methods

Review of the medical records of the Central Hospital, Aichi Prefectural Colony, Japan revealed that 130 infants with myelomeningocele were admitted to our hospital from 1970 to 1989. Of these, 125 patients received back closure operations and were subsequently followed in our clinic. Hydrocephalus was observed in 112 patients (86%) and 94 (72%) were shunted. Up to May 1990, 34 children had died, 9 were lost to follow-up, and the remaining 87 were followed-up. The sites of the myelomeningocele in the 130 children are demonstrated in Fig. 1. Of the 87 survivors, 69 patients who were aged 5 years or older were the candidates for the present study.

Initial (preshunting) CT was performed in the neonatal period after closure of the myelomeningocele. Follow-up CT was performed at the age when the IQ of the children was tested. Ventricular size on these CT scans was measured

Fig. 2. Measurement of ventricular size on CT. Anterior Evans' ratio = B/A, trigonal Evans' ratio = C/A. A, greatest transverse diameter of cerebrum; B, greatest distance between the anterior horns; C, greatest distance between the trigones

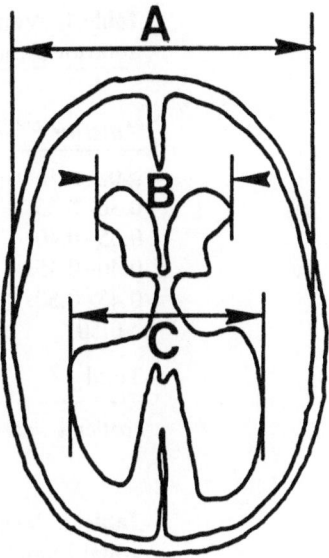

using Evans' ratio (Yamada 1983). We defined the anterior Evans' ratio and trigonal Evans' ratio as follows: Anterior Evans' ratio = greatest distance between the anterior horns/greatest transverse diameter of cerebrum; trigonal Evans' ratio = greatest distance between the trigones/greatest transverse diameter of cerebrum (Fig. 2).

IQ was evaluated using the Tanaka-Binet Intelligence Scale (Japanese version of the Binet Test created by K. Tanaka, Taken Shuppan, Tokyo)

Results

Shunting and Ventricular Size

Shunt diversion of cerebrospinal fluid was performed in 54 (78%) of the 69 infants studied. Initial CT was obtained for the 36 infants who were born in the CT era; one of these infants was excluded from the study because of ventriculitis. Follow-up CT scans were available for 62 children; 4 of these were excluded from this investigation owing to CNS infection. Ventricular sizes on initial CT (35 infants) and those on follow-up CT (58 children) are shown in Tables 1, 2, and 3. Fifty five percent (26 out of 47) of the children who had received a shunt showed slit-like ventricles.

Intelligence Quotient

IQ testing was done on 59 children: 10 were not shunted and 49 were shunted. Three patients with low IQ (23, 45, and 57) caused by ventriculitis were excluded from this study. The mean IQs of the subgroups were as follows:

Table 1. Ventricular size, measured by anterior Evans' ratio, on initial CT

Anterior Evans' ratio	No. of patients[a] (n)	
	Shunt	No shunt
≦0.3	1	8
0.30–0.35	3	2
0.35–0.40	7	0
0.40–0.45	5	1
0.45–0.50	7	0
>0.50	1	0
Total	24	11

[a] patients with CNS infection were excluded

Table 2. Ventricular size, measured by trigonal Evans' ratio, on initial CT

Trigonal Evans' ratio	No. of patients[a] (n)	
	Shunt	No shunt
≦0.55	0	7
0.55–0.60	4	4
0.60–0.65	7	0
0.65–0.70	6	0
0.70–0.75	2	0
>0.75	5	0
Total	24	11

[a] patients with CNS infection were excluded

Table 3. Ventricular size, measured by anterior Evans' ratio, on follow-up CT

Anterior Evans' ratio	No. of patients[a] (n)	
	Shunt	No shunt
Slit ventricle	26	0
≦0.3	4	7
0.30–0.35	7	2
0.35–0.40	7	1
0.40–0.45	2	1
0.45–0.50	1	0
Total	47	11

[a] patients with CNS infection were excluded

Table 4. Summary of IQ testing

Subgroup	No.	IQ	IQ ≧ 80
All children	59	88.8 ± 21.3	71%
Children without CNS infection	56	91.3 ± 18.5	75%
Without shunt	9	105.8 ± 14.4	89%
Normal ventricle	5	112.6 ± 7.8	100%
Ventriculomegaly	4	97.3 ± 16.1	75%
With shunt	46	88.5 ± 18.1	72%
Slit ventricle	26	87.2 ± 18.4	69%
Non-slit	20	90.2 ± 17.6	75%

Nonshunted with normal ventricle, IQ = 113; nonshunted with mild to moderate ventriculomegaly, IQ = 97; shunted with mild to moderate ventriculomegaly, IQ = 90; shunted with slit ventricle, IQ = 87. These results of IQ testing are shown in Table 4.

Relationship Between IQ and Ventricular Size

Excluding children with incomplete IQ testing or incomplete CT and those with CNS infection, or with a severe form of symptomatic Arnold-Chiari malformation, the relationship between IQ and the initial CT was analyzed in 32 patients and the correlation between IQ and the follow-up CT was investigated in 55 children. There was a tendency for IQ to decrease as the ventricular size on initial CT increased. In other words, the percentage of children with normal intelligence decreased with increasing ventricular size on initial CT (Tables 5 and 6, Fig. 3). However, there was no correlation between IQ and ventricular size on the follow-up CT (Table 7).

Discussion

Hydrocephalus occurs with a frequency of between 70% and 95% in children with myelomeningocele (Ames and Schut 1972; Laurence 1964; McLone et al.

Table 5. Anterior Evans' ratio on initial CT vs intelligence quotient

Anterior Evans' ratio	No.[a]	IQ	IQ ≧ 80
≦0.3	7	108.9 ± 10.4	7/7 (100%)
0.30–0.35	5	96 ± 15.5	4/5 (80%)
0.35–0.40	6	87.7 ± 23.5	4/6 (67%)
0.40–0.50	6	92.7 ± 20.1	4/6 (67%)
0.45–0.50	7	85.4 ± 18.1	3/7 (43%)
>0.50	1	53	0/1 (0%)
Total	32	93.0 ± 20.9	22/32(69%)

[a] patients with CNS infection were excluded

Table 6. Trigonal Evans' ratio on initial CT vs intelligence quotient

Trigonal Evans' ratio	No.[a]	IQ	IQ ≧ 80
≦0.55	5	102.2 ± 7.0	5/5 (100%)
0.55–0.60	8	97.6 ± 22.4	6/8 (75%)
0.60–0.65	6	98.2 ± 16.3	5/5 (83%)
0.65–0.70	6	81.3 ± 22.4	3/6 (50%)
0.70–0.75	2	80 ± 18	1/2 (50%)
>0.75	5	89.2 ± 22.3	3/5 (60%)
Total	32	93.0 ± 20.9	22/32(69%)

[a]patients with CNS infection were excluded

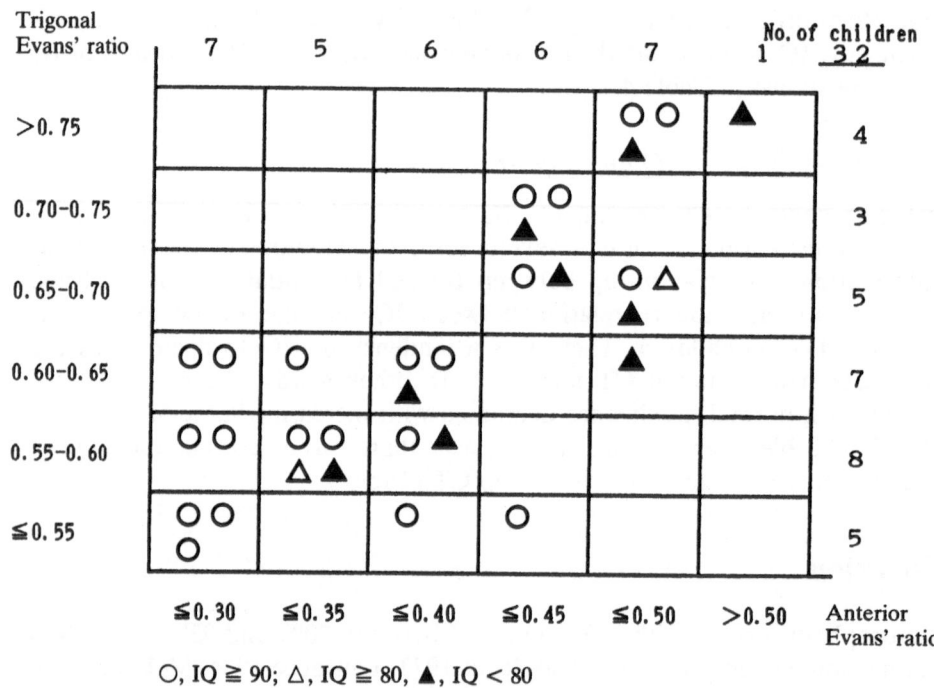

O, IQ ≧ 90; △, IQ ≧ 80, ▲, IQ < 80

Fig. 3. Intelligence quotient by initial ventricular size

1982; McLone and Naidich 1989; Nagasaka et al. 1989; Storrs 1988), and its presence has been reported to be an unfavorable factor in the intellectual development of these patients (Mapstone et al. 1984; McLone and Naidich 1989; Nagasaka et al. 1989; Soare and Raimondi 1977). Therefore the proper management of hydrocephalus is necessary for infants with myelomeningocele. So far, many variables (Hunt and Holmes 1975; Kojima et al. 1988; Laurence 1964; Mapstone et al. 1984; McLone et al. 1982; Nagasaka et al. 1989;

Table 7. Anterior Evans' ratio on follow-up CT of shunted patients vs intelligence quotient

Anterior Evans' ratio	No.[a]	IQ	IQ ≧ 80
Slit ventricle	26	87.2 ± 18.4	18/26(69%)
≦0.3	4	87 ± 21.3	2/4 (50%)
0.30–0.35	7	87.9 ± 18.9	5/7 (71%)
0.35–0.40	6	96.3 ± 12.6	6/6 (100%)
0.40–0.45	2	89 ± 17	1/2 (50%)
0.45–0.50	1	84	1/1 (100%)
Total	46	88.5 ± 18.1	33/46(72%)

[a] patients with CNS infection were excluded

Laurence 1964; Mapstone et al. 1984; McLone et al. 1982; Nagasaka et al. Raimondi and Soare 1974; Soare and Raimondi 1977; Storrs 1988) relating to hydrocephalus in terms of intellectual development have been analyzed retrospectively. Raimondi and Soare (1974) pointed out that the variables which seemed to have a large impact were shunt function, race or socioeconomic level, and age at first shunt, while the variables that seemed to be less important were number of revisions and degree of hydrocephalus at initial shunt. However, in our series, as the ventricular size of the initial preshunt CT in the neonatal period increased in size, the number of children with low IQ increased. This result corresponded with the finding of Hunt and Holmes (1975) that intelligence was significantly related to the thickness of the pallium when the shunt was inserted during the first 4 weeks of life. Hence, the larger ventricles, seen on initial CT in the neonatal period, might have an adverse effect on the future intellectual development of children with myelomeningocele. Storrs (1988) showed that there was no correlation between ventricular size after shunting and intellectual performance, except in cases with persistent severe ventricular enlargement. This result agreed with our finding that there was no relationship between IQ and ventricular size on the follow-up CT. Many investigators have proven that central nervous system (CNS) infection and associated CNS anomalies have a significant negative effect on intelligence (Kojima et al. 1988; Mapstone et al. 1984; McLone et al. 1982). In our series, children with CNS infection also had low IQs.

It is obvious that early shunting is necessary for myelodysplastic infants with severe ventriculomegaly, large head, and high intracranial pressure. However, shunt procedure and the subsequent control of hydrocephalus have the potential hazards of shunt infection, malfunction, slit-like ventricle and shunt dependency (McLone and Naidich 1989; Rekate 1985, 1989). Moreover, it is well known that some survivors of untreated stable hydrocephalus have normal intelligence (Laurence 1964; McLone and Naidich 1989; Nagasaka et al. 1989; Storrs 1988). In our series the nonshunted patients with stable ventriculomegaly had better IQs (mean IQ = 97) than the shunted patients (mean IQ = 89). Therefore it is difficult to determine whether infants with mild to moderate ventriculomegaly should be shunted in early infancy. Rekate (1985, 1989) proposed a close observation approach, using serial ultrasound, for patients with mild to moderate ventriculomegaly. As far as IQ is concerned, myelo-dysplastic infants with mild to moderate ventriculomegaly would be properly managed by this approach.

References

Ames MD, Schut L (1972) Results of treatment of 171 consecutive myelomeningoceles — 1963 to 1968. Pediatrics 50: 466–470

Hunt GM, Holmes AE (1975) Some factors relating to intelligence in treated children with spina bifida cystica. Dev Med Child Neurol 17(Suppl 35): 65–70

Kojima N, Tamaki N, Matsumoto S (1988) Evaluation of shunt treatment in hydro-cephalus with myelomeningocele: Some factors relating to mental prognosis (in Japanese). No To Shinkei 40: 1181–1187

Laurence KM (1964) The natural history of spina bifida cystica, detailed analysis of 407 cases. Arch Dis Child 39: 41–57

Mapstone TB, Rekate HL, Nulsen FE, Dixon MS Jr, Glaser N, Jaffe M (1984) Relationship of CSF shunting and IQ in children with myelomeningocele: A retro-spective analysis. Childs Brain 11: 112–118

McLone DG, Czyzewski D, Raimondi AJ, Sommers RC (1982) Central nervous system infection as a limiting factor in the intelligence of children with myelomeningocele. Pediatrics 70: 338–342

McLone DG, Naidich TP (1989) Myelomeningocele: Outcome and late complications. In: McLaurin RL, Venes JL, Schut L, Epstein F (eds) Pediatric neurosurgery 2nd Ed, WB Saunders, Philadelphia, pp 53–70

Nagasaka M, Tanaka Y, Yamada H, Nakamura S (1989) Long-term follow-up results of infants with myelomeningocele (in Japanese). Shoni no Noshinkei 14: 95–101

Raimondi AJ, Soare P (1974) Intellectual development in shunted hydrocephalic chil-dren. Am J Dis Child 127: 664–671

Rekate HL (1985) To shunt or not to shunt: Hydrocephalus and dysraphism. Clin Neurosurg 32: 593–607

Rekate HL (1989) Treatment of hydrocephalus. In: McLaurin RL, Venes JL, Schut L, Epstein F (eds) Pediatric neurosurgery 2nd Ed. WB Saunders, Philadelphia, pp 200–218

Soare PL, Raimondi AJ (1977) Intellectual and perceptual-motor characteristics of treated myelomeningocele children. Am J Dis Child 131: 199–204

Storrs BB (1988) Ventricular size and intelligence in myelodysplastic children. In: Marlin AE (ed) Concepts in pediatric neurosurgery, Vol. 8. Karger, Basel, pp 51–56

Yamada H (1983) Pediatric cranial computed tomography. Igaku-shoin, Tokyo, pp 115–120

58 — Continuous Cerebral Blood Flow Velocity (CBFV) and Simultaneous Intraventricular Pressure Measurements During Sleep in Hydrocephalic Children

Day-eel Goh[1], Robert A. Minns[1], Steven D. Pye[2], and A. James W. Steers[1]

Summary. Transcranial Doppler ultrasonography (TCD) can be used to study cerebral blood flow velocity (CBFV) changes during episodic increases in intracranial pressure (ICP) which occur during sleep in hydrocephalic patients. Eight studies of continous ICP with simultaneous middle cerebral artery blood flow velocity measurements were recorded during sleep in seven children (age range 12–118 months). The Resistance Index, $RI = (S - D)/s$, where S is peak systolic velocity and D is end diastolic velocity, and mean flow velocity (MFV) were used to characterise the CBFV change. ICP was measured directly from a frontal reservoir. There were two main patterns of CBFV response to raised ICP. The "ischemic-type" response with progressive decrease in MFV ($r = -0.46$, $P < .001$) and increase in RI ($r = +0.7$, $P < .001$) as ICP increased was seen in three patients with craniocerebral disproportion, suggesting reduced circulatory reserve in patients with limited intracranial compliance. The "hyperemic-type" response of increased MFV with rise in ICP ($r = +0.63$, $P < .001$) seen in four studies suggests that appropriate cerebrovascular increase in blood flow occurs to maintain adequate cerebral perfusion in those with sufficient circulatory reserve. Change in RI can be variable in those with a "hyperemic-type" response. Simultaneous CBFV and ICP measurements may help to identify those patients with reduced circulatory reserve and limited intracranial compliance who are at greater risk of ischemic insult from increased ICP.

Keywords. Hydrocephalus — Sleep — Intraventricular pressure — Cerebral blood flow velocity response — Transcranial Doppler Ultrasonography

[1]Department of Paediatric Neurology, Royal Hospital for Sick Children, Edinburgh, EH9 1LF Scotland, UK
[2]Department of Medical Physics and Medical Engineering, Western General Hospital, Edinburgh, EH4 2XU Scotland, UK

Introduction

Cerebral blood flow increases during rapid-eye-movement (REM) sleep (Ingvar 1971) and this is felt to be the underlying cause of the spontaneous episodic increases in intracranial pressure (ICP) known to occur in patients with hydrocephalus. Sustained plateau A and B waves are thought to occur in those patients with reduced compliance while autoregulation remains intact (Rosner and Becker 1984). The major concern is of ischemic insult from significant reduction of cerebral perfusion pressure with prolonged raised ICP. Sleep can be used as a physiological challenge to detect intermittent active from compensated hydrocephalus (Di Rocco et al. 1975; Minns 1990).

Transcranial Doppler ultrasound techniques, described by Aaslid et al. (1982) now allow us to noninvasively measure cerebral blood flow velocity (CBFV) repeatedly in the basal cerebral arteries, in all age groups. Age-dependant normal values in childhood have been reported (Bode and Wais 1988). With very close time resolution, this technique is ideally suited for evaluating simultaneous cerebral hemodynamic changes while monitoring ICP during sleep. Other presently available methods of cerebral blood flow determination, e.g., those involving radioisotopes are not continously repeatable, or are too invasive, e.g., those employing the Kety-Schimdt method. Change in transcranial Doppler CBFV in response to hypercapnia correlates closely with change in cerebral blood flow measured with xenon 133, although correlations with absolute measurements are less reliable due to wide inter-patient variations (Bishop et al. 1986). Aaslid et al. (1986) compared an estimated cerebral perfusion pressure (CPP) derived from middle cerebral artery (MCA) flow velocity and arterial blood pressure waveforms which correlated closely with true CPP measured in ten patients with hydrocephalus undergoing ventricular infusion tests. Klingelhofer et al. (1988) reported a decrease of mean flow velocity (MFV) and increase in Pourcelot's Resistance Index (RI) with increased ICP in a mixed group of adult patients with severe cerebral disease in whom there was assumed impaired autoregulation.

The aim of this study was to investigate the cerebrohemodynamic effects of ICP increases during sleep in children with hydrocephalus when we suspected reduced compliance, progressive hydrocephalus, or shunt malfunction.

Patients and Methods

Seven patients (five males and two females), age range 12–118 months, had eight sleep studies of simultaneous ICP/CBFV recordings performed. All but one had pre-existing ventricular peritoneal shunts; their underlying etiology and clinical details are described in Table 1. Three patients had clinically suspected craniocerebral disproportion, with slit ventricles on the CT scan. One of them had a repeat study performed after skull morcellation.

Direct intraventricular pressure was measured in all patients, using a non-displacement method connecting a strain gauge pressure transducer (Gaeltec)

Table 1. Demographic and clinical details

Patient	Age	Sex	Diagnosis	Indication
1.	37 months	M	Post-meningitis	Increased vent size
2.	14 months	M	Post-hemorraghic, not shunted	Dilated vent
3.	34 months	M	Post fossa cyst	Dilated vent
4.	12 months	M	Myelomeningocele	Increased vent size
5.	25 months	F	PHH, slit vent, CCD	Vomiting
6.	118 months	F	Post-meningitis, slit vent, CCD	Ataxia
7.	108 months	M	Myelomeningocele, CCD	Headaches

CCD, craniocerebral disproportion; PHH, posthemorraghic hydrocephalus; vent, ventricle

to a 25-gauge butterfly needle inserted into a frontal ventriculostomy. A separate reservoir is inserted routinely in almost all our patients with hydrocephalus to access ICP measurement or drainage as required (Leggate et al. 1988). The pressure transducer was calibrated with a sphygmomanometer before each proceedure and continous ICP measurements were charted by a pen recorder.

CBFV was measured in the middle cerebral artery (MCA) with pulsed- wave Doppler (Decoder — Doptek Ltd, Chichester, UK) with a hand-held 2 MHz probe placed in the temporal position. The spatial peak temporal average intensity of the ultrasound beam measured in water was less than 100 mW cm−2. MCA identification and depth selection (typically 3.5–5cm) of optimal signals was carried out as described by Aaslid et al. (1982). The MCA was chosen for accessibility, easy identification, and reliability (Maeda et al. 1990). CBFV recordings were made at 10–15 min intervals while ICP was stable, and more frequently during changing ICP states. Doppler signals were stored on audiotape. This was later reviewed separately and only good quality consecutive waveforms were analyzed, with a mean value obtained from at least ten waveforms. Incorporated computer calculation of Resistance Index (RI = (S − D)/S where S is peak systolic velocity and D is end diastolic velocity) and MFV (= time mean of maximum velocity envelope) was used to characterise the waveforms. RI has been described as an index of cerebrovascular resistance (Pourcelot 1976; Bada et al. 1979) while MFV serves as an index of mean CBF assuming no change in vessel diameter (Bishop et al. 1986). When it was possible to do so without disturbing the children's sleep, blood pressure was measured, using the oscillometric method with a Dinamap machine.

Results

Table 2 summarizes the results of recorded ICP and correlation with MFV and RI in individual studies. There were two main patterns of CBFV response, associated with episodic increased ICP occurring during sleep. In four studies increased ICP was associated with a progressive decrease in MFV ($r = -0.46$,

Table 2. Recorded ICP and correlations with MFV and RI in individual studies

Patient	ICP (mmHg)		ICP/MFV		ICP/RI	
	Baseline	Max	r	P	r	P
A.D.	12	55	−0.64	<.001	+0.89	<.001
L.Hl	8	37	−0.46	<.05	+0.70	<.001
H.S (pre)	18	37	−0.24	ns	+0.61	<.001
I.S.	12	29	−0.13	ns	+0.41	<.01
C.M.	9	26	+0.37	<.01	+0.69	ns
K.P.	15	22	+0.64	<.001	+0.13	ns
H.S (post)	15	20	+0.58	<.001	+0.03	<.001
P.B.	16	33	+0.63	<.001	−0.8	<.001

RI, Resistance Index; MFV, time-averaged mean of maximum velocity curve; ICP, intracranial pressure; r, correlation coefficient; P, significance value; ns, not significant; max, maximum

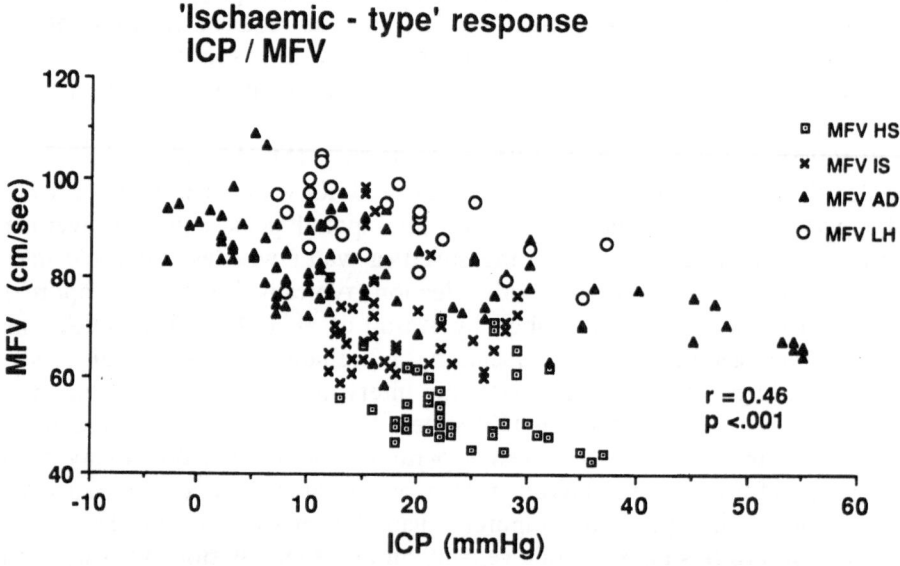

Fig. 1. Plot of mean flow velocity (*MFV*) versus intracranial pressure (*ICP*) in four studies with an "ischemic-type" cerebral blood flow velocity (*CBFV*) response where MFV decreased ($r = -0.46$, $P < .001$) as ICP increased. Each patient is represented by a different symbol

$P < .001$: Fig. 1) and increase in RI (r = +0.7, $P < .001$; Fig. 2) which we have termed an "*ischemic — type*" CBFV response. Three of these patients had craniocerebral disproportion, with small ventricles on CT scan. Plateau A and B waves were recorded during sleep in these three patients. A graphical plot of a plateau wave with corresponding ICP, RI, and MFV in patient AD (Fig. 3) shows increased MFV with low RI just before onset of the rapid ICP rise, followed by a steadily decreasing MFV with increasing RI as ICP increased; the trend reversing as ICP fell. Figure 4 shows a graphical plot of B

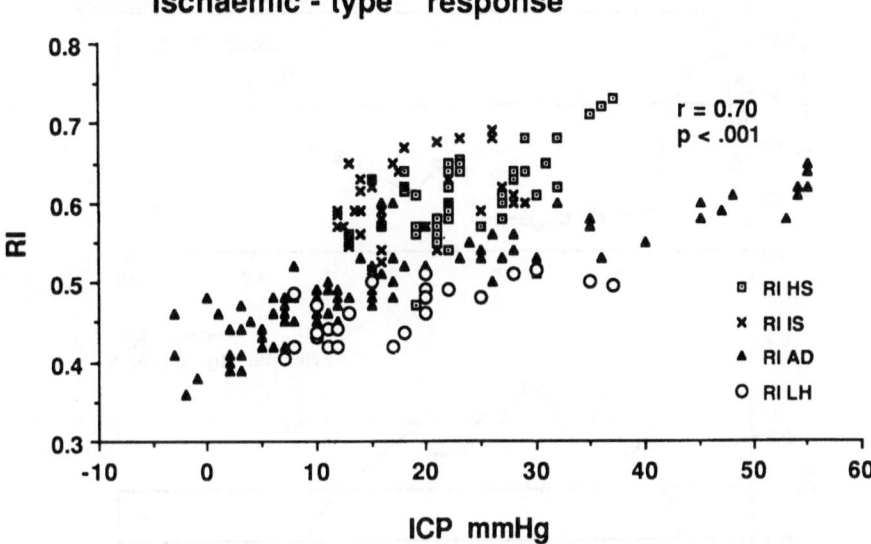

Fig. 2. Plot of Resistance Index (*RI*) versus intracranial pressure (*ICP*) in four studies with an "ischemic-type" CBFV response shows significant positive correlation ($r = +0.7$, $P < .001$) of RI with increase in ICP. Each patient is represented by a different symbol

waves from patient LH, showing a similar pattern to that of the A waves. This Doppler waveform pattern suggests that in these patients raised ICP, which may be initiated by a small increase in cerebral blood volume, can lead to a significant rise in cerebrovascular resistance and can result in reduced cerebral blood flow. Patient IS who showed only a weak "ischemic-type" response had deteriorating shunt function although he was asymptomatic at the time the sleep recording was performed. He returned 4 months later with acute symptoms of raised ICP with vomiting and lethargy. ICP was elevated (25 mmHg) and he required early shunt revision at that stage.

However, even when peak ICP was greater than diastolic blood pressure with a calculated cerebral perfusion pressure of 30 mmHg during the plateau wave, there was no cessation of diastolic blood flow velocity, as seen in young infants with hydrocephalus (Hill and Volpe 1982). In older children RI does not seem to rise as significantly as in younger infants, even when ICP is markedly elevated.

A second pattern of "hyperemic-type" CBFV response with correspondingly increased MFV when ICP increased ($r = +0.63$, $P < .001$; see Fig. 5) was seen in 4 studies. However, the "hyperemic-type" response was associated with a variable change in RI (Fig. 6). Figure 7 shows an illustrative graphical plot from patient CM, with increased MFV and RI as ICP increased. A different cerebrovascular resistance result was seen in one patient (PB) with a "hyperemic-type" response where MFV increase when ICP increased was associated with a corresponding decrease in RI (Fig. 8). None of these studies

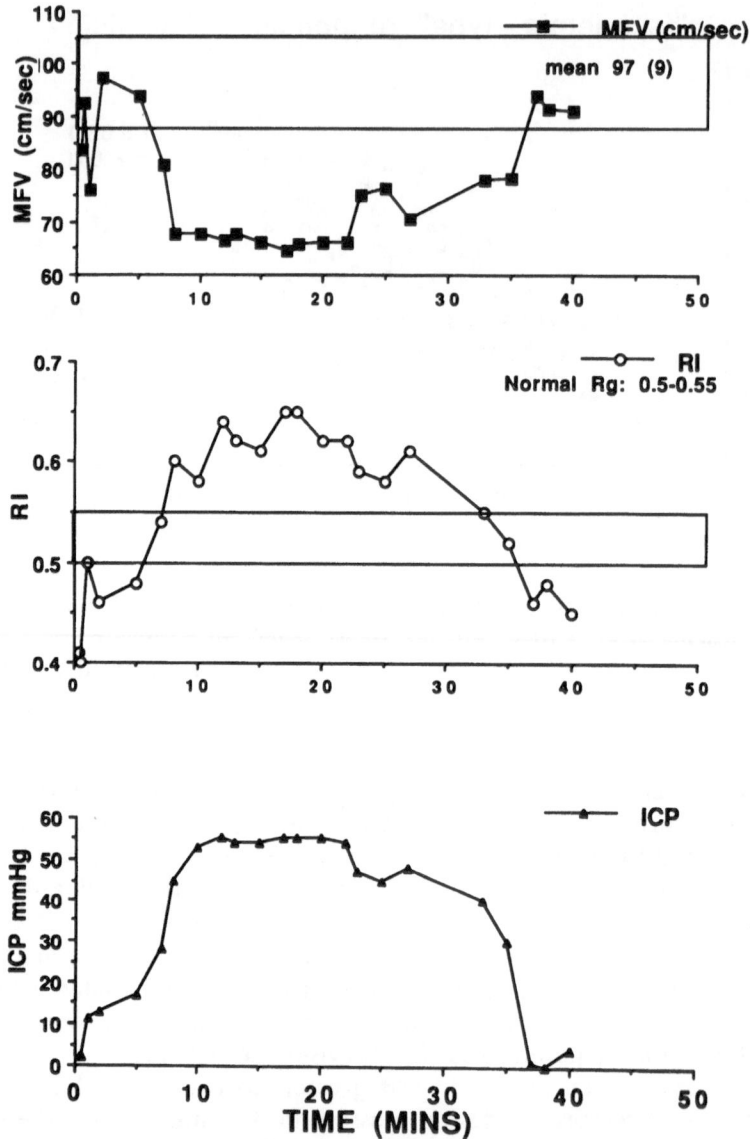

Fig. 3. A graphical plot of simultaneous ICP, RI, and MFV during an A-wave recorded in patient AD, showing an "ischemic-type" CBFV response with progressive decrease in MFV and increase in RI as ICP increased. Range of mean (±SD) RI and MFV for age (Bode and Wais 1988) is indicated on graphs

with a "hyperemic-type" response had prolonged elevated ICP recorded; maximum were pre-plateau waves of 25–30 mmHg for 5–6 min. One was a repeat study in patient HS after skulll morcellation was performed, when ICP recorded was significantly improved from the preoperative study. The previous "ischemic type" CBFV response was not present postoperatively.

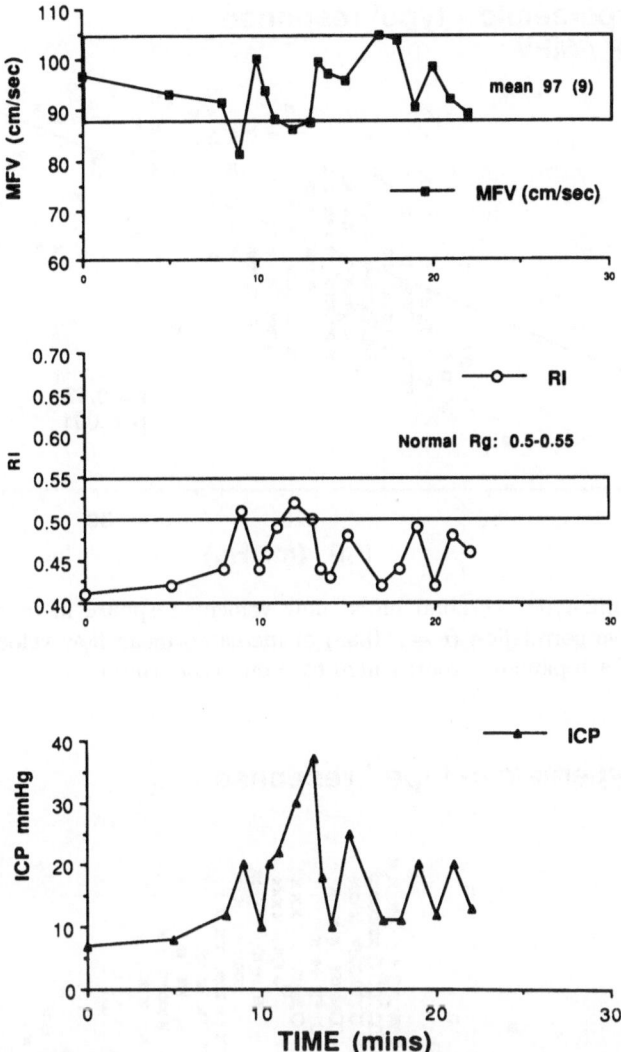

Fig. 4. Plot of simultaneous ICP, RI, and MFV during B waves recorded in patient LH, showing "ischemic-type" CBFV response with decreased MFV and increased RI as ICP increased. Range of mean (±SD) RI and MFV for age (Bode and Wais 1988) is shown

Discussion

A significant correlation has been reported for Doppler velocity indices and CBF in neonates, measured using the well established xenon 133 method (Greisen et al. 1984). In particular, CO_2-induced percentage change shows reliable correlation with MFV as an index of flow (Bishop et al. 1986) and RI as an index of distal cerebrovascular resistance in individual patients (Archer et al. 1986). In our study, measurement error of CBFV due to varying angle

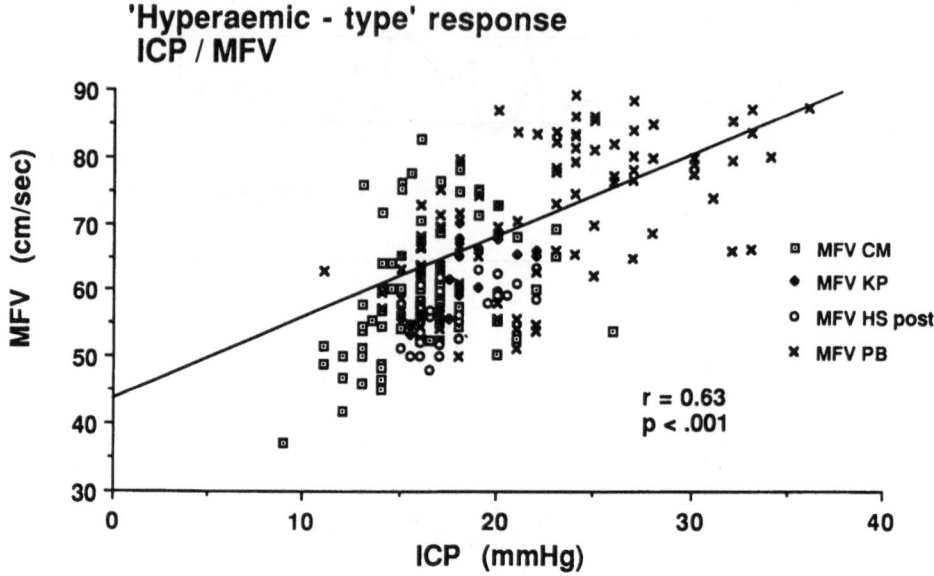

Fig. 5. "Hyperemic-type" cerebral blood flow velocity response in four studies with significant positive correlation ($r = +0.63$) of increased mean flow velocity (*MFV*) as ICP increased. Each patient is represented by a different symbol

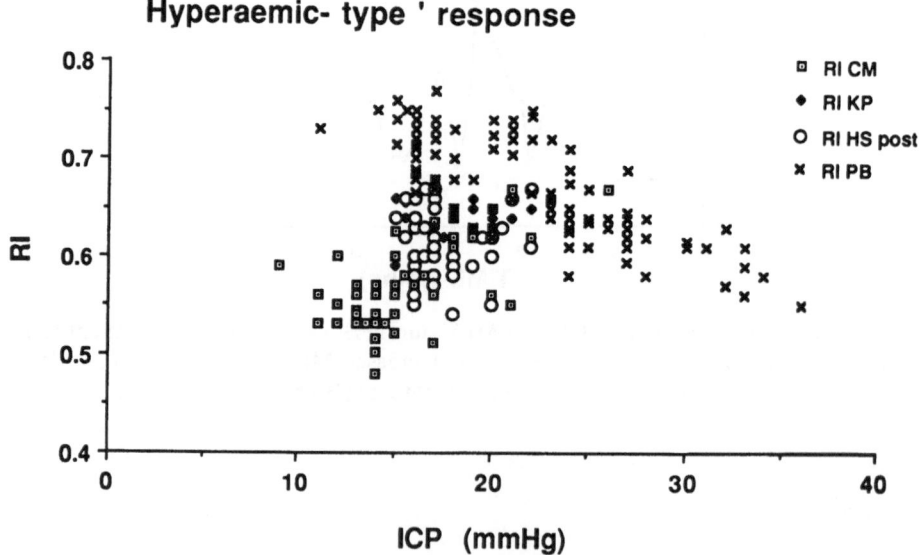

Fig. 6. Shows a variable Resistance Index (*RI*) change with increased ICP in four studies with a "hyperemic-type" response, i.e., increased MFV as ICP increased. Each patient is represented by a different symbol

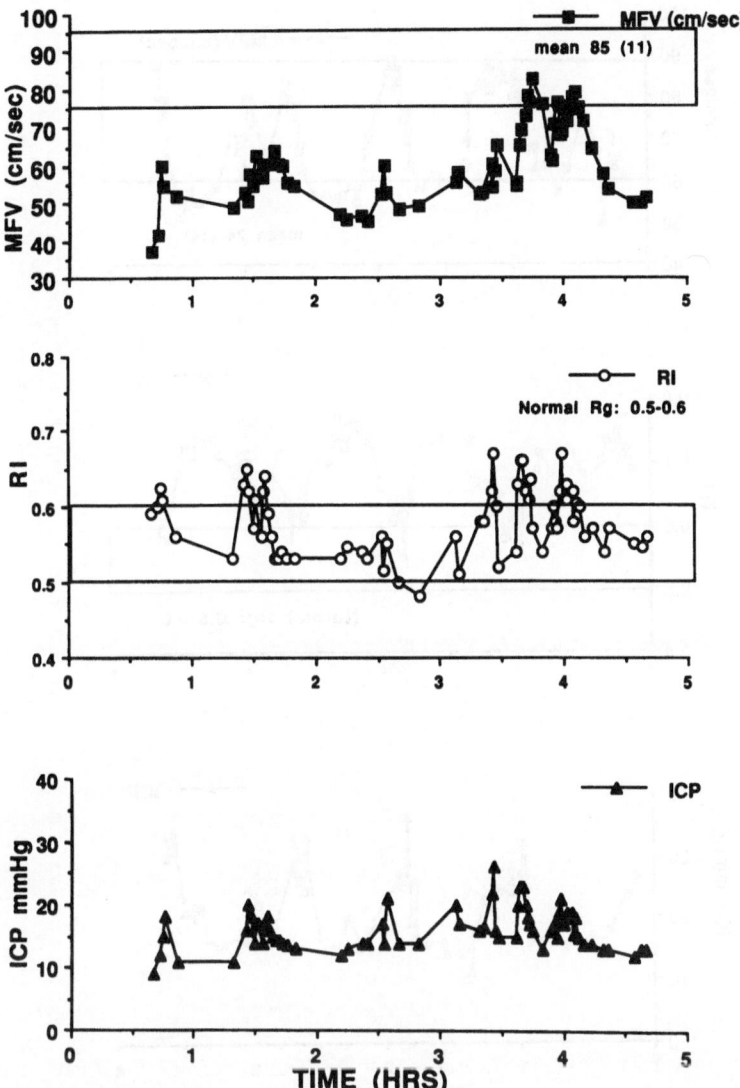

Fig. 7. Plot of simultaneous ICP, RI, and MFV in patient CM, illustrating "hyperemic-type" CBFV response with increased MFV and increased RI as ICP increased. Range of mean (±SD) RI and MFV for age (Bode and Wais 1988) is shown

of insonation was minimized, as very frequent or continous recording was performed throughout an individual study from a constant position and depth when the optimal signal was determined at the beginning. We have assumed that it is unlikely that there would be any significant change in MCA diameter to significantly affect CBFV in our study, as firstly, there was no evidence of cerebral vascular disease in our young patients and secondly, autoregulatory response occurs mainly through alteration of caliber in distal resistance vessels rather than in a major artery such as the MCA.

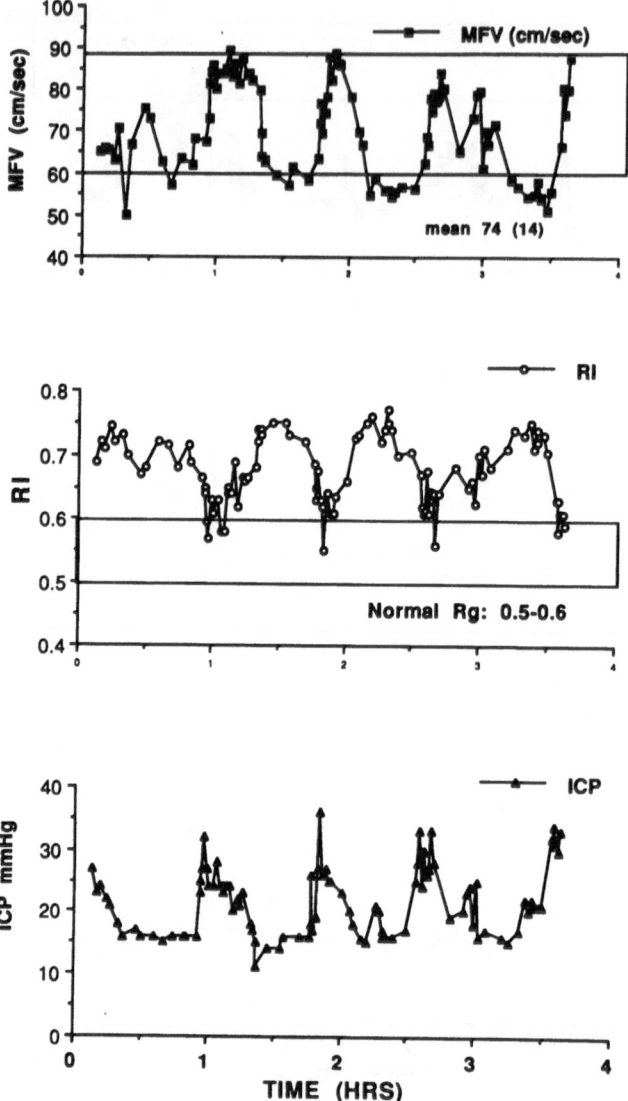

Fig. 8. Plot of simultaneous ICP, RI, and MFV in patient PB who showed a "hyperemic-type" response with increased MFV as ICP increased, but associated with corresponding decrease in RI. The range of mean (±SD) RI and MFV for patient's age (Bode and Wais 1988) is shown

Minns and Merrick (1989) have shown that a prolonged nett cerebral mean transit time representing reduced circulatory reserve correlates significantly with reduced perfusion pressure due to raised intraventricular pressure in hydrocephalic children. Cerebrovascular response to increased cerebrospinal fluid pressure occurs by collapsing cerebral veins and by pial arterial dilatation of 40% when ICP is increased from 13 to 45 mmHg with, however, no marked further arterial dilatation occurring with further rises in ICP (Kato and Auer 1989). Our results suggest that in the studies with a "hyperemic-type" CBFV response, arterial dilatation and increased cerebral blood flow occurred with increased ICP in sleep to maintain an adequate perfusion pressure. This is more likely to occur in patients who have adequate circulatory reserve. The RI response may be variable, as change in distal cerebrovascular resistance will depend on other factors such as existing transmural pressure, vascular compliance, and cerebral blood volume. In some patients increased flow may be associated with a decrease in distal cerebrovascular resistance (e.g., patient PB) possibly due to a significant reduction in CPP with impaired autoregulation, although in other patients increased flow may result in little or further increase in distal resistance. Doppler flow velocities cannot quantitate absolute CBF nor its ratio to blood volume and hence it may be difficult from this technique alone to reliably predict the overall effect on cerebrovascular resistance and nett perfusion.

In cases with craniocerebral disproportion where intracranial compliance is likely to be more significantly reduced, a clear "ischemic-type" CBFV response seen during A and B waves suggests that circulatory reserve may be critical during these episodes. Further increase of ICP beyond 45 mmHg did not significantly increase pial arterial dilatation (Kato and Auer 1989), thus maximum autoregulatory response of increased CBF has already occurred and any subsequent further increase in ICP will be likely to result in reduced perfusion with increased resistance. Our results suggest that this is more likely when intracranial compliance is critical, hence small increases in any intracranial compartment, such as in the vascular compartment, during sleep (REM or stage II nREM sleep) can cause a significant rise in resistance, resulting in reduced CBF. This "ischemic-type" response was abolished in patient HS after skull morcellation, which would have improved intracranial compliance by enhancing total intracranial volume; consequently circulatory reserve should also have improved.

Doppler techniques cannot, as we have indicated, provide a true measure of CBF, hence it is not possible to determine if critical levels of perfusion (Jones et al. 1981) occurred. Although we have indicated reported normal ranges of MFV (mean + SD) from Bode and Wais (1988) in our illustrations, this cannot be interpreted as higher or lower than normal CBF, because without knowing individual true cerebral artery cross-sectional area, CBFV cannot accurately be equated as CBF between individuals. Changes in Doppler waveforms may also reflect factors other than those occurring within the cerebral circulation, factors such as the cardiac output. Satisfactory simultaneous true arterial pressure was not available as we felt that an indwelling arterial catheter was not justified for overnight monitoring purposes in children. Heart rate and oscillometric measurement of blood pressure, however, showed no significant change over each study period. End-tidal pCO_2 was also not measured, as our patients would not have tolerated a face mask throughout a normal sleep period. However none of the patients had any chronic or intercurrent respiratory complications.

Studies which have reported a consistent increase only in pulsatility of Doppler waveforms where RI increased and MFV decreased during major increase in ICP have been performed in severely ill adult patients when auto-regulation was assumed to be impaired (Hassler et al. 1988; Klingelhofer et al. 1988). Circulatory reserve would most likely also be critical in these cases. Although our study numbers are small, our results suggest that in hydrocephalic children during sleep, appropriate increased CBF response generally occurs during episodic increase of ICP, but when compliance is limited circulatory reserve may be critical and this may result in an "ischemic-type" response during a sustained rise of ICP. Simultaneous transcranial Doppler monitoring of CBFV response to ICP changes during sleep may help to further determine the patients whose intracranial compliance renders them less able to respond adequately to increased ICP and thus more liable to suffer subsequent ischemic damage.

Acknowledgment. We are grateful to the Earl of Elgin and the TSB Foundation for supporting research into hydrocephalus at the Neurology Unit, Royal Hospital for Sick Children, Edinburgh.

References

Aaslid R, Markwalder TM, Nornes H (1982) Noninvasive transcranial Doppler ultrasound recording of flow velocity in basal cerebral arteries. J Neurosurg 57: 769–774

Aaslid R, Lundar T, Lindegaard KF, Nornes H (1986) Estimation of cerebral perfusion pressure from arterial blood pressure and transcranial Doppler recordings. In: Miller JD, Teasdale GM, Rowan JO, Galbraith SL, Mendelow AD (eds) Intracranial pressure VI. Springer, Berlin Heidelberg New York, pp 226–229

Archer LNJ, Evans DH, Paton JY, Levene MI (1986) Controlled hypercapnia and neonatal cerebral artery Doppler ultrasound waveforms. Pediatr Res 20: 218–221

Bada HS, Hajjar W, Chua C, et al. (1979) Noninvasive diagnosis of neonatal asphyxia and intraventricular hemorrhage by Doppler ultrasound. J Pediatr 95: 775

Bishop CCR, Powell S, Rutt D, et al. (1986) Transcranial Doppler measurement of middle cerebral artery blood flow velocity: A validation study. Stroke 17: 913–915

Bode H, Wais U (1988) Age dependance of flow velocities in basal cerebral arteries. Arch Dis Child 63: 606–61

Di Rocco C, McLone DG, Shimoji T, Raimondi AJ (1975) Continous intraventricular cerebrospinal fluid pressure recording in hydrocephalic children during wakefulness and sleep. J Neurosurg 42: 683–689

Greisen G, Johansen K, Ellison PM, et al. (1984) Cerebral blood flow in the newborn infant: comparison of Doppler ultrasound and 133 Xenon clearance. J Pediatr 104: 411–418

Hassler W, Steinmetz H, Gawlowski J (1988) Transcranial Doppler ultrasonography in raised intracranial pressure and in intracranial circulatory arrest. J Neurosurg 68: 745–751

Hill A, Volpe JJ (1982) Decrease in pulsatile flow in the anterior cerebral arteries in infantile hydrocephalus. Pediatrics 69: 4–7

Ingvar DH (1971) Cerebral blood flow and metabolism related to EEG and cerebral functions. Acta Anaesthesiol Scand [Suppl] 45: 110–113

Jones TH, Morawetz RB, Crowell RM, et al. (1981) Thresholds of focal cerebral ischemia in awake monkeys. J Neurosurg 54: 773–782

Kato Y, Auer LM (1989) Cerebrovascular response to elevation of ventricular pressure. Acta Neurochir (Wien) 98: 184–188

Klingelhofer J, Conrad B, Benecke R, et al. (1988) Evaluation of intracranial pressure from transcranial Doppler studies in cerebral disease. J Neurol 235: 159–162

Leggate JRS, Baxter P, Minns RA, et al. (1988) Role of a separate subcutaneous cerebrospinal fluid reservoir in the management of hydrocephalus. Br J Neurosurg 2: 327–338

Maeda H, Etani H, Handa N, et al. (1990) A validation study on the reproducibility of transcranial Doppler velocimetry. Ultrasound Med Biol 16: 9–14

Minns RA (1991) Infectious and parainfectious encephalopathies. In: Minns RA (ed) Problems of intracranial pressure in childhood — clinics in developmental medicine. MacKeith Press, London, pp 233–248

Minns RA, Merrick MV (1989) Cerebral perfusion pressure and nett cerebral mean transit time in childhood hydrocephalus. J Pediatr Neurosci 5: 69–77

Pourcelot L (1976) Diagnostic ultrasound for cerebral vascular diseases. In: Donald I, Levi S (eds) Present and future of diagnostic ultrasound. Kooyker, Rotterdam, pp 141–147

Rosner MJ, Becker DP (1984) Origin and evolution of plateau waves. J Neurosurg 60: 312–324

V. Normal-Pressure Hydrocephalus

59 — Lumboperitoneal Shunt for Communicating Hydrocephalus

Joong Uhn Choi, Young Soo Kim, Sang Sup Chung, and Kyu Chang Lee[1]

Summary. In the last 6 years a series of 70 lumboperitoneal shunts for communicating hydrocephalus were performed at our institute. Causes of communicating hydrocephalus were various: 24 subarachnoid hemorrhage, 23 posttraumatic, 7 spontaneous intracerebral hemorrhage, 6 postmeningitic, 5 idiopathic normotensive hydrocephalus, 3 external hydrocephalus, and 2 infantile hydrocephalus. Complications were found in 11 patients. We encountered nine obstructions of shunt catheters (13%), four migrations (6%), and one infection (1.4%). Ventricular size was compared on brain computed tomography (CT) scans taken before and after shunting. Only 15 cases (21%) showed moderately or markedly reduced ventricular systems after shunting. Changes of ventricular size were not related to clinical course or outcome.

About 59 patients (84%) were clinically improved after lumboperitoneal shunts.

Keywords. Lumboperitoneal shunt — Communicating hydrocephalus — Isotope cisternography

Introduction

Jackson and Snodgrass first reported a lumboperitoneal shunt, using a polyethylene tube, in 1955. Since that time this procedure has been used not only for communicating hydrocephalus, but also for benign intracranial hypertension, cerebrospinal fluid fistula, and bulging craniectomy (Selman et al. 1980; James and Tibbs 1981). In the last 6 years the authors have treated 70 patients with communicating hydrocephalus, using lumboperitoneal shunts. The following is a report on those cases, together with a review of the literature.

---

[1] Department of Neurosurgery, Yonsei University College of Medicine, Seoul, Korea

Table 1. Causes of communicating hydrocephalus

Causes	No. of patients (n)
Subarachnoid hemorrhage	24
Posttraumatic	23
Intracerebral hemorrhage	7
Postmeningitic	6
NPH of unknown cause	5
External hydrocephalus	3
Infantile hydrocephalus	2
Total	70

NPH, normal pressure hydrocephalus

Patients and Methods

The communicating hydrocephalus in our 70 patients was due to various causes (Table 1). Communicating hydrocephalus after subarachnoid hemorrhage was the most common cause (24 cases), followed by 23 posttraumatic, 7 intracerebral, 6 postmeningitic, 5 normotensive hydrocephalus of unknown cause, 3 external hydrocephalus, and 2 infantile hydrocephalus.

We performed radioisotope cisternography using Tc^{99m} in all patients suspected of communicating hydrocephalus. If the ventricular reflex persisted over 24 h, we selected those patients as candidates for lumboperitoneal shunt.

In most cases in our series the percutaneous method was used. The patient was placed in the right lateral recumbent position, and left abdomen and lower back were prepared and draped in the usual manner. A small midline incision (1 cm) was made at the L4–5 space and a spinal tap was done using a 14-gauge Touhey needle.

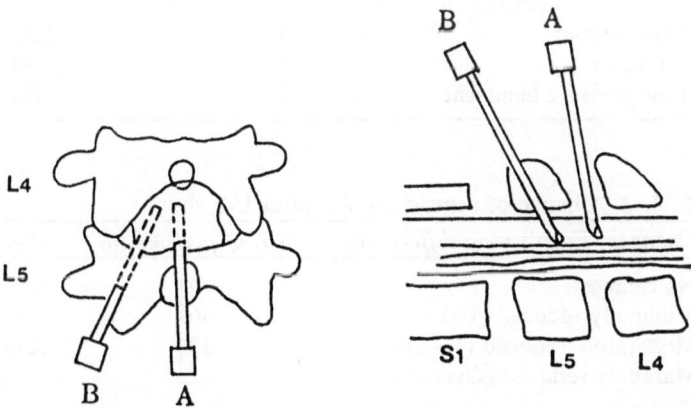

Fig. 1. Methods of spinal tap during lumboperitoneal shunt. A, Classical midline approach; B, Lateral approach 1 cm lateral from midline at L5 spinous process level

The spinal side of the shunt catheter was introduced into the spinal sub-arachnoid space through the needle. About 5–10 cm of catheter was introduced into the spinal canal. An abdominal incision was made in the left lower lateral part of abdomen. The tip of the abdominal side of the catheter was passed subcutaneously from the back wound and inserted into the peritoneal cavity. The shunt catheter was encircled with a fixation sleeve and this was sutured to the fascia of the lower back. The wound was closed in layers. Sometimes we failed to introduce the catheter through the tapped needle. On those occasions we tried to do the spinal tap from 1 cm lateral from the L5 spinous process (Fig. 1). We found out that this approach was much more successful for introducing the shunt catheter through the tapped needle.

In three young children below the age of 6 months we used a T-tube catheter (Hoffman et al. 1976) after the laminectomy of L4. We let the patients sit up from the day following surgery.

Results

Complications

Sixteen complications were found in 11 patients after shunting (Table 2). Obstructions were found in nine patients; six of them were revised and ventriculoperitoneal shunts were performed in three patients.

There were migrations in four cases; two migrated into the spinal canal and two into the peritoneal cavity. In none of these four patients had a fixation sleeve been used, as they were operated at the beginning of our series of

Table 2. Complications of lumboperitoneal shunt

Complications	No. of patients (n)		(%)
Migration of shunt	4		(6)
Spinal		2	
Peritoneal		2	
Obstruction	9		(13)
Infection	1		(1.4)
Low pressure headache	2		(3)

Table 3. Change of ventricular size after L-P shunt

Changes (Evan's ratio difference)	No. of patients (n)	(%)
No change	9 ⎤	(79)
Minimally reduced (1–10)	46 ⎦	
Moderately reduced (11–20)	13 ⎤	(21)
Markedly reduced (Over 20)	2 ⎦	
Total	70	

L-P, lumboperitoneal

Table 4. Patient outcome after L-P shunt

Outcome	No. of patients (n)	(%)
Normal at first	8 ⎤	
Recovered to normal from some deficits	16 ⎬	(84)
Improved with some deficits	35 ⎦	
Not improved, with deficits	11	(16)
Total	70	

L-P, lumboperitoneal

lumboperitoneal shunts. Two patients had low pressure headache after shunting, but they gradually tolerated this without specific management. There was only one infection, in a 5-year-old boy. This patient needed revision after infection control.

Changes of Ventricular Size

We compared ventricular size on brain CT scans taken preoperatively and at 2 weeks after shunting. We measured ventricular size using Evan's ratio and we graded postoperative changes into four categories (Table 3). Fifty five patients (79%) showed no change in, or minimally reduced (Evan's ratio change less than 10) ventricular size. Only 15 patients (21%) showed moderately or markedly reduced (Evan's ratio change more than 11) ventricular size. Changes of ventricular size were not related to clinical improvement.

Outcome of Patients After Shunting

Neurological deficits mainly depended on the primary diseases of the patients; however, we tried to compare changes of neurological condition before and after lumboperitoneal shunt (Table 4).

Eight patients had no deficits before or after shunting. Sixteen patients had some minor deficits, such as ataxic gait, preoperatively but recovered to normal after lumboperitoneal shunt. Thirty five patients had some neurological deficits which improved after shunting. Eleven patients (16%) did not show any improvement postoperatively.

Discussion

Shunting into the peritoneal cavity in hydrocephalus was first performed by Ferguson in 1889. He placed a silver wire in a canal drilled through a lumbar vertebra, connecting the subarachnoid space with the abdominal cavity, but the patient died within 24 h of the procedure. In 1908, Cushing used a silver cannula for transvertebral lumboperitoneostomies in 12 patients, but had poor results.

In 1955 Jackson and Snodgrass described lumboperitoneal shunting using a polyethylene tube; they reported that only 22 out of 62 patients were alive after 4 years.

In 1967 Murtaugh and Lehman described their percutaneous procedure, using a 16-gauge Touhey spinal needle to introduce a polyethylene catheter into the lumbar subarachnoid space. The tubing was then tunneled subcutaneously around the flank and inserted through a small muscle-splitting incision into the peritoneal cavity. Complications of kinking, adhesive arachnoiditis, and migration were reported.

The good results of Eisenberg et al. (1971) with lumboperitoneal shunts in which silastic tubing was placed into the lumbar subarachnoid space by way of hemilaminectomy, established lumboperitoneal shunting as an effective treatment for communicating hydrocephalus. Subsequently Spetzler et al. (1975) reported their use of the percutaneous lumboperitoneal shunt employing silastic tubing and its advantage over polyethylene as a biologically inert material.

Previous reports have cited complication rates as high as 44% for ventriculoatrial or ventriculoperitoneal shunts, with 9% shunt-related deaths (Wood et al. 1974) and a 20% incidence of subdural hematoma (Samuelson et al. 1972). In 1980 Black reported a series of 62 patients with idiopathic normal pressure hydrocephalus. Fifty seven of these patients had ventriculoatrial shunts installed and five had ventriculoperitoneal shunts. The complication rate was 35.4%, including six patients who had chronic subdural hematoma and four patients who developed seizures of new onset.

Selman et al. (1980) reported a series of 130 patients who underwent percutaneous lumboperitoneal shunting. The morbidity in this series was 18%, the infection rate was 0.8%, and the subdural hematoma rate was 0.8%. There were no shunt — related mortalities. We encountered nine obstructions (13%), four migrations (6%) and one infection (1.4%) among our 70 patients. Migrations were found after we began to use fixation sleeves.

Selman et al. (1980) reported a series of 98 patients with communicating hydrocephalus who were treated with lumboperitoneal shunts. Of these cases, 26 were secondary to known causes such as subarachnoid hemorrhage, tumor, or meningitis. Seventy two cases were defined as idiopathic. Of the patients with communicating hydrocephalus secondary to known causes, 92% improved after shunting, compared to a 51% improvement rate in cases classified as idiopathic. Our results clearly followed this outcome. Most of the patients in our series had communicating hydrocephalus secondary to known causes such as trauma, subarachnoid hemorrhage, spontaneous intracerebral hematoma, and meningitis. Eighty four percent were improved after shunting.

We compared ventricular sizes on brain CTs taken before and after shunting. Only 15 cases (21%) showed moderately or markedly reduced ventricular size after shunting. However, reduction rates of ventricular size were not related to clinical courses or to outcome.

These findings could be suggested as possible factors in the low rate of intracranial complications, such as subdural hematoma or slit ventricle syndrome after lumboperitoneal shunts.

Since the report of Eisenberg et al. (1971) the lumboperitoneal shunt has become established as an effective procedure for the treatment of communicating hydrocephalus. The great advantage of this shunt is that it is completely extracranial and thus eliminates the need to further invade an already compromised brain and ventricular system, thereby significantly reducing morbidity and mortality.

References

Black PM (1980) Idiopathic normal pressure hydrocephalus. Results of shunting in 62 patients. J Neurosurg 52: 371–372

Cushing H (1908) The cerebral envelopes: Meninges and ependyma. In: Keen WW (ed) Surgery: Its principles and practice. Philadelphia, WB Saunders, pp 101–149

Eisenberg HM, Davidson RI, Shillito J Jr (1971) Lumboperitoneal shunts, review of 34 cases. J Neurosurg 35: 427–431

Ferguson AH (1889) Intraperitoneal diversion of the cerebrospinal fluid in cases of hydrocephalus. NY State J Med 67: 902

Hoffman JH, Hendrick EB, Humphrey RP (1976) New lumboperitoneal shunt for communicating hydrocephalus. J Neurosurg 44: 258–261

Jackson IJ, Snodgrass SR (1955) Peritoneal shunts in the treatment of hydrocephalus and increased intracranial pressure: A 4 year surgery of 62 patients. J Neurosurg 12: 216–222

James HE, Tibbs PA (1981) Diverse clinical applications of percutaneous lumboperitoneal shunts. Neurosurgery 8: 39–42

Murtagh F, Lehman R (1967) Peritoneal shunts in the management of hydrocephalus. JAMA 202: 98–102

Samuelson S, Long DM, Shou SN (1972) Subdural hematoma as a complication of shunting procedures for normal pressure hydrocephalus. J Neurosurg 37: 548–551

Selman WR, Spetzler RF, Wilson CB, Grollmus JM (1980) Percutaneous lumboperitoneal shunt: Review of 130 cases. Neurosurgery 6: 225–257

Spetzler RF, Wilson CB, Grollmus JM (1975) Percutaneous lumboperitoneal shunt. J Neurosurg 43: 770–773

Wood JH, Bartlet D, James AE Jr, Udvarhelyi GB (1974) Normal pressure hydrocephalus: Diagnosis and patient selection for shunt surgery. Neurol (Minneapolis) 24: 517–526

60 — Properties of Interstitial Fluid in the Cerebral White Matter of Patients with Normal Pressure Hydrocephalus

Norihiko Tamaki, Tatsuya Nagashima, Kazumasa Ehara,
Takayuki Shirakuni, Masahiro Asada, Katsuzo Fujita, and
Satoshi Matsumoto[1]

Summary. The properties of interstitial fluid in the periventricular white matter in normal pressure hydrocephalus (NPH) were evaluated by measurement of the relaxation times of brain water protons. Patients with NPH were divided into two groups: Shunt responders and shunt non-responders. In the shunt responder group both T1 and T2 values of the periventricular white matter were significantly prolonged compared to those of the controls, and were shortened after shunting. Both T1 and T2 values of the white matter were significantly longer than those of the gray matter, while the reverse relationship was seen in normal controls. However, in the shunt non-responder group, although T1 of the white matter was significantly prolonged, T2 of the same area was not. There was no change in either T1 or T2 of this region after shunting. Both T1 and T2 were almost the same in white and gray matter in shunt non-responders. It is suggested that the periventricular abnormalities seen in various diseases may be distinguished on the basis of the varying relaxation behavior of tissue water.

Keywords: Normal pressure hydrocephalus — Interstitial edema — Water proton relaxation times — Cerebrospinal fluid shunting — Dementia

Introduction

There has been no single investigation to establish the diagnosis of normal pressure hydrocephalus (NPH) or to distinguish patients with NPH from patients with dementia of other causes. Computed tomography (CT) scans and magnetic resonance (MR) images may reveal similar abnormal density or intensity suggesting increased water content in the periventricular white matter not only in NPH patients, but also in other dementia patients.

In the present study, the properties of the interstitial fluid in the white matter in NPH patients were determined by measurement of the relaxation

---

[1] Department of Neurosurgery, Kobe University School of Medicine, Kobe, 650 Japan

times of the brain water protons. The possibility of distinguishing interstitial edema from other white matter abnormalities was also investigated.

Materials and Methods

Twenty one patients with a mean age of 64, diagnosed as having NPH, underwent ventriculoperitoneal shunting. The diagnosis was made on the basis of clinical findings.

Patients were classified into three groups: The first group consisted of 14 patients with true NPH, who responded to shunting, the second consisted of 7 patients with suspected but false NPH, who did not respond to shunting, and the third group consisted of 17 control patients, with a mean age of 64, who had no proven intracranial organic diseases.

The causes of suspected NPH included idiopathic origin in 13 patients, head injury in 5, and intracranial bleeding in 3.

MR imaging was performed on a total of 38 patients for obtaining T1 and T2 images of the brain. A 0.15 tesla, resistive MRI unit was used for the study. The relaxation times were read directly from calculated T1 and T2 images produced from a two-point method by computer algorithms using a combination of two different pulse sequences. The T1 and T2 were measured in the regions of interest; the periventricular white matter and the cortical gray matter. Post-shunt MR imaging was performed, and T1 and T2 measurements were made in the same fashion, on an average of 51 days after ventricular shunting, varying from 15 to 134 days.

Results

A comparison between T1 and T2 in both the cortical gray matter and the periventricular white matter was made. Both T1 and T2 were significantly longer in the gray matter than in the white matter in the control group. Conversely, in the true NPH group, however, they were longer in the white matter than in the gray matter. In the false NPH group, there was no significant difference between the gray and the white matter in either T1 or T2.

A comparison of T1 and T2 of the regions of interest among the three groups is shown in Fig. 1.

The preshunt T1 of white matter in the true NPH group was significantly prolonged when compared to that in the controls and in the false NPH group. The T1 of white matter in the false NPH group was also significantly longer than that in the control group. However, there was no difference among the three groups in T1 of the gray matter.

As far as the pre-shunt T2 is concerned, the T2 of white matter in the true NPH group was significantly prolonged when compared to that in the control and false NPH groups. There was no significant difference in T2 of white matter between the false NPH and the control group. However,

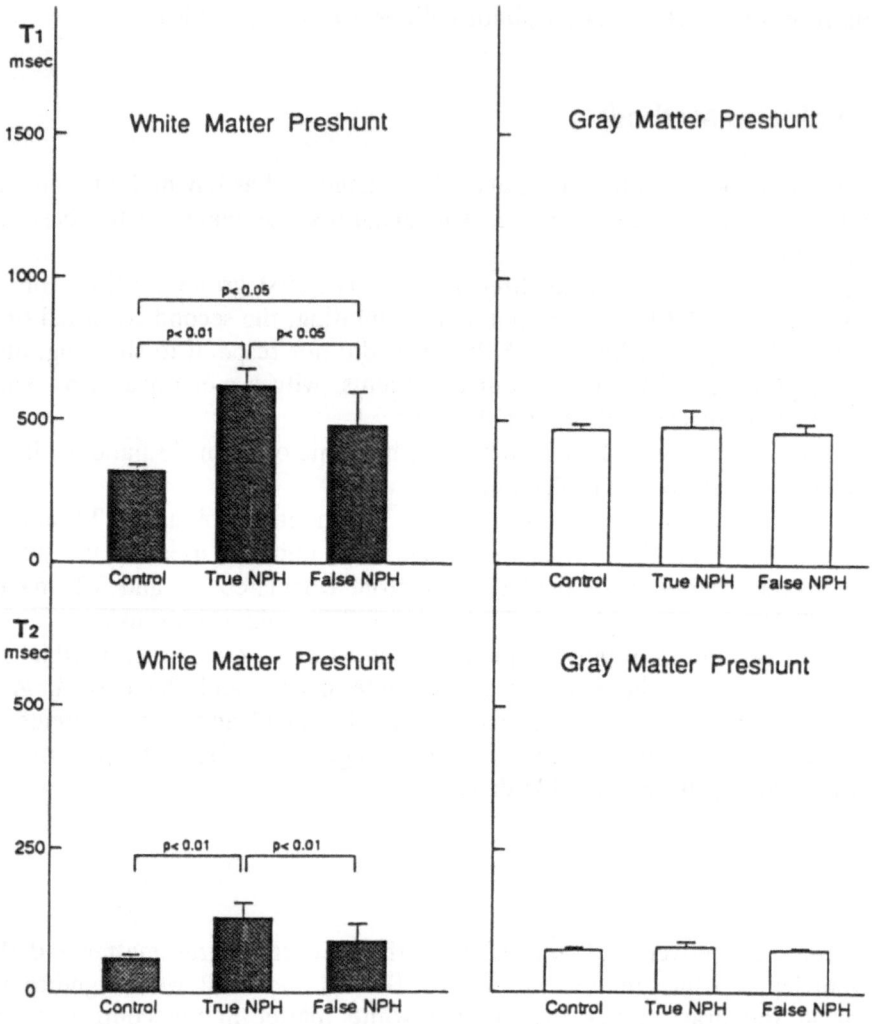

Fig. 1. Comparison of T1 and T2 among control, true NPH, and false NPH groups

there was no difference in the pre-shunt T2 of the gray matter among the three groups.

Changes in T1 and T2 after shunting are shown in Figs. 2 and 3. While there was no change in T1 and T2 of the gray matter after shunting, both T1 and T2 of the white matter in the true NPH group shortened significantly after shunting. In the false NPH group, however, after shunting the T1 and T2 did not change in either area.

A comparison of T1 and T2 in the post shunt true NPH group and the control group is shown in Fig. 4. Both T1 and T2 of white matter in the true NPH group were significantly prolonged, even an average of 51 days after

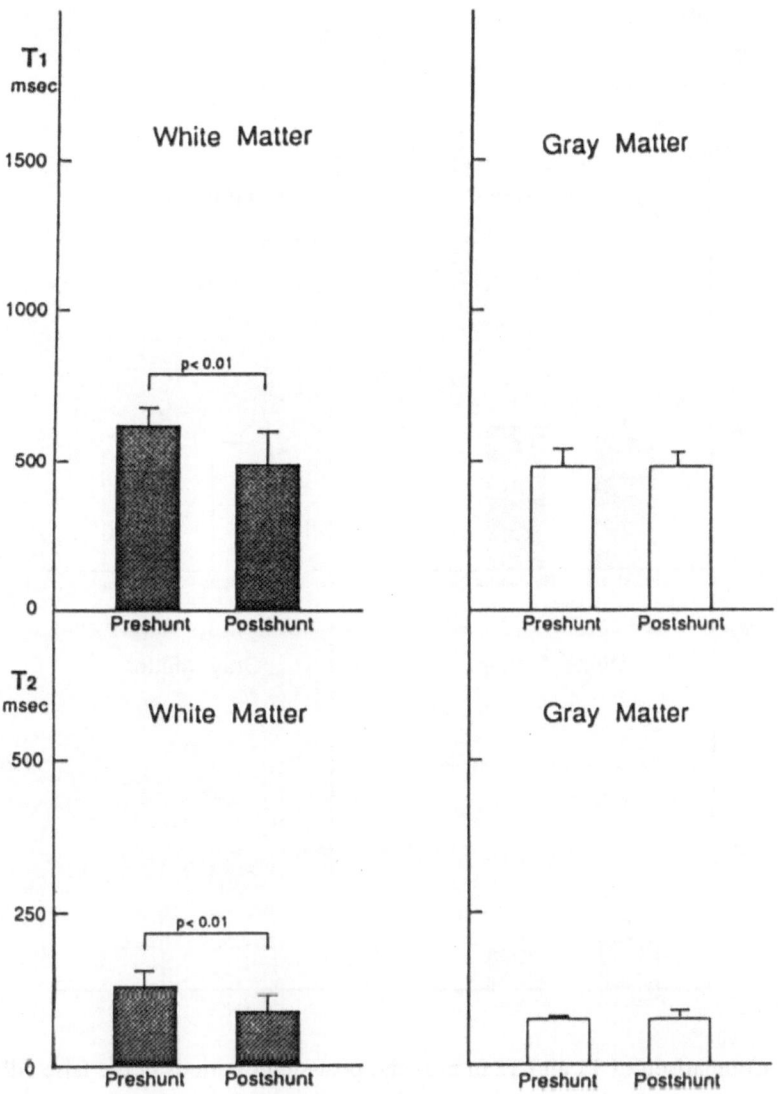

Fig. 2. Comparison of T1 and T2 in pre- and post-shunt periods in the true NPH group

shunting. There was no difference between the postshunt true NPH and the control group in T1 and T2 of the gray matter.

Discussion of Results

The interstitial edema seen in the periventricular white matter of the true NPH group is produced by increased free water content due to CSF migration. This

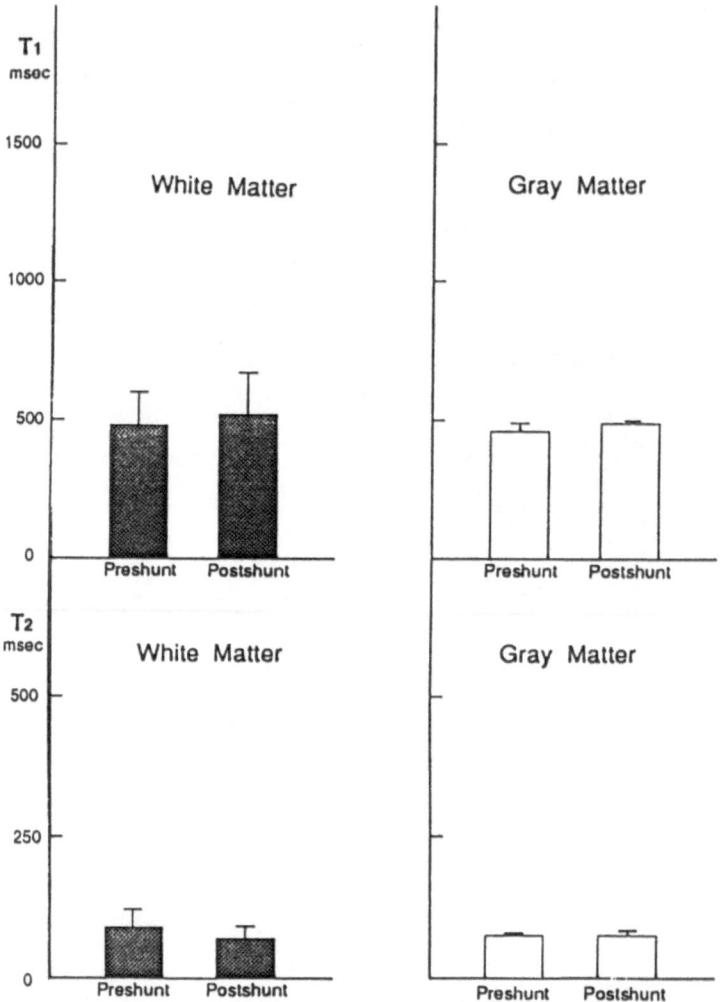

Fig. 3. Comparison of T1 and T2 in pre- and post-shunt periods in the false NPH group

is associated with a proportional prolongation of T1 and T2. In the true NPH group, the free water content in the periventricular white matter appeared to be higher than that in the cortical gray matter. After cerebrospinal fluid (CSF) shunting, the periventricular interstitial edema regressed over a period of several months.

Periventricular CSF edema in NPH may be distinguised from other white matter pathologies. Other white matter pathologies are associated with a significantly prolonged T1 and no significant change in T2 and have very similar T1 and T2 in both the cortical gray matter and the periventricular white matter.

The difference in the relaxation behavior of water protons in true and false NPH patients may be explained by the higher molecular mobility and

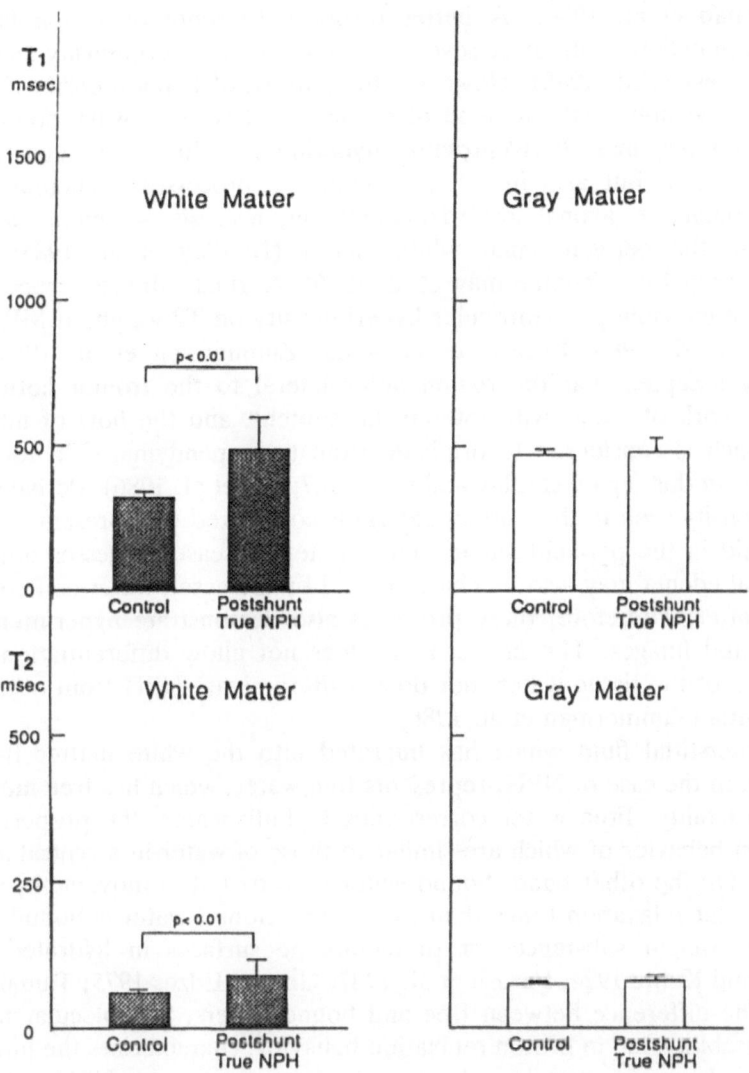

Fig. 4. Comparison of T1 and T2 in post-shunt true NPH patients and controls

diffusibility of the free water proton which exists in the periventricular white matter of the true NPH group.

General Discussion

Hydrated tissue such as periventricular white matter accompanied by interstitial cerebrospinal fluid edema is demonstrated as a high signal intensity on T2-weighted MR images. On the basis of its extent and distribution, a grading system of periventricular hyperintensity on T2-weighted images is now available (Gerard and Weisberg 1986; Kertesz et al. 1988; Tamaki et al. 1985; Zimmerman et al. 1986). A better response to shunt operation has been reported in patients with more severe periventricular hyperintensity (Jack et al. 1987; Kertesz et al. 1988). However, the pattern of hyperintensity alone has proved to be nonspecific to type of disease, and is not always predictive of good shunt response. Periventricular hyperintensity has been seen not only in CSF edema, but also in other pathological processes: Ischemia, gliosis, encephalomalacia, axonal loss, demyelination, necrosis, softening, and lipid change in the periventricular white matter (Bradley et al. 1984; Gerard and Weisberg 1986; Zimmerman et al. 1986). Normal subjects, especially the elderly, often show periventricular hyperintensity on T2-weighted MR images (George et al. 1986; Kertesz et al. 1988; Zimmerman et al. 1986). It is generally accepted that the region anterolateral to the frontal horns has a loose network of axons with low myelin content, and the flow of interstitial fluid, which is considered to originate from transependymal CSF formation, converges in this region (Pollay and Curl 1967; Sze et al. 1986). Periventricular hyperintensity seen in the normal elderly is considered to represent this interstitial fluid in the periventricular white matter. Disease processes other than interstitial edema may also be characterized by increased water content in the white matter. Therefore, these processes also demonstrate hyperintensity on T2-weighted images. The image alone does not allow differentiation of the properties of the tissue water, nor does it discriminate NPH from other types of dementia (Zimmerman et al. 1986).

The interstitial fluid which has migrated into the white matter from the ventricle, in the case of NPH, represents free water, which has free movability and diffusability. Free water corresponds to bulk water, the properties and relaxation behavior of which are similar to those of water in a typical aqueous solution. On the other hand, bound water is restricted in movement, and has much shorter relaxation times than free water. Bound water is bound to high molecular weight substances or to membrane surfaces in hydrated tissues (Cooke and Kuntz 1974; Furuse et al. 1987; Go and Edzes 1975; Tamaki et al. 1990). The difference between free and bound waters, in molecular mobility and diffusability and in proton relaxation behavior, characterizes the interstitial edema of the periventricular white matter in patients with NPH. Thus, the exact measurement of the relaxation times of periventricular white matter appears to be a useful method of characterizing the properties of water in hydrated tissue, and further, it appears to be useful in differentiating patients with NPH from patients with other types of dementia.

References

Bradley WG Jr, Waluch V, Brant-Zawadzki M, Yadley RA, Wycoff RR (1984) Patchy, periventricular white matter lesions in the elderly: A common observation during NMR imaging. Noninvas Med Imag 1: 35–41

Cooke R, Kuntz LD (1974) The properties of water in biological systems. Annu Rev Biophys Bioeng 3: 95–126

Furuse M, Gonda T, Inao S, Kuchiwaki H, Hirai N, Kageyama N (1987): Thermal analysis of water components in brain tissue. Quantitative determination of free and bound water fractions. No to Shinkei 39: 761–767

George AE, de Leon MJ, Kalnin A, Rosner L, Goodgold A, Chases N (1986) Leucoencephalopathy in normal and pathologic MRI of brain lucencies. AJNR 7: 567–570

Gerard G, Weisberg LA (1986) Magnetic resonance imaging in adult white matter disorders and hydrocephalus. Semin Neurol 6: 17–27

Go KG, Edzes HT (1975) Water in brain edema. Observations by the pulsed nuclear magnetic resonance technique. Arch Neurol 32: 462–465

Jack CR, Mokri B, Laws ER, Houser OW, Baker HL, Peterson RC (1987) MR findings in normal-pressure hydrocephalus: Significance and comparison with other forms of dementia. J Comput Assist Tomogr 11: 923–931

Kertesz A, Black SE, Tokar G, Benke T, Carr T, Nicholson L (1988) Periventricular and subcortical hyperintensities on magnetic resonance imaging. "Rims, caps, and unidentified bright objects". Arch Neurol 45: 404–408

Pollay M, Curl F (1967) Secretion of cerebrospinal fluid by the ventricular ependyma of the rabbit. Am J Physiol 213: 1031–1038

Sze G, De Armond SJ, Brant-Zawadzki M, Davis RL, Norman D, Newton TH (1986) Foci of MRI signal (pseudo lesions) anterior to the frontal horns: Histologic correlations of a normal finding. AJNR 7: 381–387

Tamaki N, Shirakuni T, Kojima N, Masumura M, Matsumoto S (1985) Nuclear magnetic resonance study of periventricular edema in hydrocephalus. In: Inaba Y (ed) Brain edema. Springer, Berlin, pp 584–593

Tamaki N, Yamashita H, Kimura M, Ehara K, Asada M, Matsumoto S, Hashimoto M (1990) Changes in the components and content of biological water in the brain of experimental hydrocephalic rabbits. J Neurosurg 73: 274–278

Zimmerman RA, Fleming CA, Lee BCP, Saint-Louis LA, Deck MDF (1986) Periventricular hyperintensity as seen by magnetic resonance. Prevalence and significance. AJNR 7: 13–20

61 — Quantitative Criteria for Successful Outcome in Shunting Operations

Jaan M. Eelmäe, Juri G. Tjuvajev, T. Talvik, and A. Tikk[1]

Introduction

Dilatated cerebrospinal fluid (CSF) spaces can be found by pneumoencephalography (PEG), computed tomography (CT), sonography, and magnetic resonance imaging. The pathogenesis of ventriculomegaly needs to be specifically determined in each individual patient, so that the most appropriate treatment method can be selected.

Patients with hydrocephalus of primary atrophic genesis cannot be improved after shunting procedures. Patients with ventriculomegaly of secondary genesis, caused by disturbances of the CSF circulation, usually improve after correction of the CSF circulation. The results of shunting procedures depend upon the timing and the indications of the operation. Especially important is the fact that sometimes in hydrocephalus of secondary genesis one can be faced with a situation in which the ventricular system is enlarging but the intracranial pressure (ICP) does not increase (Arnold and Laas 1983); shunting procedures are not indicated in such cases.

In the last 10–20 years many investigations reporting the successful shunting of patients with hydrocephalus of primary atrophic genesis have been published. It can be presumed that among these patients were cases with concealed CSF circulation disturbances (Gado et al. 1983; Guidetti and Galiardi 1980; Fox et al. 1973).

For the successful treatment of hydrocephalus a complete investigation, both of the CSF volume and of pressure-volume response compensation mechanisms in the craniospinal system (CSS), must be performed. Such investigations involve the measurement of ventricular system size and the quantitative analysis of CSF dynamics (Sainte-Rose et al. 1987; Tans and Poortvliet 1983, 1984, 1985; Marmarou et al. 1975, 1976, 1978; Ekstedt 1975, 1977).

Keywords. Hydrocephalus — CSF shunt — CSF circulation — CSF pressure

---

[1] Department of Neurosurgery, Tartu University Hospital, Tartu, Estonia

Clinical Material and Methods

This prospective study was carried out in two different groups of patients. The first group consisted of 184 patients with several different types of hydrocephalus. The second group consisted of 64 persons who underwent shunting procedures. All of them were treated either in the intensive care unit or in the neurosurgical and neurological departments of Tartu University Hospital.

Computed tomography studies (CT) were performed on the "Delta-Scan −190" (Ohio Nuclear, USA). The thickness of the slices was 10 mm. To achieve maximum objectivity, a modified Evans index (EI) was used for the evaluation of ventricular dimensions (Fig. 1). Four groups were formed according to the enlargement of ventricular size: hydrocephalus — EI > 0.3; encephalopathy — EI = 0.2–0.3; normal size — EI 0.1–0.2; brain edema — EI < 0.1.

The investigation of CSF dynamics by repeated bolus injection technique was carried out as follows (Fig. 2): After inserting a spinal needle into the lumbar subarachnoid space the CSF pressure was measured by a registering system (Transducer MP-4 and Amplifier RP-3, Nihon-Kohden, Japan, and chartwriter PS-1-02, USSR). Then 20 ml of saline was injected in 2 ml boluses (mean injection rate was 1.7 ± 0.2 ml/min). After every bolus the pressure was measured. CSF pathway obstruction was excluded by the Queckenstedt maneuver. The mean test time was 24.0 ± 5.9 min. From the curves obtained (Fig. 3) a complex of CSF dynamics parameters was calculated: Initial intracranial pressure (ICP), pulsatile amplitude (A), elastance (E), compliance (C),

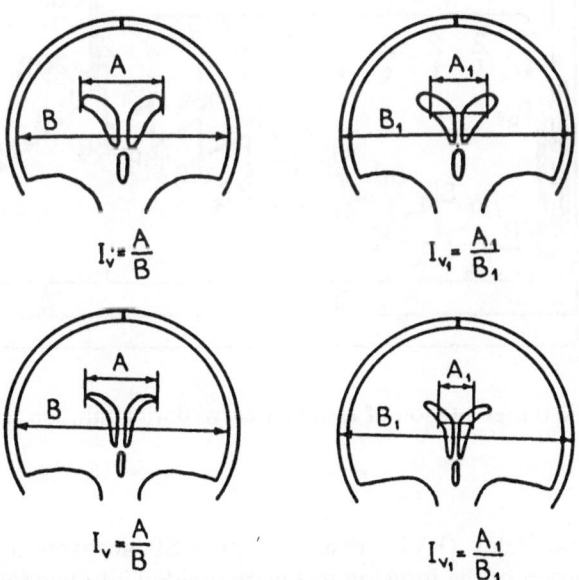

Fig. 1. Measurement of ventricular size by Evans and modified Evan's index. I_v, Evans index; I_{v1}, modified Evan's index; A, ventricular width; B, cranial width

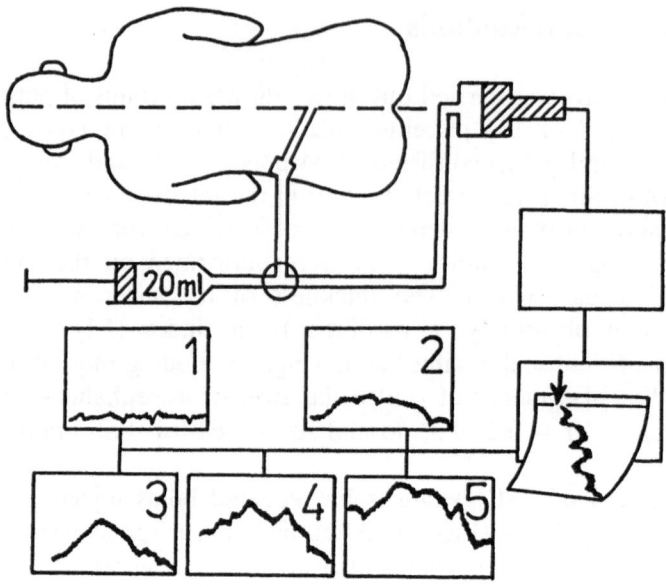

Fig. 2. Scheme of infusion test and types of pressure curves. 1, atrophic curve; 2, normal curve; 3, compensated curve; 4, decompensated curve; 5, hypertensive curve

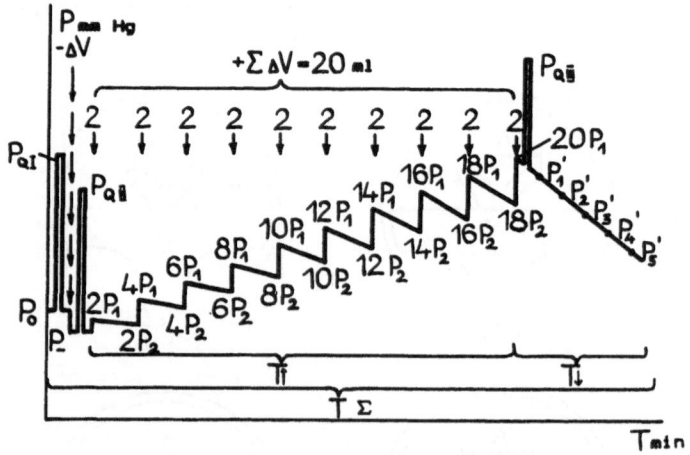

Fig. 3. Schematic representation of resultant curve during infusion test

pressure-volume index (PVI), resistance to CSF absorption (R), and Ayala index (AI). Curves of the infusion test were divided into five types: (1) atrophic, (2) normal, (3) compensated, (4) decompensated, and (5) hypertensive (see Figs. 4, 5, 6, 7 and 8).

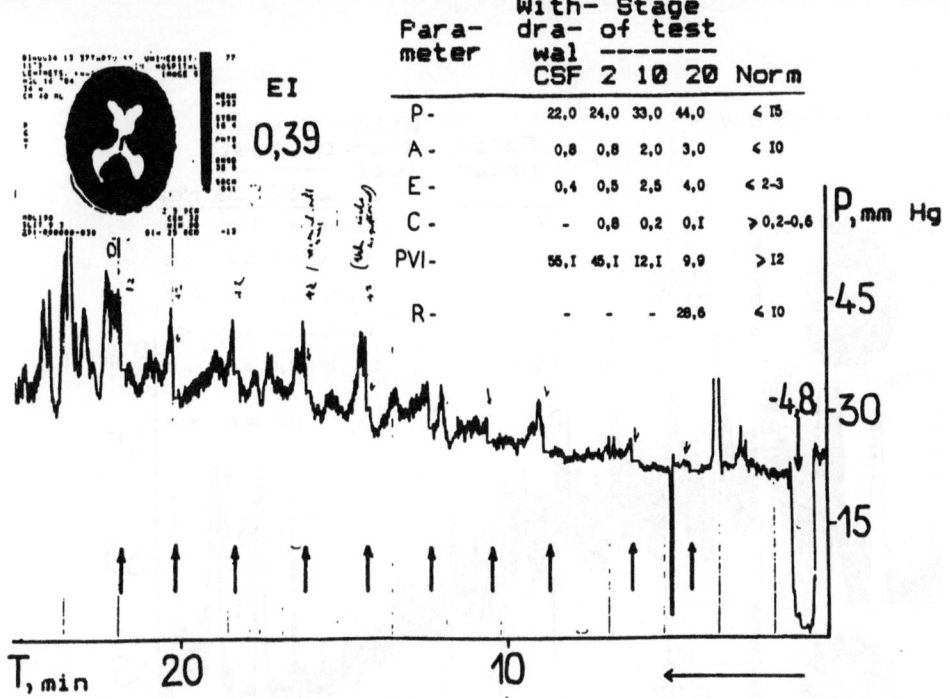

Parameter	Withdrawal CSF	Stage of test 2	10	20	Norm
P-	22,0	24,0	33,0	44,0	< 15
A-	0,8	0,8	2,0	3,0	< 10
E-	0,4	0,5	2,5	4,0	< 2-3
C-	-	0,8	0,2	0,1	> 0,2-0,6
PVI-	55,1	45,1	12,1	9,9	> 12
R-	-	-	-	28,6	< 10

EI 0,39

Fig. 4. Preoperative hypertensive type of pressure curve during infusion test and quantitative parameters of CSF dynamics in a 39-year-old patient with communicative hydrocephalus of unknown etiology. Evans index (*EI*) 0.39. P, pressure; A, pulsatile amplitude; E, elastance; C, compliance; PVI, pressure-volume index; R, resistance to cerebrospinal fluid absorption

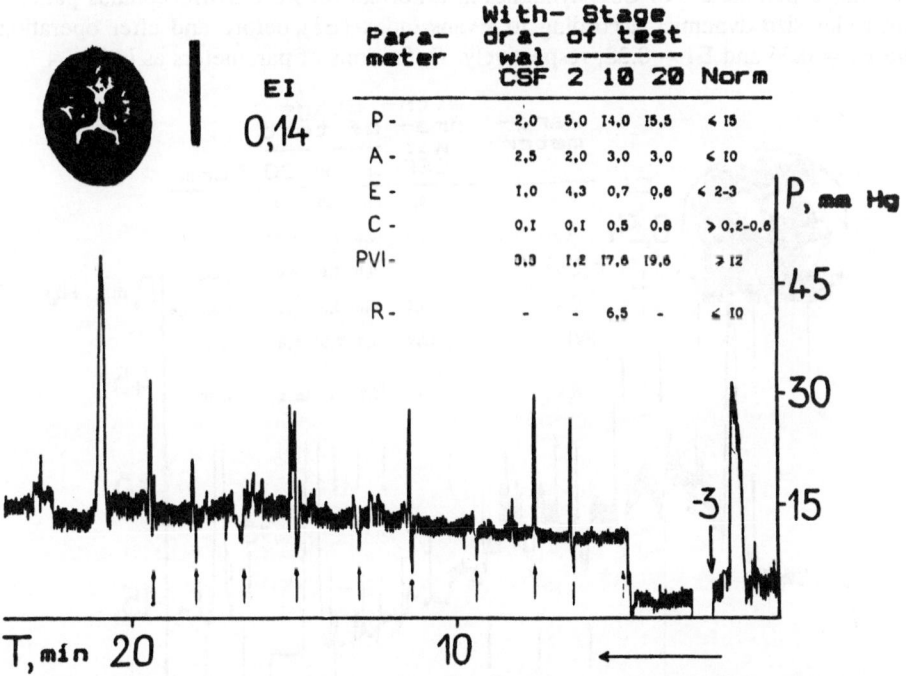

Parameter	Withdrawal CSF	Stage of test 2	10	20	Norm
P-	2,0	5,0	14,0	15,5	< 15
A-	2,5	2,0	3,0	3,0	< 10
E-	1,0	4,3	0,7	0,8	< 2-3
C-	0,1	0,1	0,5	0,8	> 0,2-0,6
PVI-	3,3	1,2	17,6	19,6	> 12
R-	-	-	6,5	-	< 10

EI 0,14

Fig. 5. Normal type of pressure curve during infusion test and quantitative parameters of CSF dynamics after shunting procedure in the patient presented in Fig. 4. Evans index (*EI*) 0.14. Definitions of parameters as in Fig. 4

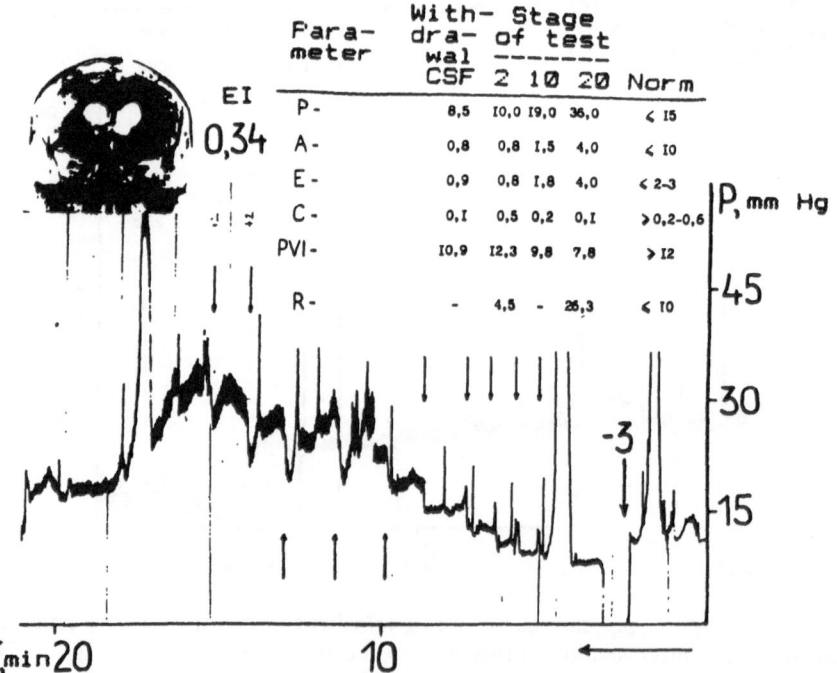

Parameter	Withdrawal CSF	Stage of test			Norm
		2	10	20	
P-	12,5	14,0	36,0	51,0	≤15
A-	4,0	4,0	10,0	12,0	≤10
E-	0,4	0,75	5,0	5,5	≤2-3
C-	0,2	0,61	0,1	0,1	>0,2-0,6
PVI-	30,0	17,6	6,1	8,2	>12
R-	-	-	51,7	25,2	≤10

EI 0,36

EI 0,28

P, mm Hg

3,4

T, min   20   10

Fig. 6. Preoperative decompensated type of pressure curve during infusion test and quantitative parameters of CSF dynamics in a normal pressure hydrocephalus patient. Ventricular size dynamics according to Evans index (*EI*) before and after operation were EI = 0.36 and EI = 0.28, respectively. Definitions of parameters as in Fig. 4

Parameter	Withdrawal CSF	Stage of test			Norm
		2	10	20	
P-	8,5	10,0	19,0	35,0	≤15
A-	0,8	0,8	1,5	4,0	≤10
E-	0,9	0,8	1,8	4,0	≤2-3
C-	0,1	0,5	0,2	0,1	>0,2-0,6
PVI-	10,9	12,3	9,8	7,8	>12
R-	-	4,5	-	25,3	≤10

EI 0,34

P, mm Hg

-3

T, min 20   10

Fig. 7. Compensated type of pressure curve during infusion test and quantitative parameters of CSF dynamics in a patient with mental disorders. Evans index (*EI*) 0.34. Definitions of parameters as in Fig. 4

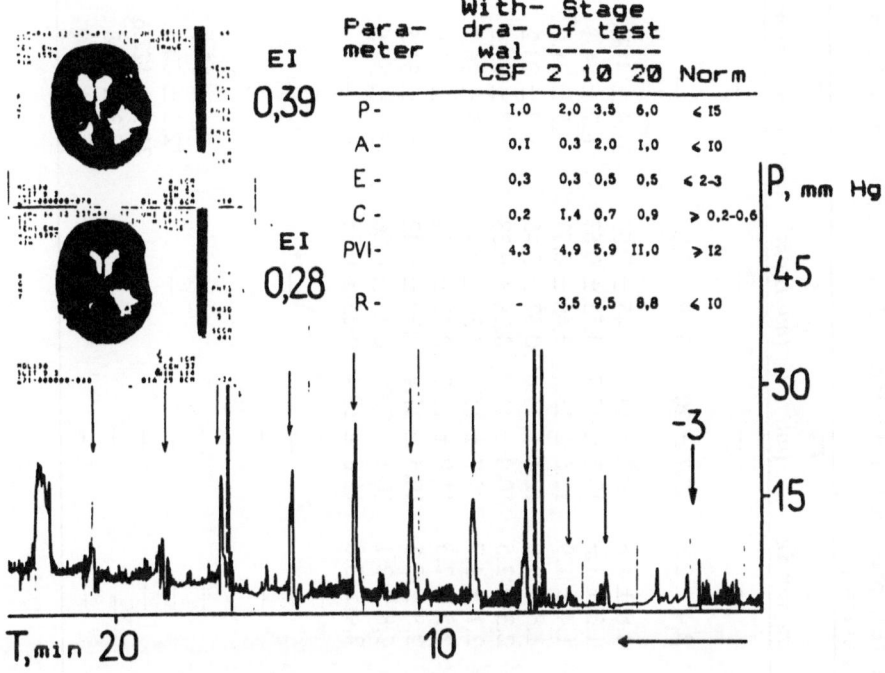

Para-meter	With-dra-wal CSF	Stage of test 2	10	20	Norm
P-	I,0	2,0	3,5	6,0	< 15
A-	0,I	0,3	2,0	1,0	< 10
E-	0,3	0,3	0,5	0,5	< 2-3
C-	0,2	1,4	0,7	0,9	> 0,2-0,6
PVI-	4,3	4,9	5,9	II,0	> 12
R-	-	3,5	9,5	8,8	< 10

Fig. 8. Atrophic type of pressure curve during infusion test and quantitative parameters of CSF dynamics in a patient with hemispheric glioma. Ventricular size by Evans index (*EI*) was 0.39 before shunting. After operation size had reduced to EI = 0.28. Definitions of parameters as in Fig. 4

Results

CSF dynamic parameters after every bolus injection were calculated in the first group (Table 1). The normal values of CSF dynamic parameters were: ICP < 15 mmHg, A < 10 mmHg, E = 2–3 mmHg/ml, C = 0.2–0.3 ml/mmHg, PVI > 12 ml, R < 10 mmHg/ml per min, and AI > 2.3 ml/mmHg. These data correspond to values published by other authors. A correlation matrix of these CSF dynamics parameters and ventricular size was composed (Table 2). A positive correlation between ventricular size and C was found ($r = 0.300$). Tendency to negative correlation between EI and E was observed ($r = -0.232$).

The criteria for shunting procedures on the infusion test were decompensated or hypertensive curves. The preoperative quantitative parameters for a 34-year-old patient with communicative hydrocephalus of unknown etiology can be seen in Fig. 4. This patient had an EI of 0.39 and a hypertensive type of infusion test curve. His ICP, E, and R values were higher than normal, but PVI and C values were lower than normal. The postoperative infusion test curve and CSF dynamic parameters are shown in Fig. 5. A normal type of curve was found and all the CSS visco-elastic property values were normalized.

Table 1. Mean value of pressure (P), pulsatile amplitude (A), elastance (E), pressure-volume index (FVI), compliance (C), and resistance to cerebrospinal fluid absorbtion (R) at various stages of the infusion test ($\bar{x} + \delta$)

Stage of investigation	P_1 (mmHg)	P_2 (mmHg)	A (mmHg)	E (ml/mmHg)	PVI (ml)	C (mmHg/ml)	R (mmHg/ml per min)
Opening values (P$_o$, A$_o$)	10.5 ± 7.4	—	1.6 ± 1.6	—	—	—	—
Parameters after withdrawal of							
CSF (P__, A__, E__, PVL__, C__)	8.2 ± 6.0	—	1.2 ± 1.4	2.4 ± 2.3	18.7 ± 20.8	0.19 ± 0.23	—
During injection of saline:							
2 ml	11.7 ± 7.8	11.3 ± 7.7	1.6 ± 1.7	1.8 ± 1.6	10.2 ± 11.7	0.45 ± 0.56	31.4 ± 418.0
4 ml	13.6 ± 8.7	12.6 ± 7.8	1.8 ± 1.8	1.3 ± 1.6	13.1 ± 15.7	0.53 ± 0.63	8.7 ± 34.1
6 ml	15.2 ± 8.5	13.8 ± 7.6	2.0 ± 1.7	1.4 ± 1.9	12.6 ± 13.1	0.48 ± 0.67	9.8 ± 28.0
8 ml	17.3 ± 9.8	15.4 ± 8.4	2.3 ± 1.8	1.8 ± 1.9	12.1 ± 13.0	0.37 ± 0.45	9.7 ± 23.2
10 ml	20.0 ± 10.9	17.0 ± 9.2	2.6 ± 1.9	2.3 ± 2.5	10.0 ± 11.2	0.28 ± 0.38	17.7 ± 65.6
12 ml	21.3 ± 10.7	18.3 ± 9.6	3.1 ± 2.5	2.1 ± 1.7	9.7 ± 15.7	0.30 ± 0.46	9.5 ± 26.7
14 ml	23.1 ± 11.7	18.4 ± 8.6	3.4 ± 2.5	2.5 ± 2.3	11.0 ± 11.2	0.32 ± 0.34	10.0 ± 17.0
16 ml	23.6 ± 11.0	19.4 ± 9.1	3.5 ± 2.4	2.8 ± 2.1	10.5 ± 11.4	0.30 ± 0.42	15.1 ± 31.5
18 ml	25.1 ± 11.7	20.9 ± 12.7	3.8 ± 2.6	2.8 ± 2.1	10.1 ± 7.9	0.25 ± 0.26	15.1 ± 31.5
20 ml	25.7 ± 12.1	—	3.9 ± 2.6	2.4 ± 5.0	11.8 ± 10.4	0.25 ± 0.36	—
I Queckenstedt's probe	34.0 ± 13.4	—	3.7 ± 2.1	—	—	—	—
II	32.8 ± 13.5	—	3.3 ± 2.0	—	—	—	—
III	42.2 ± 12.2	—	4.9 ± 2.4	—	—	—	—
After injection of saline:							
1 min	23.5 ± 12.9	—	3.5 ± 2.6	—	—	—	9.6 ± 37.3
2 min	21.3 ± 12.1	—	3.0 ± 2.4	—	—	—	12.2 ± 60.3
3 min	20.2 ± 11.2	—	2.6 ± 2.2	—	—	—	21.9 ± 122.6
4 min	20.1 ± 11.6	—	2.7 ± 2.1	—	—	—	19.3 ± 52.8
5 min	19.7 ± 11.3	—	2.6 ± 2.2	—	—	—	19.1 ± 55.0

Table 2. Correlation matrix of ventricular size and CSF dynamics parameters

	EI	ICP	A	E	PVI	C
ICP	−0.160					
A	−0.65	0.990*				
E	−0.232	0.874*	0.869*			
PVI	0.094	−0.388	−0.370	−0.667		
C	0.300*	−0.908*	−0.873*	−0.896	0.645	
R	−0.074	−0.434	−0.420	0.481	−0.413	0.228

$^* - P < 0.05$

EI, Evans index; ICP, initial intracranial pressure; A, pulsatile amplitude; E, elastance; PVI, pressure-volume index; C, compliance

Figure 6 shows the correct indications for shunting. The curve was decompensated and CSF dynamics parameters had abnormal values after the last 2 ml bolus injection; ICP (51 mmHg), A (12 mmHg), E (5.5 mmHg/ml), and R (25.2 mmHg/ml per min) were increased, but C (0.1 ml/mmHg) and PVI (8.2 ml) were decreased. After shunting, the headache and gait disturbances disappeared and, on CT investigation, EI was found to have decreased from 0.36 to 0.28. The compensated curve (Fig. 7) of a patient with mental disorders and large ventricles on PEG did not justify shunting, as 5 min after the last injection ICP decreased to normal values (16 mmHg). The infusion test was also used for detecting shunt function (Fig. 8). A patient with a cyst after the removal of hemispheric glioma was shunted as she showed CSF circulation disturbances, based on clinical and CT signs (large ventricles and midline shift). The infusion test was not performed. The patient improved initially after shunting, but two months later mental disorders, vomiting, and stupor developed. As the curve of the infusion test was of the atrophical type and quite normal ventricular size without midline shift was found on CT, the worsening of patients' condition was probably due to tumor growth, not to shunt occlusion.

Changes in ventricular size before and after operation were analyzed in 31 out of 64 patients. The ventricular size had not decreased in 4 cases (Fig. 9), but in 27 other cases a successful result of shunting was observed, together with decrease of the ventricles. It was found that good results were obtained in cases with an EI > 0.45 before the operation (Fig. 10).

Discussion

Numerous investigations have shown the usefulness of the infusion test in determining indications for shunting operations. Hussey et al. (1970) stated that patients with rapid elevation of the CSF curve need shunting procedures, but Alberti (1977) was of the opinion that the main importance was the decreasing part of the curve after injection. In our opinion, both parts of the

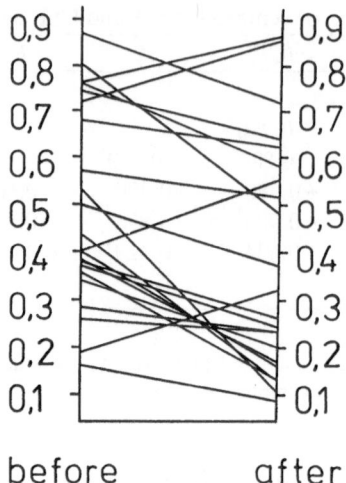

Fig. 9. Changes of ventricular size according to Evans index in 31 patients before and after shunting operation

curve are important. The rate of elevation of ICP after injection characterizes the visco-elastic quality of the craniospinal compartment, while the decrease of the curve indicates craniospinal system (CSS) ability to absorb CSF. Our data are in accordance with the findings of Lamas and Lobato (1979) who, in 92.5% of their cases, found it possible to determine the effectiveness of shunting procedures from the type of infusion test curve.

The pressure-volume index (PVI) is one of the main parameters which characterizes the volumic compensation of the CSS (Shapiro and Marmarou 1982; Tans and Poortvliet 1983). But there are some difficulties in the interpretation of this index, especially regarding its correlation vith ventricular size. Shapiro and Marmarou (1982) and Kosteljanez (1985) found that PVI depended on the volume of the CSS; however, in a later study Shapiro et al. (1985) did not find a correlation between PVI and ventricular size. We agree with Tans and Poortvliet (1983), who recommended investigating the visco-elastic parameters of the CSS in complex, preferably by the bolus technique.

The real parameter of CSF dynamics is R (resistance to CSF absorption) and there are no problems with its interpretation: patients whose R value is more than 10 mmHg/ml per min need a shunting operation. At the same time, R is more sensitive than PVI because, when $R > 20$ mmHg/ml per min, the decrease in PVI stopped (Tans and Poortvliet 1985). Our data support their opinion.

In conclusion, the indications for shunting procedures in different types of hydrocephalus are based on the type of infusion test curve and on CSF dynamics parameters. The hydrocephalic patients selected must be operated as early as possible before ventricular enlargement (EI > 0.45) develops.

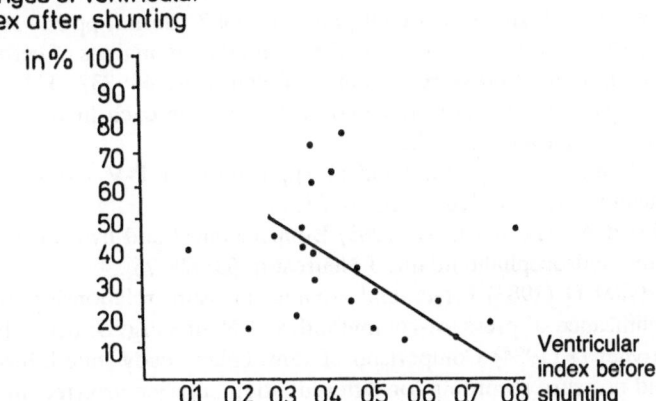

Fig. 10. Relative decrease of ventricular size, according to Evans index, in 21 shunted patients

References

Alberti E (1977) Differentiation of communicating hydrocephalus and presenile dementia by continuous recording of cerebrospinal fluid pressure. J Neurosurg 40: 680–540

Arnold H, Laas R (1983) Extracellularraum und Liquorreabsorbtion. In: Hydrocephalus im fryhen Kindersalter. H von Voght, Stuttgart, pp 46–48

Ekstedt J (1975) CSF hydrodynamics studied by means of constant pressure infusion technique. In: Intracranial pressure, vol 2. Berlin, pp 35–41

Ekstedt J (1977) CSF hydrodynamic studies in man: Method of constant pressure CSF infusion. J Neurol Neurosurg Psychiatry 41: 105–119

Fox J, McCullough D, Green R (1973) Effects of cerebrospinal fluid shunts on intracranial pressure and cerebrospinal fluid dynamics. 2: A new technique of pressure measurement: Result and conception. 3: A concept of hydrocephalus. J Neurol Neurosurg Psychiatry 36: 211–216

Gado M, Patel J, Hughes C, Danziger W, Berg L (1983) Brain atrophy in dementia judged by CT scan ranking. Am J Neurol Radiol 4: 699–702

Guidetti B, Gallardi F (1980) Dementia due to normal pressure hydrocephalus. In: Barbagallo-Songiorgi G, Exton-Smith AN (eds) Aging brain: Neurological and mental disturbances. New York, pp 161–177

Hussey F, Schanzer B, Katzman R, (1970) A simple constant infusion manometric test for measurement of CSF absorption: II clinical study. J Neurol (Minneapolis) 20: 665–680

Kosteljanetz M (1985) Pressure-volume conditions in patients with subarachnoidal and/or intraventricular hemorrhage. J Neurosurg 63: 398–403

Lamas E, Lobato R (1979) Intraventricular pressure and CSF dynamics in chronic adult hydrocephalus. Surg Neurol 12: 287–295

Marmarou A, Shulman K, LaMorgese J (1975) Compartmental analysis of compliance and outflow resistance of the cerebrospinal fluid system J Neurosurg 43: 523–534

Marmarou A, Shapiro K, Shulman K (1976) Isolation of factors leading to sustained elevation of the ICP. In: Intracranial pressure, vol 3. Berlin, pp 33–36

Marmarou A, Shulman K, Rosende R (1978) A nonlinear analysis of cerebrospinal fluid system and intracranial pressure dynamics. J Neurosurg 48: 332–344

Sainte-Rose C, Hooven M, Hirsch J (1987) A new approach in treatment of hydro-cephalus. J Neurosurg 66: 213–226

Shapiro K, Marmarou A (1982) Clinical application of P-V index in treatment of pediatric head injuries. J Neurosurg 56: 819–825

Shapiro K, Fried A, Marmarou A (1985) Biomechanical and hydrodynamic character-ization of the hydrocephalic infant. J Neurosurg 63: 69–75

Tans J, Poortvliet D (1983) Intacranial volume- pressure relationship in man. Part 2: Clinical significance of pressure-volume index. J Neurosurg 59: 810–816

Tans J, Poortvliet D (1984) Comparison of ventricular steady-state infusion with bolus infusion and pressure recording for differentiation between arrested and non-arrested hydrocephalus. Acta Neurochir (Wien) 72: 15–29

Tans J, Poortvliet D (1985) CSF outflow resistance and pressure-volume index deter-mined by steady-state and bolus infusion. Clin Neurol Neurosurg 87: 159–165

62 — The Implications of Shunt Surgery in the Intracranial Hydrodynamics of Normal Pressure Hydrocephalus (NPH)

Kiyoaki Tanaka, Hirotsune Naruse, Hideaki Hayashi, Yoshiyasu Iwai, and Shuro Nishimura[1]

Summary. In order to elucidate the mechanics of shunt functioning in normal pressure hydrocephalus (NPH), intracranial pressure (ICP), pressure volume index (PVI) and outflow resistance (Ro) measured by Marmarou's bolus injection technique (Marmarou et al. 1975), and other ICP parameters were measured. Out of 27 patients who underwent shunt surgery, symptomatic improvement was observed in 24. Twenty-eight shunt operations in these 24 patients were analyzed. The mean ICP (mICP) dropped to 6.0 ± 2.2 mmHg from the pre-opening value of 10.3 ± 2.0 mmHg. The peak pressure of B-waves (BPp) decreased from 20.7 ± 5.6 to 11.9 ± 3.7 mmHg. Ro decreased from 5.82 ± 4.67 to 1.40 ± 0.78 mmHg/ml/min and PVI increased from 26.9 ± 10.4 to 42.6 ± 20.2 ml. The post-operative mICP did not correlate with the shunt valve closing pressure at all, but the reduction of mICP and BPp significantly correlated with the reduction of Ro. The Ro(gross), the post-operative Ro, significantly correlated with the Ro(gross) calculated by the following equation: $1/Ro(gross) = 1/Ro(h) + 1/Ro(shunt)$, where Ro(h): Ro of the patient before shunt and Ro(shunt): Ro of the shunt system. The shunt installation lowers mICP and BPp by reducing Ro and increases intracranial buffering capacity, as noted by the increase in PVI. The reduction in Ro seems to play a key role in alleviating the abnormal hydrodynamic situation in NPH patients.

Keywords. Normal pressure hydrocephalus — Shunt surgery — Intracranial hydrodynamics — Outflow resistance — Pressure volume index

Introduction

Shunt surgery has been accepted as a mode of treatment for normal pressure hydrocephalus (NPH). Reports on pre-operative intracranial pressure (ICP) and resistance to outflow (Ro) of cerebrospinal fluid (CSF) are available, but there are only a few studies regarding these ICP parameters after shunt surgery

---

[1] Department of Neurosurgery, Osaka City University Medical School, Osaka, 545 Japan

(Symon and Dorsch 1975; Gücer et al. 1980). In order to elucidate the actual mechanism of shunt functioning in operated patients with NPH, ICP, Ro and pressure volume index (PVI) measured by Marmarou's bolus injection technique (Marmarou et al. 1975), and other ICP parameters were measured before and after installation of a CSF diversion device.

Clinical Material and Methods

Twenty-seven patients with NPH underwent shunt surgery performed using Heyer-Schulte's on-off flushing reservoir with anti-siphon device (Cat. No. 850–0155, American V. Mueller Ill. USA) attached to a low pressure Pudenz's peritoneal catheter (Cat. No. 850–1390, American V. Mueller, Ill., USA). A ventricular catheter was inserted into the lateral ventricle, opposite the shunted side, for continuous monitoring of ICP and for CSF manipulation. ICP was monitored for 24 h before and after opening the on-off valve. The highest and the lowest values of the ICP fluctuation were sampled every 30 min throughout the period of recording, except for the period when pressure waves appeared. The mathematical mean of all these readings was arbitrarily defined as the mean ICP for 24 h ($mICP_{24}$). Two prominent B-waves were also sampled every 30 min; the peak (BPp) and trough pressures (BPo) of the B-waves were measured and the magnitude of each B-wave ($Bmag = BPp - BPo$) was calculated. Out of all the B-waves sampled, the percentage of B-waves with a peak pressure exceeding 14.7 mmHg, %B(shunt), was also calculated. Ro and PVI measurements were periodically carried out several times pre- and post-opening the on-off valve, and the mean of these measurements was calculated. Theoretically, Ro(gross), post-opening Ro, can be calculated by the following equation:

$$1/Ro(gross) = 1/Ro(h) + 1/Ro(shunt), \qquad (1)$$

where Ro(h): Ro of the patient before the on-off valve is opened, and Ro(shunt): Ro of the entire shunt system installed. The ideal value of Ro(gross) which is necessary to decrease BPp below 14.7 mmHg, Ro(gross)id, was calculated in each patient, as previously reported (Tanaka and Nishimura 1989).

Results

In these 27 patients, 34 shunt operations were performed. Twenty-four patients showed improvement. Twenty-eight shunt operations in these 24 patients were analyzed.

Post-Operative Changes in ICP Parameters

After the on-off valve was opened, the $mICP_{24}$ dropped to 6.0 ± 2.2 mmHg (mean ± SD) from the pre-opening value of 10.3 ± 2.0 mmHg (Fig. 1). The

Fig. 1. After the on-off valve was opened, the $mICP_{24}$ decreased to 6.0 ± 2.2 mmHg (mean ± SD) from the pre-opening value of 10.3 ± 2.0 mmHg. The mean value of % reduction was 40.4 ± 22.6%

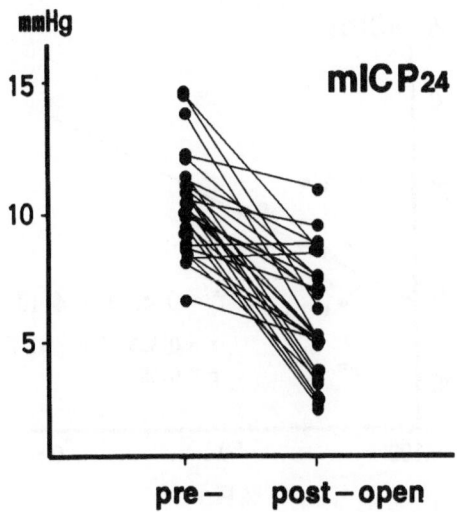

BPp and Bmag decreased by 39% from their pre-opening values of 20.7 ± 5.6 and 4.0 ± 2.4 mmHg, respectively. The %B(shunt) also decreased from 84.5 ± 16.9% to 13.4 ± 19.0%. The Ro decreased from 5.82 ± 4.67 to 1.40 ± 0.78 mmHg/ml/min. The value of Ro in all patients, except two, ranged below 8.5 mmHg/ml/min. On the other hand, the PVI increased post-operatively, from 26.9 ± 10.4 to 42.6 ± 20.2 ml.

Correlations among ICP Parameters

Post-Operative $mICP_{24}$ vs Closing Pressure of Shunt

In all patients, only the low-pressure Pudenz peritoneal catheter was used as a differential pressure valve. The values of the shunt valve closing pressure,

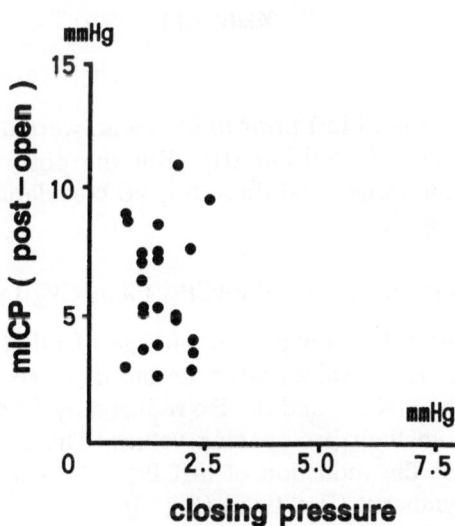

Fig. 2. The post-opening $mICP_{24}$ (Y-axis) did not correlate at all with the closing pressure of the shunt valve (X-axis)

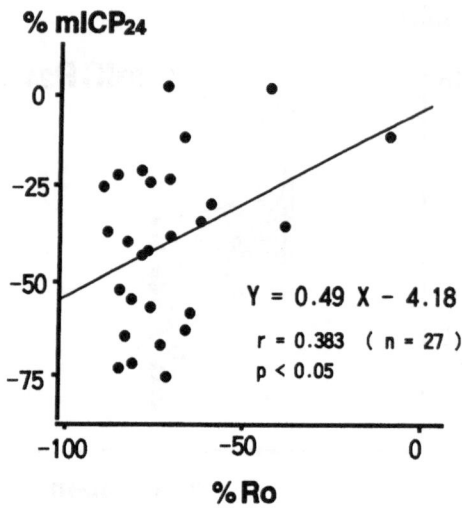

% mICP$_{24}$

$$Y = 0.49 X - 4.18$$

$r = 0.383$ (n = 27)

$p < 0.05$

% Ro

Fig. 3. The mICP$_{24}$ and the Ro reduced by 40.4 ± 22.6% and 71.3 ± 17.3%, respectively, from their pre-opening values, and there was a significant correlation between these parameters. The greater the reduction of Ro, the greater was the reduction of mICP$_{24}$

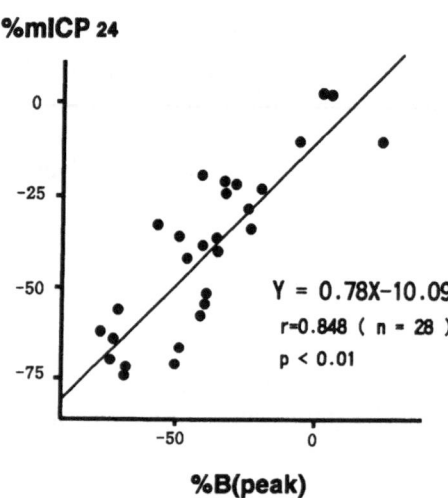

%mICP $_{24}$

$$Y = 0.78X - 10.09$$

$r = 0.848$ (n = 28)

$p < 0.01$

%B(peak)

Fig. 4. The correlation between the percent change of mICP$_{24}$ and the peak pressure of the B-wave was highly significant ($P < 0.01$)

measured just prior to insertion, were distributed within a narrow band ranging from 2.6 to 0.7 mmHg. But the post-operative mICP$_{24}$ was scattered over a wide range, and there was no correlation at all between these two parameters (Fig. 2).

Percent Change of mICP$_{24}$ (%mICP$_{24}$) vs Percent Change of Ro (%Ro)

The values for percent change of mICP$_{24}$ and Ro were calculated, comparing the mean values after the on-off valve was opened to the pre-opening values. The mICP$_{24}$ and the Ro reduced by 40.4 ± 22.6%, 71.3 ± 17.3%, respectively, from their pre-opening values. The greater the reduction of Ro, the greater was the reduction of mICP$_{24}$. The correlation between these parameters was significant (P < 0.05) (Fig. 3).

Fig. 5. The actual value of Ro measured after the on-off valve was opened (Y-axis), was plotted against the Ro calculated by equation (1). There was highly significant correlation between these values ($P < 0.01$)

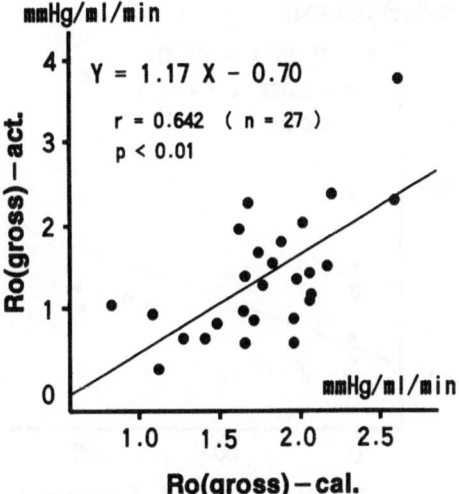

%mICP$_{24}$ vs Percent Change of the BPp (%BPp)

The BPp reduced by $38.3 \pm 24.6\%$ from its pre-opening values. There was a highly significant correlation between these parameters ($P < 0.01$) (Fig. 4). The more the %mICP$_{24}$ reduced, the greater was the percent reduction of BPp.

Analysis of Ro(Gross)

Correlation between Post-Operative Ro and Calculated Ro

In order to calculate the outflow resistance of CSF in the shunted patient, Ro(gross), using equation (1), the values for Ro(h) and Ro(shunt) are necessary. The Ro value for each patient before the on-off valve is opened should be used as Ro(h). In our laboratory, we measured the resistance to outflow of mock CSF through three complete sets of shunt systems with a peritoneal catheter of 80 cm in length. These systems were identical to those which were installed in the patients. The mean value of Ro(shunt) was 2.96 mmHg/ml/min. The Ro(gross), calculated using equation (1), Ro(gross)cal, was compared with the actual post-opening value of Ro for the patient, Ro(gross)act. There was highly significant correlation between these values, and the slope of the correlation line was close to 1 ($P < 0.01$) (Fig. 5).

Correlation between Percent Difference of Ro(gross) and Percent Change of %B(Shunt)

The percent difference of the Ro(gross)act from its ideal value, Ro(gross)id, was calculated such that if the values were positive, the Ro(gross)act values were not sufficiently small compared to the Ro(gross)id, and if the values turned out to be negative, all values were allotted to zero (see Fig. 6). There

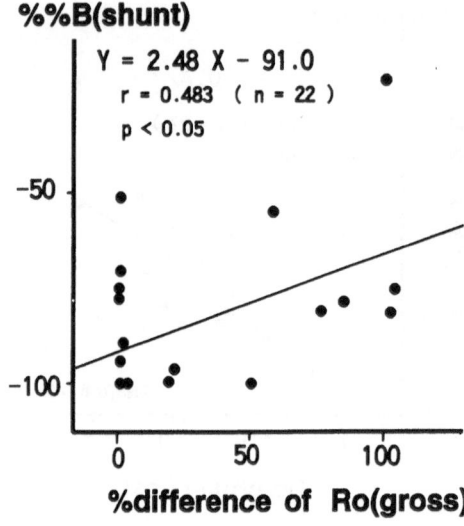

%%B(shunt)

$Y = 2.48\ X - 91.0$

$r = 0.483$ ($n = 22$)

$p < 0.05$

-50

-100

0   50   100

%difference of Ro(gross)

Fig. 6. The percentage of B-waves sampled which exceeded the normal ICP range was designated as %B (shunt). The percent change of %B (shunt) (Y-axis) was plotted against the percent difference between the post-shunt actual Ro and the ideal Ro, which was obtained by calculation to eliminate B-waves (X-axis). The closer the actual Ro to the ideal Ro, the more completely were B-waves eliminated

was a significant correlation between these parameters ($P < 0.05$), indicating that the closer the Ro(gross)act was to the Ro(gross)id, the more completely were B-waves eliminated.

Discussion

Although there are many studies which have reported the effectiveness of shunt surgery correlated with presence of B-waves in ICP recordings (Chawla et al. 1974; Lamas and Lobato 1979; Cardoso et al. 1989) or with low conductance to the outflow of CSF (Børgesen and Gjerris 1982), only a few studies have reported the resultant ICP changes after shunt installation. As expected, the mean ICP, the peak pressure, the amplitude of B-waves, and the resistance to outflow of CSF significantly reduced after the on-off valve was opened. The %B(shunt), the percentage of B-waves which need CSF diversion, also decreased after shunt installation. Although there are reports showing a significant correlation between mICP and Ro (Kosteljanetz 1986; Børgesen and Gjerris 1987), we did not observe such a correlation between these parameters, either in the pre- or in the post-opening period. But there was a significant correlation between the percent changes of mICP and Ro (Fig. 3). The percent changes of BPp and Bmag were also significantly correlated with the percent change of Ro. These observations imply that the reduction in Ro after shunt seems to play a key role in alleviating the abnormal hydrodynamic situation in NPH patients. Børgesen reported a flow-chart for the management of NPH patients and stated that patients with B-waves during 5%–50% of the recording time should be shunted only when the conductance to CSF outflow is below 0.08 ml/min/mmHg (Børgesen and Gjerris 1982). Because the conductance is a reciprocal of the resistance, a conductance value below 0.08 ml/min/

mmHg equals a resistance value above 12.5 mmHg/ml/min. The resistance to CSF outflow in 22 out of 24 patients in this study was in a range below 8.5 mmHg/ml/min; 4.62 ± 1.89 (mean ± SD) mmHg/ml/min. Even if the report that the Ro obtained by bolus injection technique will result in smaller values than those obtained by the constant infusion technique is taken into consideration (Kosteljanetz 1985), the flow-chart suggested by Børgesen may still miss a group of patients who are likely to benefit from shunt surgery. The $mICP_{24}$ did not correlate at all with the closing pressure of the differential pressure valve of the shunt system (Fig. 2), but the percent change of $mICP_{24}$ did correlate significantly with the percent change of Ro brought about by shunt installation. The post-opening Ro correlated significantly with the Ro calculated by equation (1), with the slope of the correlation line equalling 1.17 ($P < 0.01$). This result implies that with this calculation the post-operative Ro might be obtained with a high probability. Portnoy et al. (1976) measured the flow characteristics of various commercially available shunt systems and stated that the pressure-flow curve of the low pressure Pudenz valve simulated that of a low resistance valve like the Hakim valve. Because of the long slits at the tip of the low pressure Pudenz peritoneal catheter, the slit valve adds very little resistance over the resistance of the catheter alone. This may be the reason why we saw no correlation at all between the post-opening $mICP_{24}$ and the closing pressure of the shunt valve. As long as a shunt system with a low pressure slit valve is used for the treatment of hydrocephalus, as is the case in the treatment of NPH, the outflow resistance of the shunt system itself may be far more important than the closing pressure. Therefore the supply of shunt catheters of various calibers, i.e., of various Ro(shunt), with low differential pressure valves should be considered by manufacturers. In summary, shunt installation lowers mICP by reducing outflow resistance and increases intracranial buffering capacity as shown by the increase in PVI.

References

Børgesen SE, Gjerris F (1982) The predictive value of conductance to outflow of CSF in normal pressure hydrocephalus. Brain 105: 65–86

Børgesen SE, Gjerris F (1987) Relationships between intracranial pressure, ventricular size, and resistance to CSF outflow. J Neurosurg 67: 535–539

Cardoso ER, Piatek D, Del Bigio MR, Stambrook M, Sutherland JB (1989) Quantification of abnormal intracranial pressure waves and isotope cisternography for diagnosis of occult communicating hydrocephalus. Surg Neurol 31: 20–27

Chawla JC, Hulme A, Cooper R (1974) Intracranial pressure in patients with dementia and communicating hydrocephalus. J Neurosurg 40: 376–380

Gücer G, Viernstein L, Walker AE (1980) Continuous intracranial pressure recording in adult hydrocephalus. Surg Neurol 13: 323–328

Kosteljanetz M (1985) Resistance to outflow of cerebrospinal fluid determined by bolus injection technique and constant rate steady state infusion in humans. Neurosurgery 16: 336–340

Kosteljanetz M (1986) CSF dynamics and pressure-volume relationships in communicating hydrocephalus. J Neurosurg 64: 45–52

Lamas E, Lobato RD (1979) Intraventricular pressure and CSF dynamics in chronic adult hydrocephalus. Surg Neurol 12: 287–295

Marmarou A, Shulman K, LaMorgese J (1975) Compartmental analysis of compliance and outflow resistance of the cerebrospinal fluid system. J Neurosurg 43: 523–534

Portnoy HD, Tripp L, Croissant PD (1976) Hydrodynamics of shunt valves. Childs Brain 2: 242–256

Symon L, Dorsch NWC (1975) Use of long-term intracranial pressure measurement to assess hydrocephalic patients prior to shunt surgery. J Neurosurg 42: 258–273

Tanaka K, Nishimura S (1989) The importance of outflow resistance of the shunt system for elimination of B-waves. In: Hoff JT, Betz AL (eds) Intracranial pressure VII. Springer, Berlin Heidelberg, pp 368–373

63 — Preoperative Evaluation of Normal Pressure Hydrocephalus by Transcranial Doppler Sonography

Katsuzo Fujita, Xingbin Lin, Kazumasa Ehara, Norihiko Tamaki, and Satoshi Matsumoto[1]

Summary. In spite of recent developments in diagnostic procedures, there are, as yet, no absolute criteria for making a definitive diagnosis of NPH. Transcranial Doppler (TCD) data concerning vascular reactivity obtained by hypercapnia, together with temporary external lumbar drainage, is useful for screening the NPH patients. Twenty patients with a clinical picture suggestive of NPH were studied by TCD to evaluate the autoregulatory reserve of brain perfusion, using the CO_2 inhalation method. In 12 patients, clinical symptoms and flow velocity changes in the basal cerebral arteries were also evaluated after temporary lumbar drainage. With symptomatic improvement after external lumbar drainage and good vascular reactivity in the basal cerebral arteries, the prognosis after shunt placement is good, but without symptomatic improvement after lumbar drainage and with bad vascular reactivity, a shunting procedure is contraindicated.

Keywords. Normal pressure hydrocephalus — CO_2 Reactivity — Transcranial Doppler sonography

Introduction

A remarkable recovery of cerebral function can be achieved by the performance of a shunting procedure in normal pressure hydrocephalus (NPH) patients (Adams et al. 1965; Hann and Thomeer 1988; Vorstrup et al. 1987; Wikkelso et al. 1986), but the clinical triad of gait disturbance, dementia, and urinary incontinence is often incomplete and the radiological picture may not be pathognomonic, especially in idiopathic NPH which is usually associated with cerebrovascular diseases. This study was undertaken to screen NPH patients by vascular reactivity testing, examined by transcranial Doppler sonography (TCD) during CO_2 inhalation.

---

[1] Department of Neurosurgery, Kobe University School of Medicine, Kobe, 650 Japan

Table 1. Clinical summary of 20 NPH patients

1. Sex		2. Age	
Male	8	From 19 to 72 years, mean age 67.5	
Female	12	years	
Total	20		
3. Etiology of NPH	**No. of cases**	**4. Initial symptoms**	
Idiopathic	8	Gait disturbance	19
Post SAH	7	Dementia	17
Post traumatic	2	Urinary incontinence	12
Post infectious	1		
Other	2		

Clinical Materials and Methods

From April 1988 through November 1990, 20 patients (8 males and 12 females, aged 19–72 years) with a clinical picture suggestive of NPH were studied by TCD (TC2-64, Eden Medizinische Elektronik) to evaluate the autoregulatory

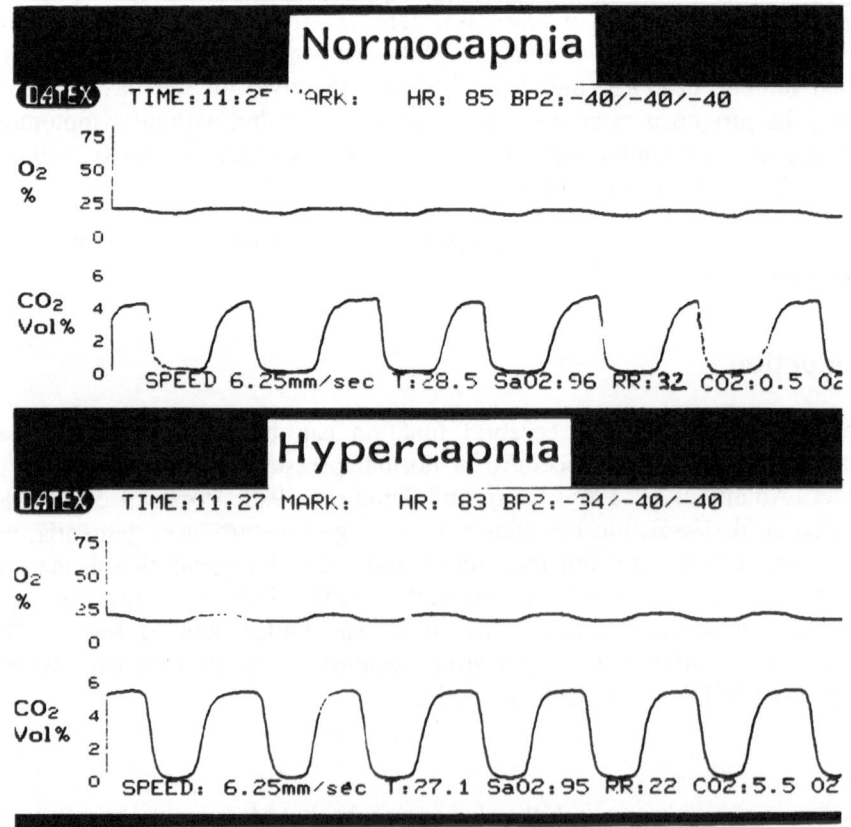

Fig. 1. CO_2 Reactivity of middle cerebral artery (*MCA*) in a normal adult

reserve of brain perfusion, using the CO_2 inhalation method. The diseases underlying the NPH were idiopathic in eight cases, post subarachnoid hemorrhage (SAH) in seven, post-traumatic in two, and postinfectious in one case (Table 1). Vascular reactivity was evaluated from the flow velocity changes of the basal cerebral arteries during hypercapnia and in 12 of these patients, clinical symptoms and flow velocity changes were also evaluated after temporary lumbar drainage. Examination by TCD was performed using an EME TC2–64. For hypercapnia, a mask with a hose (1 m in length) was fitted to the patient's mouth for 3 min. Using this method, carbon dioxide pressure was increased from 37% to 45% without changes of oxygen concentration.

Temporal lumbar drainage was performed at the level of L4–5 or S1 using a lumbo-peritoneal (L-P) shunt tube; this was continued for 5 days. During lumbar drainage, symptom changes and neurological findings were carefully studied; daily monitoring of flow velocity changes in the basal cerebral arteries and CO_2 reactivity was also carried out in 12 patients. Response to the shunt was evaluated from the patients' neurological findings 3 months after shunt placement.

Results

CO_2 Reactivity in Normal Adults

CO_2 reactivity was examined in seven normal adults. During hypercapnia, the mean flow velocity of the basal cerebral arteries was increased from 23%–32%, with a mean value of 25% (Fig.1). From this result, an increase of more than 25% in the mean flow velocity in the basal cerebral arteries during hypercapnia was judged as normal in the CO_2 reactivity test.

CO_2 Reactivity in NPH Patients

Of the 20 patients, 11 showed an increase of more than 25% in blood flow velocity during hypercapnia. In six of seven post SAH patients, CO_2 reactivity was maintained at normal levels, but in most idiopathic NPH patients,

Table 2. Correlation of etiology with carbon dioxide reactivity

	No. of cases (n)	Preoperative vascular status	
		CO_2 reactivity	CO_2 reactivity
		>25%	<25%
Idiopathic	8	2	6
Post NPH	7	6	1
Post trauma	2	1	1
Post infectious	1	1	0
Other	2	1	1
Total	20	11	9

Table 3. Correlation of surgical results with carbon dioxide reactivity

	No. of cases (n)	Preoperative vascular status	
		CO_2 reactivity	CO_2 reactivity
		⩾25%	<25%
Improved			
Marked improvement	8	7	1
Slight	6	4	2
No improvement	6	0	6
Total	20	11	9

Table 4. Correlation of surgical results with mean MCA velocity changes after lumbar drainage

	No. of cases (n)	Mean MCA velocity changes	
		⩾10%	<10%
Improvement			
Marked improvement	6	5	1
Slight	3	2	1
No improvement	3	0	3
Total	12	7	5

MCA, middle cerebral artery

CO_2 reactivity was disturbed because of possible coexistent cerebral vascular diseases; only two out of eight of these patients showed normal CO_2 reactivity (Table 2). Of the 14 patients who showed symptomatic improvement after shunt placement, 11 (78%) had an increase in blood flow velocity of less than 25%, and only 3 had improved at follow up (Table 3).

Change of CO_2 Reactivity and Flow Velocity After Temporary Lumbar Drainage

Of the 12 patients who underwent temporary lumbar drainage, 7 had an increase in blood flow velocity of more than 10% and showed good CO_2 reactivity after this procedure. All these patients showed symptomatic improvement after shunt placement (Table 4).

Surgical Results

When the etiology of NPH patients was correlated with the surgical results, post SAH patients showed good response to shunt placement and six out of seven of these patients were improved after the shunting operation. In contrast, only three out of the eight idiopathic NPH patients showed symptomatic improvement after the shunting operation (Table 5).

Two illustrative cases are presented:

Table 5. Surgical results

	No. of cases (n)	Improvement	No improvement	Deteriorated
Idiopathic	8	2	6	0
Post SAH	7	6	1	0
Post trauma	2	2	0	0
Post infection	1	1	0	0
Other	2	2	0	0
Total	20	13	7	0

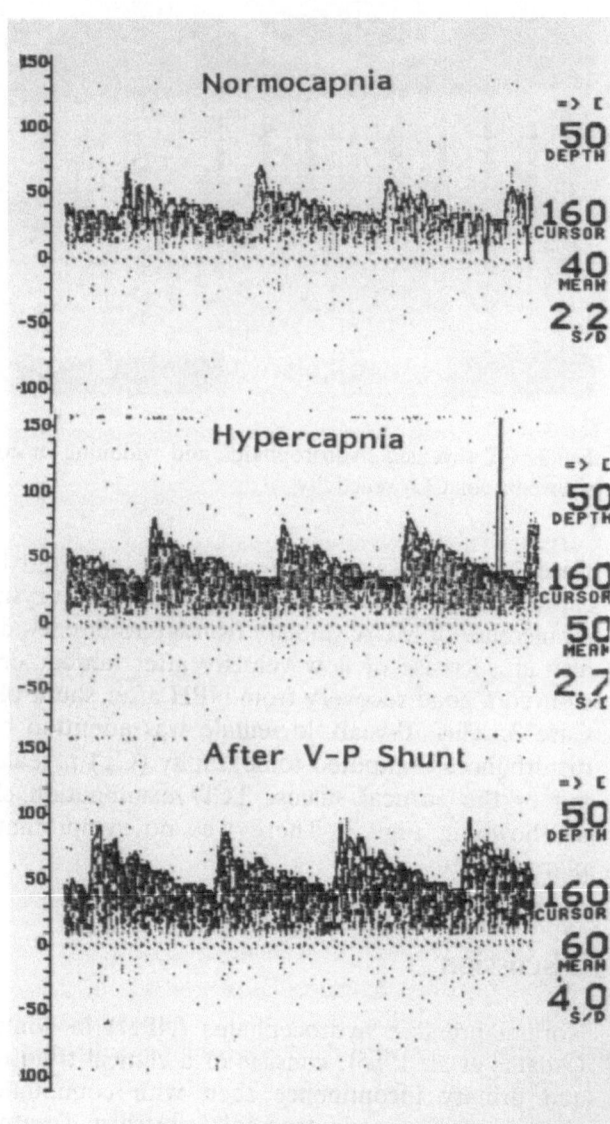

Fig. 2. TCD examination showed an increase of middle cerebral artery (*MCA*) flow velocity from 40 to 50 cm/s during hypercapnia (63 female)

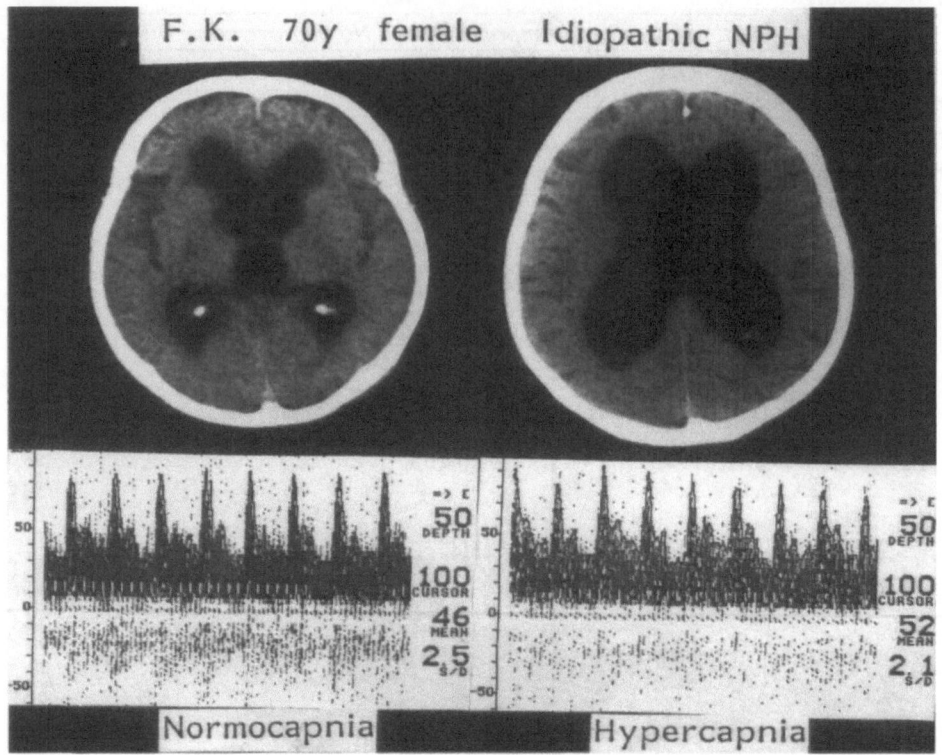

Fig. 3. CT revealed hydrocephalus and widening of cortical sulcus. TCD examination showed poor CO_2 reactivity

Case 1. This 63 year-old-female was admitted because of SAH following a ruptured middle cerebral artery (MCA) aneurysm. TCD examination showed an increase of MCA velocity from 40 to 50 cm/s during hypercapnia; there was also an increase of flow velocity after lumbar drainage (Fig. 2). This patient showed a good recovery from NPH after shunt placement.

Case 2. This 70-year-old female was admitted because of dementia and gait disturbance. Computed tomography (CT) revealed hydrocephalus and widening of the cortical sulcus. TCD examination showed poor CO_2 reactivity, as shown in Fig. 3. There was no symptomatic improvement after shunt placement.

Discussion

Normal pressure hydrocephalus (NPH) in adults, as first described in 1965 (Adams et al. 1965), consists of a clinical triad of dementia, gait disturbance, and urinary incontinence seen with communicating hydrocephalus in the absence of increased intracranial pressure. Treatment with shunting procedures

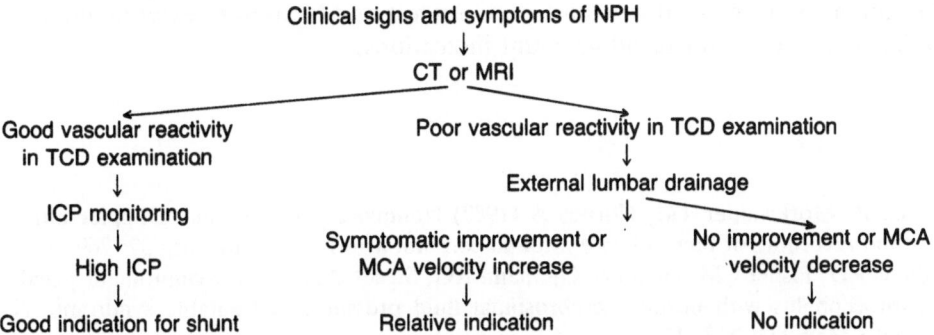

Fig. 4. A Method for selecting patients to be shunted in NPH Clinical signs and symptoms of NPH

can improve the clinical symptoms in NPH. Nevertheless, in certain patients, treatment fails without recognizable shunt problems. In spite of recent developments in diagnostic procedures, confusion still exists concerning indications for surgery; there are no absolute criteria for making a definitive diagnosis. With increase in life expectancy, the prevalence of dementia is increasing. Alzheimer's disease, Pick's disease, and multi-infarct dementia, which all cause the same clinical symptoms, must be differentiated from NPH. Most perfusion studies in NPH patients (Mamo et al. 1987; Meyer et al. 1984, 1985; Vorstrup et al. 1987) were carried out to screen for possible pathogenic mechanisms. Xe contrast CT scanning examination of patients with NPH (Meyer et al. 1985) reveals characteristic patterns of cerebral perfusion and changes in tissue integrity which are indicated by reduced local partition coefficients for Xe gas; phenomena suggesting a reduced autoregulatory brain perfusion reserve. However, this complicated method is not available to every hospital or practice. Transcranial Doppler sonography (Aaslid et al. 1982; Fritz et al. 1989) is a new diagnostic tool developed by Aaslid and co-workers. TCD data concerning vascular reactivity obtained by hypercapnia is useful for screening NPH patients, especially those with idiopathic NPH, which is often associated with co-existent vascular disease. Improvement of symptoms after external lumbar drainage is strongly suggestive of NPH and findings of increased blood flow velocity in the basal cerebral arteries after external lumbar drainage are also useful when deciding shunt indications.

After a presumptive CT diagnosis of NPH, the vascular reactivity during CO_2 inhalation is measured using the transcranial Doppler method. Thereafter, external lumbar drainage is performed for 5 days. If there is symptomatic improvement after external lumbar drainage and an increase in blood flow velocity of more than 25% during CO_2 inhalation, the prognosis after shunt placement is good. If there is an increase in blood flow velocity of less than 25% during CO_2 inhalation without symptomatic improvement after external lumbar drainage, a shunting procedure is contraindicated (Fig. 4).

This is still a preliminary report and more studies are needed before definitive conclusions can be drawn; however, because of its simplicity, we recommend this noninvasive cerebral vascular reactivity test and temporary external lumbar drainage as a basis for deciding shunt indications.

References

Aaslid R, Morkwalder TM, Nornes A (1982) Noninvasive transcranial Doppler ultrasound recording of flow velocity in basal cerebral arteries. J Neurosurg 57: 769–774

Adams RD, Fisher CM, Hakin S, Ojemann RG, Sweet WH (1965) Symptomatic occult hydrocephalus with normal cerebrospinal fluid pressure: A treatable syndrome. N Engl J Med 273: 117–126

Fritz W, Kalbarczyk H, Schmidt K (1989) Transcranial Doppler sonographic identification of a subgroup of patients with normal pressure hydrocephalus with coexistent vascular disease and treatment failure. Neurosurgery 25: 777–780

Hann J, Thomeer RTWM (1988) Predictive value of temporary external lumbar drainage in normal pressure hydrocephalus. Neurosurgery 22: 388–391

Mamo HL, Meric PC, Ponsin JC (1987) Cerebral blood flow in normal pressure hydrocephalus. Stroke 18: 1074–1080

Meyer JS, Tachibana H, Hardenberg JP, et al. (1984) Normal pressure hydrocephalus, influences on cerebral hemodynamic and CSF pressure chemical autoregulation. Surg Neurol 21: 195–203

Meyer JS, Kitagawa Y, Tanahashi N, et al. (1985) Evaluation of treatment of normal pressure hydrocephalus. J Neurosurg 62: 513–521

Vorstrup S, Christensen J, Gjerris F (1987) Cerebral blood flow in patients with normal pressure hydrocephalus before and after shunting. J Neurosurg 66: 379–387

Wikkelso C, Andersson H, Blomstrand C, Lindquist G, Svendsen P (1986) Normal pressure hydrocephalus, Predictive value of the cerebrospinal fluid tap test. Acta Neurol Scand 73: 566–573

64 — Reversibility of Dementia in Hydrocephalus After Shunt Surgery: A Comparative Study of Elderly and Non-Elderly Patients

Takashi Matsumoto[1], Hideo Mabe, and Hajime Nagai[2]

Summary. In general, dementia is one of the characteristic symptoms of normal pressure hydrocephalus (NPH); however, it is well known that it occurs even in acute or obstructive hydrocephalus. Seventy-two patients who had hydrocephalus were examined neuropsychologically before and after a ventriculoperitoneal (VP) shunt operation. To evaluate the reversibility of the dementia, a comparative study of the elderly group (over 65 years old, 29 cases) and the non-elderly group (under 64 years old, 43 cases) was carried out. Before the shunt operation, dementia had been recognized in 23 of the 29 elderly patients (73.9%), and in 19 patients of the 43 non-elderly patients (44.2%). VP shunt operations were performed on all 42 patients in whom dementia was recognized. Dementia was evaluated at the time of discharge and at the most recent visit to an outpatient clinic. In conclusion, the present investigation confirms that (1) elderly hydrocephalus patients, as compared with the non-elderly, easily reach a state of dementia, (2) shortly after the operation, there is not much difference between the effects of the shunt procedure on dementia in the elderly and the non-elderly, (3) in the elderly group, some patients showed exacerbation of symptoms during the follow up period, and (4) the final evaluation showed that the prognosis for dementia was less favorable in the elderly group.

Keywords. Hydrocephalus — Dementia — Elderly — Surgical outcome

Introduction

Hydrocephalus is regarded as one of the representative neurosurgical diseases in which dementia is a symptom (Black 1980; Gustafson and Hagberg 1978; Thomsen et al. 1986). In general, dementia is a characteristic symptom of normal pressure hydrocephalus (NPH); however, it is well known that it occurs

---

[1] Department of Neurosurgery, Meitetsu Hospital, Nagoya, 455 Japan
[2] Department of Neurosurgery, Nagoya City University, Nagoya, 467 Japan

Table 1. Primary diseases and initial signs and symptoms of elderly group

Initial signs & symptoms	ICP*elevation sign	Dementia	Incontinence	Gait disturbance
Total (29 cases)	9 cases (31.0%)	7 cases (24.1%)	9 cases (31.0%)	4 cases (13.8%)
Tumor (7 cases)	4 cases (57.1%)	2 cases (28.6%)	1 case (14.3%)	
CVD** (13 cases)	5 cases (38.5%)	3 cases (23.1%)	5 cases (38.5%)	
NPH*** (9 cases)		2 cases (22.2%)	3 cases (33.3%)	4 cases (44.4%)

* ICP : intracranial pressure
** CVD: cerebrovascular disease
*** NPH: normal pressure hydrocephalus

even in acute or obstructive hydrocephalus (Levine et al. 1985). Meanwhile, it is apparent that there is some mental deterioration that comes with advanced age, even in the face of perfect health (Rinn 1988). Therefore we must know when to suspect NPH in people over 75 years old, knowing that in this population almost 50% of people have some problems of mobility, 10%–40% have problems with incontinence, and 15%–20% have dementia syndrome (St-Laurent 1988). These facts lead us to the presumption that the potential for recovery in elderly patients with dementia caused by hydrocephalus is also less than that in non-elderly patients. However, little comprehensive study has been carried out in this area. In order to make this point clear, we carried out a study comparing the reversibility of this type of dementia in the elderly (over 65 years old) and the non-elderly (under 64 years old).

Clinical Data

From 1977 to 1989, 72 patients underwent ventriculoperitoneal (VP) shunt operations for hydrocephalus in Nagoya City University Hospital. In this series, there were 29 (40.3%) elderly and 43 (59.7%) non-elderly patients. The mean age of the elderly group was 70.0 years and that of the non-elderly was 44.8 years (children were excluded to avoid confusion). As shown in Table 1, the primary diseases of patients in the elderly group were brain tumor in 7, cerebrovascular disease (CVD) in 13, and idiopathic NPH in 9. In patients of the non-elderly group (Table 2) brain tumor was present in 20, CVD in 18, idiopathic NPH in 4, and aqueduct stenosis in one.

Table 2. Primary diseases and initial signs and symptoms of non-elderly group

Initial signs & symptoms	ICP elevation sign	Dementia	Incontinence	Gait disturbance
Total (43 cases)	29 cases (67.4%)	9 cases (20.9%)	2 cases (4.7%)	3 cases (7.0%)
Tumor (20 cases)	19 cases (95.0%)	1 case (5.0%)		
CVD (18 cases)	9 cases (50.0%)	5 cases (27.8%)	2 cases (11.1%)	2 cases (11.1%)
NPH (4 cases)	1 case (25.0%)	2 cases (50.0%)		1 case (25.0%)
Other (1 case)		1 case (100%)		

Clinical Signs and Symptoms

Initial signs and symptoms are summarized in Tables 1 and 2. In this paper, dementia is defined as progressive intellectual deterioration sufficient to interfere with social or occupational functioning (Martin and Guthrie 1988). Dementia had been recognized in 7 of the 29 elderly patients (24.1%) [2 (28.6%) of the 7 brain tumor cases, 3 (23.1%) of the 13 CVD cases, and 2 (22.2%) of the 9 NPH cases]. Nine of the 43 non-elderly patients (20.9%) suffered from dementia [1 (5%) of the 20 brain tumor cases, 5 (27.8%) of the 18 CVD cases, and 2 (50.0%) of the 4 NPH cases]. AS an initial symptom, there was no significant difference between the incidence of dementia in the elderly and the non-elderly group. Tables 3 and 4 summarize the signs and symptoms at the time of the shunt operation. During the period between onset and operation, the incidence of dementia increased markedly in the elderly group. By the time of the shunt operation, 23 of the 29 elderly patients (79.3%) presented with dementia [5 (71.4%) of the 7 brain tumor cases, 9 (69.2%) of the 13 CVD cases, and 9 (100%) of the 9 NPH cases]. On the other hand, in the non-elderly group, the number of patients who suffered dementia remained relatively unchanged. In this group, dementia had been recognized in 19 of the 43 patients (44.2%), [7 (35.0%) of the 20 brain tumor cases, 7 (38.9%) of the 18 CVD cases, and 4 (100%) of the 4 NPH cases] before the shunt operation. These data reveal that the elderly hydrocephalus patients, as compared with the non-elderly, quickly reached a state of dementia.

VP shunt operations were performed on all 42 patients (23 elderly and 19 non-elderly) who showed dementia.

Table 3. Signs and symptoms at shunt operation (elderly group)

Preoperative signs & symptoms	ICP elevation sign	Dementia	Incontinence	Gait disturbance
Total (29 cases)	14 cases (48.3%)	23 cases (79.3%)	21 cases (72.4%)	12 cases (41.4%)
Tumor (7 cases)	6 cases (85.7%)	5 cases (71.4%)	7 cases (100%)	4 cases (57.1%)
CVD (13 cases)	6 cases (46.2%)	9 cases (69.2%)	7 cases (53.8%)	1 case (7.7%)
NPH (9 cases)	2 cases (22.2%)	9 cases (100%)	7 cases (77.8%)	7 cases (77.8%)

Table 4. Signs and symptoms at shunt operation (non-elderly group)

Preoperative signs & symptoms	ICP elevation sign	Dementia	Incontinence	Gait disturbance
Total (43 cases)	34 cases (79.1%)	19 cases (44.2%)	13 cases (30.2%)	8 cases (18.6%)
Tumor (20 cases)	20 cases (100%)	7 cases (35.0%)	5 cases (25.0%)	3 cases (15.0%)
CVD (18 cases)	11 cases (61.1%)	7 cases (38.9%)	5 cases (27.8%)	2 cases (11.1%)
NPH (4 cases)	2 cases (50.0%)	4 cases (100%)	2 cases (50.0%)	3 cases (75.0%)

Effects of Shunt Surgery on Dementia

Dementia was evaluated at the time of discharge, for the elderly, 37.4 (mean) days; for the non-eldery, 42.8 (mean) days after the shunt procedure and at the most recent visit to an outpatient clinic, for the elderly, 7.0 (mean) months; for the non-elderly, 25.1 (mean) months. Results were classified as death, deteriorated, unchanged, barely improved, moderately improved, and remarkably improved. Results showing "barely improved," "moderately improved," and "remarkably improved" were regarded as good surgical outcomes. At the time of discharge, of the 23 elderly patients with dementia, the condition

Table 5. Surgical outcome of dementia at discharge (elderly group)

Outcome at discharge	death	deterio-rated	un-changed	barely improved	moderately improved	remarkably improved
Total (23 cases)			10 cases (43.5%)	7 cases (30.4%)	3 cases (13.0%)	3 cases (13.0%)
Tumor (5 cases)			2 cases (40.0%)	2 cases (40.0%)	1 case (20.0%)	
CVD (9 cases)			4 cases (44.4%)	2 cases (22.2%)	1 case (11.1%)	2 cases (22.2%)
NPH (9 cases)			4 cases (44.4%)	3 cases (33.3%)	1 case (11.1%)	1 case (11.1%)

Table 6. Surgical outcome of dementia at discharge (non-elderly)

Outcome at discharge	death	deterio-rated	un-changed	barely improved	moderately improved	remarkably improved
Total (19 cases)			6 cases (31.6%)	2 cases (10.5%)	8 cases (42.1%)	3 cases (15.8%)
Tumor (7 cases)			1 case (14.3%)	1 case (14.3%)	5 cases (71.4%)	
CVD (7 cases)			1 case (14.3%)	1 case (14.3%)	3 cases (42.9%)	2 cases (28.6%)
NPH (4 cases)			3 cases (75.0%)			1 case (25.0%)

remained unchanged in 10 (43.5%), was barely improved in 7 (30.4%), moderately improved in 3 (13%), and remarkably improved in 3 (13%) (Table 5). In the non-elderly group (19 patients) at discharge, the dementia remained unchanged in 6 patients (31.6%), was barely improved in 2 (10.1%), moderately improved in 8 (42.1%), and remarkably improved in 3 (15.8%) (Table 6). In the elderly group at the time of the final evaluation, 2 of the 23 patients (8.7%) had died. The dementia had deteriorated in 2 patients (8.7%), remained unchanged in 11 (47.8%), was barely improved in 4 (17.4%), moderately improved in 2 (8.7%), and remarkably improved in 2 (8.7%) (Table 7). In the non-elderly group, 2 of the 19 patients (10.5%) had died by

Table 7. Final surgical outcome of dementia (elderly group)

Final outcome	death	deterio-rated	un-changed	barely improved	moderately improved	remarkably improved
Total (23 cases)	2 cases (8.7%)	2 cases (8.7%)	11 cases (47.8%)	4 cases (17.4%)	2 cases (8.7%)	2 cases (8.7%)
Tumor (5 cases)	2 cases (40.0%)		2 cases (40.0%)		1 case (20.0%)	
CVD (9 cases)			6 cases (66.7%)	1 case (11.1%)		2 cases (22.2%)
NPH (9 cases)		2 cases (22.2%)	3 cases (33.3%)	3 cases (33.3%)	1 case (11.1%)	

Table 8. Final surgical outcome of dementia (non-elderly group)

Final outcome	death	deterio-rated	un-changed	barely improved	moderately improved	remarkably improved
Total (19 cases)	2 cases (10.5%)		5 cases (26.3%)	2 cases (10.5%)	7 cases (36.8%)	3 cases (15.8%)
Tumor (7 cases)	2 cases (28.6%)		1 case (14.3%)	1 case (14.3%)	3 cases (42.9%)	
CVD (7 cases)			1 case (14.3%)	1 case (14.3%)	3 cases (42.9%)	2 cases (28.6%)
NPH (4 cases)			3 cases (75.0%)			1 case (25.0%)

the time of the final evaluation. The dementia remained unchanged in five patients (26.3%), was barely improved in two (10.5%), moderately improved in seven (36.8%), and remarkably improved in three (15.8%). Figures 1 and 2 indicate the outcome in each disease category. In the brain tumor group, during the period between discharge and the final evaluation, the number of "good outcomes" was reduced for both elderly (from 60% to 20%) and non-elderly patients (from 85.7% to 57.2%). "Death" patients were regarded as ineffective. If these "death" patients were excluded, then in the final evaluation, the "good outcome" in elderly was 33.3% and in non-elderly patients it was 80%. During the follow up period in the CVD group, the number of

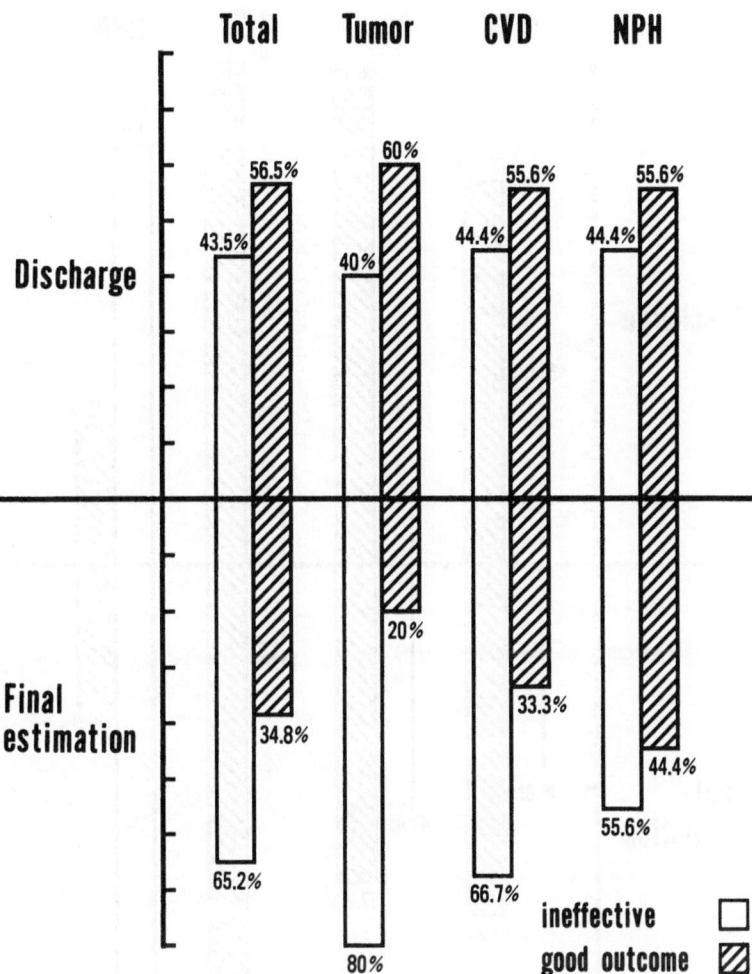

Fig. 1. Outcome for each disease category (elderly group) CVD, cerebrovascular disease; NPH, normal pressure hydrocephalus

"good outcomes" was reduced in elderly patients (from 55.6% to 33.3%), but there was no change in the non-elderly patients (from 85.8% to 85.8%). During the follow up period in the NPH group, the number of "good outcomes" was relatively unchanged for both elderly (from 55.6% to 44.4%) and non-elderly patients (from 25% to 25%). However, the shunt operation was less effective in the idiopathic NPH patients than in those with other diseases.

Discussion

In the literature, dementia is generally defined for convenience as progressive intellectual deterioration sufficient to interfere with social or occupational

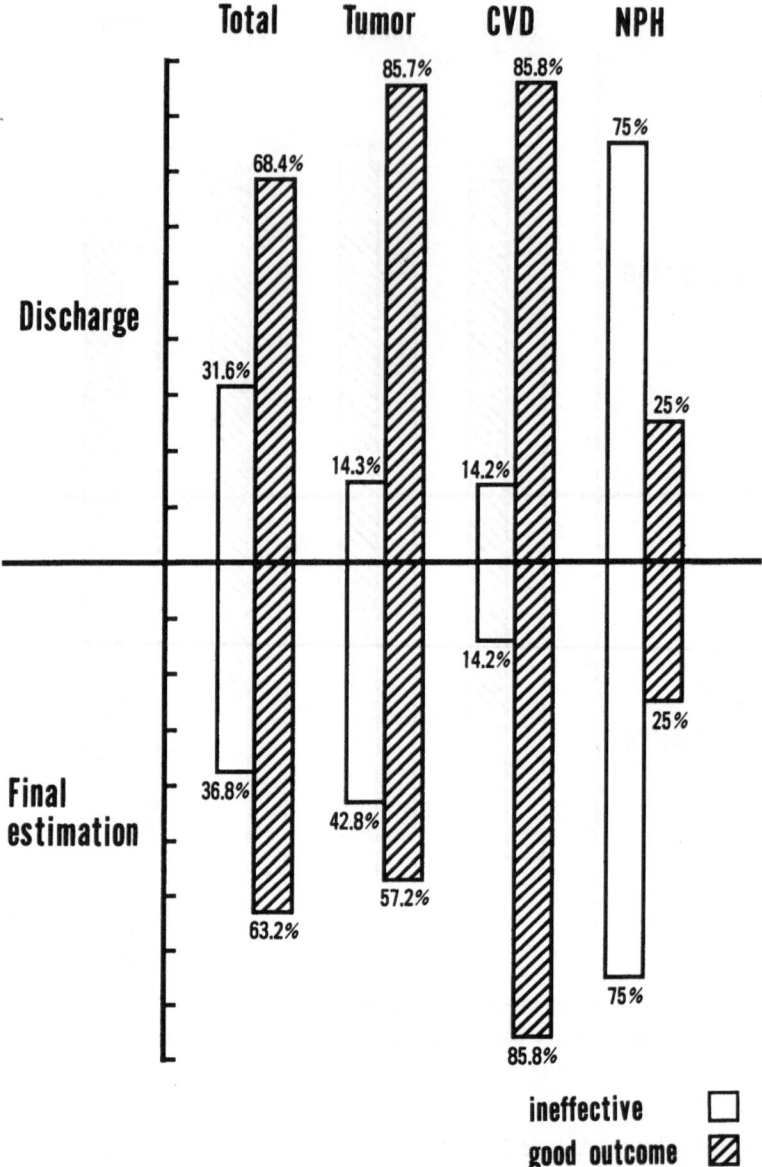

Fig. 2. Outcome for each disease category (non-elderly group) CVD, cerebrovascular disease; NPH, normal pressure hydrocephalus

functioning (Martin and Guthrie 1988). Maletta (1990) defined it as a complex clinical symptom in an alert individual, characterized by the onset of an acquired, persistent, and global loss of cognitive and behavioral function. In addition to these, many other definitions for dementia have been offered. As there is no absolute definition of dementia itself, the meaning of "treatable dementia" is, of course, obscure. However, Maletta (1990) has attempted to classify treatable dementia into several groups. The best recognized are the "reversible dementias" a group which consists of a variety of disease-specific dementias, e.g., those caused by vitamin B12 deficiency, chronic hypothyroidism, heavy metal intoxication, normal pressure hydrocephalus, chronic subdural hematoma, and so on. They are also referred to as "secondary dementias" to distinguish them from the clearly irreversible primary degenerative dementias (PDD) — Alzheimer's disease and Pick's disease. With the secondary dementias, the progression of cognitive and functional decline is often effectively arrested with proper treatment. It is a well known fact that some of the hydrocephalic dementias are treatable by shunt procedure (Black 1980; Gustafson et al. 1978; Meyer et al. 1985; Thomsen et al. 1986; Turner and McGeachie 1988; Vassilouthis 1984). Features of hydrocephalic dementia are described as slowness and poverty of ideation, lack of perception, and poor performance on vigilance tasks (Levine et al. 1985). Many studies have addressed the reversibility of hydrocephalic dementia after shunt surgery, without reference to age (Black 1980; Gustafson et al. 1978; Meyer et al. 1985; Thomsen et al. 1986). However, little attention has been given to the surgical outcome of the elderly patient (Lehman 1980; Petersen et al. 1985). Petersen and co-workers' data (1985) indicate that, even if the patients were elderly, there was about a 75% chance of some improvement in hydrocephalic dementia after shunt procecdure and a 40% chance of an enduring satisfactory result. However, the median duration of improvement was only 24 months (range, 1–147 months) and the mode was 10–19 months. Lehman (1986) reported a 78-year-old patient whose CT scan revealed moderately dilated ventricles with little evidence of cortical atrophy. A medium-pressure VP shunt was placed and the patient showed dramatic improvement in mental capacity. As these reports in the literature show, it is true that some hydrocephalic dementia in the elderly is treatable and curable. So far as we know, however, there is no study comparing the reversibility of hydrocephalic dementia after shunt surgery in elderly and non-elderly patients. Some new features have been elucidated in our present study. The first point to the noticed is that elderly hydrocephalic patients, as compared with the non-elderly, quickly reach a state of dementia. This is probably due to many of the elderly patients having some subclinical brain damage. Therefore their brains are very vulnerable to hydrocephalic damage and progress easily to a state of decreased brain function.

Secondly, shortly after the operation, there was not much difference between the effect of the shunt procedure in the elderly and non-elderly. However, in the elderly group, some patients showed exacerbation of symptoms during the follow up period and the final prognosis was less favorable for this group. There is no satisfactory explanation as to why the symptoms of elderly patients were so readily exacerbated during the follow up period. However, as a matter of course, a considerable degree of mental decline is evident in most persons of advanced age (Rinn WE 1988). This natural mental decline might have been synchronous with the follow up period after shunt surgery. Also, it is likely that most elderly persons have some medical disorder, whether they know it or not. There is some possibility that the exacerbation was produced by small pathological changes (e.g., atherosclerosis, lacuna stroke, and so on) which occurred after the shunt surgery (Rinn 1988). In addition, it might be mentioned that the shunt system itself is more likely to become dysfunctional in elderly patients than in the non-elderly.

Finally, it bears re-emphasizing that elderly hydrocephalus patients quickly reach a state of dementia and that the final outcome of shunt surgery is less favorable for these patients than for non-elderly patients.

References

Black PM (1980) Idiopathic normal-pressure hydrocephalus. Results of shunting in 62 patients. J Neurosurg 52: 371–377

Friedland RP (1989) "Normal"-pressure hydrocephalus and the saga of the treatable dementias. JAMA 262: 2577–2581

Gustafson L, Hagberg B (1978) Recovery in hydrocephalic dementia after shunt operation. J Neurol Neurosurg Psychiatry 41: 940–947

Lehman LB (1986) Two elderly men with reversible dementia. Hosp Pract 15: 36A–36H

Levine DN, Grek A, Calvanio R (1985) Dementia after surgery for cerebellar stroke: An unrecognized complication of acute hydrocephalus? Neurology 35: 568–571

Maletta GJ (1990) The concept of "Reversible" dementia. How nonreliable terminology may impair effective treatment. J Am Geriatr Soc 38: 136–140

Martin RA, Guthrie R (1988) Office evaluation of dementia. How to arrive at a clear diagnosis and choose appropriate therapy. Post-grad Med 84: 176–187

Meyer JS, Kitagawa Y, Tanahashi N, Tachibana H, Kandula P, Cech DA, Clifton GL, Rose JE (1985) Evaluation of treatment of normal-pressure hydrocephalus. J Neurosurg 62: 513–521

Petersen CR, Mokri B, Laws ER (1985) Surgical treatment of idiopathic hydrocephalus in elderly patients. Neurology 35: 307–311

Rinn WE (1988) Mental decline in normal aging: A review. J Geriatr Psychiatry Neurol 1: 144–158

St-Laurent M (1988) Normal pressure hydrocephalus in geriatric medicine: A challenge. J Geriatr Psychiatry Neurol 1: 163–168

Thomsen AM, Borgesen SE, Bruhn P, Gjerris F (1986) Prognosis of dementia in normal-pressure hydrocephalus after a shunt operation. Ann Neurol 20: 304–310

Turner DA, McGeachie RE (1988) Normal pressure hydrocephalus and dementia — Evaluation and treatment. Clin Geriatr Med 4: 815–830

Vassilouthis J (1984) The syndrome of normal-pressure hydrocephalus. J Neurosurg 61: 501–509

65 — Clinical Evaluation of Sophisticated Mental Tests and ^{123}I-IMP SPECT in Normal Pressure Hydrocephalus (NPH) Patients

Katsushi Taomoto, Akihiro Ijichi[1], Michio Yamaguchi and Isao Kinoshita[2]

Summary. We examined the mental functions and intelligence, as well as the dynamics of cerebrospinal fluid and cerebral blood flow pre- and post-shunting in NPH patients.

Three kinds of mental and intelligence tests, Seiken's dementia screening test, the Bender-Gestalt test, and the Benton Visual Retention test were administered to 20 NPH patients before and after treatment.

Single photon emission computed tomography scans (SPECTs) with ^{123}I-iodoamphetamine (^{123}I-IMP) were examined in 17 NPH patients. Although all NPH patients complained of mild mental and intelligence disorders, Seiken's test revealed normal values for almost all the patients before shunt operations; however, half of the patients had abnormal values on the Bender-Gestalt and Benton tests. Although clinical symptoms such as gait disturbance and urinary incontinence were improved in many patients after shunt operation, mental symptoms such as disorientation and poor comprehension still remained in about two-thirds of the patients. Of the three kinds of clinical tests for evaluating the sophisticated mental functions and intelligence of NPH patients before and after treatment, the Benton Visual Retention Test was the most sensitive. Finally, there was no significant correlation between the improvement of cerebral blood flow, examined by ^{123}I-IMP SPECT, and the improvement of mental symptoms assessed by the three kinds of mental tests.

Keywords. NPH — Seiken's Dementia Screening Test — Bender-Gestalt Test — Benton Visual Retention Test, ^{123}I-IMP SPECT

Introduction

With increases in life expectancy, the prevalence of mental disorders and dementia is gradually increasing. The original definition of normal pressure

[1] Department of Neurosurgery, Hyogo Medical Center for Adults, Akashi Hyogo, 673 Japan
[2] Allied Medical Science, Kobe University, Kobe, 650 Japan

hydrocephalus (NPH), as first described by Adams and co-workers 1965, is a triad consisting of dementia, apraxia, or gait disturbance, and urinary incontinence, seen in adults (Ojemann et al. 1969). These symptoms are associated with communicating hydrocephalus in the absence of increased intracranial pressure and there have been remarkable improvements of these symptoms after shunt operations. However, besides the many reports of improvement after shunting, there are a considerable number of patients who did not improve after shunt operations, in spite of the presence of typical clinical symptoms (Bannister 1972; Salmon 1972; Wood 1974).

As many neurosurgeons have pointed out, confusion still exists concerning the diagnosis of NPH and the subsequent need for surgery. The clinical triad of mental disorder, gait disturbance, and urinary incontinence is not a pathognomonic factor in predicting the success of a shunt operation. As there is no precise diagnosis for NPH before surgery, some shunt operations are performed which result in no improvement in clinical symptoms.

We present the results of our study of the relationship between assessment by sophisticated mental tests and quantitative cerebral blood flow monitoring by SPECT. In this report, we use the term "NPH" as a broad definition which constitutes the clinical triad without the results of shunt operation.

Clinical Materials and Methods

Between July 1987 and August 1990, 20 patients were selected from among 36 possible NPH patients as subjects for sophisticated mental tests and continuous CSF pressure monitoring. This monitoring was performed with a Gaeltec transducer, by the spinal drainage route. Seventeen patients received ^{123}I-iodoamphetamine — single photon emission computed tomography (^{123}I-IMP SPECT) so that changes of cerebral blood flow could be determined. In several patients, we tried a CSF dynamic study with cine magnetic resonance imaging (MRI) (1.5 Tesla superconducting type MRI-200RX, Toshiba Co., Japan)

Each patient underwent serial neurological examinations, neuroradiological studies such as computed tomography (CT) scans, MRI, CT cisternography, and three kinds of mental tests. All mental tests were performed by Dr. Kinoshita, professor of psychology and allied medical science at Kobe University. The results on the pre-shunting tests were compared with those on the post-shunting tests. The three Kinds of Mental Tests were:

1. Seiken-shiki dementia screening test (Ootsuka et al. 1987) (See Table 1). Although this test is somewhat influenced by the patient's memory or background experience, it is easier to administer than the other two tests.

2. Bender-Gestalt test (Bender L 1938). This has been used as a clinical and psychological tool for some considerable time. In this test the patient draws

Table 1. Seiken-shiki dementia screening test (a dementia scale produced and standardized by the Japanese National Institute for Mental Health)

Name	(M,F) Date	Examiner	
Question	Type of answer	Correct answer	Score
1. What is your date of birth?	Year, month, day	If correct	1
2. What day is it today?	Month, day	If correct	1
3. What day of the week was it yesterday?			
4. What is May 5?		Children's day	1
5. When is Seijin-no-hi? (a Japanese national holiday)		Jan. 15	1
6. You can walk on the crossroad when the traffic light is ------?		Green	1
7. Who is the sister of (your) mother?		Aunt	1
8. Who is the daughter of your sister?		Niece	1
9. The sun rises in the ------?		East	1
10. When the wind blows from the west, a balloon flies to the ------?		East	1
11. When you face north, your right arm will point ------?		East	1
12. Please repeat as I read a short sentence: "We pull the rope together."		No mistake	1
13. Add 18 and 19		37	1
14. Subtract 16 from 32		16	1
15. Please repeat in the right order: 3-6-4-8		3-6-4-8	1
16. Please repeat in reverse order: 9-2		2-9	1
17. The same task (reverse order): 2-4-6		6-4-2	1
18. The same task (reverse order): 7-1-6-5		5-6-1-7	1
		Total score	

Score: 0–10 Dementia is strongly suspected. Consult specialist
        11–15 Border-line. Dementia should be ruled out
        16–20 Normal. No further examination is needed at this time

copies of 9 test cards and these copies are interpreted indicating the state of mind of the patients. On this point, this test is different from routine intelligence tests.

3. Benton visual retention test (Benton 1974). This test was originally designed to distinguish brain disorders from other inorganic abnormalities, so it is not actually a general intelligence test. It is a non-verbal test which is closely correlated to the level of intelligence and aging; it can also be used in the evaluation of comprehension ability. We used 10 test cards of the C-type and listed scores for correct answers from 0 to 10, and scores for incorrect answers from 0 to 25.

Table 2. Clinical summary of NPH patients

Case No.	Age (years)	Sex	Etiology of NPH	Duration of symptoms	Risk Factors for dementia	Type of shunt
1.	65	M	Idiopathic	6 Months	Hypertension	V-P
2.	74	M	Post-SAH	2 Years	None	V-P
3.	57	M	Idiopathic	1 Year	Hypertension	V-P
4.	76	F	Idiopathic	2 Years	Cerebral infarction	V-P
5.	74	F	Idiopathic	6 Months	None	V-P
6.	75	M	Idiopathic	3 Years	None	V-P
7.	78	M	Idiopathic	2 years	Alzheimer's disease?	Not done
8.	72	M	Idiopathic	6 Months	None	V-P
9.	66	M	Idiopathic	3 Years	Hypertension	V-P
10.	73	M	Idiopathic	3 Years	D.M.? Hypertension	V-P
11.	70	M	Idiopathic	5 Years	Hypertension	V-P
12.	76	M	Idiopathic	4 Years	Hypertension	V-P
13.	59	F	Idiopathic	2 Years	Alzheimer's disease?	Not done
14.	76	M	Idiopathic	5 Years	Alzheimer's disease?	Not done
15.	66	F	Post-SAH	5 Months	None	V-P
16.	52	F	Post-SAH	6 Months	Hypertension	V-P
17.	62	F	Post-SAH	6 Months	Hypertension	V-P
18.	76	M	Idiopathic	3 Years	Hypertension	Not done
19.	59	F	Post-intra tumoral bleeding	6 Months	None	V-P
20.	58	M	Removal of huge tentorial meningioma	4 Months	None	V-P

SAH, sub-arachoid hemorrhage; V-P, ventriculo-peritoneal; D.M., diabetes mellitus

^{123}I-IMP SPECT

3mci of ^{123}I-IMP was intravenously injected in each patient and early images were obtained with a universal gamma camera (GCA-90A2 type Toshiba Co., Japan) with an attached low energy/high resolution collimeter. Axial and sagittal images were obtained using a 10mm slice thickness.

Results

Table 2 is a clinical summary of NPH patients. The etiology of NPH was mainly idiopathic, with some post-subarachnoid hemorrhages. Background disorders which are risk factors for dementia include: hypertension, infarction, diabetes mellitus, and so on. Preoperative functional grades using Stein and Langfitts' classification (Stein and Langfitt 1974) were Grade III in 60% of cases, Grade IV in 20%, and Grade II in 20%. No patients were considered to be Grade I, functioning independently at home. Ventricular-peritoneal (V-P) shunts were performed in 16 patients and 69% of these improved by one grade.

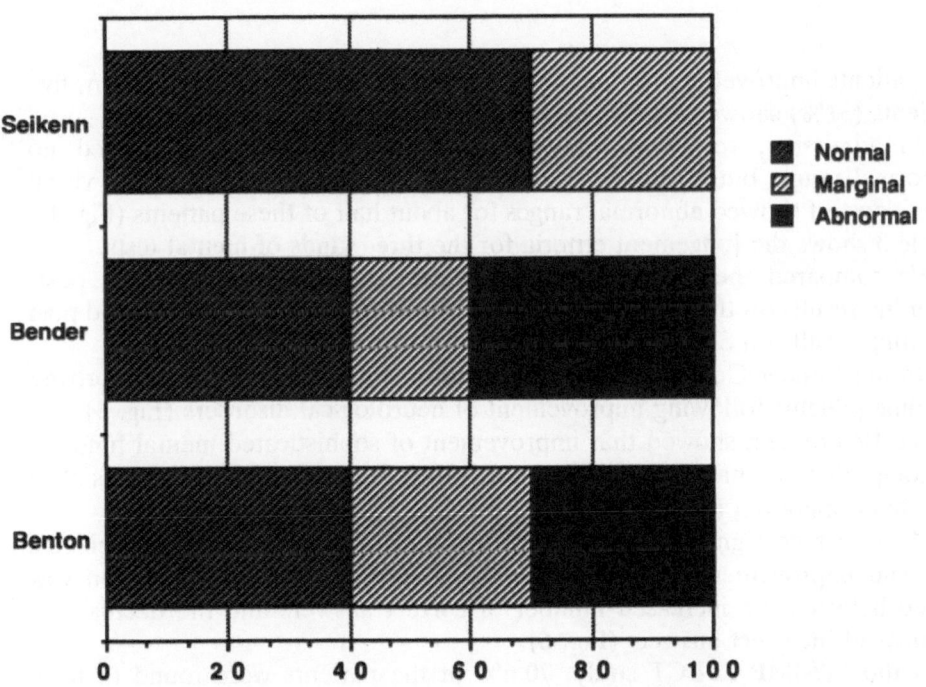

Fig. 1. Abnormalities on three types of mental test on admission

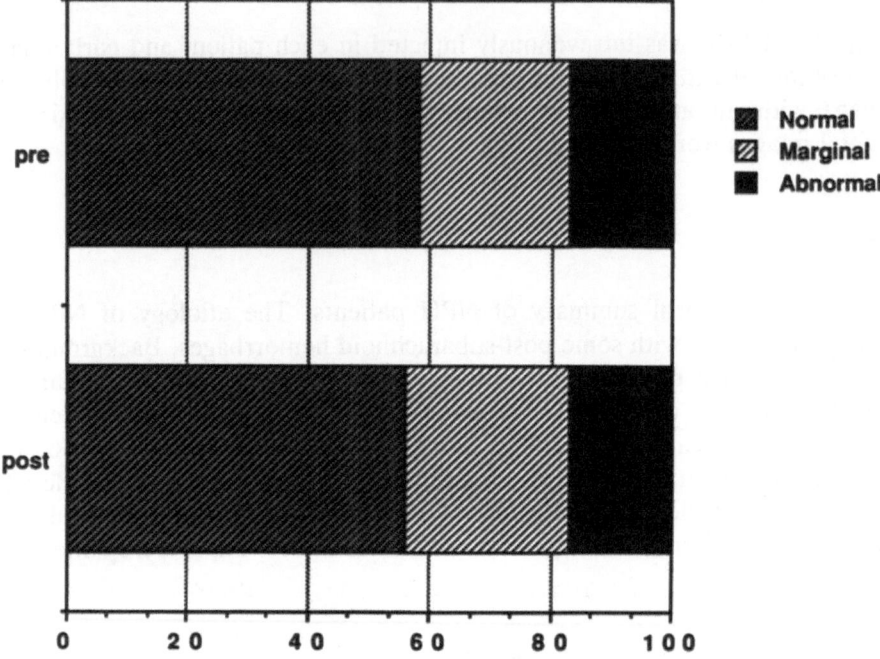

Fig. 2. Pre- and post-shunting results on Seiken's dementia screening test

No patients improved more than one grade. On neurological examination, five patients (31%) showed no change at all.

On admission, results of Seiken's dementia screening test showed no abnormal range, but results of the Bender-Gestalt test and the Benton visual retention test showed abnormal ranges for about half of these patients (Fig. 1). Table 3 shows the judgement criteria for the three kinds of mental tests.

We compared the pre-shunting results on the three tests with the post-shunting results on these tests. There was no change between the pre- and post shunting results on Seiken's dementia screening test (Fig. 2).

On the Bender-Gestalt tests, sophisticated mental functions were improved in some patients following improvement of neurological disorders (Fig. 3).

The Benton test showed that improvement of sophisticated mental function or comprehension had occurred in a remarkable number of NPH patients after the shunt operation (Fig. 4).

There was no significant correlation between the improvement on Seiken's test and improvement on the Benton test (Fig. 5). A good correlation was noted between the increased number of correct answers and the decrease in number of incorrect answers (Fig. 6).

In the ^{123}I-IMP SPECT study, 70.6% of the patients were found to have hypoperfusion, mainly in the frontal and front-temporal white matter and

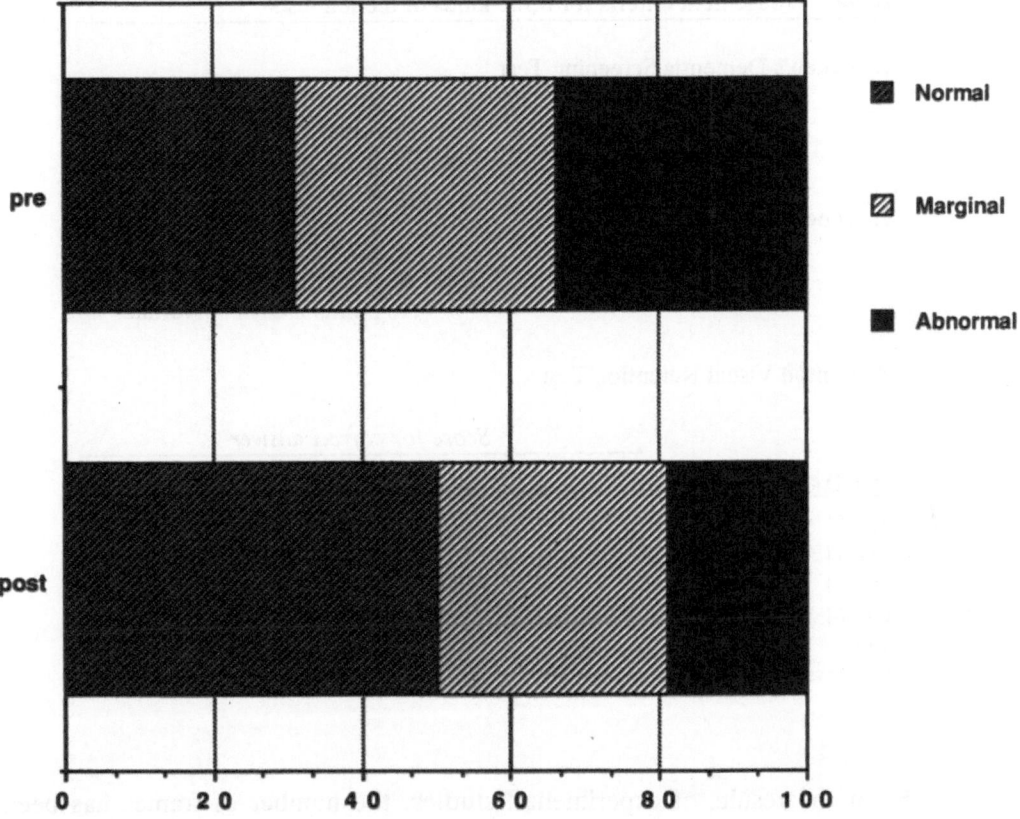

Fig. 3. Pre- and post-shunting results on the Bender-Gestalt test

cortex. After shunting, 41.2% of the patients showed slight improvements and remaining 58.8% of the patients showed no changes. However, this was a qualitative, not a quantitative finding. It was very difficult to analyze cerebral blood flow (CBF) quantitatively before and after shunting with our gamma camera, because of limits of analytic capability and limitations in the quality of the equipment.

The summary of the SPECT study is shown in Table 4. There was no significant correlation between the improvement of cerebral blood flow and the improvement of mental symptoms as shown by the results of the three kinds of mental tests. We have attempted to study the dynamics of CSF in various neurosurgical diseases, using MRI. Although this is a preliminary study, CSF flow was visualized with cine MRI by the single planar multi-phase (SPMP) method, with an electron cardiogram gating under a pulse sequence of repetition time (TR) = 50 ms, echo time (TE) = 15 ms, and 20 degrees of flip angle, and combining the flow compensation method.

Table 3. Judgement criteria for three kinds of mental tests

1. Seiken's Dementia Screening Test

0–10 points --------	Abnormal
11–15 points --------	Border-line
16–20 points --------	Normal

2. Bender-Gestalt Test
   Total score

>60 points --------	Abnormal
41–60 points --------	Border-line
<40 points --------	Normal

3. Benton Visual Retention Test

	Score for correct answer		
Age (years)	Abnormal	Border-line	Normal
15–44	<5	6	7<
45–54	<4	5	6<
55–64	<3	4	5<
65–74	<2	3	4<
75<	<1	2	3<

From the results of experimental studies, the number of frames has been found to be dependent on the R wave-R wave (R-R) interval of the patient's ECG. In this method, CSF flow was visualized as a high intensity signal, just as T2 weighted images are visualized.

Case Presentations

Case 12, a 76-year-old male, had been evaluated for idiopathic NPH and had shown typical progressive dementia, ataxic gait, hypertension, and urinary incontinence. This patient's Benton tests pre- and post-shunting are shown in Fig. 7. After V-P shunt placement, this patient's clinical symptoms were remarkably improved and correct answers were obtained on the Benton tests.

Case 20, a 58-year-old male, had typical clinical symptoms of NPH after the removal of a huge left sphenoidal ridge meningioma.

Pre- and post-shunting Benton tests, as shown in Fig. 8, show that remarkable improvements occurred post-shunting, following significant clinical improvement.

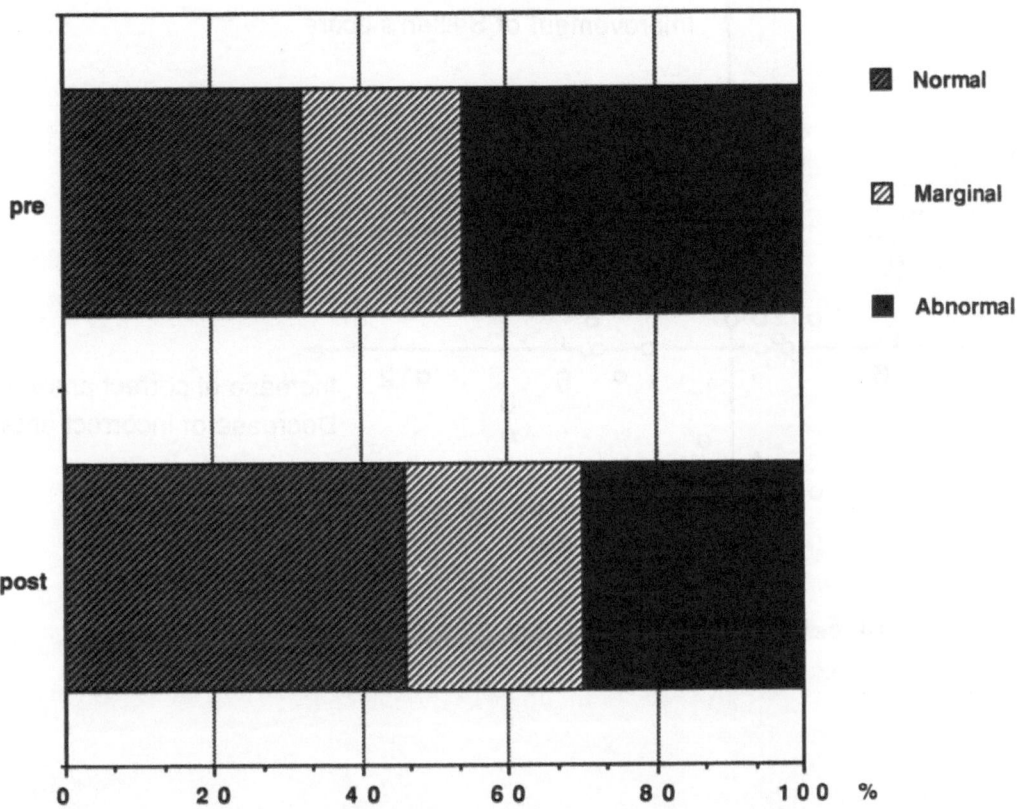

Fig. 4. Pre- and post-shunting results on the Benton Visual Retention test (*BVRT*)

Discussion

Although the pathophysiology and cerebral blood flow of patients with normal pressure hydrocephalus have been reported in many papers (Di Rocco et al. 1977; Mamo et al. 1987; Matthew et al. 1975; Meyer et al. 1983, 1985; Nuft et al. 1983; Tamaki et al. 1984), there are few quantitative analyses of their mental disorders (Jinpo and Baba 1979; Nakamura and Kanda; Rice and Gendelman 1973). One of the reasons why quantitative analysis of dementia in NPH is difficult is the lack of suitable mental tests for patients. Up till now, considerable numbers of mental tests have been reported (American Psychiatric Association 1987; Bender 1938; Benton 1974; Folstein et al. 1975; Hasegawa 1974; Ootsuka et al. 1987; Wechsler 1955); however, many of these mental or intelligence tests contain too much material and are too complicated for aged handicapped patients to perform routinely.

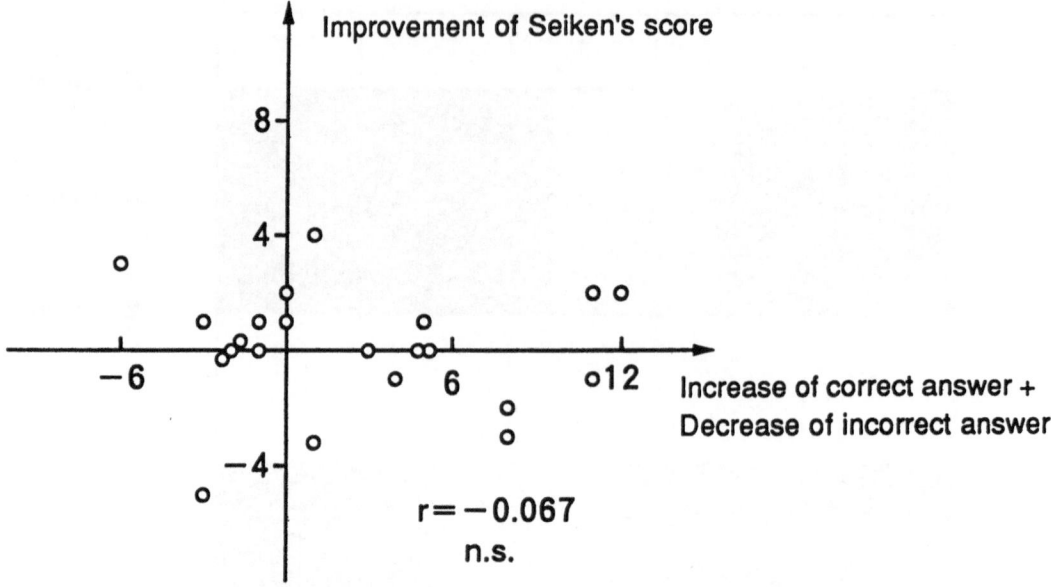

Fig. 5. Correlation of improvement in the Benton and Seiken-shiki tests

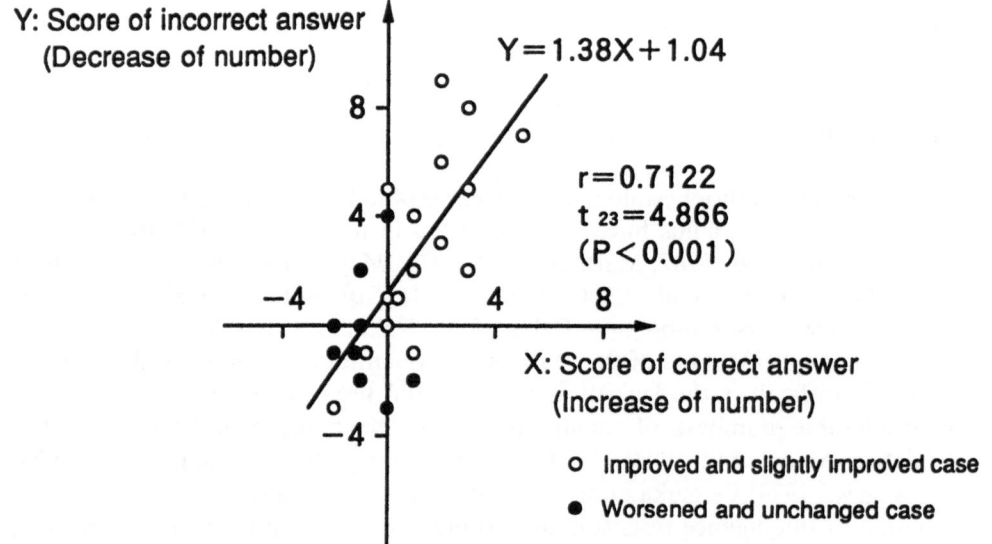

Fig. 6. Correlation between the increase in correct answers and the decrease in incorrect answers on the Benton Visual Retention test (*BVRT*)

Table 4. Summary of ^{123}I-IMP SPECT study of NPH

Case No.	Age (years)	Sex	Pre-shunting	Post-shunting
1.	65	M	Not examined	
2.	74	M	Frontal hypoperfusion	Improved
3.	57	M	Not examined	
4.	76	F	Diffuse hypoperfusion	Unchanged
5.	74	F	Frontal hypoperfusion	Improved
6.	75	M	Within normal limit	Unchanged
7.	78	M	F-T hypoperfusion	Unchanged
8.	72	M	Frontal hypoperfusion	Unchanged
9.	66	M	F-T hypoperfusion	Improved
10.	73	M	Within normal limit	Unchanged
11.	70	M	Frontal hypoperfusion	Improved
12.	76	M	Frontal hypoperfusion	Improved
13.	59	F	F-T hypoperfusion	Deteriorated
14.	76	M	F-T hypoperfusion	Unchanged
15.	66	F	Frotal hypoperfusion	Improved
16.	52	F	F-T hypoperfusion	Unchanged
17.	62	F	Frontal hypoperfusion	Unchanged
18.	76	M	Not examined	
19.	59	F	F-T hypoperfusion	Unchanged
20.	58	M	F-T hypoperfusion	Improved

We chose three tests, (Seiken's screening test, the Bender-Gestalt test, and the Benton Visual Retention test (BVRT) because of their quantitative nature and their relative simplicity. Of the three tests, BVRT was the most sensitive and reliable for evaluating mental and intellectual functions in NPH patients before and after shunt operations.

As Karasawa has pointed out (Karasawa et al. 1980), BVRT has some advantages for the examination of the aged in comparison with other tests, e.g., it can be administered even to aged people who have hearing and/or speech disturbances. Due to its simplicity, the test can be done even by patients who have hand tremors or some difficulty of hand movement, and even by aged people whose motivation for doing the test is low. Because it is non-verbal, this test also can be used with aged people of different social and educational backgrounds. Finally, this test can evaluate the capacity for attention, which is an important factor considering intelligence in the aged.

The Wechsler Adult Intelligence Scale (WAIS) is the most precise intelligence test which includes both verbal and emotional analysis (Wechsler 1955). However, this test does not seem practical as a routine measure because it needs much time to perform. In addition, it is often difficult to complete, especially for aged post-operative neurosurgical patients. As there is no single test available for the evaluation of all sophisticated mental functions, we must judge those functions by combining the results on several kinds of mental and intelligence tests.

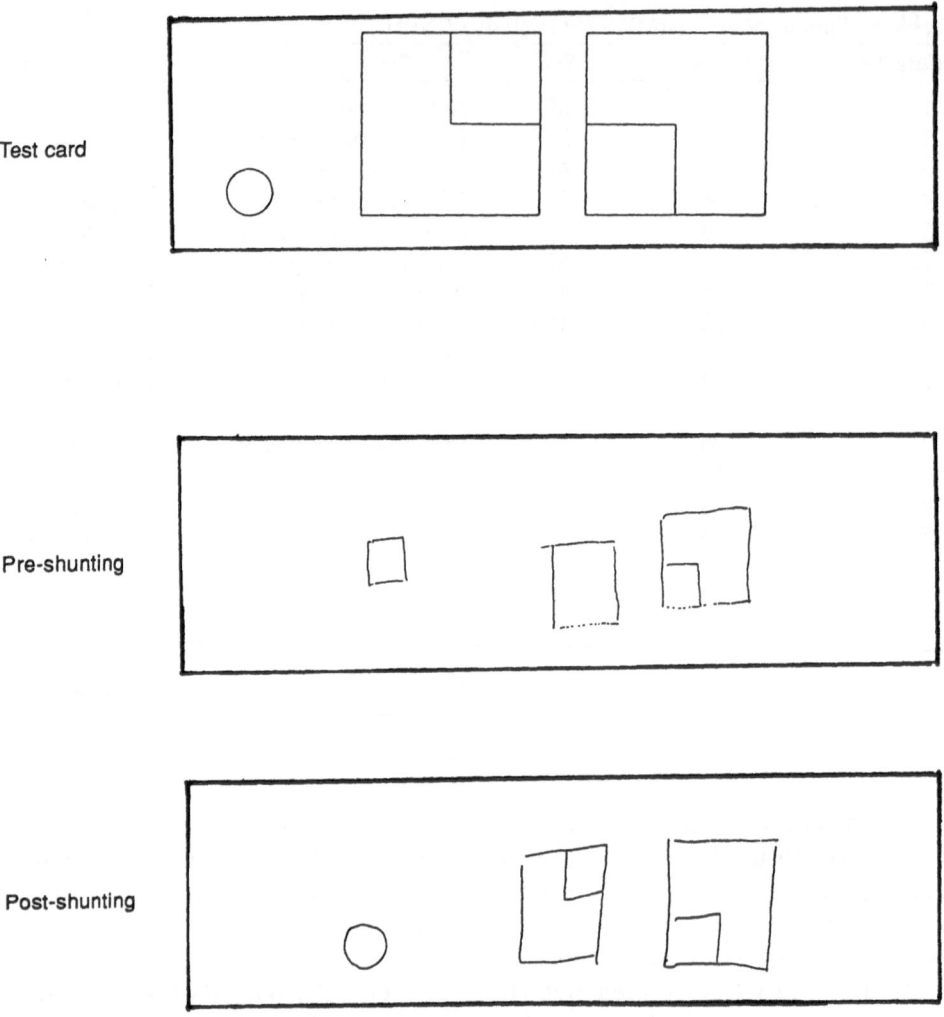

Fig. 7. Benten tests, pre- and post-shunting (case 12)

It has been suggested that measurements of cerebral blood flow (CBF) may prove helpful for differentiating NPH from other forms of dementia, such as multi-infarct dementia and senile dementia of the Alzheimer type. Abnormalities of CBF values in patients with NPH have been reported using both CT and ^{133}Xe CBF monitoring methods (Meyer et al. 1983; Ootsuka et al. 1987). ^{133}Xe-CT abnormalities in NPH were different from those seen in cases of senile dementia of the Alzheimer type or seen in cases of multi-infarct dementia (Meyer et al. 1983).

Recently, CBF measurements by [123]IMP-SPECT (Matsuda et al. 1987) and positron emission tomography (PET) (Frackowiak et al. 1981; Thomas

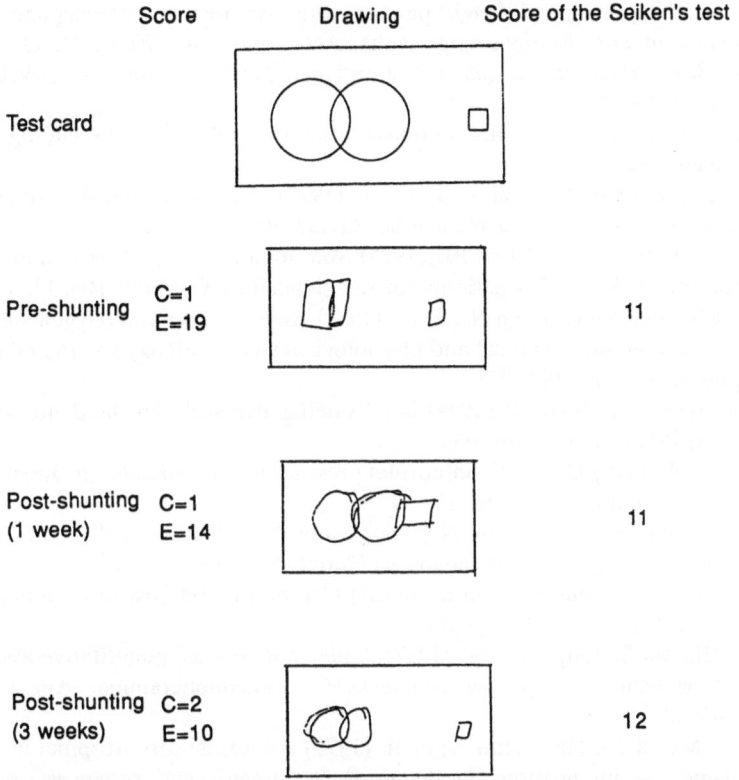

Fig. 8. Benton tests, pre- and post-shunting. NPH occurred after removal of a huge sphenoidal ridge meningioma (case 20)

et al. 1984) methods have been reported in cerebrovascular diseases and brain tumors, but there are few reports of hemodynamic studies using SPECT in NPH patients (Shose et al. 1990). In our study, reduced CBF values in the frontal lobe were noted in half of the NPH patients pre-shunting; their CBF revealed a moderate improvement after shunting. However, there was no significant correlation between the improvement of cerebral blood flow and the improvement of mental symptoms as shown by the three kinds of mental tests. It was very difficult to quantitatively analyze CBF before and after shunting because of limitations in the quality of our equipment.

References

Adams KD, Fisher CM, Hakim S, et al. (1965) Symptomatic occult hydrocephalus with "Normal" cerebrospinal-fluid pressure. A treatable syndrome. N Engl J Med 273: 117–126

American Psychiatric Association: Diagnostic and Statistical Manual of Mental Disorders (DSM-III-R) (1987) American Psychiatric Association, Washington, pp 103–109

Bannister CM (1972) A report of eight patients with low pressure hydrocephalus treated by CSF diversion with disappointing results. Acta Neurochir (Wien) 27: 11–15

Bender L (1938) A visual motor gestalt test and its clinical use. Am Orthopsychiatr Ass Res Monogr 3: 1–176

Benton AL (1974) Revised Visual Retention test (4th edn). The Psychological Corporation, New York

Di Rocco C, DiTrapani G, Maira G, et al. (1977) Anatomo-clinical correlations in normotensive hydrocephalus. J Neurol Sci 33:437–452

Folstein MF, Folstein SE, McHugh PR (1975) Mini-mental state, a practical method for grading the cognitive state of patients for the clinician. J Psychiatr Res 12: 189–198

Frackowiak RSJ, Pozzilli C, Legg NJ, et al. (1981) Regional cerebral oxygen supply and utilization in dementia. A clinical and physiological study with oxygen-15 and positron tomography. Brain 104: 753–778

Hasegawa K, Inoue K, Moriya K (1974) Brief Intelligence Scale for the demented aged. (in Japanese) Psychiatr Med 16: 965

Jinpo M, Baba M (1979) Dementia in normal pressure hydrocephalus. (in Japanese) No To Shinke, (Brain and Nerve) 31: 19–29

Karasawa A, Kobayashi M, Yatomi N (1980) Clinical Evaluation of the Benton Visual Retention Test in the Aged. (in Japanese) Geriatr Soc Sci 2: 82–97

Mamo HL, Meric PC, Ponsin JC, et al. (1987) Cerebral blood flow in normal pressure hydrocephalus. Stroke 18: 1074–1080

Matsuda H, Higashi S, Tsuji S, et al. (1987) A new noninvasive quantitative assessment of blood flow using N-isopropyl-(Iodine-123) P-iodoamphetamine. Am J Physiol (Imag) 2: 49–55

Matthew NT, Meyer JS, Hartmann A, et al. (1975) Abnormal cerebrospinal fluid-blood flow dynamics — implications in diagnosis, treatment, and prognosis in normal pressure hydrocephalus. Arch Neurol 32: 657–664

Meyer JS, Shaw TG, Okayasu H, et al. (1983) Multi-infarct Alzheimer dementia differentiated from normal aging by xenon contrast CT/CBF measurements. J Cereb Blood Flow Metab 3 (Suppl 1): 506–507

Meyer JS, Kitagawa Y, Tanahashi N, et al. (1985) Pathogenesis of normal-pressure hydrocephalus — preliminary observations. Surg Neurol 23: 121–133

Nakamura N, Kanda R (1981) Dementia in normal pressure hydrocephalus. (in Japanese) Adv Neurol Sci 25: 1235–1242

Nuft A, Namo H, Meric P, et al. (1983) Cerebral blood flow measurments in the diagnosis of normal pressure hydrocephalus. J Cereb Blood Flow Metab 3: 65–66

Ojemann RG, Fisher CM, et al. (1969) Further experience with the syndrome of "normal" pressure hydrocephalus. J Neurosurg 31: 279–294

Ootsuka T, Shimonaka J, Kitamura T, et al. (1987) A new screening test for dementia. (in Japanese) Psychiatr Med 29: 395–402

Rice E, Gendelman S (1973) Psychiatric aspects of normal pressure hydrocephalus. J A MA 223: 409–412

Salmon JH (1972) Adult hydrocephalus. Evaluation of shunt surgery in 80 patients. J Neurosurg 37: 423–428

Shose Y, Kawaguchi T, Hosoda H, et al. (1990) ^{123}I-IMP SPECT in hydrocephalus (abstract) Perfusamin Res 6: 10

Stein SC, Langfitt TW (1974) Normal-pressure hydrocephalus: Predicting the results of cerebrospinal fluid shunting. J Neurosurg 4: 463–470

Tamaki N, Kusunoki T, Wakabayashi T, et al. (1984) Cerebral hemodynamics in normal-pressure hydrocephalus. Evaluation by ^{133}Xe inhalation and dynamic CT study. J Neurosurg 61: 510–514

Thomas DGT, Beaney RP, Brooks DJ (1984) Positron emission tomography in the study of cerebral tumors. Neurosurg Rev 7: 257–258

Wechsler D (1955) Wechsler adult Intelligence Scale. The Psychological Corporation, New York

Wood JH, Bartlet D, James AE JR, et al. (1974) Normal pressure hydrocephalus: Diagnosis and patient selection for shunt surgery. Neurology 24: 517–526

VI. New Concepts and Future Aspects

66 — Serotonergic Effects on Cerebrospinal Fluid Production

Saburo Nakamura, Koji Maeda, Jun Sasaki, and Takashi Tsubokawa[1]

Summary. In an attempt to elucidate the participation of serotonin in CSF production, the effects of 5-hydroxytryptophan (5-HTP) on the dynamics of CSF production and on carbonic anhydrase (CA) activity in the choroid plexus were examined in mongrel dogs. Examination was by electron microscopy. CSF dynamics were studied by the ventriculocisternal perfusion method developed by Pappenheimer and by an automatic continuous measurement technique devised by the authors. Administration of 10–30 mg/kg 5-HTP reduced CSF production by 35%–40%, showing no correlation with dose. On the other hand, after administration of 100 mg/kg acetazolamide (Diamox), CSF production decreased by 57%. Following administration of 20 mg/kg 5-HTP, the CA activity fell to 43.3% of the control value. That is, approximately 56% of the CA activity in the choroid plexus was affected by serotonin. These results suggest a serotoninergic reducing effect on CSF production which derives from a reduction of the CA activity in the choroid plexus.

Keywords: Acetazolamide — Carbonic anhydrase activity — Choroid plexus — CSF production — Serotonin

Introduction

Although several hypotheses have been proposed concerning the production of cerebrospinal fluid (CSF) (Ames et al. 1964; Brightman 1968; Maren and Broder 1970; Segal 1974; Johanson 1984), the details still remain controversial. Lindvall et al. (1978) reported that electrical stimulation of the cervical sympathetic nerves suppressed CSF production and Edvinsson et al. (1974) noted the presence of adrenergic nerve terminals in the choroid plexus. Nakamura and Milhorat (1978) identified stromal and vascular nerve endings in the choroid plexus by electron microscopy. Moreover, suppressive effects of

---

[1] Department of Neurological Surgery, School of Medicine, Nihon University, Itabashi-ku, Tokyo, 173 Japan

noradrenaline and serotonin on CSF production have been reported by several authors (Lindvall et al. 1979; Maeda 1983). The above findings indicate the participation of monoamines in CSF production.

On the other hand, it is thought that the active transport in the choroid plexus depends on Na^+, K^+-ATPase (Milhorat et al. 1975) and carbonic anhydrase (CA). The existence of CA in the choroid plexus has been demonstrated previously in biochemical (Fisher and Copenhaver 1959; Giacobini 1962) and morphological studies (Atkinson and Ward 1958; Korhonen et al. 1964; Roussel et al. 1979), and the fact that acetazolamide (Diamox) decreases CSF formation (Knopp et al. 1957; Davson and Pollay 1963; Holladay and Cassin 1972; Smith et al. 1974), as shown clinically, supports the above hypothesis.

In the present study, the authors employed the ventriculocisternal perfusion method developed by Pappenheimer (Pappenheimer et al. 1962) and examined the involvement of 5-hydroxytryptophan (5-HTP) in CSF-producing dynamics by applying an automatic and continuous measurement technique to monitor CSF production. Further, in an attempt to elucidate the participation of serotonin in CSF production, the effects of 5-HTP on CA activity in the choroid plexus were investigated by electron microscopy.

Materials and Methods

Measurement of CSF Production

Thirty-one adult mongrel dogs of both sexes, weighing 7.0–12.0 kg, were anesthetized by intravenous injection of Nembutal (30 mg/kg). After intratracheal intubation, the animals were placed on a stereotaxic operation apparatus in the prone position. They were then given generalized anesthesia with N_2O, O_2, and halothane and their respiration was controlled. Intraventricular puncture was made into the lateral ventricles on both sides. Of the two punctures, one was used for infusion of the perfusion fluid, and the other was connected with a transducer to monitor the intaventricular pressure. During the measurements, 100 ml/kg per day of Haltoman's solution was given by drop infusion and the arterial pressure was monitored.

Perfusion Methods

Blue Dextran (molecular weight 2 000 000) was dissolved in the perfusion fluid, consisting of Elliot-B artificial cerebrospinal fluid, to a concentration of 100 mg/dl. The resultant solution was gassed with a mixture of 95% O_2 and 5% CO_2, and the pH was adjusted to 7.4. The osmotic pressure of the perfusion liquid was 190–300 mOsm/l.

Perfusion was carried out with a Harvard infusion pump at the rate of 0.21 ± 0.001 ml/min. At the time of perfusion, the temperature of the liquid was maintained at 37°C with a warmer. A 21G needle was inserted into the cisterna magna at a height of 15 cm from the heart, to form the outlet. The needle was was connected to a continuous measurement system for monitoring CSF production (Nakamura et al. 1983).

Administration of Drugs

Pretreatment control values for CSF production were obtained about 2–2.5 h after starting perfusion of the Blue Dextran-Elliot-B perfusion fluid, when the values reached a plateau. Once data for the control had been obtained, administration of drugs was commenced. With a view to examining the control mechanism of CSF production by monoamines, intravenous administration of 10–30 mg/kg 5-HTP, 50 mg/kg tetrabenazine (TBZ), and 50 and 100 mg/kg acetazolamide (Diamox) in distilled water was carried out. In order to confirm the actions of the drugs, the blood concentrations of adrenaline, noradrenaline, and serotonin was determined by high-speed liquid chromatography after administration.

Electron Microscopic Examination of CA Activity

Twelve healthy adult mongrel dogs of both sexes, each weighing between 6.5 and 12.0 kg, were anesthetized with 30 mg/kg i.v. pentobarbital sodium, intubated, and given generalized anesthesia with N_2O, O_2, and halothane and their respiration was controlled. The dogs were divided into four experimental groups: Group 1 dogs ($n = 3$) formed the controls and received no drugs; group 2 dogs ($n = 3$) received an intravenous injection of 50 mg/kg Diamox in distilled water; group 3 dogs ($n = 3$) received 20 mg/kg i.v. 5-HTP in distilled water; and group 4 dogs ($n = 3$) received 50 mg/kg i.v. TBZ in distilled water. All the dogs were sacrificed painlessly by perfusion with fixative (0.5% glutaraldehyde, 2% paraformaldehyde with 8% sucrose, buffered with 0.1 M cacodylate buffer to pH 7.2) through the heart at the time when changes in CSF production were at their maximum, that is, at 30 min after the injection of 5-HTP in group 3, and 60 min after the injection of each other drug in groups 2 and 4.

Preparation of Materials for Electron Microscopy

The choroid plexuses were removed from the fourth ventricle. After additional fixation in the same fixative for 1 h, the tissue samples were rinsed with cacodylate buffer and incubated for 20 min at room temperature in a solution containing 0.1 M $CoSO_4$, 0.5 M H_2SO_4, 1/15 M KH_2PO_4, 0.75 M $NaHCO_3$, and 8% sucrose. They were then prepared by Yokota's method (Yokota 1969). The samples were postfixed in 2% osmium tetroxide buffered with cacodylate sodium for 60 min, dehydrated in a methanol series, and embedded in epoxy resin. After ultrathin sections were prepared, electron staining with uranyl acetate and lead citrate was carried out before observation.

Morphometric Quantification of CA Activity

Electron microscopic examinations were performed under an electron micro-scope (HU-12 model, Hitachi Tokyo) with a filament voltage of 75 kV. Electron micrographs of the apical surface of epithelial cells of the choroid plexus at 1000 times original magnification were taken at random. The pictures were enlarged to 25000 times prints. The spotty reaction products were counted within an area of 25 square cm (4 μm square originally), predominantly over the microvilli.

Fifty pictures from each group were analyzed and the levels of CA activity were evaluated statistically by Student's *t*-test for uncorrelated pairs.

Results

CSF Production

Control Values

The control values for CSF production determined in 31 mongrel dogs ranged from 17.53 to 47.63 μl/min, with a mean of 33.02 ± 8.42 μl/min.

5-HTP Treated Group (Fig. 1)

The mean levels of CSF production before and after administration of 10 mg/kg 5-HTP ($n = 5$) were 28.14 ± 8.32 μl/min and 17.96 ± 6.51 μl/min, respectively. The reduction in CSF production after this administration was thus 10.18 ± 2.00 μl/min (37.1% ± 5.4%) as the mean. This change represented a significant difference by Student's *t*-test, the level of significance being 5%. On

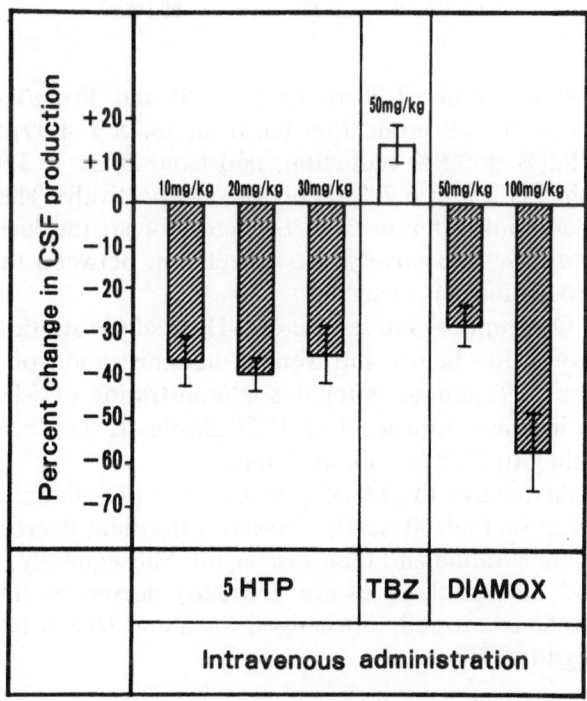

Fig. 1. Percent changes in CSF production. Control value = 33.02 ± 8.42 μl/min

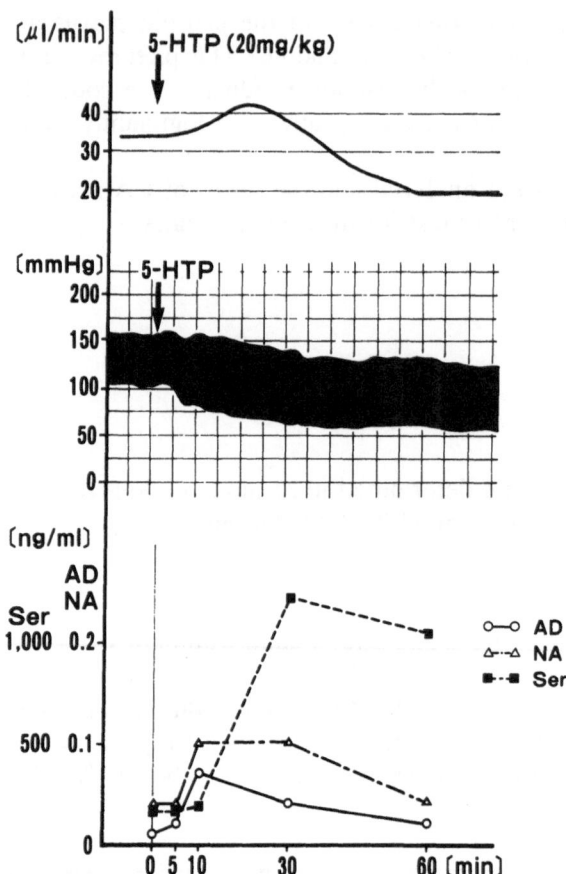

Fig. 2. Changes of CSF production rate, blood pressure, and blood concentration of monoamines after intravenous administration of 20 mg/kg 5-hydroxytryptophan (*5-HTP*). *Upper*, CSF production rate; *middle*, blood pressure; *lower*, blood concentration of monoamines. AD, adrenaline; NA, noradrenaline; Ser, serotonin

administration of 20 mg/kg ($n = 5$) and 30 mg/kg ($n = 5$) 5-HTP, the mean levels of CSF production fell from $36.75 \pm 4.99 \,\mu$l/min to $22.06 \pm 2.75 \,\mu$l/min (39.9% ± 3.8% reduction) and from $38.51 \pm 3.01 \,\mu$l/min to $24.82 \pm 0.96 \,\mu$l/min (35.2% ± 6.7% reduction), respectively. These changes also represented significant differences by Student's *t*-test, the levels of significance being 2% and 5%, respectively. No correlation between the doses of 5-HTP and CSF production was observed.

One representative case of 5-HTP administration is illustrated in Fig. 2. CSF production before intravenous administration of 20 mg/kg 5-HTP in a bolus was 32.93 μl/min. After this administration of 5-HTP, CSF production tended to increase, to a level of 41.70 μl/min. It then underwent a gradual decrease, falling to 19.10 μl/min at 70 min.

As regards the blood pressure, the pre-administration systolic and diastolic levels of 150/100 mmHg showed a transient decrease immediately after 5-HTP administration and then rose again. Subsequently, the pulse pressure expanded and the systolic pressure gradually decreased. However, the pulse pressure remained virtually unchanged for about 60 min after the systolic pressure had begun to fall.

Fig. 3. Changes of CSF production rate, blood pressure, and blood concentration of monoamines after intravenous administration of 50 mg/kg tetrabenzine (*TBZ*). *Upper*, CSF production rate; *middle*, blood pressure; *lower*, blood concentration of monoamines. AD, adrenaline; NA, noradrenaline; Ser, serotonin

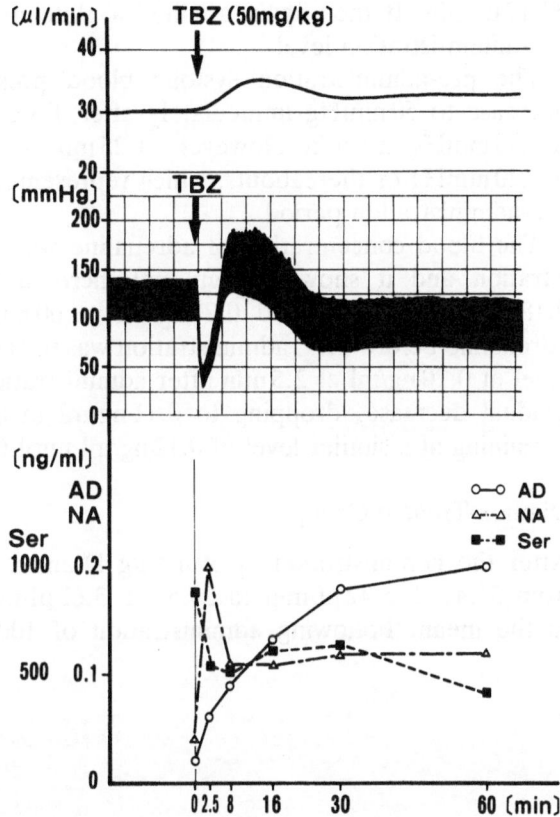

The blood concentration of serotonin, which was at a level of 328 ng/ml before the administration of 5-HTP, maintained a similar level for 10 min. It then increased strongly, to reach 1270 ng/ml in 30 min, and remained at a high level, 1080 nl/ml, at 60 min after 5-HTP administration. However, the concentrations of noradrenaline and adrenaline revealed transiently high levels for 10–30 min and then gradually decreased to pre-administration levels within 30–60 min.

TBZ Treated Group (Fig. 1)

The levels of CSF production on intravenous administration of 50 mg/kg TBZ in a bolus ($n = 6$) changed from 34.99 ± 9.25 µl/min to 39.71 ± 10.05 µl/min (13.7% ± 4.4% increase) as the mean. This change represented a significant difference by Student's *t*-test, the level of significance being 0.1%

In one of the representative cases of TBZ administration, the volume of CSF production before TBZ administration was 29.94 µl/min (Fig. 3). In view of the time lag, the volume increased at an early stage after TBZ administration, reaching a maximum of 34.94 µl/min in about 5 min. However, at 10 min after TBZ administration, the level underwent a slight decrease and fell to

32.19 µl/min. It then again attained a plateau, showing an increase from the pre-admin-istration level.

The pre-administration systolic blood pressure of 140 mmHg began to decrease to 50 mmHg immediately after TBZ administration, but rose again to 180 mmHg in 6 min. However, at 25 min, the systolic pressure had dropped to 120 mmHg or thereabouts, which represented a lower level than that in the pre-administration period.

The blood concentration of adrenaline was 0.02 ng/ml before TBZ admin-istration and it showed a gradual increase after administration, reaching 0.18 ng/ml in 30 min and 0.20 ng/ml in 60 min. The concentration of nor-adrenaline before TBZ administration was 0.04 ng/ml and it reached a maximal level of 0.20 ng/ml at 2.5 min after administration. However, it then showed a gradual decrease, dropping to 0.11 ng/ml at 8 min after administration and remaining at a similar level of 0.12 ng/ml until 60 min afterwards.

Diamox-Treated Group

After the administration of 50 mg/kg Diamox ($n = 5$), CSF production fell from 34.41 ± 5.42 µl/min to 24.53 ± 3.63 µl/min (28.5% ± 4.1% reduction) as the mean. Following administration of 100 mg/kg Diamox ($n = 5$), the

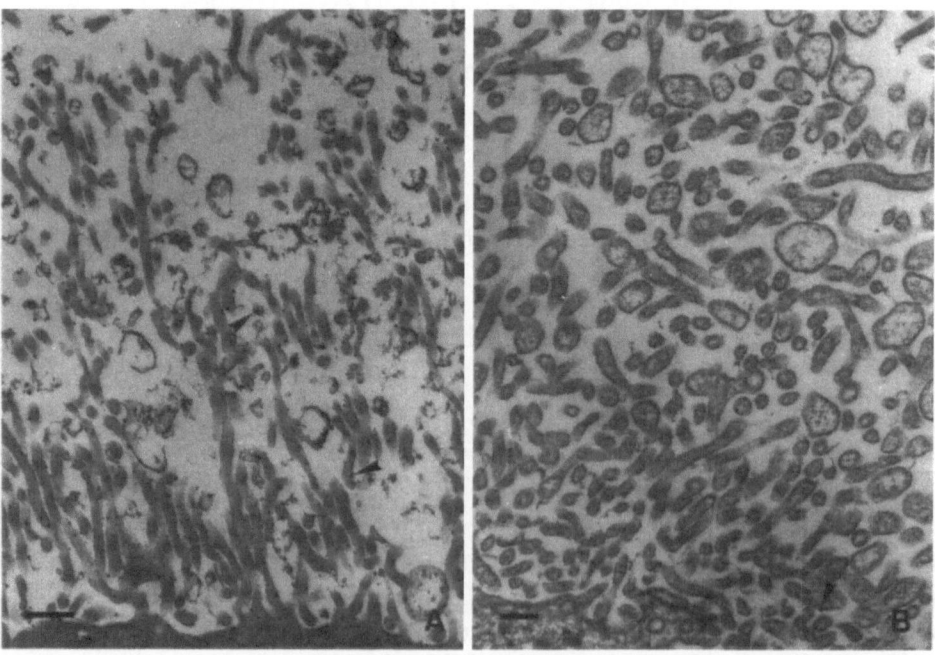

Fig. 4. Electron micrographs **A** showing CA activity as spotty reaction product (*arrowheads*) in the microvilli of the choroid plexus of a normal dog, and **B** showing scanty reaction products (*arrowhead*) in the microvilli of the choroid plexus of a dog treated with acetazolamide (Diamox). *Bar* = 0.2 µm

level fell from a pre-administration value of 36.35 ± 13.50 µl/min to 16.08 ± 8.40 µl/min as the mean, the decrease in CSF production being 57.2% ± 8.1% as the mean.

CA Activity

Group 1 (Control)

CA activity detected in the control dogs was located in the choroid epithelial cells as spotty reaction products (Fig. 4a). CA activity was observed mostly in the membrane and was scarce in the cytoplasm of the microvilli. Activity was also detected in the apical plasmalemma but not in the vesicles in cytoplasm adjacent to microvilli. Some activity was located in the basal and lateral apposed plasmalemma of epithelial cells.

Group 2 (Administration of Diamox)

Following administration of Diamox, the microvilli of the choroid plexus became elongated, some reaching 4 µm in length, and were swollen at their tips (Fig. 4b). CA activity was so significantly decreased as to be barely

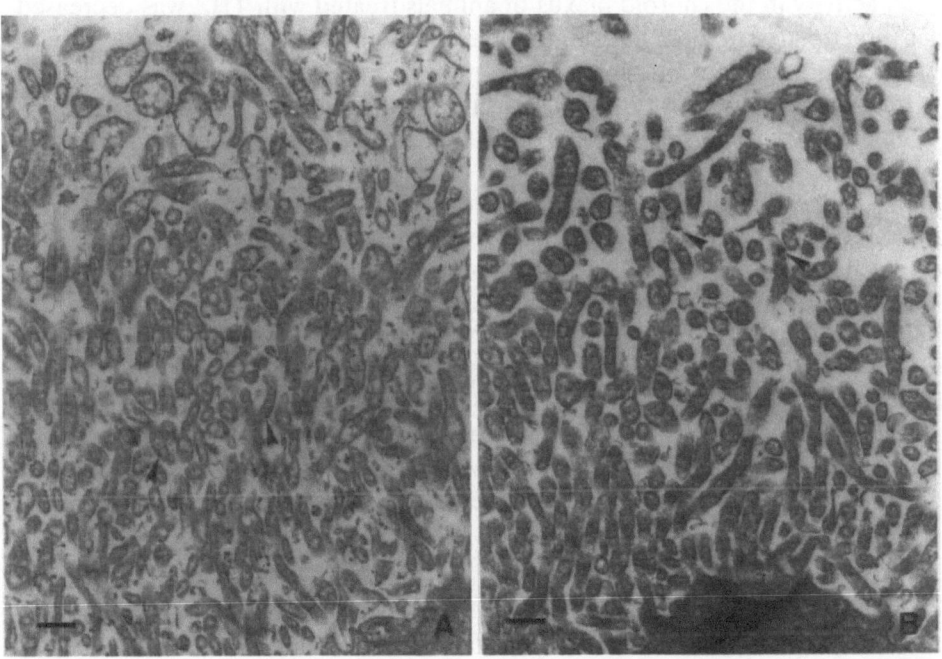

Fig. 5. Electron micrographs **A** showing markedly decreased reaction products (*arrowheads*) in the microvilli of the choroid plexus of a dog treated with 5-hydroxytryptophan (*5-HTP*), and **B** showing more markedly decreased reaction products (*arrowheads*) in the microvilli after treatment with tetrabenazine (*TBZ*) than after treatment with 5-HTP. *Bar* = 0.2 µm

observable in the choroid plexus. Activity in the microvilli was also markedly diminished.

Group 3 (Administration of 5-HTP)

No remarkable morphological changes were observed in the epithelial cells of the choroid plexus following administration of 5-HTP. However, the microvilli did show slight changes in their contours (Fig. 5a). CA activity in the choroid plexus was distributed in almost the same fashion as in the control. However, CA activity was generally decreased in the epithelium, especially in the microvilli.

Group 4 (Administration of TBZ)

When TBZ was administered the choroid plexus underwent some small changes, including dilatation of the extracellular space at the basal infolding and lateral interdigitations (Fig. 5b). The intracellular structure and organellae did not exhibit any remarkable changes. However, the vesicles at the apical plasmalemma were increased in number, and most of the microvilli were elongated and swollen, giving rise to the polypoid shape observed in animals treated with 5-HTP.

CA activity in the choroid plexus of animals treated with TBZ was decreased to a greater extent than in animals treated with 5-HTP. Slight activity was observed in the shafts and bases of the microvilli but not at their tips.

Quantitative studies of the control choroid plexus yielded values of 27.0–34.3/μm^2, with an average of 30.9 ± 1.9 (mean ± SD)/μm^2 (Table 1, Fig. 6). This value included both membranous and intrinsic activity. Following the administration of Diamox, the reaction products in the choroid plexus amounted to 0–1.5/μm^2, with an average of 0.6 ± 0.5/μm^2. This value corresponded to only 1.9% of the control, so this represented a definite decrease of nearly 98% of the control value. Following the administration of 5-HTP, the spotty reaction products in the choroid plexus amounted to as much as 11.3–17.0/μm^2, with an average of 13.5 ± 1.6μm^2. This value indicated a definite decrease ($P < 0.01$) of as much as 56% of the control value. Following the administration of TBZ, the reaction products in the choroid plexus amounted to as much as 4.5–9.0/μm^2, with an average of 7.0 ± 1.4/μm^2. This value represented a more significant decrease than that observed in animals

Table 1. Monoamines and carbonic anhydrase activity

| | Carbonic anhydrase activity | | | |
	Control	Diamox	5-HTP	TBZ
Range (/μm^2)	27.0–34.3	0–1.5	11.3–17.0	4.5–9.0
Mean	30.9	0.6	13.5	7.0
SD	1.9	0.5	1.6	1.4

5-HTP, 5-hydrocytryptophan; TBZ, tetrabenzine

Fig. 6. Carbonic anhydrase activity. *Line*, SD

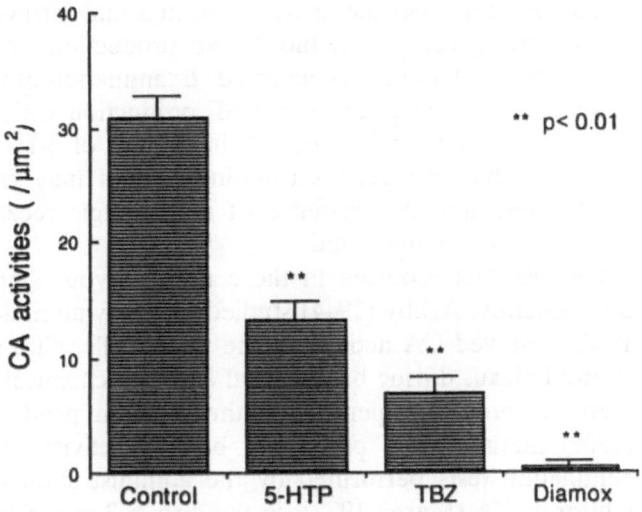

treated with 5-HTP ($P < 0.01$) and in the controls ($P < 0.01$), down to 22.4% of the control value.

Discussion

Participation of the nervous system in CSF production was first reported by Benedikt (1874), who discovered nerve fibers in the choroid plexus and designated them as the 13th cranial nerve. Subsequently, other researchers, including Stöhr (1922), Clark (1928), and Schapiro (1931), also recognized such fibers by light microscopy. More recently, Nakamura and Milhorat (1978) reported nerve endings containing dense core vesicles in the vascular wall and stroma of the choroid plexus. They proposed that their findings could provide a morphological basis on which to justify a role for biogenic amines in CSF production.

Lindvall et al. (1978) found that bilateral electrical stimulation of the cervical sympathetic nerves markedly reduced the production of CSF, whereas sympathetic denervation enhanced the rate of formation, concomitant with a marked reduction in noradrenaline concentration. Lindvall et al. (1979) also reported a decrease in CSF formation following intravenous or intraventricular administration of noradrenaline.

Based on the results of fluorescence microscopy, Edvinsson et al. (1974) proposed that each choroid plexus was innervated by a substantial number of noradrenaline-containing axons. Further, examination of the effects on CSF production of specific agonists and antagonists of neurotransmitters of the autonomic nervous system by Haywood and Vogh (1978), and examination of the effects nialamide, an MAO inhibitor, by Lindvall and Owman (1980), confirmed an association between monoamines and CSF production.

The present experiments demonstrated that intravenous injection of 5-HTP, a serotonin precursor, reduced CSF production by 35%–40%; however, no correlation with dose was observed. Examination of the blood concentration of serotonin revealed changes in CSF production which corresponded well with those of serotonin following administration of 5-HTP. From these data, it is proposed that increased serotonin function may cause a reduction of CSF production, and the existence of serotonergic receptors and neurons in the choroid plexus is suggested.

CA was first reported in the central nervous system by van Goor (1940). Subsequently, Ashby (1944) studied this enzyme in detail and Giacobini (1961, 1962) observed CA activity in the nerve cells, glia, and epithelial cells of the choroid plexus during biochemical and histochemical investigations.

In the present experiments, the reaction products revealed by Yokota's (1969) method were proven to be CA activity. This proof was based on elimination tests performed by the administration of Diamox, a specific inhibitor of CA (Maren 1977), in the Group 2 experiments.

This enzyme activity has been demonstrated previously in the basal infoldings, the apical plasmalemma, and predominantly, in the microvilli, of choroid epithelial cells in rats (Shimabukuro et al. 1982). Although the choroid plexus of the dog was examined in the present study, the localization of the enzyme was found to be almost the same as that reported in the rat.

In the choroid plexus the CA localized in the microvilli and plasmalemma catalyzes the reaction from CO_2 and H_2O to H^+ ion and HCO_3^- ion and releases HCO_3^- into the CSF, controlling its pH. Hydrogen ion is exchanged at the basal plasmalemma when sodium ion is taken up into the epithelial cells from the stroma of the choroid plexus. Release of sodium ion is thought to be performed by active transport involving Na^+, K^+-ATPase (Milhorat et al. 1975; Masuzawa et al. 1980).

The present data indicated that CA activity fell to 43.3% of the control value following administration of 5-HTP. That is, approximately 57% of the CA activity in the choroid plexus was affected by serotonin. This confirms a suppressive effect by serotonin on CA in the choroid plexus, and also supports the possibility of the participation of serotonin in CSF production.

The present experiments also revealed that intravenous injection of TBZ (50 mg/kg), which denervates monoaminergic neurons in the central nervous system, increased CSF production by approximately 14% from the pre-administration level. However, the fact that CA activity in the choroid plexus was found to fall to 22.4% of the control value following the administration of TBZ strongly suggests a reduction of CSF production in the choroid plexus by TBZ.

Lindvall et al. (1978) reported that the formation of CSF was increased when the cervical sympathetic nerve trunks were blocked and the blood concentration of noradrenaline declined. In the present studies, the increase in CSF production following TBZ administration was considered to reflect a continuous reduction of the blood concentration of serotonin. The mechanism whereby the CA activity in the choroid plexus was reduced by about three-quarters of the control value following TBZ administration remains to be clarified.

However, the data suggest that CA activity in the choroid plexus is markedly suppressed when the nervous control of the choroid plexus is disturbed by the administration of a monoamine denervator such as TBZ. The increase of CSF production after TBZ administration demonstrated in the present study is therefore thought to reflect some unclarified influence of the monoaminergic pathways on extrachoroidal CSF production mechanisms.

The fact that CA activity is inhibited by noradrenaline has been demonstrated previously by Lindvall et al. (1978) and Edvinsson et al. (1974). The present data show that serotonin also inhibits CA activity, but its inhibitory effect is weaker than that of acetazolamide. The mechanism of inhibition by serotonin is therefore thought to differ essentially from that of acetazolamide, but the detailed mode of action remains to be clarified in the future.

References

Ames A 3rd, Sakanoue M, Endo S (1964) Na, K, Ca, Mg and Cl concentrations in choroid plexus fluid and cisternal fluid compared with plasma ultrafiltrate. J Neurophysiol 27: 672–681

Ashby W (1944) On the quantitative incidence of carbonic anhydrase in the central nervous system. J Biol Chem 155: 671–679

Atkinson JR, Ward AA (1958) Effect of Diamox on intracranial pressure and blood volume. Neurology 8: 45–50

Benedikt M (1874) Über die Innervation des Plexus choroideus inferior. Arch Path Anat Physiol Klin Med 59: 395–400

Brightman ME (1968) The intracerebral movement of proteins injected into blood and cerebrospinal fluid of mice. Progr Brain Res 29: 19–37

Clark SL (1928) Nerve endings in the choroid plexus of the fourth ventricle. J Comp Neurol 47: 1–21

Davson H, Pollay M (1963) The turnover of ^{24}Na in the cerebrospinal fluid and its bearing on the blood brain barrier. J Physiol (Lond) 167: 245–255

Edvinsson L, Nielsen KC, Owman CH, West KA (1974) Adrenergic innervation of mammalian choroid plexus. Am J Anat 139: 299–308

Fisher RG, Copenhaver JH (1959) The metabolic activity of the choroid plexus. J Neurosurg 16: 167–176

Giacobini E (1961) Localization of carbonic anhydrase in the nervous system. Science 134: 1524–1525

Giacobini E (1962) A cytochemical study of the localization of carbonic anhydrase in the nervous system. J Neurochem 9: 169–177

Haywood JR, Vogh BS (1978) Some measurements of autonomic nervous system influence on production of cerebrospinal fluid in the cat. J Pharmacol Exp Ther 208: 341–346

Holladay LS, Cassin S (1972) Effect of acetazolamide and ouabain on CSF production rate in the newborn dog. Am J Physiol 22: 503–506

Johanson CE (1984) Differential effects of acetazolamide, benzolamide and systemic acidosis on hydrogen and bicarbonate gradients across the apical and basolateral membranes of the choroid plexus. J Pharmacol Exp Ther 231: 502–511

Knopp LK, Atkinson JR Ward AA (1957) Effect of Diamox on cerebrospinal fluid pressure of cat and monkey. Neurology 7: 119–123

Korhonen LK, Näätänen E, Hyyppä M (1964) A histochemical study of carbonic anhydrase in some parts of the mouse brain. Acta Histochem (Jena) 18: 336–347

Lindvall M, Edvinsson L, Owman CH (1978) Sympathetic nervous control of cerebrospinal fluid production from the choroid plexus. Science 201: 176–178

Lindvall M, Edvinsson L, Owman CH (1979) Effect of sympathomimetic drugs and corresponding receptor antagonists on the rate of cerebrospinal fluid production. Exp Neurol 64: 132–145

Lindvall M, Owman CH (1980) Evidence for the presence of two types of monoamine oxidase in rabbit choroid plexus and their role in breakdown of amines influencing cerebrospinal fluid formation. J Neurochem 34: 518–522

Maeda K (1983) Monoaminergic effect on cerebrospinal fluid production. Nihon Univ J Med 25: 155–117

Maren TH (1977) Use of inhibitors in physiological studies of carbonic anhydrase. Am J Physiol 232: F291–F297

Maren TH, Broder LE (1970) The role of carbonic anhydrase in anion secretion into cerebrospinal fluid. J Pharmacol Exp Ther 172: 197–202

Masuzawa T, Saito T, Sato F (1980) Cytochemical study of the electronmicroscopical localization of K^+-dependent p-nitrophenyl-phosphatase activity on choroidal ependymal epithelium in normal rat brain-comparing with the activity of Mg^+-ATPase and alkaline phosphatase. Acta Histochem Cytochem 13: 394–403

Milhorat TH, Davis DA, Hammock MK (1975) Localization of ouabain sensitive Na^+, K^+-ATPase in frog, rabbit and rat choroid plexus. Brain Res 99: 170–174

Nakamura S, Milhorat TH (1978) Nerve endings in the choroid plexus of the fourth ventricle of the rat: Electron microscopic study. Brain Res 153: 285–293

Nakamura S, Maeda K, Tsubokawa T (1983) Automatic and continuous measurement of CSF production. J Nihon Univ Med Assoc 42: 277–281

Pappenheimer JR, Heisey SR, Jordan EF, Downer J de C (1962) Perfusion of the cerebral ventricular system in unanesthetized goats. Am J Physiol 203: 763–774

Roussel G, Delaunoy JP, Nussbaum JL, Mandel P (1979) Demonstration of a specific localization of carbonic anhydrase C in the glial cells of rat CNS by an immunohistochemical method. Brain Res 160: 47–55

Schapiro B (1931) Über die Innervation des Plexus choroideus. Z Ges Neurol Psychiat 136: 530–546

Segal MB (1974) A combined physiological and morphological study of the secretory process in the rabbit choroid plexus. J Cell Sci 14: 339–350

Shimabukuro H, Masuzawa T, Sato F (1982) Enzyme histochemistry of ventricular choroid plexus (Part II): The localization of carbonic anhydrase activity. Neurol Med Chir (Tokyo) 22: 181–184

Smith RV, Roberts PA, Fisher RG (1974) Alteration of cerebrospinal fluid production in the dog. Surg Neurol 2: 267–270

Stöhr P (1922) Über die Innervation der Pia mater und des Plexus choroideus des Menschen. Arch Ges Anat (Abt 1) 63: 562–607

van Goor H (1940) Die Verbreitung und Bedeutung der Carboanhydrase. Enzymologia 8: 113–128

Yokota S (1969) Electron microscopic demonstration of carbonic anhydrase activity in mouse liver cells. Histochemie 19: 255–261

67 — Alterations of Atrial Natriuretic Peptide Receptors in the Choroid Plexus of Rats with Kaolin-Induced Hydrocephalus

Kazuo Mori, Keisuke Tsutsumi, Masaki Kurihara, Tsutomu Kawaguchi, Teruaki Kawano[1], and Masami Niwa[2]

Summary. Relatively little is known about the central regulation of cerebrospinal fluid (CSF) production. The present experiments show that atrial natriuretic peptide (ANP) administered intraventricularly inhibits the rate of CSF production. Separate experiments also show a dramatic increase in the number of specific ^{125}I-ANP binding sites in the choroid plexus of rats with kaolin-induced hydrocephalus and a significant decrease in these sites after continuous ventricular drainage of CSF for 7 days. These results may be explained by the up-regulation and compensation of ANP receptors which interrupts the production of CSF. New therapeutic approaches for hydrocephalus can be considered.

Keywords. Atrial natriuretic peptide — Hydrocephalus — Choroid plexus — CSF production

Introduction

Several lines of evidence have suggested that atrial natriuretic peptide (ANP) plays a significant role in the regulation of water and electrolyte fluxes across the blood-brain and blood-cerebrospinal fluid (CSF) barriers (Lynch et al. 1986; Steardo and Nathanson 1987). We recently found a dramatic increase in the number of specific ^{125}I-ANP binding sites in the choroid plexus of rats with kaolin-induced hydrocephalus as compared to the number of these sites in age-matched control Wistar rats (Mori et al. 1990; Tsutsumi et al. 1988). To further clarify the role of ANP in the regulation of CSF production, two series of experiments were performed in kaolin-induced hydrocephalic rats. In one series, the altered numbers of radiolabeled ANP receptor sites in the choroid plexus were continuously observed. In the other series, the effect of intraventricular ANP on CSF production was measured.

Departments of [1]Neurosurgery and [2]Pharmacology, Nagasaki University School of Medicine, Nagasaki, 852 Japan

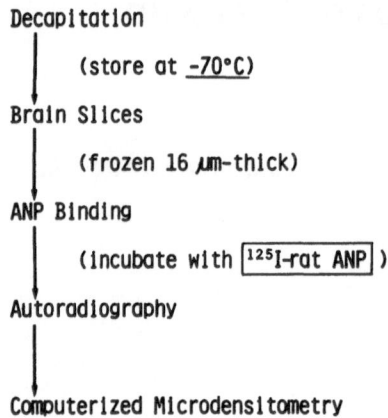

Fig. 1. Flow chart of in vitro quantitative autoradiography

Material and Methods

ANP Receptor Binding Assay

Male 7-day-old Wistar rat pups were used. One group was given 50 µg of kaolin (hydrated aluminum silicate) suspended in physiological saline in a volume of 100 µl, intracisternally. The other group of pups was given the same volume of physiological saline and was used as a control group. Three days or 3 weeks after the kaolin injection, animals were killed by decapitation. The brain was removed rapidly and immersed in isopentane at $-30°C$. Within 24 h, frozen 16-µm-thick sections were cut in a cryostat at $-20°C$, thaw-mounted onto gelatin-coated glass slides, and stored overnight under vacuum at $4°C$. The ANP binding sites were labeled by incubation with ^{125}I-rANP (spec. act., 1850 Ci/mmol, Amersham International, UK) by the method of Saavedra et al. (1986). Non-specific binding was determined in adjacent brain slices in the presence of excess unlabeled ANP (Fig. 1). Statistical differences between kaolin-induced hydrocephalic rats and rats in the control group were analyzed by using Student's t-test.

CSF Production Study

Three weeks after the kaolin injections, 10 µl of ^{3}H-inulin (MW: 5000 and about 40 000 cpm/µl) was stereotactically injected into the right lateral ventricle under pentobarbital anesthesia. In approximately half the rats, 100 pmol of ANP or 100 pmol of ouabain was incorporated in the labelled inulin. A dialysis probe (CMA/10: φ0.5 mm, 2 mm membrane, Carnegie Medicin, Stockholm, Sweden) was then inserted stereotactically into the left ventricle and the ventricle was perfused with Krebs-Ringer bicarbonate (KRB) buffer solution at a flow rate of 2 µl/min (Fig. 2).

After a 30-min equilibration period, dialysis perfusion with KRB buffer was continued and dialysates (intraventricular CSF) were collected every 30 min for 2 consecutive hours. Then, in order to estimate the extent of CSF production

Fig. 2. In vivo microdialysis system. LV, left ventricle

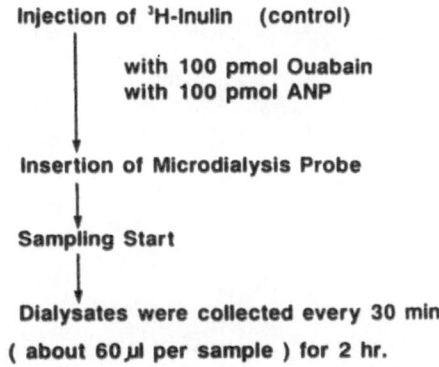

Injection of ³H-Inulin   (control)

with 100 pmol Ouabain
with 100 pmol ANP

Insertion of Microdialysis Probe

Sampling Start

Dialysates were collected every 30 min
(about 60 µl per sample) for 2 hr.

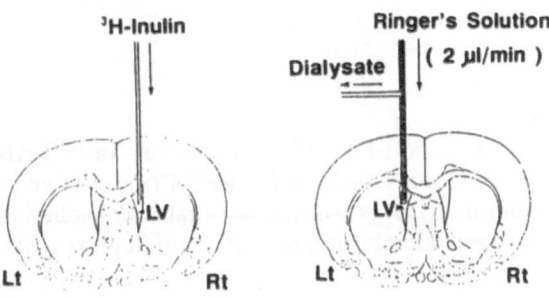

by observing the decline in radioactivity, the ³H content of each dialysate sample was determined using a scintillation counter.

Results

Binding Assay

In rats with kaolin-induced hydrocephalus, a clear dilatation of the lateral and third ventricles was observed. High numbers of ^{125}I-ANP binding sites were concentrated in the choroid plexus and subfornical organ, the distribution being similar to that observed in the controls (Fig. 3). However, Scatchard analysis indicated that maximum binding capacity (B_{max}) was increased significantly in rats with kaolin-induced hydrocephalus as compared to that in age-matched control rats. The increase in the B_{max} of rats 3 days after injection (at 10 days of age) was higher than in rats 3 weeks after injection (at 28 days of age). On the other hand, the binding affinity constant (Ka) showed no apparent difference between controls and hydrocephalic rats (Fig. 4). Also of special interest was the observation that in hydrocephalic rats, ventricular CSF drainage carried out for 7 days resulted in a significant decrease in the number of ANP receptors in the choroid plexus (Fig. 5).

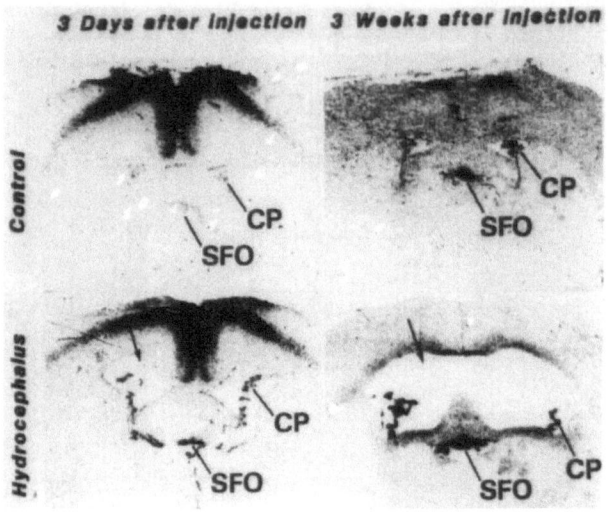

Fig. 3. Autoradiographic localization of ^{125}I-ANP binding sites in the rat choroid plexus, 3 days (*left*) and 3 weeks (*right*) after kaolin injection. *Upper panel*, from a control rat; *lower panel*, from a rat with kaolin-induced hydrocephalus. *Arrows* indicate enlarged lateral ventricle. CP, choroid plexus; SFO, subfornical organ

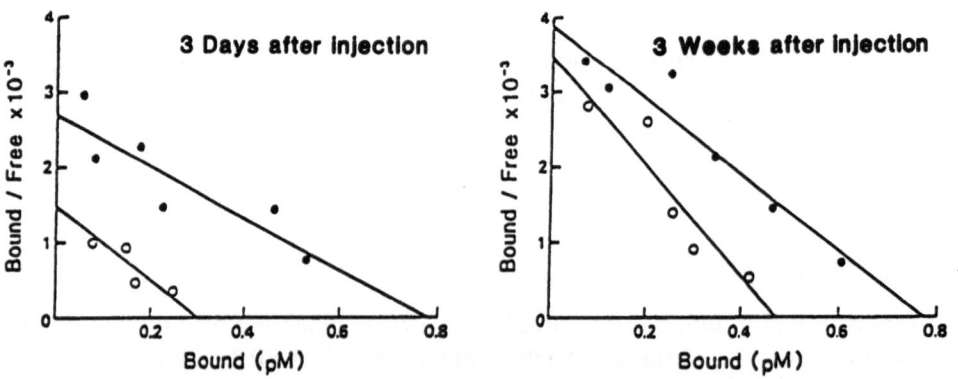

Fig. 4. Typical Scatchard plots of specific ^{125}I-ANP binding to the choroid plexus of a rat with hydrocephalus (*closed circles*) and a control rat (*open circles*). Correlation coefficients (*r*): 3 days after injection, 0.958 for controls and 0.890 for hydrocephalus; 3 weeks after injection, 0.948 for controls and 0.959 for hydrocephalus. (Data from Tsutsumi et al. [1988], with permission). ○, control; ●, hydrocephalus

Fig. 5. Changes in number of ^{125}I-ANP specific binding sites. Note that the binding sites decrease and return to control (baseline) levels after ventricular drainage of CSF

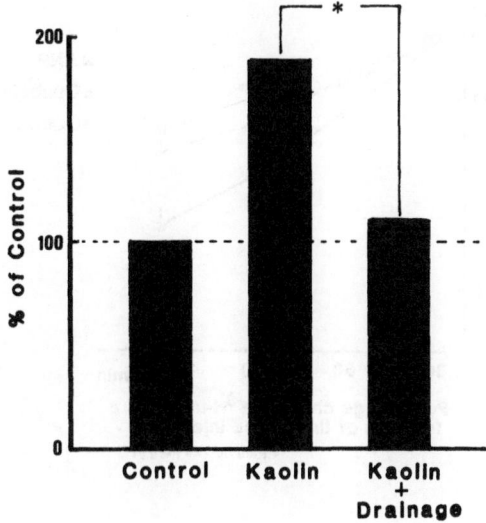

Fig. 6. Changes in radioactivity of ^{3}H-inulin in CSF collected through a dialysis probe located in the lateral ventricle

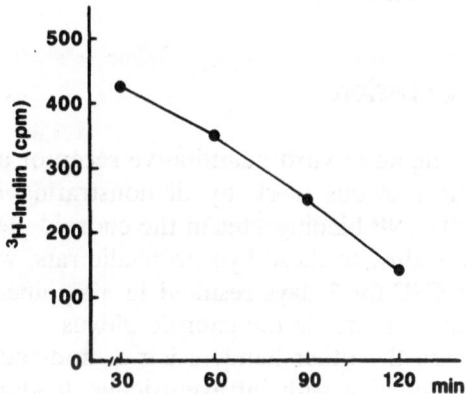

In Vivo Microdialysis Assay

Figure 6 shows one example. Radioactivity recovered in dialysate samples (CSF) declined almost linearly as time passed. This result indicates that the radioactivity of the dialysate presumably reflects the amount of inulin surrounding the dialysis tip in the ventricle; this technique opens up a new method for the quantitative study of CSF formation rates in animals which have ventricular systems of limited size, in which repeated perfusion (Pappenheimer et al. 1962) is technically difficult.

In Figure 7, the amount of radioactivity obtained from the first sample was used as a control and expressed as one hundred. The activities of consecutive samples were then expressed in terms of percentage of the control. Without intraventricular ANP, radioactivity dropped by 40% within a 2-h period. With 100 pmol of ANP, the decreased activity was prevented by a factor of 72%

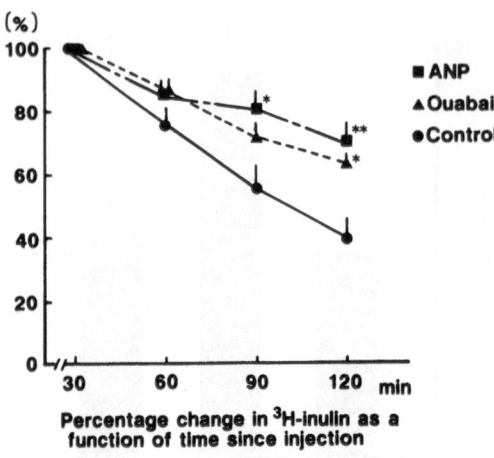

Fig. 7. Effects of intraventricular ANP and ouabain on CSF production rate, estimated from changes in radioactivity of ^{3}H-inulin

within the same period. The effect of 100 pmol of intraventricular ouabain was equivalent to the effect of ANP.

Discussion

Using an in vitro quantitative receptor autoradiographic method, we extended our previous work by demonstrating a significant increase in the B_{max} of ^{125}I-ANP binding sites in the choroid plexus of rats with kaolin-induced hydrocephalus. In these hydrocephalic rats, we also found that continuous drainage of CSF for 7 days resulted in a significant decrease in the number of specific receptor sites in the choroid plexus.

On the other hand, using a modified technique of in vivo microdialysis in conjunction with intraventricular loading of ^{3}H-inulin, we demonstrated that ANP injected into the lateral ventricle decreased the rate of CSF production to the same extent as ouabain.

Steardo and Nathanson (1987) also reported that ANP, when administered intraventricularly to rabbits, reduced the rate of CSF production in vivo. By observing changes in the optical density of blue dextran in a ventricular-cisternal perfusion model, they demonstrated that intraventricular ANP resulted in CSF production decreasing by 30%–40% from starting baseline levels. They also demonstrated elevation of the activity of membrane-bound guanylate cyclase in intraparenchymal cerebral microvessels and in epithelial cells isolated from the choroid plexus (Steardo and Nathanson 1987). We also reported evidence for a significant increase in cGMP, a biological marker for peptide action (Hamet et al. 1986), in freshly prepared rat choroid plexus, in the presence of ANP, in vitro (Tsutsumi et al. 1987).

Taken together, our present experiments lend support to the idea that ANP plays a significant role in the control of CSF production. In rats with kaolin-induced hydrocephalus, intraventricular ANP resulted in a marked reduction in the rate of CSF production. The dramatic increase in specific ANP receptor sites in the choroid plexus may result from an up-regulation and compensatory mechanism which interrupts the production of CSF.

ANP could have therapeutic application to disorders of water balance in the brain such as hydrocephalus, brain edema, and so on.

References

Hamet P, Trembly J, Pang SC, Skuherska R, Schiffrin EL, Garcia R, Cantin M, Genest J, Palmour R, Ervin FR, Martin S, Goldwater R (1986) Cyclic GMP as mediator and biological marker of atrial natriuretic factor. J Hypertens 4(Suppl.2): S49–S56

Lynch DR, Braas KM, Snyder SH (1986) Atrial natriuretic factors in rat kidney, adrenal gland, and brain: Autoradiographic localization and fluid balance dependent changes. Proc Natl Acad Sci USA 83: 3557–3561

Mori K, Tsutsumi K, Kurihara M, Kawaguchi T, Niwa M (1990) Alteration of atrial natriuretic peptide receptors in the choroid plexus of rats with induced or congenital hydrocephalus. Nerv Syst Child 6: 190–193

Pappenheimer JR, Heisey SR, Jordan EF, Downer J C (1962) Perfusion of the cerebral ventricular system in unanesthetized goats. Am J Physiol 203: 763–774

Saavedra JM, Correa FMA, Plunkett LM, Israel A, Kurihara M, Shigematsu K (1986) Binding of angiotensin and atrial natriuretic peptide in brain of hypertensive rats. Nature 320: 758–761

Steardo L, Nathanson JA (1987) Brain barrier tissues: End organs for atriopeptins. Science 235: 470–473

Tsutsumi K, Niwa M, Kawano T, Ibaragi M, Ozaki M, Mori K (1987) Atrial natriuretic peptides elevate the level of cyclic GMP in the rat choroid plexus. Neurosci Lett 79: 174–178

Tsutsumi K, Niwa M, Himeno A, Kurihara M, Kawano T, Ibaragi M, Ozaki M, Mori K (1988) Atrial natriuretic peptide binding sites in the rat choroid plexus are increased in the presence of hydrocephalus. Neurosci Lett 87: 93–98

68 — Effects of Atrial Natriuretic Peptide on Intraventricular Pressure in Rats with Congenital Hydrocephalus

Masatsune Ishikawa, Haruhiko Kikuchi, Kenji Hashimoto, Jun Minamikawa, Kunio Yamamura, and Kameyoshi Mitsuno[1]

Summary. Using congenitally developed hydrocephalic rats, the functional effect of intraventricularly administered atrial natriuretic peptide (ANP) on intraventricular pressure and brain water and sodium content was investigated. Physiological saline and 0.2 µg of ANP did not induce any change in these three parameters. In contrast, 2 µg of intraventricular ANP induced a significant decrease of intraventricular pressure. Brain water and sodium content were also decreased, but not to a statistically significant extent.

The present study thus revealed a beneficial effect of central ANP on lowering intraventricular pressure. This effect might be due to an inhibitory effect on CSF production in the choroid plexus; however, the precise mechanism is not known.

Keywords. Hydrocephalus — ANP — CSF production — Water — Sodium

ANP in Congenital Hydrocephalus

Atrial natriuretic peptide (ANP), a potent natriuretic diuretic and vasorelaxant hormone, is released from mammalian heart atria (de Bold 1979). This peptide has been implicated in the regulation of systemic water and electrolyte balances and blood pressure. Recent studies have revealed the existence of ANP-containing neurons (Morii et al. 1985; Skofitsch et al.) and receptors (Roques and Beaument 1990; Tsutsumi et al. 1987) in the brain. Since ANP does not pass the blood-brain barrier (Marumo et al. 1988), and regulation of the ANP level in the brain differs from that in the heart (Morii et al. 1985), the existence of a separate central ANP system which may regulate ion and volume homeostasis in the central nervous system is hypothesized. To investigate its regulatory effect on brain water and cerebrospinal fluid (CSF), we measured intraventricular pressure and brain sodium and water content in congenitally developed hydrocephalic rats after intraventricular administration of ANP.

---

[1] Department of Neurosurgery, Faculty of Medicine, Kyoto University, 606 Japan

Materials and Methods

In this study, 40 HTX strain rats, 14, 21, and 28 days old (body weight, 30–100 g), were used. It has been reported that congenital hydrocephalus developed in half of a litter of newborn HTX rats (Wada 1988). The survival period of hydrocephalic rats was 4–5 weeks. Congenitally developed hydrocephalus was easily diagnosed by the 3rd week after birth, as disproportional bulging of the skull (hydrocephalic group), in contrast to rats with non-bulging skulls (non-hydrocephalic group). Hydrocephalic rats were placed on a stereotaxic frame and the intracranial pressure was measured with pressure transducer via a 26-gauge fine needle which was inserted directly into the left ventricle through the thin skull. CSF leakage around the canula was sealed by adhesive. This procedure allowed for precise continuous measurement of CSF pressure. Another needle of the same size was implanted in the right lateral ventricle for intraventricular drug administration. Alpha-human ANP (0.2 or 2 µg) was dissolved in 10 µl physiological saline and injected as a single dose. Physiological saline of the same volume was used as a control. In most of our studies, CSF pressure monitoring was carried out for 40 min; in some of the studies, however, freely moving animals were monitored with a telemetric system (PhysioTel, DS Inc. Minn, USA) for 120 min.

The rats were decapitated and the whole brain was sampled for the measurement of water and sodium content. Brain water content was measured by a dry-weight method and sodium content was measured with an atomic absorption spectrophotometer (AA-670 Shimazu Corp., Kyoto, Japan).

Results

Intraventricular Pressure (IVP) (Fig. 1)

IVP before drug administration was 5.63 ± 0.54 ($n = 4$), 5.27 ± 0.36 ($n = 24$), and 7.36 ± 0.73 ($n = 8$) mmHg in 14-, 21-, and 28-day-old rats, respectively. Intraventricular administration of 10 µl of physiological saline and 0.2 µg of alpha-hANP dissolved in the same solution did not yield any change in IVP during the study period of 40 min.

Intraventricular administration of 2 µg of alpha-hAND, in contrast, gradually decreased IVP. IVP began to decrease at 20 min and the decrease became statistically significant ($P < 0.01$) at 30 min. In the 21-day-old HTX rats ($n = 10$), IVP changed from 5.25 ± 0.60 (mean $\pm$ SEM) mmHg at the start to 3.00 ± 0.35 mmHg at 40 min and in the 28-day-old HTX rats ($n = 5$), IVP changed from 7.38 ± 1.13 mmHg to 5.20 ± 1.32 mmHg.

Brain Water and Sodium Content (Figs. 2. and 3)

At 40 min after ANP administration, brain water and sodium content changed from $83.47\% \pm 0.15\%$ and 305.5 ± 9.1 mmol/kg dry weight to $83.09\% \pm$

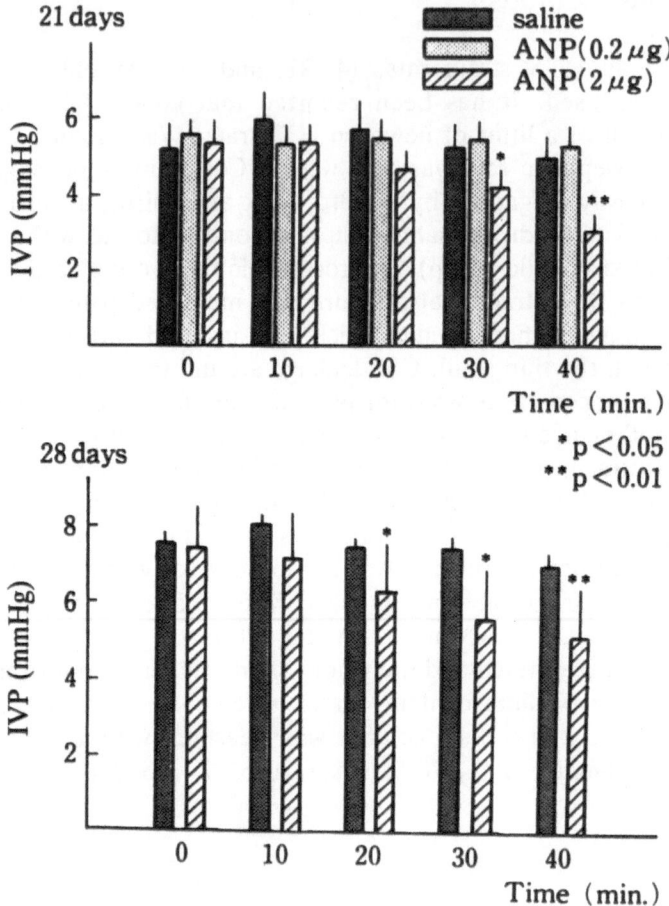

Fig. 1. Intraventricular pressure (*IVP*) in hydrocephalic rats. Note statistically significant decrease of IVP after an intraventricular administration of ANP in both 21-day-old (*upper*) and 28-day-old (*lower*) rats

0.15% and 291.2 ± 6.5 mmol/kg dry weight, respectively, in the 21-day-old HTX rats and from 81.74% ± 0.24% and 288.0 ± 14.6 mmol/kg dry weight to 81.14% ± 0.18% and 267.3 ± 9.9 mmol/kg dry weight, respectively, in the 28-day-old HTX rats. However, these changes were not statistically significant.

Duration of Lowered IVP (Fig. 4)

In a separate study carried out with conscious and freely-moving rats, 6 μg of intraventricular ANP administered as a single dose induced a decrease of IVP for up to 100 min after drug administration. In this study, 2 μg of ANP did not induce any changes in IVP.

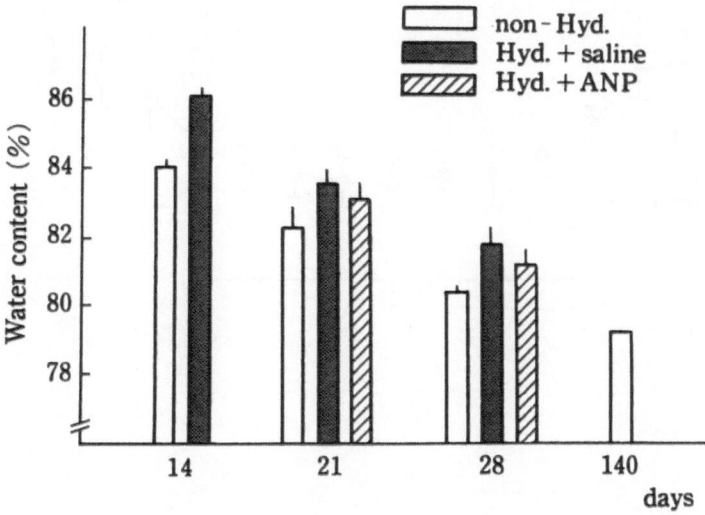

Fig. 2. Brain water content in hydrocephalic (*Hyd.*) and non-hydrocephalic (*non-hyd.*) rats. Brain water content gradually decreased as rats grew. Intraventricular ANP induced a slight, but not statistically significant decrease of brain water content

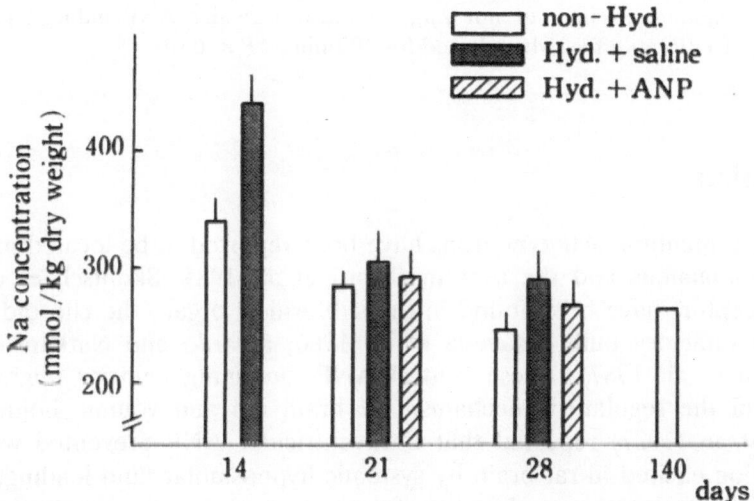

Fig. 3. Brain sodium content in hydrocephalic (*Hyd.*) and non-hydrocephalic (non-hyd.) rats. Intraventricular administration of ANP induced only a minimal decrease of sodium content in the brain

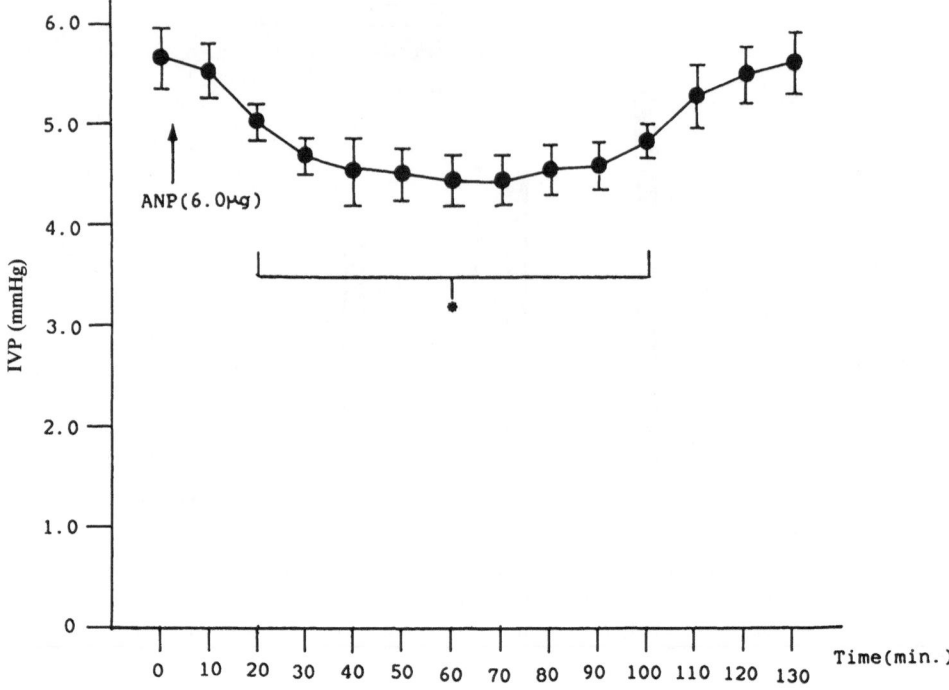

Fig. 4. Duration of lowered IVP in a freely moving rat; pressure was monitored with a telemetric system. Six μg, but not 2 μg, of intraventricular ANP induced prolonged lowering of IVP, an effect which lasted for 100 min . *$P < 0.01$

Discussion

ANP-like immunoreactive neurons have been reported to be located mainly in the hypothalamus and the septum (Morii et al. 1985; Skofitsch et al.) and their receptors have been found in the subfornical organ, the choroid plexus, and the olfactory bulb (Saaveda et al. 1986; Steardo and Nathanson 1989; Tsutsumi et al. 1987). These central ANP-containing neurons might be involved in the regulatory mechanism of brain ion and volume homeostasis. Doczi et al. (1987) reported that intraventricular ANP prevented water accumulation elicited in rat brain by systemic hypoosmolar fluid loading. Nakao et al. (1990) demonstrated a beneficial effect of intraventricular ANP on ischemic brain edema in rats. They suggested that this antiedematous effect of central ANP might be related to direct action on brain microvessels.

The distribution of ANP receptors is known to be rich in the choroid plexus (Saaveda et al. 1986; Tsutsumi et al. 1987). Further, Steardo and Nathanson (1987) demonstrated an inhibitory effect of intraventricular ANP on CSF production. In the present study, intraventricular ANP induced a significant decrease of intraventricular pressure; brain water and sodium content also decreased, but not to a statistically significant extent. This effecte of ANP on lowering IVP may be due to ANP having an inhibitory effect on CSF production, although the antiedematous effect of ANP should not be excluded.

Intraventricular ANP administered as a single injection had a prolonged effect on decreasing CSF pressure, in contrast to its rapid deactivation in plasma. In our separate study, this effect lasted for 100 min. Although a period of this magnitude is not sufficient in clinical practice, inhibitors of ANP inactivating enzyme may prolong the lowering effect on CSF pressure (Roques and Beaumont 1990).

Thus, intraventricular ANP administration has potential as a therapeutic adjunct for hydrocephalus. Further study is necessary to elucidate the functional role of the central ANP system so that this knowledge may lead to advancements in the treatment of hydrocephalus.

References

de Bold AJ (1979) Heart atria granularity effects of changes in water-electrolyte balance. Proc Soc Exp Biol Med 161: 508–511

Doczi T, Joo F, Szerdahelyi P, Bodosi M (1987) Regulation of brain water and electrolyte contents: The possible involvement of central atrial natriuretic factor. Neurosurgery 21: 454–458

Marumo F, Masuda T, Masaki Y, Ando K (1988) The presence of atrial natriuretic peptide in canine cerebrospinal fluid and its possible origin in the brain. J Endocrinol 119: 127–131

Morii N, Nakao K, Sugawara A, Sakamoto M, Suda M, Shimokura M, Kiso Y, Kihara M, Yamori Y, Imura H (1985) Occurrence of atrial natriuretic polypeptide in brain. Biochem Biophys Res Commun 127: 413–419

Nakao N, Itakura T, Yokote H, Nakai K, Komai N (1990) Effect of atrial natriuretic peptide on ischemic brain edema; changes in brain water and electrolytes. Neurosurgery 27: 39–44

Roques BP, Beaumont A (1990) Neutral endopeptidase-24.11 inhibitors: From analgesics to antihypertensives? TIPS 11: 245-249

Saaveda JM, Israel A, Kurihara M, Fuchs E (1986) Decreased number and affinity of rat atrial natriuretic peptide (6–33) binding sites in the subfornical organ of spontaneously hypertensive rats. Circ Res 58: 389–392

Skofitsch G, Jacobowitz DM, Eskay RL, Zamir N Distribution of atrial natriuretic factor-like immunoreactive neurons in the rat brain. Neuroscience 16: 917–948

Steardo L, Nathanson JA (1987) Brain barrier tissues: Endorgans for atriopeptins. Science 235: 470–473

Tsutsumi K, Niwa M, Kawano T, Ibaragi M, Ozaki M, Mori K (1987) Atrial natriuretic polypeptides elevate the level of cyclic GMP in the rat choroid plexus. Neurosci Lett 79: 174–178

Wada M (1988) Congenital hydrocephalus in HTX rats: Incidence, pathophysiology, and developmental impairment. Neurol Med Chir (Tokyo) 28: 955–964

69 — "Neuroendoscopic Third Ventriculostomy"

Charles Teo, Robert F.C. Jones,[1] Warwick A. Stening, and Bernard C.T. Kwok[2]

Summary. We have operated on 47 patients, achieving significant improvement or total shunt independence in 80% with only one major complication. We have not restricted the procedure only to those with late onset aqueduct stenosis, but rather have included 29 patients with both early and late onset aqueduct stenosis, 8 patients with associated myelomeningocoele, 7 patients with neoplastic secondary aqueduct stenosis and 3 patients with previous central nervous system (CNS) infection or hemorrhage. We believe that a procedure which carries an appreciable failure rate is acceptable if the only alternative to improve patient selection is an invasive and time-consuming investigation such as a cerebrospinal fluid (CSF) infusion study. Such a study may or may not identify those patients in whom CSF absorptive capacity is inadequate. Furthermore, this study illustrates two important principles that may improve the overall outcome of third ventriculostomy. Firstly, comprehensive preoperative structural studies will help to eliminate some of those patients anatomically unsuitable for this procedure. Secondly, an adequate period should be allowed to pass before declaring the operation unsuccessful, as head growth did not show an improved trend for several weeks in two patients. We believe that in these patients, the CSF absorptive capacity improved over that time.

Keywords. Endoscopy — Third ventriculostomy — Non-communicating hydrocephalus

Introduction

Although extracranial shunts are the mainstay of neurosurgical management for non-communicating hydrocephalus, they have a well recognized complica-

[1] Deparment of Neurosurgery, Prince of Wales Children's Hospital, Sydney, Australia
[2] Department of Neurosurgery, Institute of Neurological Sciences, Prince Henry Hospital, Sydney, Australia.

tion rate that includes blockage, overdrainage, and infection. (Griebel et al. 1985; Sayers 1976; Walters et al. 1984)

The procedure of intracranial CSF diversion by third ventriculostomy was first introduced by Dandy in 1922. Since then several techniques have been proposed. (Avman and Kanpolat 1979; Brocklehurst 1974; Dandy 1945; Griffith 1975; Hirsch 1982; Hoffman et al. 1980; Kelly et al. 1986; Mixter 1923; Perlman 1968; Stookey and Scarff 1936; Torkildsen 1960; Vries 1978; Ziedses des Plantes and Crezee 1978). In 1923, Mixter performed an endoscopically guided ventriculostomy which was popularized again in 1978 by Vries. Recently, Jack and Kelly (1989) published a series of stereotactically guided third ventriculostomies with excellent results after strict patient selection. However, in general, intracranial CSF diversion has been associated with modest success. For a procedure to be a viable alternative to extracranial shunting it should be as simple to perform and carry a low morbidity rate.

Recently, we published a series of endoscopically guided third ventriculostomies in 20 patients (Jones et al. 1990) with a 71% success or improved status. There were 4 patients out of 20 in whom endoscopy was performed but fenestration not attempted. Subsequently, only 1 further patient in a series of 28 did not have fenestration. The overall success/improved rate is now 81%. With these results and low morbidity, the procedure is now performed routinely in our unit.

Method

General Profile

At the Prince of Wales Children's Hospital and Prince Henry Hospital we have now performed 47 ventriculostomies on 52 patients who underwent neuro-endoscopy between 1979 and 1990. There were 28 males and 24 females, ranging from 2 weeks premature to 78 years of age. Forty four patients were under 16 years of age and 8 patients were over 16 years. Patients have been followed from 3 months to 11 years with an average follow up of 31 months.

Patients were classified into four major groups (Table 1): (1) Aqueduct stenosis, (2) tumor, (3) myelomeningocele, and (4) infection and hemorrhage. These major groups were further subdivided into those patients who had had previous shunt procedures or those who had never been shunted. There were 29 patients in the first group, of which 22 had primary aqueduct stenosis. Those patients with secondary aqueduct stenosis from tumors were placed in a separate category. There were seven patients in this group, six that were endoscoped pre-radiotherapy and one that was endoscoped post-radiotherapy.

The third category consisted of those patients with associated myelomeningocoele, of whom there were eight. Finally, the fourth category included those patients with previous CSF infection or intraventricular hemorrhage. There were three patients in this group.

Table 1. Patient classification

	Shunted	*Never shunted*	*Total*
Aqueduct stenosis			
Primary			
Early onset	4	6	
Late onset	4	8	
Secondary			
Congenital	0	1	
Acquired	3	3	29
Tumor			
Pre-radiotherapy	5	1	
Post-radiotherapy	1	0	7
Myelomeningocele	5	3	8
Infection/hemorrhage	1	2	3

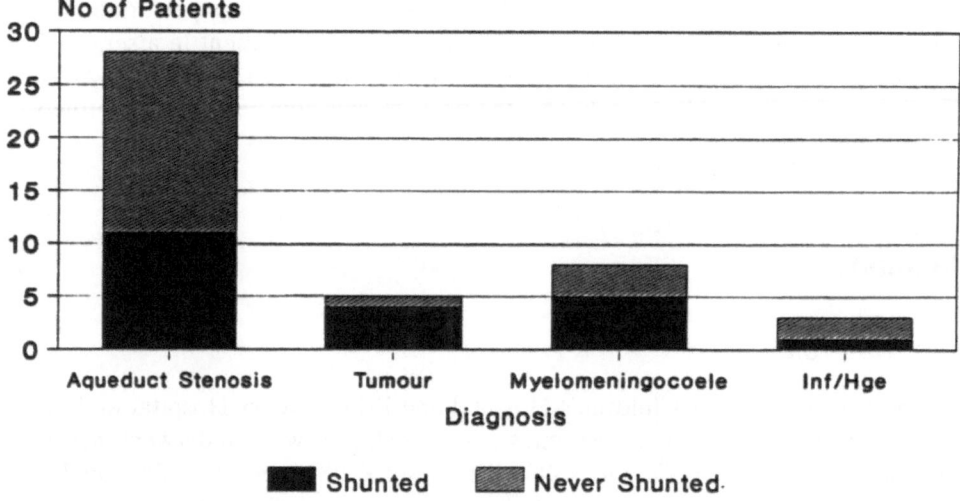

Fig. 1. Categories: Shunted vs never shunted. Most patients were in the Aqueduct Stenosis category. Inf/hge, infection/hemorrhage

Figure 1 demonstrates that most patients were in the aqueduct stenosis group and that in fact the number of shunted to unshunted patients was approximately 1 to 1.

Selection/Exclusion Criteria

Five patients underwent endoscopic examination of their third ventricles and were found to be unsuitable for ventriculostomy, three on the basis of a thickened, non-attenuated floor and one on the basis of a large massa intermedia. The fifth patient sustained prolonged episodes of bradycardia with any degree of pressure on the floor. The case of bradycardia was unpredictable, but morbidity may be reduced by eliminating those anatomically unsuitable patients with pre-operative magnetic resonance imaging (MRI) and ultrasound imaging. The patient that sustained a hemiparesis had confusing anatomical landmarks that caused bleeding to obscure the field.

Patients with apparent noncommunicating hydrocephalus on computerized tomography (CT) scan or on CT ventriculography, depending on the surgeon involved, were subjected to third ventriculostomy. If the width of the third ventricle was less than 7 mm we rejected the child for endoscopy, as one needs a larger ventricle than this to maneuver the rigid scope. If structural studies demonstrated anomalous anatomy such as a large massa intermedia, these patients were also rejected.

Technique

Although described in our previous publication, several surgical aspects need to be emphasized. The scope is passed into the lateral ventricle via a right frontal burr hole. This is made approximately 2–3 cms from the midline and immediately anterior to the coronal suture. In infants the burr hole should be made approximately 1cm anterior to the coronal suture and 2 cm from the midline. This entry point offers the best trajectory through the foramen of Monro into the interpeduncular cistern. Once in the lateral ventricle the foramen can usually be identified by choroid plexus, the septal and thalamostriate veins. Sometimes no choroid plexus is found and veins can be anomalous, in which case one must follow the contour of the ventricle to find the foramen. The optimal point for fenestration is immediately posterior to the clivus, thereby keeping well anterior to the basilar artery, its bifurcation and posteriorly directed perforators. Electrocardiographic monitoring is mandatory during the procedure as any pressure on the ventricle floor may cause episodes of bradycardia. The rigid scope is then pushed through the attenuated floor into the interpeduncular cistern. To ensure patency of the ventriculostomy, the scope may need to be passed through the fenestration several times, although once is usually enough. Pulsatile flow of CSF can be inferred by the flapping of the margins of the fenestration.

Assessment of Outcome

Patients were assessed by a minimum of two of the following three methods:

Clinical

This included the patient's symptomatology and head circumference which was plotted preoperatively and postoperatively (Fig. 2).

Structural Imaging

This included ultrasound, CT scan, and MRI. MRI also had the advantage of demonstrating a flow void through the fenestration in some cases (see Fig. 3)

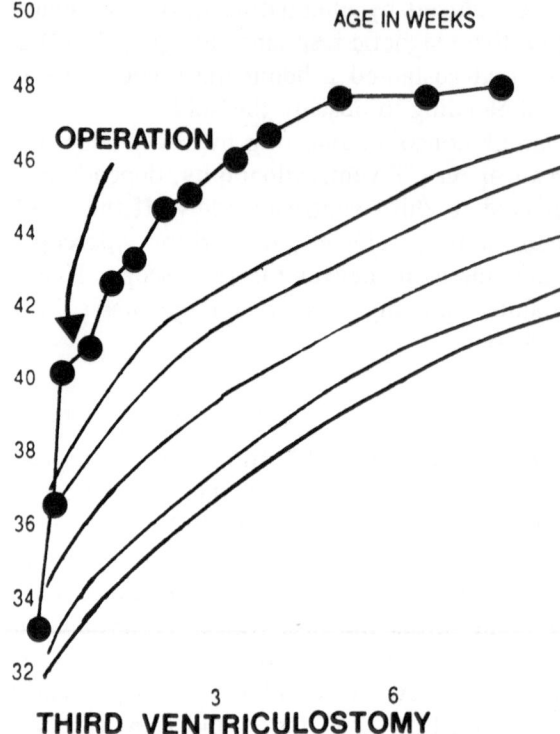

Fig. 2. Head circumference chart showing slowing of progression of hydrocephalus after third ventriculostomy. Evan's Index remained stationary but the rate of head-circumference did not stabilise for 6 months

Intracranial Pressure (ICP) Monitoring

This included 24-h monitoring via a ventricular catheter reservoir or fontanelle tension in those children with subtemporal decompression or open fontanelles.
  Patients were then graded into the following categories:

Successful

These patients had clinical evidence of normal ICP and structural evidence of improved cortical mantle (Fig. 4). If previously shunted, the shunt had to be either removed or proven to be non-functional.

Improved

Patients fell into this category if there was significant immediate reversal of their intracranial hypertensive symptoms, slowing of head growth, or an apparently "successful" outcome that was short-lived and eventually needed extracranial diversion.

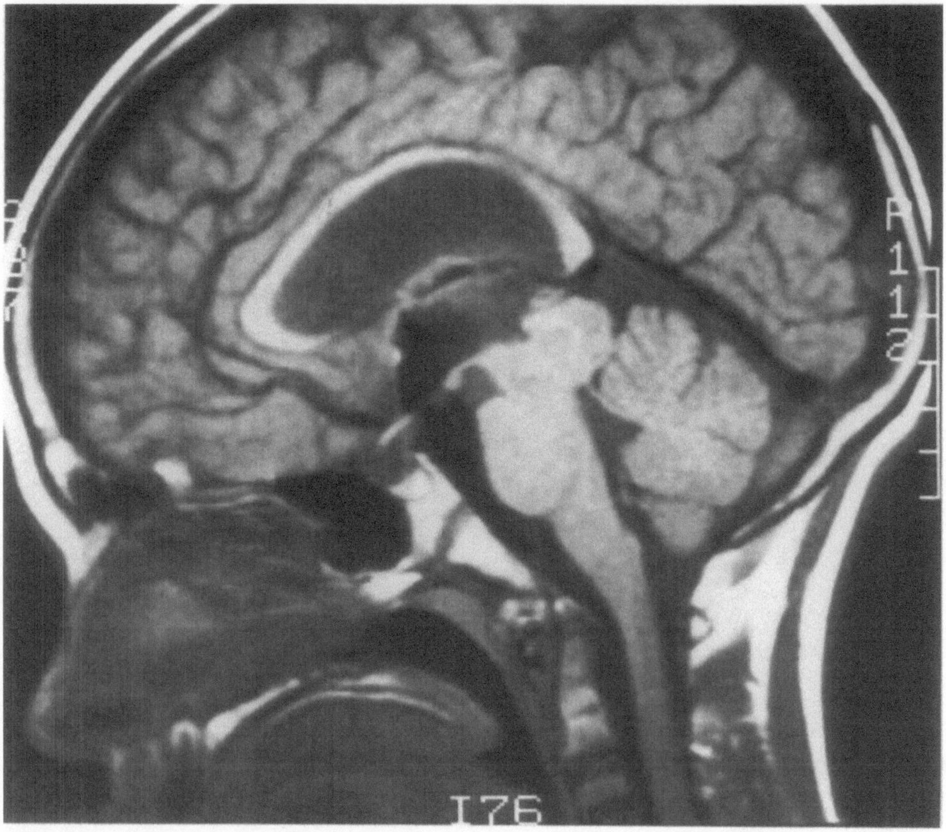

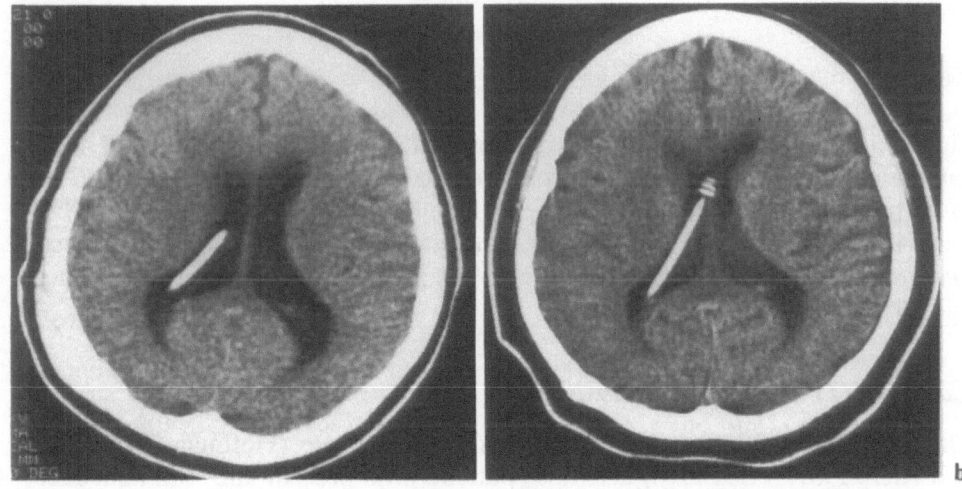

Fig. 3. Post-third ventriculostomy MRI demonstrating flow void through the floor of the third ventricle

Fig. 4. Plain CT scans of a patient **a** before and **b** after third ventriculostomy

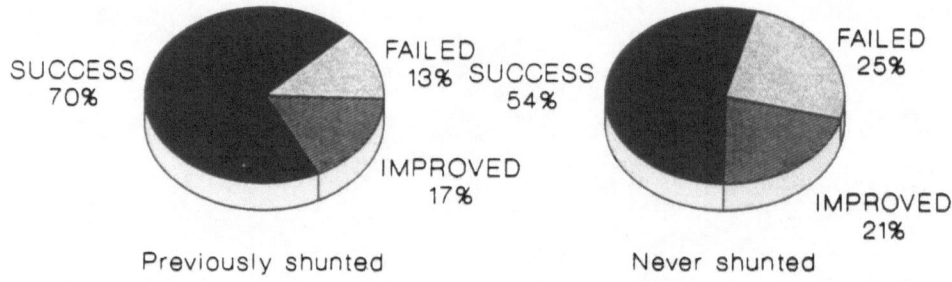

Fig. 5. Results of previously shunted patients (*n* = 23) vs never shunted patients (*n* = 24)

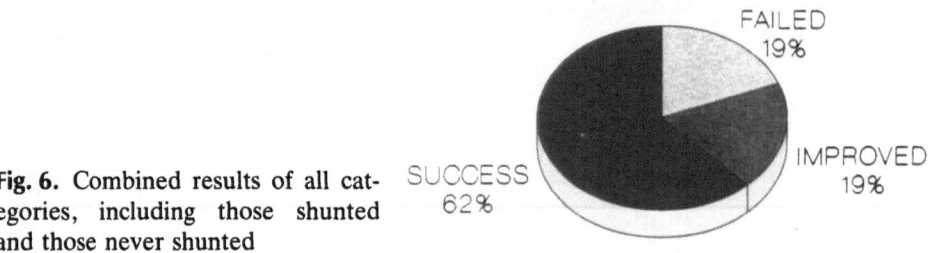

Fig. 6. Combined results of all categories, including those shunted and those never shunted

Failed

These patients had no change in their clinical progress or structural studies or they needed a shunt within 6 months of the procedure.

Results

Figure 5 demonstrates the success, improved, and failure rates in all four categories. When the figures are broken down to separate the success rates in those previously shunted and those never shunted, we see success rates of 70% and 54%, respectively (Fig. 5). There is no statistical difference between these two groups. The overall success rate was 62%, with 19% of patients improving and 19% failing (Fig. 6).

Category (1) Aqueduct Stenosis

The most successful group of patients, as in other series (Hoffman 1976; Jack and Kelly 1989; Vries 1978) are those patients who present late with aqueduct stenosis (Fig. 7) In our series, out of ten patients who fell into this category, there were seven successes and three improved, with no failures. Of the other 19 patients in this group there were 12 with early onset primary aqueduct stenosis, of whom 8 had successful outcomes, 2 improved, and 2 failed. Seven

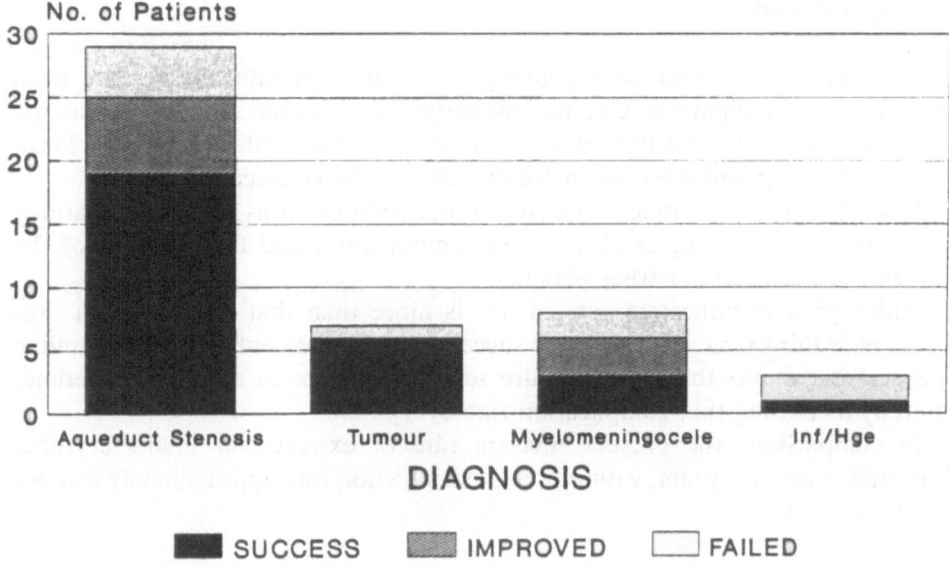

Fig. 7. Results of ventriculostomy in each category. Inf/hge, infection/hemorrhage

patients had secondary aqueduct stenosis, with four successes, one improved, and two failed. Two of these patients had acquired aqueduct stenosis secondary to long-term shunting for communicating hydrocephalus. (Foltz and Shurtleff 1966)

Category (2) Associated Myelomeningocele

The results were not so pleasing in this group, with three successes, three improved, and two failed. However, two of the previously shunted patients in this group who underwent third ventriculostomy, although not completely shunt independent, have experienced remarkable improvements in the number of shunt revisions required since operation. (see Discussion).

Category (3) Tumors

There were six successes and one failed. The child that failed had previously been given radiotherapy.

Category (4) Intraventricular Hemorrhage/Infection

The patient that had a successful outcome had been previously shunted for neonatal meningitis. When the shunt blocked, a ventriculostomy was performed and the shunt was subsequently removed. Two patients failed.

Complications

There were four complications, giving a complication rate of 8%. The most serious was a hemiparesis. One patient sustained a chronic subdural hematoma after the procedure and two patients had postoperative infection — one localized to the scalp and the other a *Staph. epidermidis* ventriculitis.

It would appear to some extent that these complications reflect the learning curve of each surgeon, as all but one complication, and this was one of the infections, occurred in earlier patients.

Although a complication rate of 8% is more than that seen in shunt procedures, a third ventriculostomy, if successful, is a once only operation, unlike extracranial shunts that often require several revisions in a patient's lifetime, thereby increasing that complication rate every time.

In comparison, the present revision rate of extracranial shunts at these hospitals is every 6 years, with our current infection rate approximately 3% per shunt revision.

Discussion

Unfortunately, 38% of our patients are still shunt dependent. There are several reasons for patients to have a communicating as well as a non-communicating hydrocephalus (NCH). Some of these will have pre-existing hypoplastic villi or, as some people believe, can develop hypoplastic villi from long-term CSF diversion (Milhorat 1972). Also, long standing NCH may cause poor absorption at the arachnoid granulation level from chronic ventricular dilatation and obliteration of the sub-arachnoid space. (Milhorat 1972). Identification of those patients with both communicating and NCH is extremely difficult. CSF infusion studies provide the best means of assessing the absorptive capacity of the arachnoid villi but require invasive and time consuming surgical techniques that are not without risks. Even then, the results can be misleading, as very often a particular infusion pressure over a short period may fail to re-establish CSF absorptive pathways that might otherwise have been re-established with a similar pressure over a longer period (see below). If one restricts the procedure to only those patients who have late onset aqueduct stenosis, as in Kelly's series (Jack and Kelly 1989), one will improve one's figures but one is denying many patients the chance to have a shunt independent life.

Furthermore, there are several patients in the *improved* category that typify the benefit of ventriculostomy, even if the patient is not totally shunt independent. Two patients who were requiring multiple shunt revisions in rapid succession have now been trouble free for several years since their ventriculostomy. We have one female patient who would present unconscious by the time she arrived in the emergency room whenever her shunt blocked. She now simply complains of headache when her shunt blocks. There are several infants whose ventriculostomies bought time for them to either gain weight or recover from other operations. It was the benefits gained by this particular group of patients that provoked Sayers, Kosnik, and Natelson to advocate third ventriculostomy for all patients with myelomeningocele and aqueduct stenosis (Sayers and Kosnik, 1976; Natelson 1981).

There are three important points that have arisen from our series of 47 procedures. Case (16) (Fig. 2) demonstrates an extremely important observation. Often the CSF resorption apparatus needs time to accommodate the increased amounts of CSF presented to it once the pathways have been re-established. To concede failure before allowing for this period may unjustly place some patients into the failed category who may otherwise have been considered successful given more time. Conversely, we consede that two of our patients who were placed in the successful category for our previous publication have since required extracranial shunting. The second point is that morbidity can be significantly reduced by comprehensive preoperative work-up. We acknowledge that triventricular hydrocephalus and a normal fourth ventricle is not necessarily a pure non-communicating hydrocephalus (Aoki and Mizutami 1985) and that in fact ventriculography can show rapid flow of contrast through the aqueduct. Also, CT and ultrasound have failings in demonstrating abnormal third ventricular anatomy where MRI may be extremely helpful. What is important, therefore, is to use as many investigative procedures as is necessary to help eliminate some of those patients who will either not tolerate neuroendoscopy or who will not benefit from third ventriculostomy. Thirdly, some authors have demonstrated the value of shunting prior to third ventriculostomy (Sayers 1976; Hoffman 1976). Their theory was that prior shunting allowed the subarachnoid space to re-open.

All our patients who were previously shunted and had successful third ventriculostomies were stabilized for many years with extracranial shunts incorporating an antisiphon device. Their success may have been related to the prevention of overdrainage by the antisiphon device and to maintenance of a normal to high CSF driving pressure, as well as to the principle that time may sometimes reestablish absorptive pathways, as is seen in that group of patients with communicating hydrocephalus who spontaneously "stabilize".

Although the differences results between the shunted and never shunted groups are statistically insignificant, they may be showing a trend that would support this theory.

In conclusion, we would like to propose the following criteria for patient selection:

1. Ventriculographic evidence of noncommunication if plain CT or MRI are equivocal.
2. A third ventricular width greater than 7 mm.
3. No structural anomalies that may hinder the procedure.
4. No previous radiotherapy.

Neuroendoscopic third ventriculostomy is a safe and effective means of definitively treating NCH, resulting in significant improvement or total shunt independence in approximately 80% of patients and carrying an 8% complication rate. Unlike stereotactic ventriculostomy (Kelly et al. 1986) it can be performed in infants with thin skulls, unlike the Stookey-Scarff technique (Stookey and Scarff, 1936) it does not require a craniotomy, and unlike the Hoffman's radiologically guided procedure (Hoffman 1976; Hoffman et al. 1980) it permits visualization of the basilar artery before perforation in many cases.

If the patient still requires a shunt, malfunction causes a less life-threatening deterioration. If successful, the patient may enjoy a shunt free life.

Acknowledgements. We wish to thank Cristina Kew for her accuracy and patience in typing the manuscript and the Department of Medical Illustrations, University of New South Wales, for the illustrations.

References

Aoki N, Mizutami H (1985) Communicating triventricular hydrocephalus and its treatment with a lumboperitoneal shunt. Neurosurgery 16: 557–561

Avman N, Kanpolat Y (1979) Third ventriculostomy by microtechnique. Acta Neurochir [Suppl] (Wein) 28: 588–595

Brocklehurst (1974) Trans-callosal third ventriculo-chiasmatic cisternostomy: A new approach to hydrocephalus. Surg Neurol 2: 109–114

Dandy WE (1922) An operative procedure for hydrocephalus. Bull Johns Hopkins Hosp 33: 189–190

Dandy WE (1945) Diagnosis and treatment of strictures of the aqueduct of Sylvius (causing hydrocephalus). Arch Surg 51: 1–14

Foltz EL, Shurtleff DB (1966) Conversion of communicating hydrocephalus to stenosis or occlusion of the aqueduct during ventricular shunt. J. Neurosurg 24: 520–529

Griebel R, Khan M, Tan L (1985) CSF shunt complications: An analysis of contributory factors. CNS 1: 77–80

Griffith HB (1975) Technique of fontanelle and persutural ventriculoscopy and endoscopic ventricular surgery in infants. Childs Brain 1: 359–363

Hirsch JF (1982) Percutaneous ventriculocisternostomies in noncommunicating hydrocephalus. Monogr Neural Sci 8: 170–178

Hoffman HJ (1976) The advantages of percutaneous third ventriculostomy over other forms of surgical treatment for infantile obstructive hydrocephalus. In: Morley TP (ed) Current controversies in neurosurgery. WB Saunders, Philadelphia, pp 691–703

Hoffman HJ, Hardwood-Nash D, Gilday, DL (1980) Percutaneous third ventriculoscopy in the management of non-communicating hydrocephalus. Neurosurgery 7: 313–321

Jack CR Jr, Kelly PJ (1989) Stereotactic third ventriculostomy: Assessment of patency with MR imagery. AJNR 10(3): 515–522

Jones RFC, Stening WAS, Bryden M (1990) Endoscopic third ventriculostomy. Neurosurgery 26: 86–92

Kelly P, Goerss S, Kall B, Kispert D (1986) Computed tomography based stereotactic third ventriculostomy: Technical note. Neurosurgery 18: 791–794

Milhorat TH (1972) Hydrocephalus and the cerebrospinal fluid. Williams and Wilkins, Baltimore.

Mixter WJ (1923) Ventriculoscopy and puncture of the floor of the third ventricle. Boston Med Surg J 188: 277–278

Natelson SE (1981) Early third ventriculostomy in myelomeningocoele infants: Shunt independence. Childs Brain 8: 321–325

Perlman BB (1968) Percutaneous third ventriculostomy in the treatment of a hydrocephalic infant with aqueduct stenosis. Int Surg 49: 443–448

Sayers MP (1976) Shunt complications. Clin Neurosurg 23: 393–400

Sayers MP, Kosnik EJ (1976) Percutaneous third ventriculostomy: Experience and technique. Childs Brain 2: 24–30

Stookey B, Scarff J (1936) Occlusion of the aqueduct of Sylvius by neoplastic and nonneoplastic processes with a rational surgical treatment for relief of the resultant hydrocephalus. Bull Neurol Inst NY 5: 348–377

Torkildsen A (1960) A follow-up study 14 to 20 years after ventriculo-cisternostomy. Acta Psychiatr Neurol Scand 35: 113–121

Vries J (1978) An endoscopic technique for third ventriculostomy. Surg Neurol 9: 165–168

Walters BC, Hoffman HJ, Hendrick EB, Hemphreys RP (1984) Cerebrospinal fluid shunt infection: Influence on initial management and subsequent outcome. J Neurosurg 60: 1014–1021

Williams B (1973) Is aqueduct stenosis a result of hydrocephalus? Childs Brain 96: 399

Ziedses des Plantes BG, Crezee P (1978) Transfrontal perforation of the lamina terminalis. Neuroradiology 16: 51–53

70 — New Surgical Therapy for Hydrocephalus: Percutaneous Flexible Endoneurosurgical Choroid Plexus Coagulation

Kazunari Oka, Shinya Ohshiro, Yoshinori Go, Yoshiaki Kin, Masamichi Tomonaga[1], Hiromichi Mannoji[2], and Norio Daikuzono[3]

Summary. A new flexible fiberoptic ventriculoscope (fiberscope) has been developed for percutaneous endoneurosurgery. This ventriculoscope has a wide channel, of 2.0 mm, allowing the use of a variety of different instruments, including an endoscopic contact Nd-YAG Laser fiber. Using our therapeutic ventriculoscope and contact Nd-YAG Laser fiber, we were successful in carrying out choroid plexus coagulation of the lateral ventricles in an infant with toxoplasmosis. After this procedure, production of cerebro-spinal fluid (CSF) diminished and its protein content gradually decreased. This ventriculoscope was applied safely to a patient in poor condition with hydrocephalus due to intra-ventricular lesions. Percutaneous endoneurosurgical choroid plexus coagulation was useful for this kind of hydrocephalus. This paper describes the device and summarizes its successful use in clinical practice.

Keywords. Flexible ventriculoscope — Endoneurosurgery — Hydrocephalus — Choroid plexus coagulation

Introduction

Use of the endoscope in the treatment of hydrocephalus has brought about a distinct advance in the surgical treatment of this condition. Using the ventriculoscope, it is possible to perform reasonable surgical procedures with minimum intervention. Dandy (1918) and Scarff (1952) attempted to decrease CSF secretion in patients with nonobstructive hydrocephalus by choroid plexus coagulation. The purpose of this article is, firstly, to present a new type of neurosurgical operating fiberscope which could be the basis of flexible endoneurosurgery, and secondly to present the results obtained by endoscopic cauterization of the choroid plexus in obstructive hydrocephalus.

[1] Department of Neurosurgery, School of Medicine, Fukuoka University, Fukuoka, 814-01 Japan
[2] Department of Neurosurgery, Yamaguchi Red Cross Hospital, Yamaguchi, 753 Japan
[3] Surgical Laser Technology Japan, Tokyo, Japan

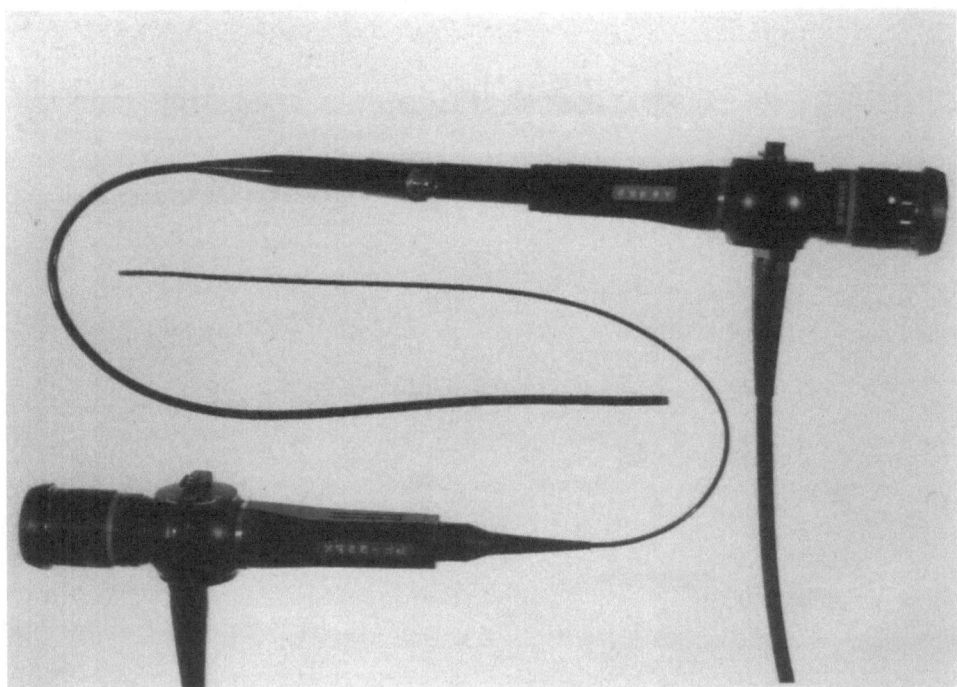

Fig. 1. Therapeutic ventriculoscope (*upper right*). Observation ventriculoscope (*lower left*)

Materials and Methods

The therapeutic ventriculoscope we used (Fig. 1) has a forward-viewing fiber-scope (XPE-41F prototype, Olympus Optical Company, Tokyo) with a field of view of 75° and tip flexion of 90° in two directions. Its diameter is 4.1 mm and it has a wide channel of 2.0 mm. Special instruments (flexible aspirating cannula, grasping forceps, puncturing needle, Seldinger wire) or endoscopic contact Nd-YAG Laser fiber (Surgical Laser Technology Japan, Tokyo) can be introduced through the channel (Fig. 2). The depth of field is 3–50 mm and the working length is 69 cm. It has automatic exposure capability when used with the appropriate cold light supply (CLV 10, Olympus Optical Company, Tokyo) and the photographic apparatus can also be connected with a TV color system (OTV-F2, Olympus Optical Company, Tokyo). A visually-monitored procedure can be recorded simultaneously.

This ventriculoscope can be introduced via ventricular needle through the fontanelle in infants, and through a burr hole in children and adults. The ventriculoscope is inserted into the anterior horn of the lateral ventricle just after the ventricular tapping procedure. The choroid plexus lies on the superior surface of the thalamus. A contact Nd-YAG Laser fiber is introduced into the channel of the ventriculoscope. Choroid plexus coagulation is carried out

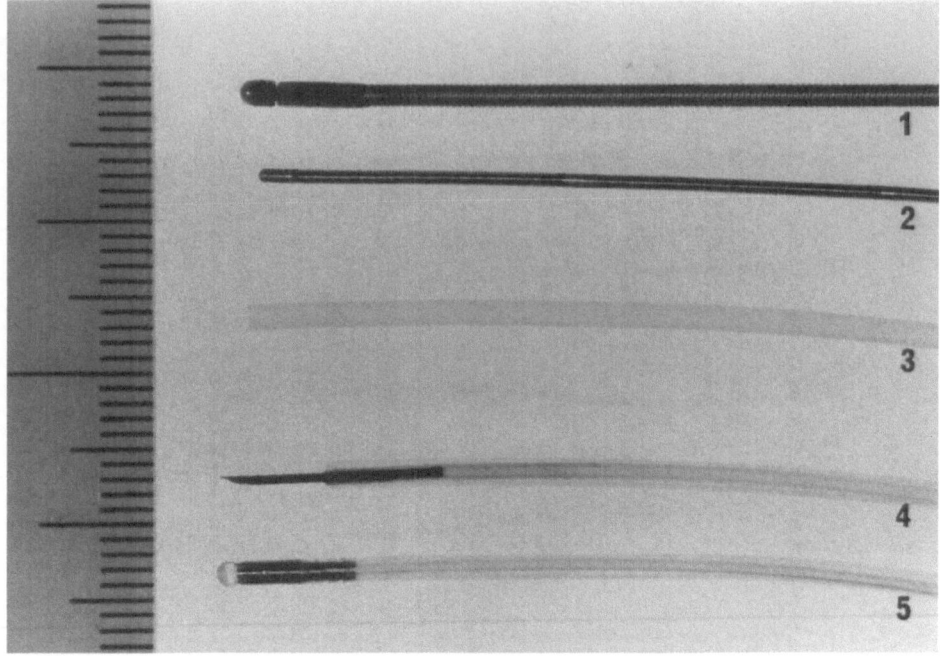

Fig. 2. Special instruments for therapeutic ventriculoscope: *1* Grasping forceps, *2* Seldinger wire, *3* flexible aspirating cannula, *4* puncturing needle, *5* Contact Nd-YAG Laser fiber

simply by touching the fronds of the choroid plexus with the contact probe of the Nd-YAG Laser fiber and by releasing short bursts of coagulation current. The choroid plexuses can often be coagulated through a single puncture, because the septum pellucidum is usually widely disrupted in hydrocephalus.

Case Report

The patient was a female infant delivered at 38 weeks on April 14, 1989. Before delivery, she had been diagnosed as hydrocephalic by echo-sonography. At birth, the circumference of the head was normal and the fontanelle was not bulging. Computed tomography (CT) scan showed hydrocephalus with calcification scattered in the paraventricular area (Fig. 3). Laboratory data revealed antenatal toxoplasmosis (Table 1). The infant's head gradually enlarged day by day. Her first ventriculo-peritoneal (V-P) shunt was carried out on April 24. She was given 120 mg/day of acetylspiramycin from May 15 to June 24, during which time her IgM-toxoplasma antibody titer was normalized. Revisions of the V-P shunt were performed twice and then external ventricular drainage was maintained from September 27 to October 23. When a V-P shunt was performed on October 23, an observation ventriculoscope (Okaetal. 1990)

Fig. 3. CT scan showing dilatation of the ventricles and intra- and paraventricular calcifications

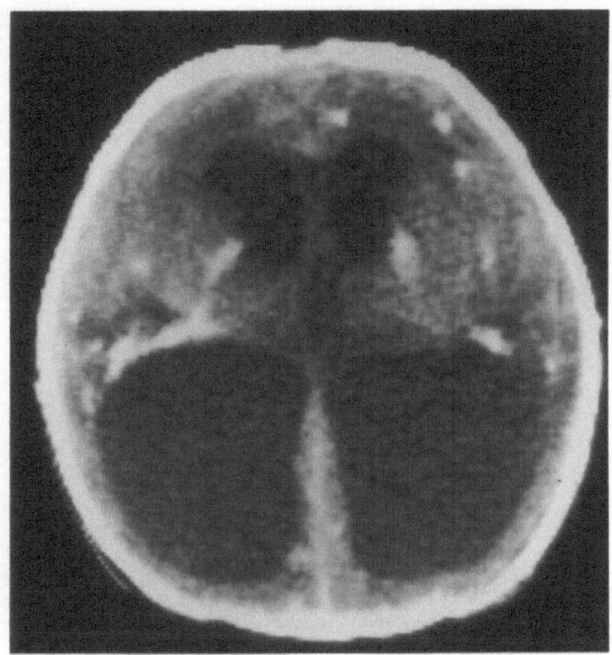

Table 1. Laboratory data of infant and its mother

Serum	Infant	Mother	Normal range
IgG toxoplasma-antibody	× 2560	× 2560	< × 20
IgM toxoplasma-antibody	× 10	× 40	< × 10
CSF			
IgG toxoplasma-antibody	× 128	n.d.	< × 2
IgM toxoplasma-antibody	× 16	n.d.	< × 2

n.d., not detected

revealed that the foramen of Monro was patent. The inner wall of the third ventricle was whitish and covered with fibrous tissue. The tuber cinereum, infundibular recess, and mamillary bodies could not be observed. Choroid plexus coagulation of the left lateral ventricle was performed, using our therapeutic ventriculoscope and contact Nd-YAG Laser fiber, and an Ommaya reservoir was placed in the anterior horn of the left lateral ventricle on December 19. Thirty seven days later, choroid plexus coagulation was performed on the right side (Fig. 4). Production of CSF diminished because the frequency of CSF aspiration from the Ommaya reservoir decreased from every two days to once in ten days. The protein content of the CSF decreased from 2300 to 66 mg/dl for about 1 year (Fig. 5). The patient is still extremely ill; she is mentally retarded and has infantile spasms, ocular toxoplasmosis, and repetitions of aspiration pneumonia.

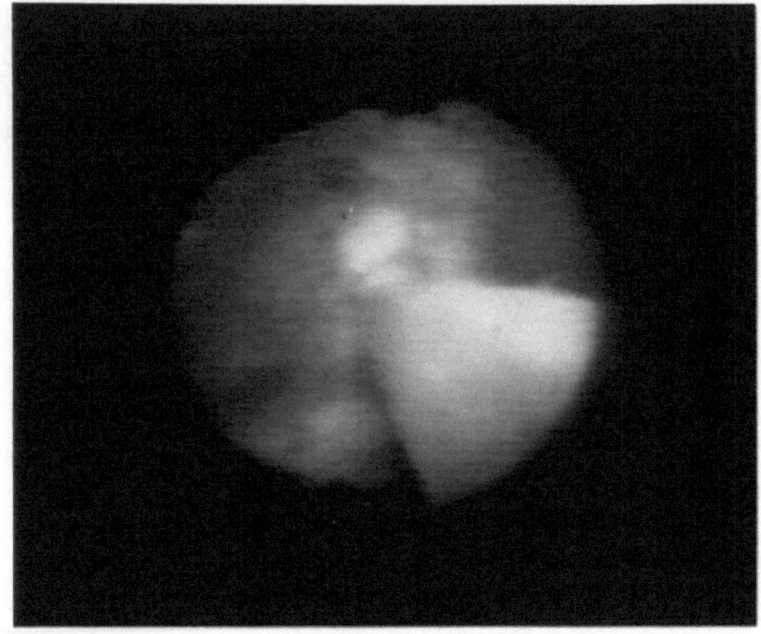

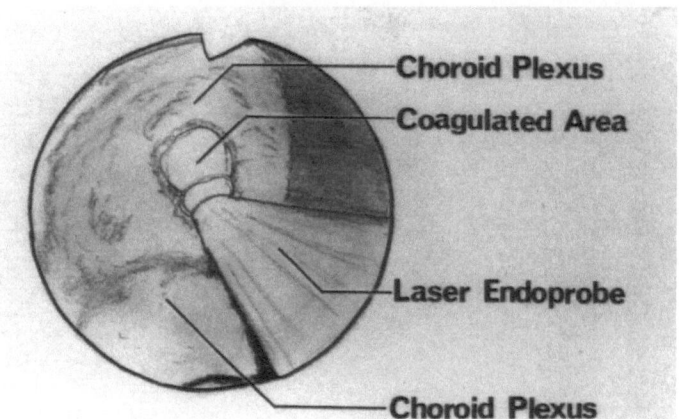

Fig. 4. Endoscopic photograph and diagram showing coagulation of the choroid plexus

Discussion

Dandy (1918) attempted to decrease CSF secretion by choroid plexus destruction. Scarff (1966) reviewed endoscopic cauterization of the choroid plexus which had been performed in 95 cases of nonobstructive (communicating) hydrocephalus, as reported by Putnam (1943), Feld (1957), and himself (1952). Fifty-five percent of those cases, followed for an average period of 8 years after operation, had resulted in arrest of the hydrocephalus. Scarff reported that serious complications occurred in only 3% of patients after endoscopic

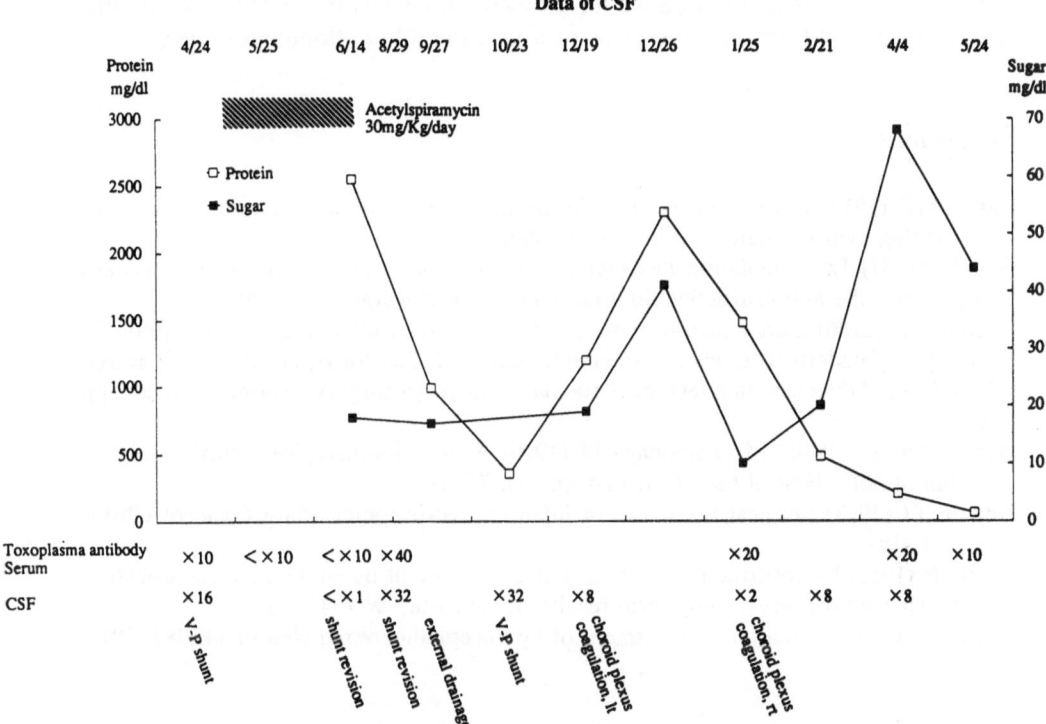

Fig. 5. Clinical summary and CSF data

cauterization of the choroid plexus, as compared to an overall reported average of 57% for 1087 cases of mechanical "shunt". However, choroid plexus coagulation for nonobstructive hydrocephalus is not popular at present.

Recently, Griffith (1986) showed that, of 35 patients with communicating hydrocephalus who were operated upon endoneurosurgically in the years 1972–1983, 34% could be controlled only with choroid plexus coagulation. Now Griffith proposes endoneurosurgical therapy in patients with communicating hydrocephalus, those with obstructive hydrocephalus, and those with myelomeningocele. He has stated that he expects rapid development in the further miniaturization of optics, improved image transmission to color camera or TV camera, and improvement and extension of operating capability for endoneurosurgery.

We have made remarkable advances in the development of this flexible fiberoptic endoscope. Firstly, the field of view is 75° and the tip flexion is 90°. Secondly, the color balance of the system has automatic exposure capability when used with the appropriate cold light supply. Thirdly, the flexible endoscope is sterilized in ethylene-oxide gas, involving a temperature of 50° degree C for 12. Fourthly, special accessories are available for the flexible ventriculoscope: A contact Nd-YAG Laser fiber, a flexible aspirating cannula, a grasping forceps, a Seldinger wire, and a puncturing needle can be accommodated in its 2.0 mm-channel.

The flexible ventriculoscope we have developed is vastly superior to the hard telescope; it could become the basis of a new flexible endoneurosurgery.

References

Dandy WE (1918) Extirpation of the choroid plexuses of the lateral ventricle in communicating hydrocephalus. Ann Surg 68: 569–579

Feld M (1957) La coagulation des plexus choroides par ventriculoscope directe dans l'hydrocephalie nonobstructive du nourrison. Neurochirurgie 3: 70–79

Griffith HB (1986) Endoneurosurgery: Endoscopic intracranial surgery. In: Symon L, Brihaye J, Guidetti B, Loew F, Miller JD, Nornes H, Pasztor E, Pertuiset B, Yasargil MG (eds) Advances and technical standards in neurosurgery. Springer, Wien, pp 2–24

Oka K, Ohta T, Kibe M, Tomonaga M (1990) A new neurosurgical ventriculoscope. Technical note. Neurol Med Chir (Tokyo) 30: 77–79

Putnam TJ (1943) Surgical treatment of infantile hydrocephalus.Surg Gynecol Obstet 76: 171–182

Scarff JE (1952) Nonobstructive hydrocephalus. Treatment by endoscopic cauterization of the choroid plexuses: Long term results. J Neurosurg 9: 164–176

Scarff JE (1966) Evaluation of treatment of hydrocephalus. Arch Neurol 14: 382–391

Subject Index